FUCHS'S
RADIOGRAPHIC EXPOSURE
AND QUALITY CONTROL

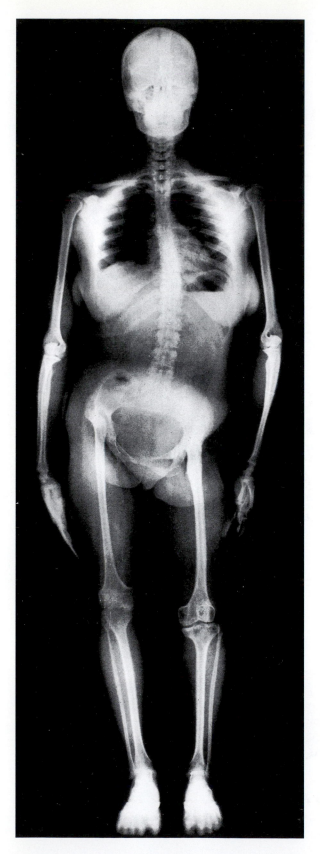

Frontispiece. X-ray film has been prepared in many sizes for medical work. The largest film (32 by 72 inches) used was for the entire body radiography of a woman, aged 33, exhibiting hip pathology. The radiograph was made with a one-second exposure, 75 kVp, 150 mA, 12 feet target-film distance, fast screens, and tissue-compensating filtration.

Seventh Edition

FUCHS'S RADIOGRAPHIC EXPOSURE AND QUALITY CONTROL

By

QUINN B. CARROLL, M.Ed., R.T.

Director
Radiography Department
Midland College
Midland, Texas

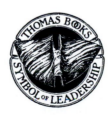

CHARLES C THOMAS • PUBLISHER, LTD.
Springfield • Illinois • U.S.A.

©2003 by CHARLES C THOMAS • PUBLISHER, LTD.

ISBN 0-398-07373-2

Library of Congress Catalog Card Number: 2002035782

First Edition, 1955
Second Edition, 1958
Third Edition, 1985
Fourth Edition, 1990
Fifth Edition, 1993
Sixth Edition, 1998
Seventh Edition, 2003

Printed in the United States of America
MM-R-3

Library of Congress Cataloging in Publication Data

Carroll, Quinn B.
   Fuchs's radiographic exposure and quality control / Quinn B. Carroll --
7th ed.
       p. cm.
   5pd. published with the title: Fuchs's radiographic exposure, processing,
and quality control.
   ISBN 0-398-07373-2 (cloth)
   1. Radiography, Medical. I. Title: Fuchs's radiographic exposure and
quality control. II. Title: Radiographic exposure and quality control. III.
Fuchs, Arthur W. (Arthur Wolfram), 1895–IV. Carroll, Quinn B. Fuchs's radiographic exposure, processing, and quality control. V. Title.

RC78.C35 2003
616.07'572--dc21   2002035782

To
WOLFRAM CONRAD FUCHS
Roentgen Pioneer
1865-1907

and

ARTHUR WOLFRAM FUCHS
1895-1962

CONTRIBUTING AUTHORS

ROBERT DEANGELIS, BSRT
Health and Allied Science Publishers
Rutland, Vermont

ROBERT J. PARELLI, MA, RT(R)
Cypress College
Cypress, California

EUCLID SEERAM, RTR, BSc, MSc
British Columbia Institute of Technology
Burnaby, British Columbia, Canada

PREFACE TO THE SEVENTH EDITION

ARTHUR W. FUCHS was a man who understood and believed in experiential learning. The philosophy is that learning obtained through hands-on experience is more likely to be understood, retained and applied than are notes from lectures. Thus, the first edition had a format of illustrated experimentation. It focused upon the real considerations of the daily practice of medical radiography rather than on physical theory. For this reason, I am honored to be able to associate my name with his in producing this updated and expanded edition on radiographic imaging.

If other educators in radiography have experienced the same kinds of frustrations in finding a comprehensive and practical text as I have, it is hoped that this edition will fill that void. While there are several excellent physics texts in the field, some of which claim by their titles to be technique books, texts on practical technique are few and far between.

It should be noted at the outset that this edition is intended to complement radiographic physics texts rather than duplicate them. It picks up where they leave off, bridges the gap between theory and practice, and therefore assumes some basic knowledge of physical principles upon which the concepts of practical technique can be built. Care was taken to include only those physics topics which directly relate to the manipulation of equipment in controlling the outcome on the image. Hence, although there is an early chapter on atomic interactions upon which much of the subsequent chapters build, there is no treatment of electricity or mechanics. This book addresses the questions of which variables must be manipulated to control image qualities and why, nothing more.

This volume also attempts to bridge the gap between quality control and technique. These two subjects have been taught and written about separately for too long. All of the concepts and rules of technique are completely dependent upon quality control for their validity. Many students have struggled with apparent contradictions in the principles of technique they have been taught simply because they were working with poorly calibrated equipment. Although some instructors cover quality control in a different course or semester, by finding these concepts alongside practical technique in the same text, the student can recognize that there are scientific explanations for techniques that do not always produce results with exactness.

Mr. Fuchs also realized that it is easier to assimilate information in small bits than in large amounts at a time. Consequently, he organized his book variable by variable, rather than image quality by image quality. There are only six essential qualities to an image. There are well over 20 fundamental variables which affect image quality. This edition holds true to the original, presenting the effects of each variable upon the six image qualities in each chapter, rather than inundating the student with twenty factors to learn about in each chapter. However, since technique courses are frequently organized by image qualities, a chapter has been added on "Analyzing the Radiographic Image," which reviews all of the material in this manner.

Unique additions to the book include chapters on technique by proportional anatomy, constructing technique charts from scratch, and how to solve multiple technique problems similar to those presented on certification examinations in radiography. Chapters covering automatic and programmed exposure controls, automatic processors, sensitometry and dark-room quality control have been added. The early chapter covering image qualities ensures that the student obtains a clear and complete concept of each of the six image components before proceeding to the effects of each variable upon them. It is easy to confuse a higher contrast image for a sharper image or a fogged image for an overexposed image. This chapter helps prevent these types of misconceptions as more and more advanced and complicated topics are presented.

The Fifth Edition was expanded in accordance with a survey of educators using the text, and contributing authors were instrumental in making improvements. Chapters were added on pathology and casts, scattered radiation, analyzing the image, minimizing patient dose, equipment quality control, and special image processing systems, along with mobile, fluoroscopic and digital imaging. The chapters on technique by proportional anatomy, technique charts and automatic exposure controls were expanded to include more detailed information. Review questions and suggested laboratory demonstrations were added at the ends of chapters.

Changes in the Fifth and Sixth Editions

were also intended to make the text even more "user-friendly" for students, with clear, concise explanations, plentiful examples, ample illustrations and practice exercises to reinforce mathematical concepts. Chapter 14 on intensifying screens and Chapter 28 on Automatic Exposure Controls were significantly expanded, not only bringing the material up to date in these essential areas of modern radiography, but presenting one of the most thorough practical treatments of these topics available.

For the Seventh Edition, contributions by Robert DeAngelis, Robert Parelli, and Euclid Seeram have updated information on fluoroscopic equipment, digital imaging, and computer radiography while preserving the focus on practical application and the resulting quality of the final image, whether conventional, fluoroscopic, or digital. Chapter review questions had been expanded, and the accompanying Instructor's Manual has also been restored with expanded multiple choice question banks and lab exercises to make this set as useful as possible to the radiography educator.

A considerable effort was made to cover all material suggested by the ASRT curriculum guide, without duplicating typical physics texts and maintaining a focus on practical application.

It is sincerely hoped that this text will contribute to the competency and fulfillment of radiographers in their career, to the professionalism and cost effectiveness of radiology departments, and ultimately to the enhancement of patient care in medical radiography.

Q.B.C.

ACKNOWLEDGMENTS

I WISH TO EXPRESS my thanks to the professional staff of Charles C Thomas, Publisher for their valuable help in developing, illustrating, and producing the text.

Special thanks to Euclid Seeram, Robert DeAngelis, and Robert Parelli for their valuable contributions to a text which remains a classic in the field, and to all of my professional colleagues who have offered suggestions for improvements, assisted with corrections, and shared their expertise and association over the years.

I am grateful to Jason, Melissa, Chad, Tiffani, Brandon, and Tyson for their patience when I am writing.

Above all, I wish to express my gratitude to my wife Margaret for her unwavering support and confidence in all that I do and for her belief in what each human being can do.

ACKNOWLEDGMENTS

CONTENTS

Part I
PRODUCING THE RADIOGRAPHIC IMAGE

Part II
VISIBILITY FACTORS

Part IV
COMPREHENSIVE TECHNIQUE

Part V
SPECIAL IMAGING METHODS

Part VI
PROCESSING THE RADIOGRAPH

FUCHS'S
RADIOGRAPHIC EXPOSURE
AND QUALITY CONTROL

Part I

PRODUCING THE RADIOGRAPHIC IMAGE

Chapter 1

X-RAYS AND RADIOGRAPHIC VARIABLES

A SATISFACTORY UNDERSTANDING of exposure and processing terms requires at least a limited knowledge of x-rays and their characteristics. X-rays are a form of invisible radiant energy and were discovered by Wilhelm Conrad Roentgen on November 8, 1895. They are quite similar to light in their general properties since they travel at the same speed and obey many of the same laws. A distinguishing feature of x-rays, however, is their extremely short wavelength—only about one ten-thousandth the wavelength of *visible* light. It is this property that is responsible for x-rays' ability to penetrate materials that ordinarily would absorb or reflect light.

GENERATION OF X-RAYS

The generation of x-rays is a complex process. Fortunately, a knowledge of only a few of the principles is necessary. The essential feature of x-ray production is the striking of matter by high-speed electrons; this may occur within or outside a vacuum but is much more efficient within a vacuum where there are no air molecules impeding the path of these electrons on their way to their target. The device in which x-rays are generated is the x-ray tube. The modern x-ray tube is a sealed glass tube with all remnants of air vacuumed out of it.

X-rays are produced in an x-ray tube when electrons, traveling at great speed, under stress of high voltage, collide with a metallic target of high molecular weight such as tungsten. The efficiency of x-ray production is very small, for only about one part in a thousand of the energy from these electrons is converted into x-rays that are penetrating enough to make a radiograph; the balance is dissipated into heat.

The x-ray tubes employed by early workers contained gas under low pressure. These tubes were known as Crookes or Hittorf tubes. Roentgen's early tubes (Fig. 1-1) were of the Crookes type which consisted of a pear-shaped glass tube filled with air under low pressure. An aluminum cathode was installed in the small end of the tube and, through a stem of glass on the side of the tube was inserted an aluminum anode.

When a high-voltage electrical current was passed between the cathode and anode, the residual gas in the tube became ionized and a stream of electrons was repelled by the cathode. Many of these electrons were attracted to the anode because of its positive charge and location in the tube, but the majority of the electrons were bombarded against the glass at the end of the tube. The sudden stoppage of the electrons against the glass produced x-rays.

When the Jackson *focus* tube was made, the electron stream was focused onto a

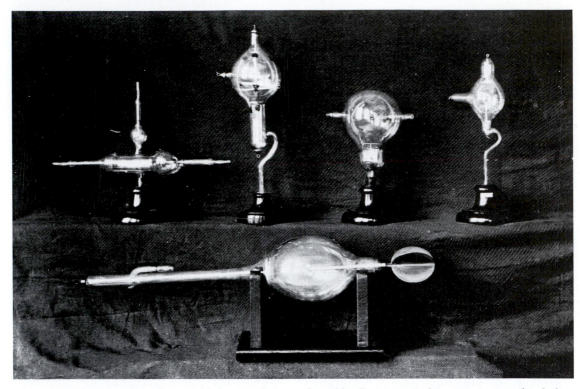

Figure 1-1. Photograph of the gas discharge tubes employed by Roentgen in his experiments that led to his discovery of the x-rays.

metal anode at the end of the tube and inclined at an angle so that a larger amount of radiation could be concentrated on a particular area.

Maintenance of a constant pressure in the early glass tubes was almost impossible for the pressure would vary with each use of the tube. These early tubes were quite erratic. The advent of the Coolidge hot cathode x-ray tube made possible the generation of a constant source of x-rays that could be easily duplicated at will. This tube was invented by Dr. W. D. Coolidge of the General Electric Company in 1913 (Fig. 1-2).

X-RAY TUBE

The modern x-ray tube consists of a highly evacuated glass bulb into which are sealed two electrodes—the *cathode*, or nega-

tive electrode (the source of electrons), and the *anode*, or positive electrode (the source of x-rays). Due to the vacuum and the arrangement of the electrodes, no discharge of electrons between the cathode and the anode is possible until the filament in the cathode is heated (Figs. 1-3 & 1-4).

Thermionic Electron Emission

Employing the principle that all *hot* bodies emit electrons, a spiral, incandescent filament of tungsten wire is incorporated in the cathode of the x-ray tube. This filament is heated by an electrical current of low amperage from a step-down transformer. The temperature of the filament, as governed by the amount of current that passes through it, controls the number of electrons emitted—the higher the filament tempera-

current and is measured in milliamperes. The electron stream is propelled by high-voltage electricity impressed on the tube electrodes by a high-voltage transformer. This voltage, which may be varied at will, regulates the *speed* with which the electrons cross the gap between the cathode and the anode. Thousands of volts (kilovolts) are normally used for this purpose. The stream of electrons forms a conducting path for the high-voltage current to reach the anode. Upon impact with the focal spot of the tube, the electrons produce a stream of x-rays which are emitted over a 180° angle from the focal spot of the target.

Rotating Anode Tube

The Coolidge tube was still limited in the quantity of x-rays it could produce.

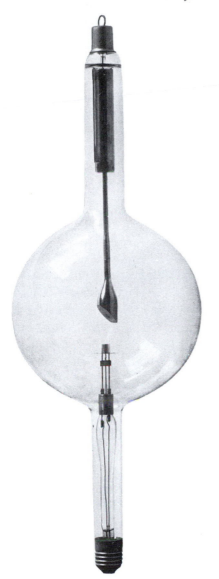

Figure 1-2. Photograph of an early Coolidge stationary anode tube in which the electrons originate in heated tungsten filament.

ture, the greater the electron emission. Because of its small mass, an electron rapidly accelerates to a high speed in an electric field. Surrounding the filament is a shield that serves to focus the electron stream from the heated filament to the *focal spot* on the tungsten target located at the end of the anode. The stream of electrons from cathode to anode constitutes the tube

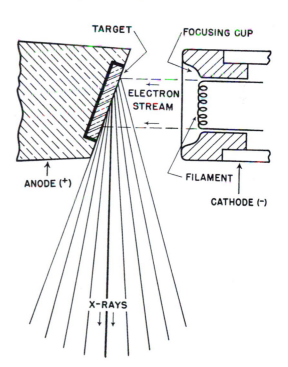

Figure 1-3. Diagram of the essential elements of an x-ray tube wherein electrons generated by a heated filament in the cathode are bombarded against a tungsten-rhenium target in the anode, resulting in x-ray production.

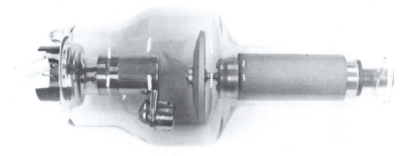

Figure 1-4. Photograph of a modern x-ray tube with the cathode visible to the lower left, the rotating anode disc in the middle, and the rotor which rotates the anode disc on the right half.

With the enhanced electron emission of a hot cathode, the stationary anode plate could be melted from the intense bombardment of electrons. To prevent this destruction of the anode surface, a better way of dissipating the heat had to be devised. In 1936, the *rotating anode tube* was developed (Fig. 1-4).

The rotating anode is shaped like a disc and composed of a metal with good heat-conducting and electron-conducting characteristics, usually molybdenum. The front surface of the disc is coated with an alloy of tungsten and rhenium. These two elements are made of "large" atoms with many orbital electrons, and are very effective at stopping the electron beam emitted from the cathode. With their high melting points, tungsten and rhenium are ideal metals for the "target" surface of the anode.

The anode disc is connected to a rotor shank (Fig. 1-4) which is actually part of a motor. Whenever the "rotor" switch is depressed on an x-ray machine, this shank spins at the same time that the filament is being heated. By spinning the anode disc, the target surface struck by the electron beam is constantly changing. The heat is distributed across a greater surface area and the anode is less likely to melt.

Thus, the three most essential components to the modern x-ray tube can be described as (1) the vacuum tube, (2) the heated cathode, and (3) the rotating anode.

X-Ray Wavelength

Despite the enormous energy in the electron stream, only a small portion is converted into x-rays; the bulk is dissipated as heat at the anode. The greater the force of impact of the electrons on the anode, the shorter is the wavelength of the x-rays produced and the more readily do they penetrate the object being examined. In other words, the higher the voltage, the greater is the speed of the electrons striking the anode. The result is an increase in both the intensity and the penetrating power of the x-rays produced, and a shortening of their wavelength. The wavelengths of x-rays (much shorter than those of visible light) are measured in *Angstrom (A) units.* An angstrom unit is equal to 10^{-6} millimeter, about one-millionth the size of a pinhead. The useful range of wavelengths for medical radiography is approximately *0.1 to 0.5 angstroms.*

INTERACTIONS IN THE ANODE

The wavelengths and the energy levels of x-rays in the beam are determined by the specific interactions of the electrons with the atoms in the anode. Atoms with a high atomic number will have much larger nuclei as well as many more orbital electrons with which the high-speed electrons from the cathode may interact. This means that more interactions will occur, and that those which do occur will result in higher-energy x-rays being produced. This is the reason why tungsten and rhenium (atomic numbers 74 and 75 respectively) are used as target material on the anode.

When a high-speed electron strikes an atom in the anode, it must interact with either the nucleus of the atom or with an orbital electron in one of the electron shells.

BREMSSTRAHLUNG

If the electron passes near the atomic nucleus, the positive attraction of the nucleus will cause it to *brake* or slow down. This deceleration in the speed of the electron represents a loss of kinetic energy, and that energy which is lost is emitted as an x-ray *photon* (Fig. 1-5). The word "photon" is often used to denote a single x-ray. X-rays produced by this interaction are called *bremsstrahlung* (braking radiation) and they account for the vast majority of the total x-ray beam.

High-speed electrons may pass by the nucleus at various distances from it. The closer an electron approaches to the nucleus, the greater will be its deceleration, due to the stronger pull of the nucleus—thus, the more energy will be lost and the higher will be the energy (keV) of the emitted x-ray. Bremsstrahlung, occurring at various distances from the nucleus, produces a wide range of x-ray energies and is thus responsible for the *heterogeneous* or poly-energetic nature of the x-ray beam. Heterogeneity contributes to the differential absorption of

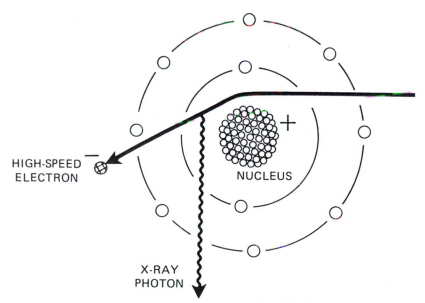

HIGH-SPEED
ELECTRON

NUCLEUS

X-RAY
PHOTON

Figure 1-5. The bremsstrahlung interaction in the x-ray tube anode. When a high-speed electron is attracted to a nearby atomic nucleus, it decelerates and changes direction, losing energy. The lost energy is emitted as an x-ray.

x-rays within the patient's body by different tissues. It is just this differential absorption which provides *subject contrast* to the image and makes the radiographic image possible. If all of the x-rays were of the same energy, the image would be extremely poor, essentially a silhouette. Subtle differences between tissues only show up on the radiograph when a variety of x-ray energies result in a wide range of densities (gray shades) in the image.

The distance at which an electron will pass a nucleus is a function of statistical probability. It is more likely that the electron will pass farther away from the nucleus, where greater areas are involved, than that it will pass very near the nucleus. Hence, more x-rays are produced at lower energies than at higher energies. A plot of this relationship between energy levels and the numbers of x-rays produced would look like Figure 1-6. However, because inherent filtration in the x-ray tube (including the glass around the tube) stops the x-rays with the lowest energies, the remaining bremsstrahlung portion of the beam is graphed like Figure 1-7.

Reviewing Figure 1-7, note that there are

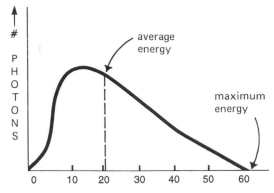

Figure 1-7. Graph of the actual bremsstrahlung x-ray beam spectrum with filtration present and the kVp set to 60. X-rays with the lowest energies are absorbed by the glass, oil, and filters through which they pass. The average energy is about 20 keV, one-third of the kV peak.

very few x-rays emitted from the x-ray tube at very low energies, because of filtration. There are also very few x-rays emitted at high energies: this is because of the statistical distribution of the bremsstrahlung interaction, that is, only a few of the electrons passed very close to the nucleus to produce these high energies. The *total* number of x-rays produced by bremsstrahlung is represented by the *total area* under the beam spectrum curve of the graph. Bremsstrahlung x-rays are produced at many different energies, making the beam *heterogeneous. Note that the average energy of these x-rays is about one-third of the maximum energy.*

CHARACTERISTIC RADIATION

The second possibility for the high-speed electron in the x-ray tube is that, instead of interacting with the nucleus of an atom in the anode, it might interact with one of the atom's orbital electrons. When it passes near an orbital electron, its repulsive negative charge will eject the orbital electron out of its orbit, leaving a vacancy in the electron shell of the atom. The atom, left with a net positive charge, will pull in another

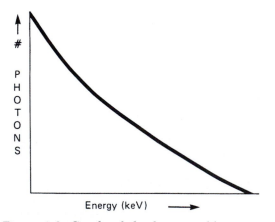

Figure 1-6. Graph of the bremsstrahlung x-ray beam spectrum as it would appear with no filtration. Most x-rays are generated at lower energy (keV) levels. Very few are produced at the highest energies.

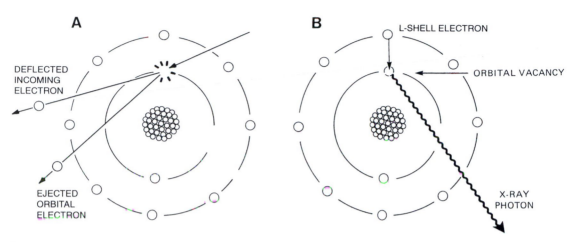

Figure 1-8. The characteristic interaction in the x-ray tube anode. In step *A*, an incoming electron from the filament collides with and dislodges an orbital electron from the atom. In step *B*, the atom "pulls" down an electron from a higher orbit to fill the vacancy left. As this electron drops into a lower orbit, it loses energy which is emitted as an x-ray.

electron, usually from an outer shell, to fill this vacancy. Energy is lost when an electron falls from an outer orbit down into an inner orbit, and that energy is emitted as a *characteristic* x-ray (Fig. 1-8). Characteristic radiation makes up only a small portion of the overall x-ray beam, but since it can possess high energies that penetrate through the patient to the film, it is still important in producing a radiographic image.

Characteristic x-rays depend entirely on the difference in energy levels between different orbital shells in the atom. Since we know what the energy levels are for each orbit in the atoms of each element, we can predict accurately what the characteristic x-ray energies will be for the tungsten and the rhenium in the anode. X-rays will be emitted at distinct energies, rather than over a range of energies like bremsstrahlung. A graph of the spectrum of characteristic x-rays produced would appear as Figure 1-9.

In tungsten atoms, characteristic x-rays will be produced in the innermost electron shell having 57, 66 and 69 kilovolts of energy. The second orbital shell will produce x-rays of 10 and 12 keV, and the third shell

will produce x-rays with about 2 keV. Inherent beam filtration will remove virtually all of the 2-kV x-rays, so these do not show on the graph in Figure 1-9. Filtration also removes most of the 10- and 12-kV x-rays, thus, the graph plots them but showing a reduced number. Those characteristic x-rays having 57, 66 and 69 kV largely escape

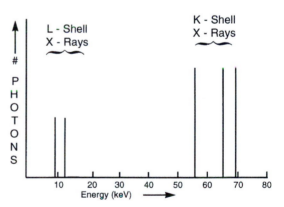

Figure 1-9. Graph of the characteristic x-ray beam spectrum for tungsten. X-rays are emitted only at discrete energy levels based upon the difference between binding energies of orbital shells in the atom. Electrons falling from various outer shells into the *K-Shell* emit x-rays having 57, 67, and 69 keV of energy. The lines to the far left represent *L-Shell* x-rays.

the x-ray tube and are considered part of the useful beam. These show up on the graph as tall spikes. Adding the predominant bremsstrahlung to the characteristic x-rays, a complete graph of the typical spectrum for a total x-ray beam appears as Figure 1-10. This graph illustrates how homogeneous characteristic radiation (the spikes) combines with heterogeneous bremsstrahlung (the bell curve) to produce a total filtered x-ray beam which is generally heterogeneous in nature and in which most of the x-rays have about one-third of the maximum energy or kilovoltage-peak (kVp).

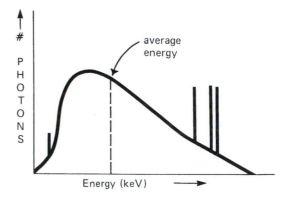

Figure 1-10. Shape of the complete diagnostic x-ray beam spectrum, representing both bremsstrahlung and characteristic interactions, with filtration present.

X-RAY BEAM SPECTRA

Graphs of the x-ray beam spectrum will be used in later chapters to demonstrate the effects of various changes, and the student must have a clear understanding of the interpretation of a spectrum such as that in Figure 1-10. An x-ray beam spectrum curve plots the *amount* of x-rays against their *energy*. Recall that an x-ray beam is heterogeneous, having a mixture of x-rays of many different energy levels. The spectrum curve depicts how many x-rays there are at each energy. The energy is usually measured in kilovolts.

This is similar to drawing a graph of a large graduating high school class, plotting the number of graduates against their height. There would be only a few very tall graduates, and a few short ones, but most of them would be of medium height, in an average range. The height distribution curve would be graphed in a "bell" shape, just as the x-ray spectrum curve is. The total number of all high school graduates would be represented by the total area under the curve.

In a similar fashion, the heterogeneous x-ray beam includes a few x-rays of very low kilovoltage (energy), and a few with very high kilovoltage, but *most* of the x-rays in the beam will have some intermediate kilovoltage. On the graph, a higher curve would indicate more x-rays being produced. A shift in the position of the spectrum curve to the right would indicate higher kilovoltages of energy, and a shift to the left would indicate lower kilovoltage levels. Thus, the height and position of the x-ray beam spectrum curve represent both the quantity and the quality of the x-ray beam.

PROPERTIES OF X-RAYS

Although many similarities between x-rays and visible light may be readily noted, the effects produced are so different that it is preferable to consider the properties of x-rays separately from other types of radiation. For example, while visible light rays behave like "waves" most of the time, x-rays behave more like a stream of "particles." For this reason, we refer to individual x-rays as *photons*, defined as small bundles or "particles" of energy. Light is refracted or "bent" by glass and is thus capable of being focused by a lens. It is also reflected by glass mirrors. X-rays, on the other hand, are essentially unaffected by lenses or mirrors and pass straight through them.

An outstanding characteristic of x-rays is their ability to penetrate through matter of any kind. Since they are also able to expose photographic film, radiography through the human body is made possible. X-rays can *ionize* atoms, effectively knocking electrons out of their shells. This ionization can lead to chemical changes which can harm cells biologically. Ionization by x-rays also excites many substances to *fluoresce* or give off light. Fluorescent screens made with these substances are used both in fluoroscopic procedures and in general radiography as intensifying screens, which help in reducing the patient's exposure to x-radiation. X-rays are a powerful agent in the treatment of cancer and other diseases. Their ability to ionize air makes possible the use of ion chambers (Geiger counters) and other devices for measurement.

THE X-RAY BEAM

Much of the x-ray beam *passes through* the human body or other object to expose a photographic film or to be detected by a computerized device. The x-ray beam may be divided into two parts, the *primary* beam and the *remnant* beam (Fig. 1-14).

Primary Radiation

The primary radiation is confined to that portion of the x-ray beam emitted by the x-ray tube which has *not* yet passed through the patient or object being studied. The quality of this primary beam is not significantly altered by its passage through atmospheric air toward the object being examined.

Remnant Radiation

The remnant radiation is that radiation that emerges from the body tissues to expose the x-ray film or otherwise record the radiographic image. It is the *image-forming* radiation. While the remnant beam includes rays from the primary beam that have passed through the object unaffected, it also contains secondary or "scattered" radiation emitted by the tissues.

At average diagnostic energy levels, about 5 percent or less of the primary radiation traverses completely through the patient's body, without interacting with any atoms in the patient, and strikes the film. In addition, about 15 percent of the primary radiation interacts with atoms in such a way that secondary photons are produced which make it out of the patient and strike the film. The remaining 80 percent of the primary beam is totally absorbed within the patient by interacting with atoms in the body.

Therefore, the total intensity of the remnant beam striking the film or detector averages about 20 percent or one-fifth of the intensity of the original primary beam. Further, it may be said that at least 75 percent (15 of the 20 percent remaining) is made up of secondary radiation produced in the patient. The actual percentage of secondary radiation constituting the remnant beam ranges from 75 percent to as much as 90 percent.

ATTENUATION

The partial absorption of the x-ray beam, properly called *attenuation*, refers to the reduction in x-ray intensity that occurs as the x-ray beam traverses the body part. Absorption is influenced by the atomic number and density of the tissue traversed as well as its thickness and the energy of the radiation employed. Soft tissues of the body are easily penetrated but produce significant amounts of secondary radiation which can fog the image. Bone contains such a large quantity of mineral matter that it absorbs much of the x-ray beam leaving light-gray densities on the image. Other very dense tissues, sometimes created by pathology, and very thick body parts can also absorb large numbers of x-rays.

ABSORPTION BY HOMOGENEOUS OBJECT

A homogeneous object is one in which the material composing it is structurally uniform such as a block of aluminum. To demonstrate the absorption character of an object of homogeneous consistency but unequal thicknesses, an aluminum step-wedge (Fig. 1-11) may be employed. X-ray

absorption by such a step-wedge is diagrammatically shown in Figure 1-12. The portion of the x-ray beam passing through the first step on the wedge is slightly absorbed and the remnant radiation produces a dark exposure on the film to represent this step. The absorption by the second step of the wedge is greater than that of the first because it is twice as thick; the intensity of the remnant beam is thereby further reduced and a "lighter" film exposure results, and so on, for the remainder of the steps. The image produced consists of a graduated scale of gray shades, called *densities*, representing the various step thicknesses of the original object.

Absorption-Density Relation

It may be seen from the above that the difference in x-ray absorption of each step

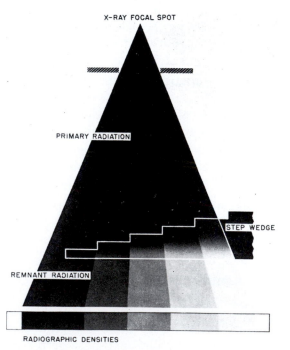

Figure 1-12. Diagram showing passage of x-rays through a homogeneous material (step wedge) that has steps of varying thickness.

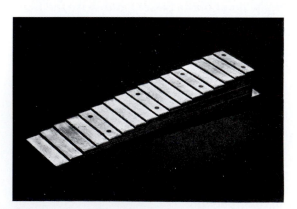

Figure 1-11. Photograph of an aluminum "step wedge" penetrometer used for experimental purposes in radiography.

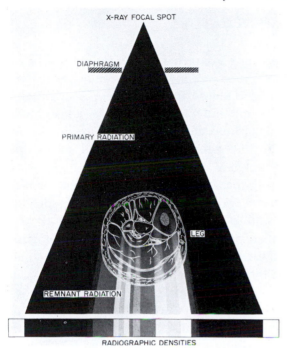

Figure 1-13. Diagram illustrating the penetration and absorption of an x-ray beam as it traverses a body part (leg) whose components absorb the x-rays in varying degree depending upon their thickness and tissue density.

of aluminum had a direct relationship to its respective radiographic density. The image density of each step was directly related to the intensity of the *remnant* radiation reaching the film.

ABSORPTION BY BODY PART

When x-rays pass through human tissue, each type of tissue absorbs its proportion of radiation according to its own tissue density and thickness. For example, as x-rays pass through one thickness of flesh, the total absorption is the sum of the various degrees of absorption exercised by the different tissues (Fig. 1-13). Radiographic delineation of human tissues cannot be predicated upon their thicknesses alone.

Their physical state (tissue density and atomic number) is of the greatest importance from the standpoint of x-ray absorption. Absorption by various tissue components introduces the element of *subject contrast* which is of major importance.

Subject Contrast

Tissue differences, sometimes called *subject contrast*, represent the differences in x-ray absorption occurring in an anatomical part. The greater the x-ray absorption of a tissue with relation to adjacent tissue, the greater the subject contrast. The lesser the difference in tissue absorption, the lower the contrast. For example, greater subject contrast is exhibited between bone and surrounding soft tissues than between kidney tissue and muscle. Also, the selective absorption of each tissue component within the leg causes different intensities within the remnant beam to produce variations in the image densities. As illustrated by the wedge (Fig. 1-12), it was possible to differentiate between the various thicknesses of metal simply by comparing the value of one density with another. The same situation in a measure holds true with the leg, but, in addition, the composite absorption of x-rays by superimposed tissues of different types at different planes also affects the image. Besides variation in thickness, variations in composition is also evidenced as small changes in radiographic density. Since these differences are to be interpreted by the radiologist as anatomical details, they should be easily visible and translucent when viewed on the illuminator. That is, all anatomical details should be depicted as a shade of gray, from light to dark, but none as "blank white" nor as "pitch black" within the anatomical part.

X-RAY BEAM NOMENCLATURE

Figure 1-14 illustrates various components of the x-ray beam and their abbreviations, with which the beginning radiography student must become familiar.

The focal spot, abbreviated *FS*, refers to the specific area on the target surface of the x-ray Tube anode which is bombarded by high-speed electrons. All of the x-rays produced emanate from this small area. It is so small (about the size of a pinhead) that in describing an x-ray beam the focal spot is considered to be a *point* from which all x-rays emerge. X-rays are actually emitted in all directions from this point, but only a small portion are allowed to escape the x-ray tube housing in a controlled direction,

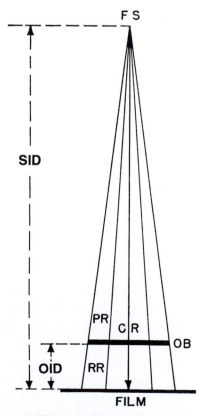

Figure 1-14. Diagram illustrating the various components of an x-ray beam with relation to an object and an x-ray film.

forming a fan-shaped beam (Fig. 1-14). X-rays traveling into the anode are absorbed by the anode material itself, and most of the remainder are absorbed by a lead housing around the tube. Those traveling in the desired direction are allowed to escape through a "window."

Primary Radiation (PR) refers to the beam projected from the focal spot or "source" to the object (OB), prior to any absorption taking place. Remnant Radiation (RR) describes the beam emanating from the object and exposing the radiographic film.

The Central Ray (CR) is the center of the x-ray beam. The term is employed in describing the direction of the x-rays in a given projection. The course of the central ray may be considered to extend from the focal spot of the x-ray tube to the film or image receptor. The entire distance traversed by the central ray is known as the source-image receptor distance or SID. The distance from the object or body part to the x-ray film is known as the object-image receptor distance or OID (Fig. 1-14).

Some electrical terms in constant use are also abbreviated. The first of these is milliamperage (mA). The milliampere is the unit for measuring the flow rate of electricity passing through the x-ray machine and across the x-ray tube. The exposure time ("s" for "seconds") delineates the amount of time in seconds during which the x-ray tube is activated for a particular exposure. The total exposure to an x-ray film is controlled by the product of the milliamperage and the exposure time, called *milliampere-seconds*, and abbreviated as mAs (mA *times* s). In common use, this term is pronounced as "mass."

Finally, the *kilovoltage-peak* refers to the energy level or "pressure" with which the electricity is being forced across the x-ray tube. In simple terms, it controls the "speed" of the electricity, and ultimately determines the *penetrating power* of the x-ray beam produced. Kilovoltage-peak is abbreviated *kVp*.

The Roentgen, and Coulombs/Kilogram

Defined and adopted in 1937, the *Roentgen* is the commonly used unit of quantity for x-rays. It is designated by the symbol *R*. This is the unit of exposure to an x-ray beam, whether by a film, detecting device, or patient. For x-rays, two other radiation terms, the *rad* and the *rem*, are quantitatively identical to the roentgen. The Coulomb per Kilogram, abbreviated C/kg, is an international unit for exposure which is equal to 2.58×10^{18} R.

THE PRIME FACTORS

Four of the variables to be studied in following chapters are considered to be under the immediate and direct control of the radiographer. These are the milliamperage (mA), the exposure time (s), the kilovoltage-peak (kVp), and the source-image distance (SID). These have come to be known as the four *prime factors* of radiography.

The prime factors are combined below with x-ray beam nomenclature to form a list of terms and their abbreviations. These should be thoroughly memorized.

Term	Symbol
1. Central Ray	CR
2. Focal Spot	FS
3. Source-Image Receptor Distance	SID
4. Kilovolts-Peak	kVp
5. Milliamperes	mA
6. Milliampere-Seconds	mAs
7. Object-Image Receptor Distance	OID
8. Primary Radiation	PR
9. Remnant Radiation	RR
10. Exposure Time in seconds	s
11. Roentgen	R

TYPES OF RADIOGRAPHIC VARIABLES

The remainder of this book will deal with the many variables which affect the radiographic image and how they are controlled and manipulated to optimize image quality. An overview of these variables is provided by categorizing them into six general types:

1. *Electrical Variables:* Electrical variables include machine phase, kilovoltage, milliamperage and exposure time—anything controlled by the technological equipment in producing the x-ray beam.

2. *Geometrical Variables:* Geometrical variables include the various distances, areas, focal spot size, angles and alignment of the x-ray beam, the part of interest and the image receptor (film). Positioning of the patient is actually a geometrical variable dealing with alignment, angles, centering and distances.

3. *Patient Status:* The condition of the patient, including gender, age and body habitus, as well as diseases and other conditions of the tissues in the patient, can cause alterations in image quality. The patient's ability and cooperation in obtaining optimum inspiration on chest radiographs, breathing or controlled movement on autotomographic procedures, and immobilization are essential to image quality.

4. *Image Receptor System:* The image receptor system includes anything which alters the condition of the remnant beam of rays after is passes through the patient, and the recording medium for the image. Grids, Potter-Bucky diaphragms, intensifying screens or film holders, radiographic films, television cameras and monitors, spotfilming devices, image intensifiers, cine cameras, electrically charged plates, and various radiation detectors coupled to computer systems are some examples. These devices are used in a number of possible combinations to provide the optimum image in the desired format.

5. *Processing Variables:* All images must be processed in some manner to allow permanent storage. Chemical concentrations, temperature and processing time, film storage and handling considerations are essential to the quality of the final image recorded. In computer systems, images are "post-processed" electronically to optimize quality before transferring them to some permanent medium such as a CD, magnetic disc, or tape.

6. *Viewing Conditions:* Even after the permanent image is recorded, variables affecting the visibility of that recorded image must be considered each time it is viewed for diagnosis. Ambient lighting, peripheral lighting around the image, adequate illumination through the film itself, and various artifacts such as smudges on the illuminators must be controlled. For computerized images, electronic noise, contrast, and brightness may need to be adjusted on the television monitor and the screen kept clean of smudges.

Every facet of radiography described in this book falls within one of these six categories of radiographic variables. It is the endeavor of every radiographer to manipulate and control them for the production of optimum quality diagnostic images.

SUMMARY

1. X-rays were discovered by Wilhelm Roentgen while he experimented with *Crookes tubes.* Refinements in the x-ray tube were made by Jackson and Coolidge, focusing the electron beam, vacuuming the tube, and heating the filament, and later the spinning anode made it more durable.

2. The three main components of the modern x-ray tube are the vacuum tube, the heated filament, and the rotating anode. X-rays are produced when high-speed electrons from the filament strike the anode and decelerate, losing energy.

3. Most of the x-ray beam is produced by *bremsstrahlung* interactions in the anode. The resulting *heterogeneous* energies in the beam allow *subject contrast* to be produced.

4. *Subject contrast* is the differential absorption of between different types of tissues, each one absorbing a different percentage or portion of the x-ray beam.

5. A portion of the beam is produced by *characteristic* interactions in the anode. These rays have discrete energies at 10, 12, 57, 66, and 69 keV.

6. The *remnant beam* which exposes the film has about one-fifth the intensity of the primary beam and carries *subject contrast.* Three-fourths or more of the remnant beam is comprised of *secondary radiation* produced within the patient.

7. The *prime factors* for radiography include

exposure time, mA, kVp, and SID.
8. All *variables* affecting radiographic image quality can be classified as: Electrical factors, geometry, patient status, image receptor systems, processing, and viewing conditions.

REVIEW QUESTIONS

1. Name the type of tube which first used a heated cathode filament wire to "boil off" a constant source of electrons:
2. As a source of free electrons with which the anode will be bombarded to produce x-rays, the cathode filament wire is heated to "boil" them off. Name this process:
3. Why are x-rays produced when electrons are slowed down or stopped in the anode?
4. Describe the bremsstrahlung interaction:
5. Sketch the characteristic interaction in two parts: 1st, the ionization of an anode atom, 2nd, the resulting orbital electron shift causing the x-ray.
6. What must you know about the orbital electron shells in an atom to be able to predict the energy of a characteristic x-ray photon produced there?
7. Why is bremsstrahlung absolutely essential for there to be any subject contrast to produce an image?
8. Draw in the graph below a beam spectrum curve for an x-ray beam with filtration, set at 68 kVp and having characteristic interactions occur at 59 kV:

9. The intensity or amount of radiation in the remnant beam is what fraction or percentage of that in the primary beam?
10. What fraction or percentage of remnant radiation reaching the film is actually primary radiation which did not interact with any atoms in the patient?
11. Define *primary beam*:
12. List the six general types of variables which affect the quality of the radiographic image:
13. X-rays are generally similar to light, but their wavelength is much _____, which enables them to penetrate matter that light cannot.
14. What are the three main components of the modern x-ray tube?
15. Why do modern x-ray tubes use rotating anodes?
16. Why are tungsten and rhenium used to coat the anode surface?
17. The average energy of a heterogeneous x-ray beam is about what fraction of its peak energy?
18. If the number of _____.
21. List the four *prime factors* of radiography:
22. What is the proper term that describes the *partial* absorption of the x-ray beam as it passes through the body?
23. Every density within the anatomy on a radiographic image should be a shade of _____.
24. What do the following abbreviations stand for:
   a. OID:
   b. CR:
   c. R:

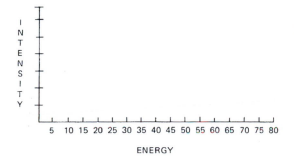

Chapter 2

RECORDING THE PERMANENT IMAGE

BEGINNINGS OF PHOTOGRAPHY

IN THE EARLY 18TH CENTURY, it became known that some silver compounds blackened when exposed to light; thus began the art of photography. In 1727, a German chemist discovered how to make black-lettered stencil images with a paste of silver carbonate mixed with chalk and exposed to light, and in 1816, a crude camera was made by exposing silver salts to light passing through a lens from a microscope, but all of these images were transient and would not last.

An Englishman named William Henry Fox Talbot discovered how to make an image permanent by treating the silver chloride paper on which it was recorded with sodium chloride. In 1840, Talbot found that he could develop a latent (invisible) image after exposure of the silver layer. He obtained a negative image and by printing on sensitized paper was able to obtain positive images. Talbot became the inventor of the *negative-positive* method of photography. A scientist friend, Sir John Herschel, coined the phrase "photography,"–drawing with light–when he wrote Talbot about his discovery.

The Frenchman Loui J.J. Daguerre recorded images in 1839 on plates covered with silver iodide, but they were faint and unsatisfactory. One day he placed one of the exposed plates in his cupboard. Upon removing it at a later date, he found that there was a well-defined positive image on the plate. Some mercury had been spilled in the cabinet and its fumes had "developed" the image completely. The unexposed silver iodide was removed by a solution of sodium chloride. Daguerre thereby discovered the phenomenon of chemical development.

In 1879, George Eastman invented a machine to coat glass plates with a gelatin containing silver bromide which were also later used in early radiography. Eastman later developed and mass-produced *American film*, which evolved into a flexible, transparent strip of nitrocellulose coated with silver halide and could hold several photographs, later to be chemically transferred onto paper as a permanent images. Thus, the stage was set for one of man's most important discoveries wherein photographic emulsion was to play a dominant role.

BIRTH OF RADIOGRAPHY

On November 8, 1895, Wilhelm Conrad Roentgen proved the existence of x-rays by exposing and processing a dry plate, thus opening to the world a vast new field of endeavor–radiography.

The moment of the actual discovery of

the x-rays proved it to be the beginning of a new era. The very nature of the x-rays was such that the whole scientific and lay world would become absorbed in it, not alone by its very spectacular nature but also by the possibility that these new rays would open the door of knowledge of the ultimate nature of matter—something that had perplexed the best scientific minds. It was the dawn of the atomic age.

After the first few months of wild exaggeration and rumor, the discovery was stripped of its sensationalism and left to the conservative experimenter who rejoiced in the possibilities of this new discovery. These efforts were based upon the sensitive dry plate which not only proved the existence of x-rays but also became the biggest factor in the development of the science of radiology.

At first, the dry plate was used to record x-ray images, but the exposures required were exceedingly long. Another disadvantage of the dry plate used in those early days was that the glass plate was easily broken. The development of an x-ray intensifying screen by Thomas Edison, which was composed of calcium tungstate fluorescent crystals, and its first use by Professor Michael Pupin of Columbia University in 1896, served to augment the exposure effect of the x-rays, extending the usefulness of the radiographic method to medicine. Until 1917, radiography was largely performed with photographic plates that were specially designed for x-ray work.

During World War I, x-ray film was produced, but the cellulose nitrate film base was highly flammable and a fire hazard. In 1924, *safety* x-ray film was introduced, made of cellulose acetate, a slower-burning material. It was found that sensitive emulsion could be coated onto both sides of the film base, both reducing its tendency to curl and increasing the film's speed. This also allowed *two* intensifying screens to be used, all of which dramatically reduced the exposure needed. The quality and uniformity of x-ray film has been greatly enhanced over the years.

MODERN X-RAY FILM

X-ray film is manufactured today with a remarkable consistency so that its exposure and processing may be standardized. Traditional x-ray film consists of an *emulsion* of finely precipitated silver bromide crystals suspended in a gelatin that is coated on both sides of a transparent blue-tinted polyester support called the *base*.

The emulsion coating is glued onto the film base with a thin layer of adhesive material. The emulsion is the functional part of the x-ray film, and consists of crystals of silver bromide suspended in gelatin. The properties of the gelatin are very important: It must be capable of suspending the crystals in a relatively even distribution, without allowing them to clump together or to settle out at the bottom layer. It must also be flexible and porous enough to allow processing chemicals to penetrate into it and reach the crystals. But, it must also not become too soft during processing or it will come off of the film base.

Finally, the emulsion is protected from scratches by a thin coating of varnish called the supercoat or T-coat (tough-coat). The four component layers of the radiographic film are illustrated in Figure 2-1. Most film is *duplitized* or coated with emulsion on both sides, as shown in Figure 2-1. This is done so that it may be effectively used in screen cassettes which usually have screens

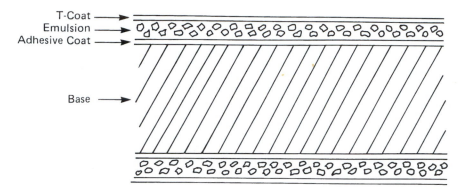

Figure 2-1. Diagram of the component layers of radiographic film: The polyester base, emulsion on either side, adhesive coats and protective T-coats.

on both the front and back covers of the cassette. Special "extremity" or "detail" cassettes sometimes have only one screen. These are best used with single-emulsion film. When a single-emulsion film is loaded into such a cassette, the film emulsion must be facing and in contact with the screen. In the dark room lighting, the radiographer can recognize the emulsion side of the film as the *dull* surface. The glossy, shiny side of

the film is the polyester plastic base and has no emulsion. The dull surface should face the screen.

Examined under a microscope, countless tiny crystals of silver bromide are seen embedded within the gelatin (Fig. 2-2). Silver bromide is a salt of silver which, when exposed to x-radiation, will begin to turn dark. The process is analogous to silverware which tarnishes from exposure to

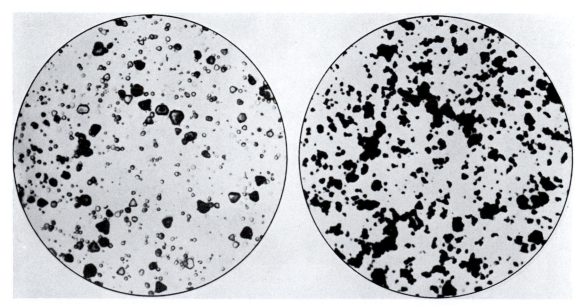

Figure 2-2. Photomicrograph (2500 X) of silver emulsion. (*Left*) Before exposure, the emulsion is seen to be made up of countless tiny crystals of silver bromide isolated from one another by gelatin. (*Right*) After exposure and development, the original crystals have been broken down to form clumps of black metallic silver.

light over long periods of time. When the film is later chemically processed, this "tarnishing" of the exposed silver bromide crystals is completed to the point that they are entirely black (Fig. 2-2).

The production and composition of x-ray film is more thoroughly described in Chapter 15, but this will serve as an introductory overview for the beginning student.

LATENT IMAGE FORMATION

As described in Chapter 1, x-rays are capable of ionizing matter, that is, they can cause orbital electrons to be "knocked out" of atoms. In the silver bromide crystals of an x-ray film, this removal of electrons can cause the molecules to break apart, separating the bromine from the silver. In simple terms, this damage may be thought of as cracks or "fractures" in the crystal at each point where an x-ray or where several light rays have struck (Fig. 2-3). Later, when the film is processed, the developing chemicals are able to penetrate and quickly "attack" those crystals already damaged by radiation, but are unable to penetrate those which are free of defects within the short time that the film is immersed in the processing solutions.

There are many hundreds of silver bromide molecules in one crystal, so these breaks caused by radiation do not immediately transform the whole crystal. Rather, they break several silver atoms from the structure. These freed silver atoms tend to clump together at special locations on the crystal called "sensitivity specks," forming small spots of metallic silver. These silver spots are not large enough to result in a visible, complete image. Therefore, upon exposure, a film will contain information which is not yet visible to the naked eye. This "invisible image" is called the *latent image.*

Although the latent image is not completely visible, the fact that a chemical change has occurred in the silver bromide

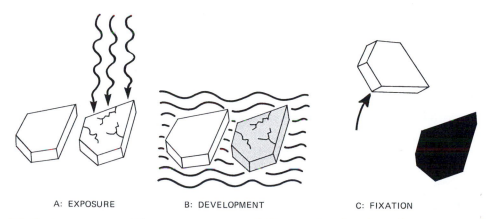

A: EXPOSURE   B: DEVELOPMENT   C: FIXATION

Figure 2-3. During exposure (A), x-rays cause several "fractures" or breaks in the structure of a silver bromide crystal. During processing (B), developer solution is able to penetrate deep into the "broken" crystals, converting them into black metallic silver. Unexposed crystals are intact and resist penetration by the developer solution. These intact crystals are later removed from the film by the fixer solution (C), while those converted into black silver remain on the film and form the visible image.

crystals can be demonstrated with the following experiment:

Experiment:

You may need someone to assist by opening doors for you. In the dark room under red lighting only, remove one small x-ray film from the film bin. Hold it between your flattened hands, placing them directly opposite each other with fingers fanned. Make sure that each finger is directly opposite its counterpart on the other hand. Keeping your hands in place, exit the dark room and immediately hold the film up next to an illuminator (view-box) for a count of about ten. Quickly step back well away from the illuminator or other lights, and have the group watch carefully as you remove both hands simultaneously. For a very brief few seconds, a lighter silhouette image of the hands will be visible. It may take some practice to get this just right—it is essential that you *not* be very close to any lights when you remove your hands.

Explanation: Those silver bromide crystals outside the hands had a latent image formed by the illuminator light. This image consisted of small spots of dark silver clumps on each crystal, making the emulsion outside the hands appear slightly darker. Upon removing your hands, the light in the room quickly causes those crystals which were previously covered to also form latent images, erasing the silhouette effect in seconds.

PROCESSING THE SILVER IMAGE

As clearly demonstrated in the foregoing experiment, the small clumps of silver which comprise the latent image are not sufficient to produce a fully visible, diagnostic image. To fully develop an image, chemical processing of the film is required.

Processing may be thought of as a chemical method of multiplying or exaggerating the effects of exposure. Those silver bromide crystals which have been "fractured" by x-rays will allow the processing chemicals to penetrate into their structure. The remaining molecules in these crystals will be broken down as the chemicals continue to separate silver atoms from bromine atoms. The free silver atoms will then adhere to the small silver spot at the sensitivity speck which was originally formed from the exposure. Thus, the small metallic silver spot is caused to grow many thousands of times larger, forming blackened areas on the radiograph which are visible to the naked eye.

The processing chemicals recognize and attack only those silver bromide crystals which have already been damaged by exposure to the x-ray beam, Figure 2-3B. Crystals that were not exposed are later washed away by "fixer" chemicals, Figure 2-3C.

A review of Figure 1-13 reminds us that under dense tissues such as bone, few x-rays reach the film. In such areas, few crystals will be damaged, and therefore not many crystals will be chemically developed into clumps of black metallic silver. Rather, these crystals are washed away by fixer chemicals, resulting in light or "white" areas on the film image. However, under soft tissue areas, many x-rays reach the film, causing "fractures" in the crystals. Those crystals are later recognized and attacked by developer chemicals, ultimately turning them into clumps of black silver which remain on the film after processing. This final image composed of black metallic silver is called the *visible image*.

The chemistry of latent image formation and of visible image formation is more fully described in Chapters 15 and 37. The following "resume" of image production, along with Figure 2-3, should serve to review and clarify the basic concepts of radiographic exposure and processing.

RESUME OF IMAGE PRODUCTION

When the exposed emulsion is considered as a whole rather than as its constituent silver bromide crystals, the various stages in the production of the silver image can be diagrammatically illustrated as in Figure 2-4. Let us assume that an aluminum step wedge (A) is exposed using an x-ray film (B) as the recording medium. When the film is represented in enlarged cross-section, a latent image of the object is produced upon exposure in the silver bromide emulsion (C). The latent image is represented by the dotted area and consists of representations of the six portions of the wedge. The radiation reaching the film is of varying intensities after its passage through the various thickness of the step wedge, and the relative absorption of each step thickness is represented.

The radiation passing through step number 1 of the object is only partially absorbed, hence more silver bromide is exposed than for that portion of the film under steps number 4 or number 6, where-in greater absorption takes place. Hence, upon development, the quantity of silver deposited in these areas is less than that under step number 1. In other words, each step is recorded as a deposit of silver that is proportionate to the intensity of the remnant radiation reaching the film.

Upon development (D), the silver bromide of the latent image is reduced to metallic silver, and the unexposed silver bromide (thin diagonal lines) is not affected. After the film has been treated by fixer solution (E), all the unexposed and undeveloped silver bromide is dissolved from the emulsion, while the metallic silver remains on the film to constitute the radiographic image of the step wedge. When the radiographic image (F) is later viewed on an x-ray illuminator, all the various deposits of silver representing the steps of the wedge are seen in their proper silver concentration with various degrees of translucency to light from the illuminator.

SUMMARY

1. Englishman William Talbot discovered modern photography, Frenchman Loui Daguerre discovered the chemical film development process, and American George Eastman developed the mass production of photographic film as well as the glass plates that were first used for radiography.

2. A *latent image* is produced on an x-ray film when incident x-ray photons *ionize* portions of a silver bromide crystal, releasing free silver atoms to collect around the *sensitivity speck*.

3. During *development*, reducing chemicals attack the crystals to complete the process of breaking all of the silver

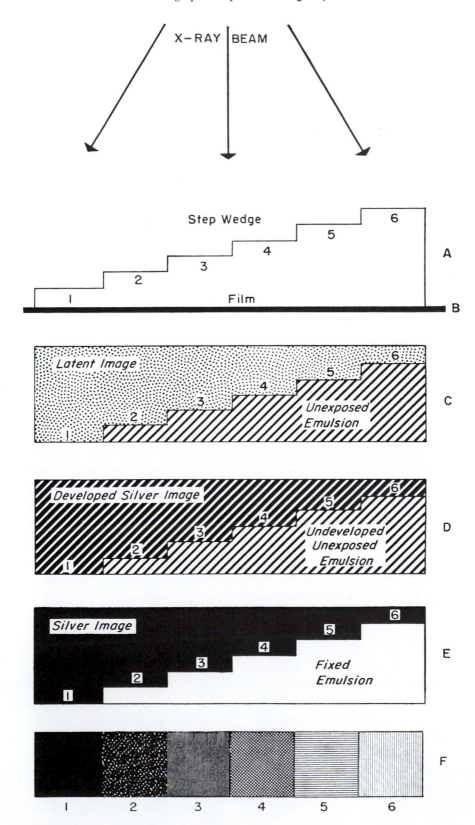

atoms free from the bromine atoms to coagulate around the sensitivity speck and form a clump of *black metallic silver.*

4. *Unexposed* crystals, having few or no

breaks in their lattice structure, resist development and are removed from the film during the *fixing* process.

REVIEW QUESTIONS

1. When x-rays were discovered, film had already been largely developed in the field of _____.
2. Instead of film, early radiographs were taken on _____.
3. What are the component layers of an x-ray film:
4. Define *latent image*:
5. What is a modern x-ray film base made of:
6. Define chemical development:
7. What are the crystals in the film emulsion made of prior to development?
8. What are the crystals left on the surface of the film after development made of?
9. What material is used to hold the film crystals in an evenly-distributed suspension?
10. Who invented the glass photographic plates which Roentgen first used to produce radiographs?
11. Define *duplitized*:

Figure 2-4. "Life cycle of a radiograph": (A) Exposure of a step wedge and x-ray film (B) creates a latent image (C). During processing, the developer solution attacks only the exposed silver bromide crystals (D), which are changed to black metallic silver. The fixer solution then removes the unexposed and undeveloped crystals (E). The final image seen as seen on the x-ray illuminator appears as various quantities of black silver on the clear base (F).

Chapter 3

QUALITIES OF THE RADIOGRAPHIC IMAGE

COMPONENTS OF THE IMAGE

WHAT ARE THE ESSENTIAL requirements for your eyes to see? The first and most obvious answer is that they need light. But, consider what light is: Light is the flow of small bundles of energy called quanta or photons–it is part of the same electromagnetic spectrum as x-rays are. In fact, the only real difference between x-rays and light is the length of their waves and the corresponding energies.

VISIBILITY

What you *see* is actually reflected light photons striking your the nerve endings in the retina of your eyes. When twice as many photons strike your eye, the image you see appears twice as bright. It is more intense. Thus, the amount of light photons flowing toward your eyes, or the number of photons striking your retina, is referred to as the *intensity* of the light. When the light intensity is very low, you cannot recognize your surroundings, because much of the information in the actual image is not visible.

However, adequate light alone does not provide vision or create and image. Suppose that everything in your field of view was the same white light and all at the same intensity or brightness. You would be just as blind seeing blank white as you would be if everything was pitch darkness. In order to see, there must be differing shades of brightness and darkness within your field of view. The greater the difference is between the shade of an object and the shade of the surrounding field of view or background, the easier it is to see the object. A pure black object against a white background, for example, is a most visible combination. This difference between intensities of reflected light is called *contrast*. For contrast to exist, and for any image at all to exist, there must be two or more different intensities present. If the differences between the intensities is great, then the image is regarded as having *high contrast*. Some contrast is required for any image to exist.

However, it is possible for an image to have *too much* contrast. This situation is illustrated by the photographs in Figure 3-1. *Photograph A* is a very high contrast image: Note that you cannot distinguish between the edges of the girl's blouse and the background wall, the edges between the stuffed animal and the girl's blouse, or the ruffles in the blouse. These details are visible in *Photograph B* which has a medium level of contrast. For *Photograph A* the contrast is too high–everything tends to be reduced to either black or white, with few intermediate shades of gray. Objects that would have been depicted as a very light gray, such as the ruffles and shadows of the blouse, are recorded instead as white and are not discernable against a background of

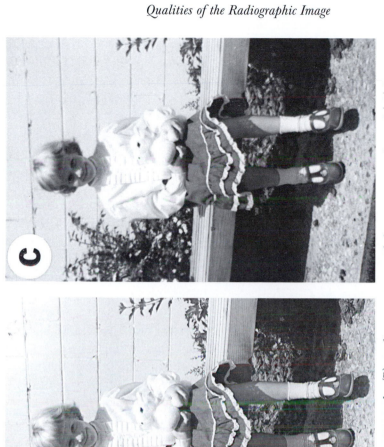

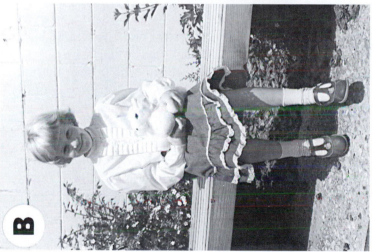

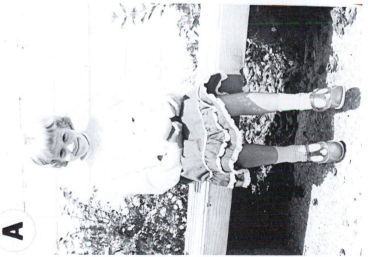

Figure 3-1. Photographs demonstrating (A) high contrast with short gray scale, (B) medium contrast with longer gray scale, and (C) low contrast with excessive gray scale. Note that details visible in the stuffed animal, blouse and sidewalk disappear with excessive contrast (A). Darker gray details in the leaves, the shadow under the bench and the girl's eyebrows disappear with excessive gray scale (C). Also, note that high contrast can deceptively mimic underexposure: Photograph A appears light at a glance, yet the shadow under the bench is actually *darker* than that in B. The overall density of Photograph A is *not* light, rather, it possesses excessive contrast.

white. Likewise, dark gray objects are depicted as black and will not stand out against a black background. This image actually has fewer visible details than *photograph B. Excessive contrast has caused a loss of useful information.*

On the other hand, insufficient contrast also leads to an image in which details are not adequately visible. If there is barely any difference between two adjacent shades of gray, it will be difficult for the human eye to detect that there are indeed two shades there. If these gray shades cannot be distinguished from each other, information is again lost. *Photograph C* in Figure 3-1 demonstrates insufficient contrast, with an overall gray appearance. Note that the subtle dark gray shades of leaves under the bench, visible in *photograph B*, are not as visible in *photograph C*, because there is little difference between them and the dark shadow of the bench.

To summarize, note that the greatest amount of information in Figure 3-1 is found in *photograph B*, where the contrast level is intermediate. If contrast is too high, gray shades are exaggerated into white or black, and information is lost. If contrast is too low, different shades of gray that lie next to each other become difficult to distinguish, and again information is lost. Excessive contrast can cause as great a loss of information as a lack of contrast. The ideal amount of contrast in an image lies in an intermediate range and is somewhat subject to personal preference.

The word *optimum* is used to describe the ideal level of contrast that an image should have. It refers to an intermediate level, a "happy medium," which is neither too much nor too little. In radiographic imaging, the goal is not to produce *maximum* contrast nor *minimum* contrast, but rather to produce *optimum* contrast. The same term should be used to describe the

intensity of light for an image: Too little light would be pitch dark, too much would blind us. The ideal amount of light is a medium amount that we would refer to as *optimum intensity.*

One more factor affects the visibility of an object in your field of view: If it is raining heavily between yourself and the object you are trying to see, you may not be able to see it well. The rain represents unwanted information which obstructs the visibility of the wanted information. Undesirable information that interferes with the subject of interest is referred to as *noise.* Interference and static on your TV screen are examples of noise in an image. In radiography, fogging of the film by heat or light, static discharges, and artifacts from foreign objects (several of which are demonstrated in Chapters 39 and 40) are forms of noise. The most common form of image noise in radiography is fogging of the film by random radiation known as *scatter.*

These three functions—intensity, contrast, and noise—are the *visibility functions* of an image. Maximum visibility is attained when light intensity and contrast are both optimum, and when noise is kept to a minimum.

RECOGNIZABILITY

In addition to the visibility functions of an image, there are what we might call *recognizability functions.* A visible image is completely worthless if we cannot recognize what it is. We depend upon the geometrical integrity of the image to recognize what real object it represents. If the image is blurry, or if its size or shape are grossly distorted, we may not be able to tell what it is, even though it is visible. Recognizability, or geometrical integrity, is made up of three components: sharpness of recorded detail, magnification and shape distortion.

Sharpness of Recorded Detail

The *sharpness of recorded detail* may be described as the *abruptness* with which the edges of a particular image *stop*. To better visualize this principle, imagine yourself moving across a black-and-white photograph, perhaps driving your microscopic sports car: You are passing from a white image onto the black background. As you cross over the edge between white and black, if you quite suddenly find yourself over the black background, then the edge of the white image was *sharp*, and stopped abruptly. If, on the other hand, you seem to pass gradually from white into black, then the edge of the white image is *blurred* and *unsharp*.

Theoretically, if shadows could be cast from a *point source* of light, such as in Figure 3-2A, there would never be any blur. There would be projected a single, pure shadow with sharp edges. But when the source of light is an *area source* such as the sun or a flashlight bulb (or an x-ray tube focal spot), there will always be partial shadows cast around the edges of the *pure* shadow. This is shown in Figure 3-2-B. These *partial shadows* occur because any given edge of the object is actually projected at several different angles from several different points within the light source.

Single point sources of light are rarely found in nature. The sun, for example, has a surface *area*, and light can be emitted from many different regions across that area. As shown in Figure 3-2, this means that the shadow of a particular edge of the object will be projected by different beams of light coming from slightly different angles. The edge of the shadow will then be projected onto the background in more

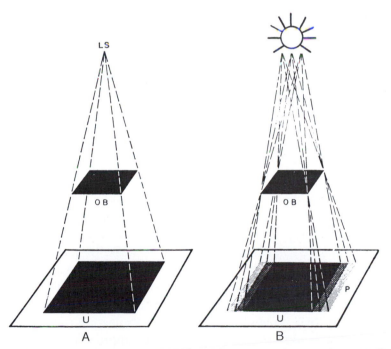

Figure 3-2. Diagram illustrating a pure umbra image from a theoretical point source of light (*A*) compared to the production of penumbra (p) at the edges of a shadow image by an area light source such as the sun or the x-ray tube anode (*B*).

than one place, resulting in an unsharp appearance called *blur.*

The *pure* projected shadow of an object is named its *umbra.* The partial shadow projected at the edge of of an object is called its *penumbra.* Penumbra is synonymous with blur–the more penumbra is present, the more blurry we would say the edge appears.

Experiment:

To demonstrate umbra and penumbra, hold your hand over an overhead projector or in front of a flashlight; Move your hand away from the light source and then back toward it, and observe the edges of the shadow that is cast. As you move your hand back and forth from the light source, you will see the blurry penumbra at the edges grow and shrink. Note that when the penumbra grows, it not only expands outward but also inward, invading the umbra, and that the umbra actually shrinks from this effect. At *extreme* distances from the light source, the pure umbra part of the shadow actually disappears and the image becomes *all* penumbra. All that is left is a nebulous, blurry density in the area of the image. If enough penumbra is present, you will not be able to recognize the image as the shadow of your hand. Even though an image may be visible, excessive blurriness can literally destroy the ability to recognize what it is, and thus render the image useless.

Now consider the problems caused with recognizability when observing the very blurry images of two objects closely adjacent to each other. (Repeat the above experiment observing two fingers held closely together.) As penumbra grows, the edges of the two shadow images will overlap and blur into each other. When two shadows overlap in this way, they may deceptively appear as one shadow of one object, even though there are really two objects.

Sharpness may be destroyed not only by a geometrical growth of the penumbra, but also by blurring due to motion. Movement of either the x-ray tube, the body part being radiographed, or the film will result in a blurred image. An example of motion blurring of a hand radiograph is found in Figure 3-14. Sharpness of recorded detail has a strong impact upon our ability to recognize an image.

Magnification

Excessive magnification of the size of an image may make it difficult to recognize what real object the image represents. Imagine standing just one inch away from the side of a rhinoceros! With just its skin filling your field of view, would you be sure it was not an elephant or a hippopotamus? When something is grossly magnified in our field of view, we may literally lose the ability to recognize what it is. In photography and in radiography, *magnification* may be defined as the difference in size between a real object and its projected image in the picture. Magnification is often referred to in radiography as *size distortion* and classified under the general heading of *distortion.* However, for the sake of clarity, the word *distortion* shall only be used in this book when referring to changes in the *shape* of an image. *Magnification* shall be consistently used to describe changes in the size of the image.

In most radiography, our goal is to minimize any magnification present in the image. Projecting the true size of an object is important to correct diagnosis. For example, one thing radiologists routinely check for on chest radiographs is possible enlargement of the heart. If the heart size is magnified because of the way the radiographer positioned the patient, the radiologist could be misled into falsely diagnosing the patient as having an enlarged heart. Magnification can lead to misinformation.

Shape Distortion

Shape distortion is defined as the difference between the shape of the real object and the shape of its projected image on a radiograph or photograph. In a given axis of direction (lengthwise or crosswise), shape distortion will consist of either a foreshortening of the image or an elongation of the image. When a square object, for example, is projected onto a two-dimensional surface or film from an angled direction as shown in Figure 3-3, its shadow is elongated into a rectangular image which does not represent

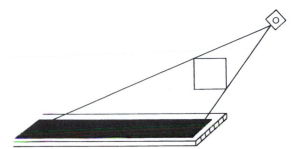

Figure 3-3. Diagram demonstrating shape distortion. Misalignment or angling of a beam of light will project the shadow of a square object as a distorted rectangular image.

the true shape of the original object. Angling or off-centering the x-ray tube, the part being radiographed or the film can lead to similar shape distortion, the true nature of the object is not recognizable, and information recorded on the film may be misleading and misinterpreted.

QUALITIES OF THE RADIOGRAPH

The image on a radiograph must have all of the same qualities as an image you visually see—intensity, contrast, noise, sharpness of detail, magnification, and shape distortion. But, since radiography works somewhat differently than your eyes, some of these qualities are given different specific names. Also, some image qualities have an "opposite," which must be named and learned in order to thoroughly critique the quality of radiographic images.

DENSITY VERSUS TONE VALUE

Standard radiographs, along with most CT, MRI, and ultrasound scans, are considered as "negative" images, white or light images on a black background, rather than dark images against a white background such as a typical photograph. The "background" of a radiograph actually consists of blackened deposits of metallic silver as described in the previous chapter. The darkest areas represent the greatest exposure of the film to the x-ray beam. In Figure 3-4, you can see that *outside* the knee, where there was nothing to absorb the x-ray beam, exposure to the film was high and the resulting background is black. The amount of blackening present at any given point on the film is referred to as its *density.* Thus, a very dark area is regarded as having high density, and a lighter area as having low density. The densities on a radiographic image indicate the intensity of the radiation that was able to penetrate the patient and strike the film there.

During their passage through a body part, the x-rays are absorbed selectively by various tissues. This absorption results in the production of a number of *different* sil-

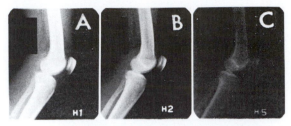

Figure 3-4. Series of radiographs demonstrating results of underexposure (A), correct exposure (B), and overexposure (C). Note the loss of visible details in the bones at both extremes.

ver deposits on the radiograph. Obviously, the greater the number of different shades of darkness present in the image, the greater the number of structural details that can be visualized in the image.

In Figure 3-4, three radiographs of a knee are demonstrated with (A) insufficient density due to underexposure to the x-ray beam, (B) optimum overall density due to correct exposure, and (C) excessive overall density due to overexposure. Comparing (A) to (B), note that details within the bones are missing in (A) because it is too light. Underexposure results in very little silver deposit, and this white silhouette image is diagnostically worthless. The same may be said for (C), where overexposure has resulted in such excessive deposits of silver as to obscure image details within the bone. Information is lost from either underexposure or overexposure. Correct exposure results in an *optimum* range of image densities in which every detail within the anatomy is depicted as a *shade of gray*.

Being negative images, standard radiographs must be viewed on an illuminator or "viewbox" that shines light through the transparent plastic base of the film from behind. The amount of light that is able to pass through the film at a given point and strike your eyes is correctly referred to as *tone value*. Tone value is the opposite of density. If there is less silver deposit in a

particular area of the film, more light will shine through it, so it will appear *whiter* or lighter than surrounding densities. This area is said to have high tone value. High tone value, then, is the same as low density. A device called a densitometer is used to measure the densities on radiographic films. What this device actually detects is the tone values, the amount of light passing through the film at different points. It then converts the tone value measurements into a density reading algebraically. The density values read off of a densitometer range from 0 to 4.0. A reading of 0 would indicate that *all* of the light from the illuminator passes through the film at that point and it would appear as a blank white area. A reading of 4.0 represents a pitch black density to the human eye, with no detectable light passing through.

Since neither blank white areas nor pitch black areas on the radiograph contain useful information, those densities that might be considered as diagnostically useful will range from a very light gray shade (slightly darker than the film base) to a very dark gray shade just short of black. *This range of useful densities extends from 0.25 to 2.5 as measured on a densitometer.*

CONTRAST VERSUS GRAY SCALE

Radiographic *contrast* is the proportional difference between two adjacent densities, measured as a ratio (not as a subtracted difference). If one density is twice as dark as the one next to it, the contrast is measured as $2/1 = 2.0$. A very contrasty radiograph appears to be more "black and white," whereas a low-contrast radiograph appears to be somewhat gray overall. Figure 3-5 shows how density levels can change without contrast being affected. Note that as long as all densities on the film increase or decrease by the same proportion, the ratios

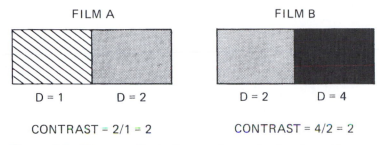

Figure 3-5. Diagram illustrating a change in density without a change in contrast. The *ratio* of difference between the two adjacent densities remains the same even though *Film B* is twice as dense overall. An image can be darker and still have high contrast.

of difference between them remain the same and contrast is equal. That is, it is possible to double all of the densities on a radiograph by doubling the exposure, and yet still have the darker ones come out twice as dark as the lighter ones. Within the range of useful densities as described above, it is possible to change the average density of an image up or down while maintaining equal contrast.

A common misconception is that anything affecting image density will also affect image contrast. This is false. Often, variables which affect image density will also change the image contrast. But, there are exceptions to this. As shown in Figure 3-5, overall density can be changed without affecting contrast, and contrast can also be changed without affecting average density.

The opposite of radiographic contrast is *gray scale*. Gray scale may be defined as the *range of different densities present in the image*. Considerable confusion has been caused by the terminology commonly used, particularly the phrase *contrast scale*. Combining the word *contrast* with the word *scale* seems indeed contradictory, since they are opposites. For the sake of clarity, this book shall consistently utilize the term *gray scale* or *scale* when referring to the range of densities in an image.

When there are many different densities,

many different shades of gray in an image, it is said to have *long scale*. Conversely, when only a few different densities are present, the radiograph is said to have *short scale*. To better understand the relationship between contrast and gray scale and why they are opposites, consider a 10-foot high staircase. This staircase may be built to have 10 individual stairs, each one being one-foot tall. On the other hand, it could be built to have only five individual stairs. If there are only five stairs, each individual stair must be two feet tall—there is a greater difference between the stairs. The greater the difference between the stairs, the fewer stairs there must be. Conversely, if there are a lot of stairs, say, 20, then there must be a smaller degree of difference from one to the next. With this staircase concept in mind, examine the *aggregate silver deposits* diagrammed in Figures 3-6 and 3-7. High contrast implies short gray scale, because when there are great differences between densities, there can only be few densities present (Fig. 3-6). With low contrast, there will be long gray scale (Fig. 3-7).

A good radiograph is one that possesses a correct balance of densities over the entire gray scale. The gray scale should be such that good differentiation is shown between tissue details portrayed over the whole area of diagnostic interest without

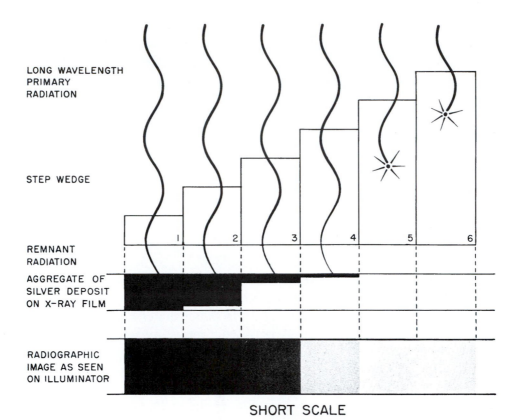

LONG WAVELENGTH
PRIMARY
RADIATION

STEP WEDGE

REMNANT
RADIATION

AGGREGATE OF
SILVER DEPOSIT
ON X-RAY FILM

RADIOGRAPHIC
IMAGE AS SEEN
ON ILLUMINATOR

SHORT SCALE

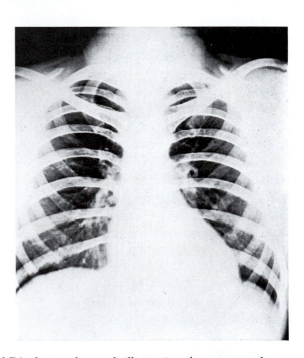

Figure 3-6. Step wedge diagram and PA chest radiograph illustrating short gray scale.

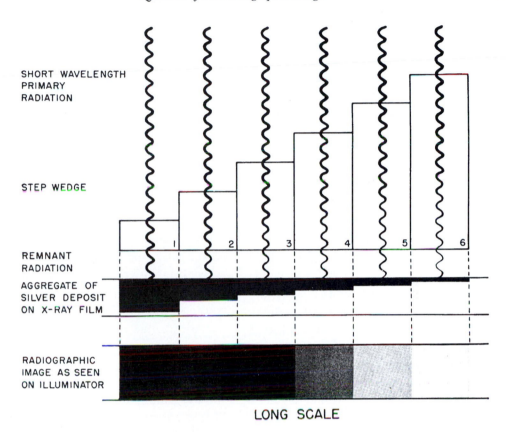

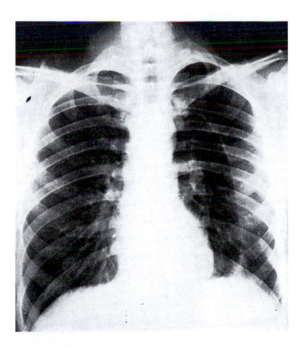

Figure 3-7. Step wedge diagram and PA chest radiograph illustrating long gray scale.

loss of details in the lighter or darker areas of the radiographic image. The scale of densities that determines the contrast and the visibility of details is directly influenced by the x-ray wavelength, which is in turn controlled by the factor of kilovoltage. This also is shown diagrammatically in Figures 3-6 and 3-7 where a cross-section of an aluminum step wedge is exposed to different wavelengths of x-rays and the resulting image as it would appear on the radiograph is depicted below.

Short Scale

In the diagram in Figure 3-6, it is assumed that long wavelength radiation produced at a low kVp is directed at the step wedge. Note that steps 5 and 6 of the wedge both remain unpenetrated by this radiation, consequently, they show up on the resulting radiographic image as having the same light density and are indistinguishable from each other. In the *aggregate silver deposit* cross-section, you can see that there are only a few steps recorded–a representative image of the entire wedge was not recorded because of an inadequacy of remnant radiation. The number of densities are too few to portray a complete image of the subject. On the other hand, note that the differences between these "steps" is relatively large–this represents high contrast. In the resulting image depicted below, note that there are only three discernable densities representing the corresponding *short gray scale* of the image: One density includes steps 1, 2, and 3, all depicted as the same dark black density, the second represents step 4 only, and the lightest density represents both steps 5 and 6.

The diagram illustrates the fact that radiographic details of an object cannot be seen in an image unless there are discernable differences in tone value between densities, and that there must be a silver deposit on the film if detail within the object is to be demonstrated. This situation is typical for *short gray scale* or for high contrast. When an image of a body part is rendered with densities that are either excessive or virtually non-existent, with a short range of widely different intermediate densities, short gray scale exists. In Figure 3-6, an actual chest radiograph demonstrating such short scale is presented. Such radiographs tend to be pleasing to the eye due to their high contrast, yet they have little diagnostic value and are economically wasteful. Note the utter lack of details in the shadows of the heart and bones on this radiograph.

Additional examples of radiographs demonstrating short scale are presented in Figure 3-8. Note that when low kilovoltage is used for thinner body parts such as the hand, greater contrast occurs between the bones and the flesh. A point is often reached in which, in order to demonstrate bone details adequately, the skin and soft tissues are obliterated by dark silver deposits. If the exposure is then reduced in order to demonstrate these soft tissue areas, details within the bones will be lost. With a short gray scale, only selected tissues may be satisfactorily demonstrated for different levels of exposure. Short scale images have their place, but only as a special procedure designed to more adequately visualize details of *small*, selected tissue areas, and then only after preliminary survey radiographs have been obtained with a fully satisfactory gray scale present.

Long Scale

Figure 3-7 portrays the same situation as shown in Figure 3-6, but using *shorter wavelength* x-rays produced at *higher kilovoltage*. In the diagram, one can see that the radia-

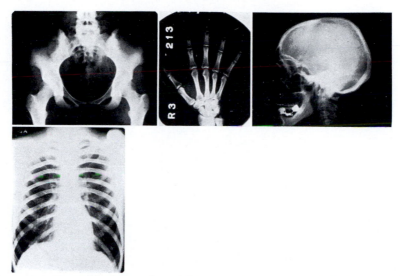

Figure 3-8. Typical radiographs exhibiting various degrees of short gray scale.

tion readily penetrates all portions of the step wedge and the selective degree of absorption by each step has permitted the remnant radiation to emerge with different intensities that are recorded as a range of densities. In the *aggregate silver deposit* diagram, the transition between between the tones is gradual. This is representative of lower contrast. Note that a distinction can now be made between steps 5 and 6 in the resulting image depicted below. Four or more distinct densities can be counted, and this image is typical of *long gray scale*. Additional examples of long gray scale radiographs are shown in Figure 3-9.

Desirable long scale is produced when the kilovoltage is high enough to penetrate and delineate all normal structures satisfactorily. More details, represented by more densities, will be present in the image. This can be clearly seen in the representative chest radiograph shown at the bottom of Figure 3-7, where additional bony details can be seen in the clavicles and ribs as well as in the vascular structures around the heart, when compared to the radiograph in Figure 3-6. Gray scale, however, should never be so long that the differentiation

between structures is difficult. If the maximum of diagnostic information is to be obtained, a compromise must be made between the radiograph with short scale and that exhibiting long scale. Just as too much contrast can cause a loss of information, too much gray scale can do the same, as was shown in Figure 3-1C. As with contrast, the correct amount of gray scale is an *optimum*, intermediate level. In the final analysis, the criterion of good diagnostic contrast and gray scale is whether one sees all one expects to see.

Figure 3-10 uses magnetic resonance images of the spine to illustrate these important concepts further: Images *A* and *B* both have too short a gray scale (excessive contrast). *A* was taken with a lighter overall density level, *B* with a much darker setting, in order to show that *the use of a lighter or darker technique does not correct the image when the gray scale is insufficient.* Images *C* and *D* were taken with long gray scale, using similar density settings. Although *C* is light and *D* is dark, *both* of these images demonstrate more details and more information than their counterparts in *A* and *B*. The ideal image would be a relatively long gray scale

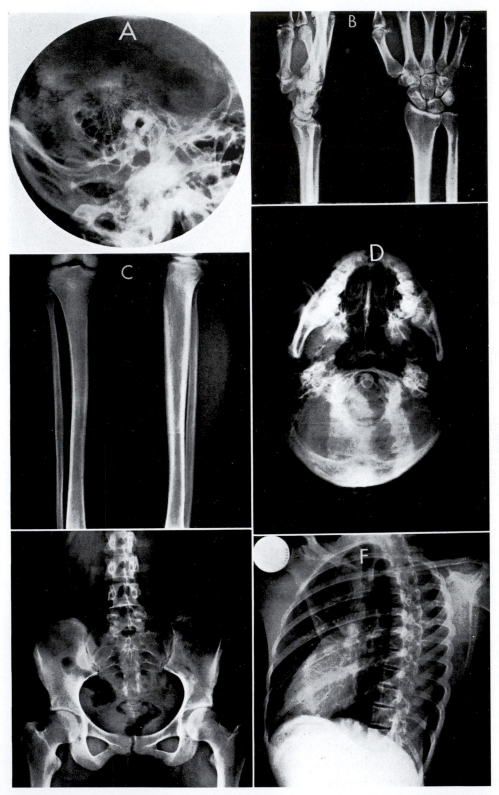

Figure 3-9. Typical radiographs exhibiting long gray scale. An abundance of details is shown because the kilovoltages used were optimum to penetrate the various tissues present.

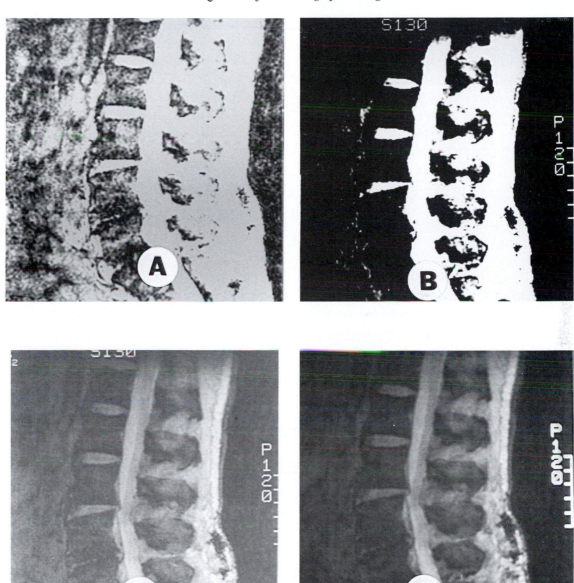

Figure 3-10. Magnetic resonance images of the lateral spine showing (A) short gray scale and light density, (B) short gray scale and dark density, (C) long gray scale and light density, and (D) long gray scale and dark density. More details are visible in the long gray scale images.

image with a density level that is intermediate between *C* and *D*.

FOG AND OTHER NOISE

On foggy days, details of the out-of-doors are obscured. The mist in the air scatters the light randomly, more or less evenly over the landscape so that it may be difficult to distinguish one object from another. However, on a clear day, the same landscape can be seen distinctly. When a beam of primary x-rays traverses through an object, some of the x-rays are completely absorbed, while others pass directly through. A considerable percentage, however, is scattered in all directions by the atoms within the material, much as light might be dispersed by a mist, Figure 3-11. These secondary x-rays comprise what is known as *scatter radiation* and affect the radiograph. Scatter radiation strikes the film from random directions and produces a fairly uniform, even deposit of silver over the entire image. This veil of silver overlays the details recorded by the controlled part of the remnant beam and is, in reality, a form of noise known as scatter *fog*. When image fog is present, the effect is as if details were being viewed through a mist. In other words, the quality of the image is degraded. Radiographic examples of image fog are shown in Figure 3-12. Observe the characteristic dull gray appearance of these images and the accompanyings absence of important details.

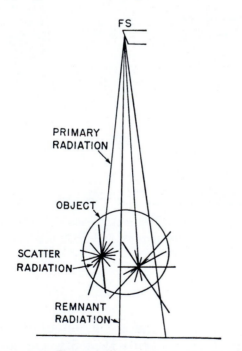

FS

PRIMARY
RADIATION

OBJECT

SCATTER
RADIATION

REMNANT
RADIATION

Figure 3-11. Diagram illustrating manner in which scatter radiation is generated when x-rays strike any form of matter. Scatter radiation is random in its direction, and destructive to the image.

Much of radiographic quality is related to the effect of scatter radiation fog on the visualization of image details. Its effect is greatest on those elements of an object that are farthest from the film. By controlling the amount of scatter radiation reaching the film during an exposure, details become more visible with a resultant improvement in image quality. Details representing small differences in tissue absorption (subject contrast) may be completely obscured by fog. Thus, reducing image fog directly results in an increase in visible information.

The intensity of scattered radiation can be reduced primarily by the use of grids and by increasing the object-image distance (OID), which are fully discussed in later chapters. Even with modern accessories, it is not always possible to control scattered radiation enough to produce a satisfactory image, particularly with large patients. Unfocused and random, scatter radiation produces a supplemental density that superimposes the entire image like a veil; it actually increases the overall density of the image and limits the ability to see radiographic details clearly. In fact, *the desirable range of densities (gray scale) is usually destroyed and important detail is obscured by this common form of image noise.*

Gray Scale, Fog and Density

It is essential to understand that every "gray" radiograph is not necessarily fogged. Long gray scale is often desirable in an image. Fog is never desirable. Yet, both make the image appear more "gray." Long gray scale can improve the image, or in excessive amounts it may degrade the image. But, *fog is always destructive.*

When gray scale is increased, contrast is reduced. But, when fogging occurs, *both gray scale and contrast are diminished.* This is

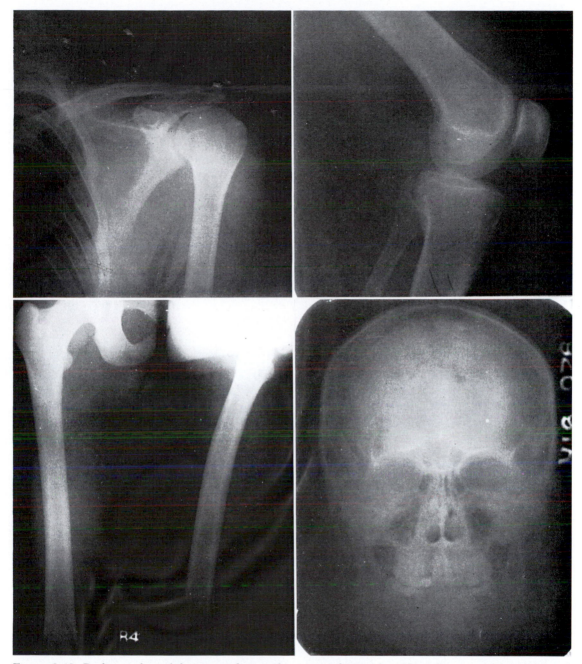

Figure 3-12. Radiographs exhibiting evidence of scatter radiation fog. Note the general loss of detail visualization because of degraded contrast.

true even though contrast and gray scale are considered to be "opposite" image qualities, and is demonstrated with a step wedge experiment in Chapter 12, Figure 12-3. After fogging of the image, fewer steps can be counted on the step wedge image. The added fog density has reduced image *gray scale*. This is possible because fog is a *blanket* of density which covers every useful density on the radiograph.

Therefore, those densities which should have been a very dark gray shade are completely lost to the image as the fog darkens them further, so there are fewer discernable densities present. Yet, there is also less difference between steps. Even though contrast and gray scale are considered opposites, they have *both* been diminished by fog. This is more fully discussed in Chapter 12.

It is quite easy to confuse an *overexposed*, "burned-out" radiograph with a fogged radiograph. It is important to understand that a darker image is not necessarily always a *fogged* image. Fogging is caused by scattered radiation. It is possible to simply overexpose a radiograph with too much radiation, without the levels of scatter changing. Figure 3-13 shows the difference between an overexposed radiograph and a fogged radiograph. The chief distinction is that on the overexposed radiograph *(A), at least some small areas in the teeth and ridges of bone still present very light densities, which are not present anywhere on the fogged radiograph (B).* Note also that a fogged radiograph is not necessarily extremely dark—the overall density can be quite light and still present a *washed-out gray*, low contrast appearance. An excessively dark image may be simply overexposed, it may be fogged, or *both*.

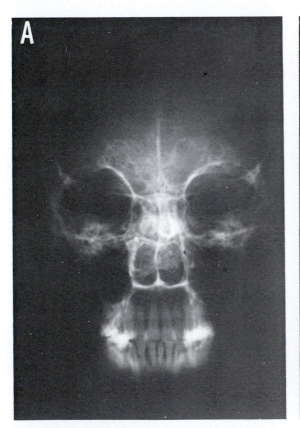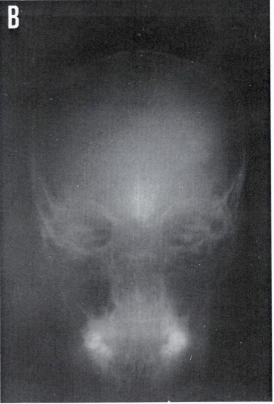

Figure 3-13. Radiographs demonstrating the difference in appearance between an overexposed image (A) and a fogged image (B). Note that a fogged image can actually be lighter in density, as within the orbits and at the top of this skull.

Artifacts

Any impertinent, useless, or false information which obscures the useful details in an image may be referred to as *noise*. Scatter fog has already been described as the most common form of image noise. In addition, a radiograph may be fogged from exposure to white light or excessive exposure to dark room safelights, or it may be *chemically* fogged from excessive temperatures, excessive development times, or improper solution concentrations during processing.

Artifacts are any extraneous images that obscure the desired information, and come from a variety of causes too numerous to attempt listing. They are all forms of image *noise*. A few examples are white marks from torn paper or dirt inside screen cassettes, iodine or barium spilled onto sponges or patient gowns; removable objects in or on the patient such as hairpins, dentures, and jewelry; scratches and splashed chemicals on the film.

Static electricity discharges on the film can be caused from rough handling, pressure from stacking boxes of film on their sides rather than on end, automatic film conveyor systems, and low humidity. These discharges cause branching or radiating black exposure marks on the finished radiograph, one of the more common and destructive types of artifacts. Another type of artifact which is often misunderstood is the *false image*. False images are images *created* by patient motion, tomographic movements or other geometrical anomalies that blur and superimpose true images into each other. Although these images are often referred to as "distorted" images, it should be clarified that they are newly *created* images which do not represent any real anatomical part at all (distorted in shape or not), and therefore are completely *false*. Further discussion and examples of these types of artifacts are found in later chapters.

Regardless of origins or causes, all of these artifacts obscure the visibility of the useful portions of the radiographic image and, therefore, constitute forms of image noise.

RECOGNIZABILITY AND GEOMETRICAL INTEGRITY

An image must have geometrical integrity with the object it represents in order to be recognizable. That is, it must have close to the same size and shape as the real object, and it must not be blurred into the surrounding details, or else it might be mistaken for some other object. Hence, recognizability refers to *geometrical integrity* the of an image.

The most important component of the recognizability of an image is the *sharpness of recorded detail.* As previously described, sharpness is the abruptness of the image edges. It may also be described as the *lack* of penumbra or blur at the edges of an image. In Figure 3-14, a radiograph demonstrating motion shows blurred edges and a consequent loss of details in the bones of the hand.

In radiography, a common misconception occurs when the *visibility* of image edges is confused with the *sharpness* of the edges. Compare the two chest radiographs in Figures 3-6 and 3-7 and see if you can determine which radiograph has sharper edges between th ribs and the background lung density. This is very difficult to do. In reality, they are both equally sharp, since they were taken using identical *geometrical* factors. High-contrast radiographs, such as the chest image in Figure 3-6, are not only deceptively appealing to the human eye but they also create the *false* impression

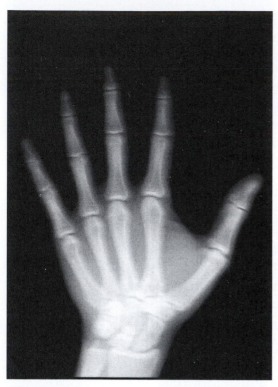

Figure 3-14. Radiograph of the hand showing blurred edges of bones and loss of details within the bones due to motion.

that they are sharper: In the longer-scale radiograph in Figure 3-7, the edges of the ribs are no more blurred than those in Figure 3-6. They "stop" just as abruptly. However, the ribs in longer gray scale Figure 3-7 have less contrast, and so they are less *visible*. The edges of an image, just as all its other portions, have both visibility and recognizability components. Edges that are more visible due to high contrast are not necessarily sharper.

Conversely, blur or penumbra must not be confused with fog. Figure 3-15 illustrates the difference between unsharpness (blur) and poor contrast. *A* shows a high contrast image which also has a sharp edge between the two densities. In *B*, the high contrast is still present, but the edge is blurry, gradually changing from one density to the other. In *C*, very poor contrast causes the edge

between the two densities to be less *visible*, but it is still sharp, because it "stops" abruptly. Blur is not present in *C*.

Geometrical penumbra and motion are the two most important causes of blur or unsharpness. Blur may also be caused by poorly constructed film or intensifying screens (called *material unsharpness*), or by absorption effects at the edges of rounded objects. These special types of blur are discussed in later chapters. To summarize, unsharpness can be caused by poor projection geometry, by motion, by recording materials, and by absorption effects.

The *magnification* of a radiographic image can be quantitatively measured by determining the difference between its size and the size of the actual object *in both dimensions or axes, lengthwise and crosswise*. If both the length and the width of an image are identical to those of the real object, then no magnification is present. In a magnified image, *both* the length and the width of the image will measure larger than the object by equal proportions. For example, if the image is both twice as long and twice as wide as the real object, this effect is due to magnification. For magnification to be present, the pure shadow, the *umbra* of the image must be larger. It is possible for the *penumbra* to spread out from blurring, yet if it expands *without the umbra being enlarged*, then magnification is not present, only blurring.

If the length of an image should measure differently than that of the real object, while its width remains unchanged, the image is *shape distorted*, it is not magnified. The shape of an object might be grossly represented as the *ratio* between its measured length and width. For example, if the length and width are equal, their ratio would be 1:1 and you might have a square or a circle shape. If the length is twice as long as the width, however, the ratio would

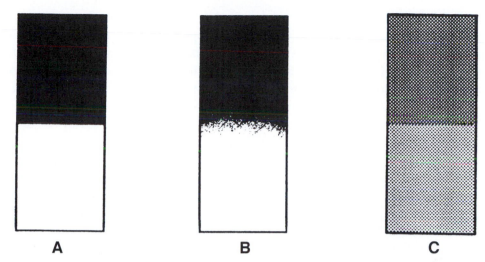

Figure 3-15. Blur versus fog. Image A shows no blur and no fog. Image B shows blurring, but with high contrast since there is no fog, while image C shows poor contrast due to fog, but with high sharpness at the edge of these densities, since there is no blur.

now be 2:1, and you might have a rectangle or an ellipse shape. The shape only changes when this ratio is altered.

These *shape ratios* can be used to help distinguish between magnification and shape distortion: In Figure 3-16A, the projected circular image has a shape ratio of 1:1. Suppose that, by changing our projection geometry (distances, angles, or centering), the result is that *both* the length and the width of this image are increase by 20 percent, as illustrated in Figure 3-16B: The shape ratio of 3-16B is now 1.2 to 1.2.

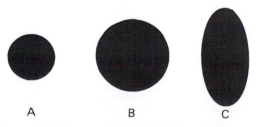

Figure 3-16. Diagram showing difference between magnification and shape distortion. If image measurement changes in *both* axes (length and width) equally, a magnified but still circular image results. Only when one axis changes *more* than the other does shape distortion occur, producing an oval shadow in this case.

Dividing these, we still get 1. The ratio of length to width is unchanged, therefore *no shape distortion is present. There is, however, 20% magnification.* The image is larger, but still maintains an identical circular shape.

For *shape distortion* to be present, one dimension or axis of the image must change by a different proportion than the other dimension. Length must change *more* than width, or vice versa. In Figure 3-16C, the *width* of this image actually measures identical to the original circle *A*, but the *length* of the image is obviously increased to perhaps 3 times that in *A*. The new shape ratio for 3-16C is 3:1 = 3. This is different than the shape ratio for *A*, and indicates that shape distortion has indeed occurred. If the length were cut in half while the width remained at 1, the shape ratio would change to 0.5 indicating distortion again. Any time one dimension of the image changes *differently* than the other, the result will be a different shape.

Suppose that *both* the length and width increase, but the *length* grows 3 times longer, while the width only doubles: The new shape ratio is 3:2 = 1.5 indicating that shape distortion has occurred. In this case, however, magnification has *also* occurred since *both* dimensions were increased. This image was both magnified and distorted.

Specifically in radiography, when the projected image measures longer than the real object, it is said to have *elongation* distortion. If it measures shorter in one axis, the image is said to have *foreshortening* distortion. If it changes *equally* in both axes, it is said to be *magnified.*

Blur, magnification, and distortion reduce the recognizability of information, can cause misleading information or even create false information, and can lead to complete loss of some details and information on the finished radiograph. It is imperative to minimize all three of these effects in standard radiography.

RESOLUTION

Finally, it is important to understand the concept of image resolution. *Resolution* is defined as the ability to distinguish two adjacent details as being separate and distinct from each other. A well-resolved image requires *both* high visibility and optimum recognizability. *All* of the image qualities affect its overall resolution. However, the two most important aspects of the resolution of a particular image detail are its *contrast* compared to other details nearby,

and its *sharpness* against background details.

Chapter 24 fully explains how contrast and sharpness are closely related to each other in affecting overall image resolution. Nonetheless, contrast and sharpness are not the same thing, and must not be confused, even though they are related. High contrast images can still have poor resolution if the edges are blurred. Further, sharp images can still have poor resolution if contrast is low, as illustrated in Figure 3-17.

Thus, the resolution of information in the image depends upon both visibility and recognizability aspects. The actual measurement of the resolution in an image can be made by exposing special metal templates (Fig. 16-1 in Chapter 16) which provide an image of alternating black and white line pairs that gradually diminish in width. The smaller the line pairs which can be visibly distinguished on the radiograph, the greater is the measured resolution. In a blurred image, the penumbral shadows at the edges of each line will spread into each other so that the smaller line pairs cannot be discerned. If the image is fogged, the visibility between the line pairs is obscured making the smaller ones harder to discern.

The smaller the lines that can be clearly recorded on the film, the more of these lines would fit into a certain area on the film. Thus, a functional unit of measurement for image resolution can be defined.

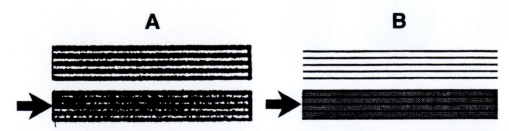

Figure 3-17. Resolution template images showing that overall image resolution can be lost by either (A, arrow) blur resulting in ragged edges that begin to run into each other, or (B, arrow) a loss of contrast, even though the edges are "sharp." In both cases the individual lines are more difficult to distinguish.

This unit is *line-pairs per millimeter*, abbreviated *LP/mm*. The more line pairs per millimeter measured, the greater is the image resolution.

The overall image quality may be defined as the total amount of diagnostic information resolved in an image. Overall image quality is dependent upon the entire imaging system—the combination of a particular type of image receptor (film, cassette, etc.) with the x-ray machine used and all of the related variables for each projection.

SUMMARY

To summarize, any image must be both visible and recognizable in order to be of value in providing information. The visibility of the image is best when its intensity (density) is adequate, its contrast and gray scale are balanced, and its noise is minimal. The image is most recognizable when its geometrical integrity is maintained with the real object it represents. This occurs when sharpness of recorded detail is maximized and when magnification and shape distortion are minimized.

HIERARCHY OF IMAGE QUALITIES

An overview of the relationship between all of the radiographic image qualities is presented in graphic form in Figure 3-18, and a concise table of definitions of imaging terms follows.

DEFINITIONS OF IMAGE QUALITIES

1. **Density:** The degree of *blackness* or darkness in an area of the image, determined by the amount of silver deposited on the film in that area.
2. **Tone Value:** The amount of light that is able to penetrate through an area on the film, or the area's *translucency*. The opposite of density.
3. **Contrast:** The ratio of *difference* between two adjacent densities in the image.
4. **Gray Scale:** The *range* or number of different densities present in the image. The opposite of contrast.
5. **Noise:** Any unwanted, *useless information* recorded in the image which obscures the visibility of the desired image details. Noise includes fog, static,

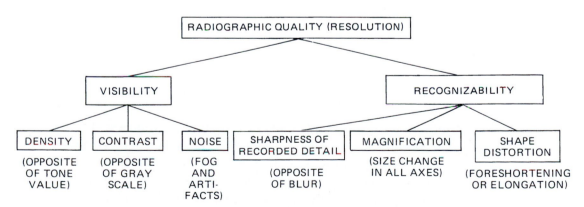

Figure 3-18. Hierarchy of radiographic image qualities.

and artifacts of various types.

6. **Fog:** A form of noise, fog is a veil of *useless density* covering portions of the desired image. It is caused by randomly scattered radiation which carries no useful signal or image.

7. **Sharpness of Recorded Detail:** The *abruptness* with which the edges of an image stop. More precisely, the *lack of penumbra* shadows at the edge of an image.

8. **Blur:** The presence of penumbra, or the lack of sharpness, at the edges of an image. See *Penumbra* below:

9. **Penumbra:** A *partial shadow* at the edges of an image, whereby its transition into the adjacent

10. **Magnification:** The *difference* between the *size* of a real object being radiographed and the size of its projected *umbral* image (measured in all dimensions).

11. **Shape Distortion:** The *difference* between the *shape* of a real object being radiographed and the shape of its projected image, consisting of either *elongation* or *foreshortening* of the image.

12. **Visibility Factors:** Those image qualities which directly affect the ability to see an image. They include density or tone value, contrast or gray scale, and noise including fog.

13. **Recognizability Factors:** Those *geometrical* image qualities which directly affect the ability to discern the nature of the real object being projected onto the image. These include sharpness of detail, magnification, and shape distortion.

14. **Resolution:** The ability to distinguish small adjacent details in the image as being *separate* from each other. Resolution is controlled by both visibility factors (primarily contrast) and recognizability factors (primarily sharpness).

15. **Radiographic Image Quality:** The total amount of diagnostically useful information resolved in an image. Image quality is controlled by the combination of all visibility and recognizability factors.

DISCREPANCIES IN TERMINOLOGY

Unfortunately for the radiography student, there are pronounced discrepancies in the imaging terminology used by different educators, authors, and organizations. Attempts have been made by certifying agencies to standardize terminology, and some progress has been made. Nonetheless, some confusion still exists. As a reference to help the student "translate" between other textbooks or sources and this text, the following discussion and *Table 3-1* are offered, listing some of the most common alternative terms used for each image quality.

The terms *density, contrast, noise,* and *fog* are widely standardized in conventional use and should pose no problem for the student. Image *gray scale* is frequently called "contrast scale." This is a very confusing practice, since gray scale and contrast are opposites as explained in this chapter. It is suggested that whenever the student sees or hears the term, "contrast scale," focus on the word *scale* and try to ignore the attachment of the word "contrast" in this context. Any phrase including the term *scale* is likely to refer to gray scale.

In the 1980s, the American Registry of Radiologic Technologists adopted the term *recorded detail* to be used on its certification examination in reference to the sharpness of the edge of an image. The single word "detail" is perhaps the most abused of all imaging terms: It has been variously defined as the overall quality of an image, the total amount of information in an image, the visibility of small images, the geometrical integrity of the image including shape distortion and magnification, and the sharpness of image edges. To make matters worse, the plural term *details* is generally used to point out the many small components of an image, as in "visibility of details." For these reasons, this text will consistently use the term *sharpness of recorded detail* in place of the ARRT's *recorded detail* when discussing the abruptness of image edges.

Note in *Table 3-1* that the ARRT term for the recognizability of an image is *sharpness of detail* and that the ARRT term for magnification is *size distortion*. The terms *recognizability* and *magnification* are straightforward terms with which most people are quite familiar, and shall be used throughout this book as they are commonly understood. A careful review of *Table 3-1* should help the student cope with the different schools of thought on image terminology.

REVIEW QUESTIONS

1. Define *density*:
2. Define *contrast*:
3. Define *gray scale*:
4. Define *noise*:
5. Define *penumbra*:
6. Describe the two types of shape distortion:
7. Define *sharpness of detail*:
8. Define *resolution*:
9. Define *radiographic quality*:
10. What are the three *visibility functions* in an image:
11. Why is very long gray scale not desirable in an image?
12. Why is penumbra present to some degree in all radiographic images?
13. Why is very high contrast not desirable in an image?
14. Explain how a radiograph could be fogged and yet light at the same time:
15. List the three image qualities which should always be *minimized*:
16. What is the useful range of image densities as measured on a densitometer?
17. List the four types of unsharpness:
18. What exposure error causes an image that is very dark, yet has some white areas in it:
19. An image that is both twice as long and twice as wide as the original object has been _____.

Chapter 4

INTERACTIONS OF X-RAYS WITHIN THE PATIENT

T HE ENDEAVOR OF EVERY radiographer is to control the six radiographic image qualities listed in the previous chapter. The *visibility* functions are completely essential to the radiographic image. All of the visibility functions are controlled by the relationship of the electrical technique variables to the patient status variables. In other words, visibility is entirely dependent upon the interactions of the x-ray beam with the atoms inside the patient, which is controlled electrically. Each visibility quality of the image is directly controlled by one of two types of atomic interactions that occur as the x-ray beam passes through the patient's body. It is important that radiographers understand these interactions well enough that they can translate the results on the radiograph into the causes within the x-ray beam and the patient.

TYPES OF INTERACTIONS

Although detailed explanations of the various atomic interactions of x-rays may be found in radiography physics texts, a simple overview will be provided here so that reference may be made effectively throughout the chapters of this book to the ultimate causes and controls of the condition of the remnant beam which exposes the film.

PHOTOELECTRIC EFFECT

The *photoelectric* effect is crucial to the formation of the radiographic image. In the photoelectric effect, an atom within the patient's body *completely* absorbs one of the x-ray photons in the x-ray beam as it passes through the body. Specifically, the x-ray photon intersects an orbital electron in one of the atom's innermost shells. This inner-shell electron absorbs *all* of the energy carried by the x-ray photon, so the photon ceases to exist, and no secondary or scatter radiation is left over. The orbital electron, now containing the additional energy of the photon, manifests that extra energy by speeding up. This results in the electron being "slung" out of its orbit and out of the atom. Such high-speed electrons that have been ejected out of atoms are called *photo-electrons*, electrons that have "captured" a photon (Fig. 4-1). The photoelectron soon collides with another atom of tissue and does not make it out of the patient's body. Therefore, it cannot reach the x-ray film and is of no consequence to the final image produced. There is also no secondary x-radiation emitted from the patient's body, since all of the original photon's energy was absorbed into the photoelectron.

Because the original x-ray photon is completely stopped within the patient's body, the radiographic film will be left blank or "white" in that area. *The photoelectric effect is*

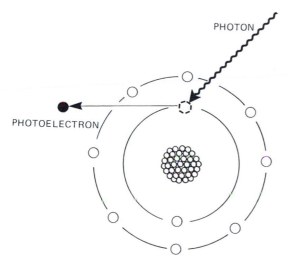

PHOTON

PHOTOELECTRON

Figure 4-1. The photoelectric effect. The impinging x-ray photon is completely absorbed by an inner-shell orbital electron, which is then ejected from the atom as a *photoelectron*. No radiation reaches the film.

responsible for the production of contrast in the radiographic image. This effect only occurs when the energy of the incoming photon is slightly higher than the binding energy with which the atom holds the electron in its orbit (the "pull" of the nucleus).

COMPTON EFFECT

The *Compton* effect occurs when the energy of the incoming x-ray photon is *much* greater than the atom's binding energy holding an electron in orbit, and occurs in the outer shells of the atom where the nuclear "pull" on the electrons is the weakest. An electron ejected from an atom by the Compton effect is called a *recoil electron.* The energy needed to eject the electron from its orbit is absorbed by that electron, but there is then considerable photon energy left over. This remaining x-ray energy is re-emitted as a secondary *Compton photon.* The Compton photon may be *scattered* in any direction (Fig. 4-2). In radiography, *scatter* refers to any x-ray photon which has

notably changed its direction from the original beam of x-rays. Scatter radiation may reach the film and expose it, causing a *fog* density in the image. Due to the random direction of scatter radiation, this fogging of the image is always destructive, as the fog is a "blanket" density which obscures details in the image.

The Compton effect may be considered synonymous with *scatter,* since 99 percent of all scattered x-ray photons originate from Compton interactions in the patient. Fog from scatter radiation reduces the contrast in an image and, therefore, works against the photoelectric interactions. Compton scatter interactions are known by several other names, including *modified scattering* and *incoherent scattering.*

THOMPSON EFFECT

When the energy of the incoming x-ray photon is less than the binding energy of an orbital electron, *Thompson* interaction may occur. The orbital electron absorbs the entire photon, but this additional energy is not sufficient to eject the electron from its orbit. Instead, the electron is raised to a heightened state of energy for just a fraction of a second, after which it re-emits the photon with its original energy. This secondary photon, even though it is unchanged in energy from the original, may be emitted in any direction and is therefore considered as *scatter* (Fig. 4-3). However, Thompson scattering accounts for only 1 percent of all scatter produced in the patient. Further, these photons have very low energy and are less likely to reach the x-ray film. Therefore, Thompson scatter is of little consequence in affecting the radiographic image. Thompson scattering is also known as *unmodified scattering, coherent scattering,* and *classical scattering.*

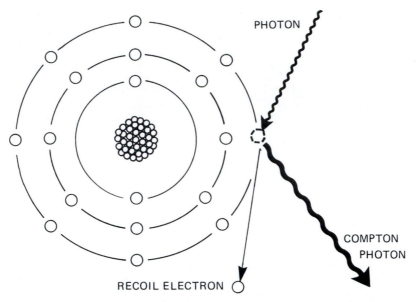

Figure 4-2. The Compton effect. The impinging x-ray photon is partially absorbed by an outer-shell orbital electron. The electron is then ejected from the atom as a *recoil* electron, and the remaining photon energy is emitted as a *Compton scatter photon* which may reach the film and fog it.

OTHER INTERACTIONS

Since primary beam photons can ionize atoms, *characteristic* interactions similar to those occurring in the anode of the x-ray tube may also occur within the patient. After any ionization event (photoelectric or Compton), the atom is left with an orbital vacancy and soon pulls another electron into that orbit to fill it. Each time an electron "falls" into an orbit, whether from a higher orbit or from outside the atom, energy is lost and is emitted in the form of electromagnetic radiation. However, the "size" of the atoms in the soft tissues of the patient is extremely small compared to the "size" of tungsten and rhenium atoms in the x-ray tube anode. The smaller an atom is, the lower are its binding energies by which electrons are held in orbit. Since the energies of characteristic photons depends on these binding energies, smaller atoms will emit only very low energy characteristic photons. These photon energies are

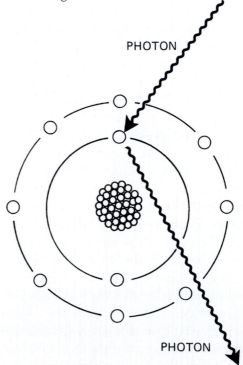

Figure 4-3. The Thompson effect. The impinging x-ray photon is *temporarily* absorbed by an orbital electron, then re-emitted with its original energy, but in a different direction as a *scatter photon* which may reach the film and fog it.

indeed so low that they will not be x-rays at all but ultraviolet or visible light rays, which will not make it out of the patient. Hence, characteristic interactions occurring within the patient cannot have any effect at all upon the radiographic film.

Physics textbooks discuss several other interactions x-ray photons can undergo when interacting with atoms, yet none of these are of significance in producing radiographs. The final quality of the radiographic image hinges upon the photoelectric, the Compton, and the Thompson interactions occurring within the patient's body.

SCATTER VERSUS SECONDARY RADIATION

Secondary radiation refers to any radiation resulting from interactions within the patient. *Scatter*, on the other hand, refers only to that secondary radiation which has been emitted in a direction different than the original x-ray beam. Some secondary radiation is emitted in directions so close to the original that it may still be considered useful in contributing to the image. This radiation would not be considered as scatter. Nonetheless, *most* secondary radiation is scattered.

Scatter radiation, traveling in random directions, becomes more or less evenly distributed across the film and cannot possess any subject contrast between one area and another. Therefore, it cannot carry any useful signal or image to the film but only fogs the film overall, destroying the visibility of that information recorded by the primary and unscattered x-rays.

It has been often stated that, generally, as much as 75 percent of the remnant radiation exiting the patient is secondary radiation. For radiography of *small* body parts, such as the hand, much of what secondary radiation is produced is scattered sideways and backward rather than toward the film; the resulting fog in the image is not significant and no special measures need be taken to prevent it. On the other hand, very *large* body parts, such as the abdomen, generate huge amounts of secondary radiation, and at the higher kilovoltages used, much more of this secondary radiation is scattered forward toward the film. The resulting image fog is severe enough that grids (Chapter 13) must be employed to remove as much of this scatter radiation as possible before it reaches the film. Although grids may eliminate the most severely scattered x-rays in the remnant beam, much of what is left is still secondary radiation which has interacted within the patient but which was not emitted at a sufficiently changed angle to be stopped by the grid. Hence, grids eliminate severely *scattered* x-rays, yet they do not come close to eliminating all of the *secondary* radiation.

PRODUCTION OF SUBJECT CONTRAST

As described in the previous chapter, *contrast* is absolutely essential to the visibility of detail in any radiographic image. The primary concern when discussing the interactions between x-ray beam photons and the atoms of tissue within the patient is their effect upon image contrast. The mechanism by which *scatter* radiation produced by the Compton interaction fogs the image and reduces image contrast will be explained later in this chapter. The most significant influence upon the overall contrast of the radiographic image is the *subject contrast* produced by the interaction of the x-ray

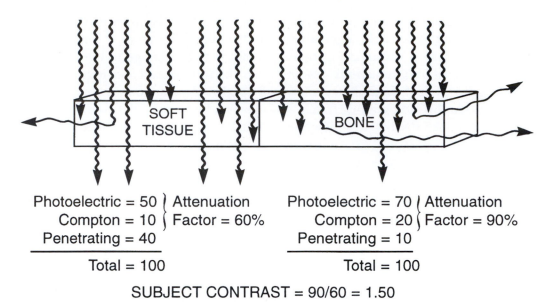

Figure 4-4. Diagram of the production of subject contrast between bone and soft tissue. In this case, photoelectric and Compton interactions in soft tissue combine to absorb 60% of the beam. In bone, all interactions combine to absorb 90% of the beam. The subject contrast produced is the *ratio* of the two attenuation factors: 90%/60% = 1.50.

beam with the various tissues of the body.

Subject contrast is produced by the *differential absorption* between various tissues of the body. The physical differences between these tissues is already present before the x-ray beam strikes them. Simply put, a tissue such as bone stands out from the "background" density of soft tissues because the bone absorbs more x-rays than soft tissue does. For the purposes of this discussion, it must be remembered that *both* the Compton interaction and the photoelectric interaction cause attenuation of the x-ray beam. Even though the Compton interaction may be considered as only a *partial* absorption event so far as the energy of a single incoming photon is concerned, bear in mind that (1) the emitted secondary photon is less likely to reach the film due to its reduced energy, and (2) the emitted secondary photon may be scattered in a direction completely missing the radiographic film; the area of film directly beneath a Compton event is likely to remain unex-

posed. Compton and Thompson interactions both result in attenuation of the x-ray beam, and may be loosely considered as "absorbing" events even though they do not produce the "total absorption" of the photoelectric effect. *All interactions within the patient, whether Compton, Thompson or photoelectric, represent some degree of absorption of the overall x-ray beam. All interactions attenuate the x-ray beam.*

The differential absorption of the x-ray beam by different tissues is a direct consequence of the *percentage* of the x-ray beam absorbed by all interactions, versus the penetration of that beam. Subject contrast is represented by the *ratio* of absorption between two adjacent structures or tissues. For example, let us examine the subject contrast of bone against soft tissue, and then determine how this might change if some disease caused the soft tissue to double in its physical density: Suppose that 100 x-rays per square inch are incident upon the body. Let us assume that, of these 100 x-ray pho-

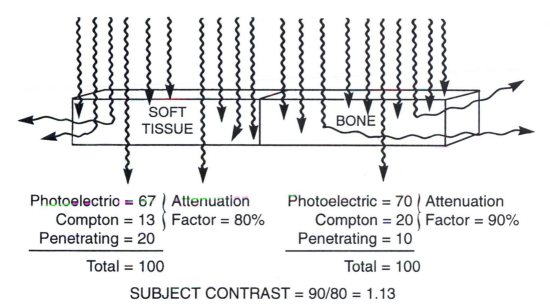

Photoelectric = 67 } Attenuation
Compton = 13 } Factor = 80%
Penetrating = 20
_____
Total = 100

Photoelectric = 70 } Attenuation
Compton = 20 } Factor = 90%
Penetrating = 10
_____
Total = 100

SUBJECT CONTRAST = 90/80 = 1.13

Figure 4-5. Diagram of the change in subject contrast from Figure 4-4 if a disease increases the physical density of the soft tissue by some 30%. Both photoelectric and Compton interactions increase in number, and the attenuation factor rises to 80%, with only 2 out of 10 photons penetrating through the soft tissue. The subject contrast between the soft tissue and the adjacent bone is now reduced to 90%/80% = 1.13.

tons, the soft tissue absorbs 50 by photoelectric interaction, and scatters 10 by Compton interaction. This leaves 40 x-rays penetrating through to the film. The overall attenuation factor would be 60 percent (photoelectric plus Compton), as shown in Figure 4-4. The nearby bone, which is much denser, will be expected to cause more of both interactions: It absorbs 70 x-rays by photoelectric interaction and scatters 20 by Compton interaction. Of the original 100, only 10 x-rays have penetrated completely through the bone. The overall attenuation for the bone is 90 percent. The bone has a much higher attenuation (90%) than the soft tissue (60%). Now, the *ratio* between the attenuation factors for the bone and the soft tissue is 90/60 = 9/6 = 1.5. As shown in Figure 4-4, the *subject contrast* for this image is 1.5 This is a fairly high ratio; the bone is absorbing 50 percent more radiation than the soft tissue. We expect the bone image to stand out with high contrast against the background of soft tissue.

Now, suppose the patient has a disease which causes soft tissues to harden, increase mineral content, and tend to calcify. We would expect this hardening of the soft tissue to increase its overall physical density. There will simply be more atoms per cubic millimeter for x-rays to "run into." Some of these events will result in photoelectric interactions and some in Compton interactions. Let us assume that both types of interactions increase by some 30 percent in the soft tissue, Figure 4-5. There are now occurring 67 photoelectric interactions and 13 Compton interactions. This leaves only 20 x-rays from the original 100 that will penetrate through to the film. The attenuation factor of the diseased soft tissue then increases to a factor of 80 percent, instead of the normal 60 percent. How does this change the *subject contrast* between the bone and the soft tissue? The attenuation factor for the normal bone is still 90 percent as before. The new *ratio* between the two tissues, the new *subject contrast*, is now $90/80 = 9/8 = 1.13$. The bone is now absorbing only 13 percent more radiation than the diseased soft tissue. There is much less difference between the two tissues, much less subject contrast.

In this hypothetical case, the hardening of the soft tissue caused the subject contrast between bone and soft tissue to decrease from 1.5 to 1.13. Accordingly, there will be less difference between the two radiographic densities of these tissues produced in the radiographic image. Image contrast will be reduced.

Note that to measure the contrast between these two tissues, a *ratio* is used, dividing one factor into the other, rather than simply subtracting the difference. In his text, *The Physical Principles of Diagnostic Radiology*, Dr. Perry Sprawls clearly defines image contrast. He states, "Actually, it is the ratio of the penetration factors, rather than the difference, which determines the amount of contrast." Dr. Sprawls provides the mathematical formula for subject contrast as:

$$C_s = \left\{ 1 - \left(\frac{P_o}{P_t} \right)^x \right\} \times 100$$

where P_o and P_t are the penetration factors for the two tissues. Note that these two factors are not subtracted one from the other, but divided to form a ratio. (The other portions of this formula are simply designed to result in an answer which is a percentage figure.)

There are three essential aspects of tissues which determine their attenuation properties and the resulting subject contrast: the thickness of each tissue area, the physical density of each tissue, and the average atomic number of each tissue.

TISSUE THICKNESS

As a tissue area becomes thicker, its attenuation of the x-ray beam is naturally greater. This attenuation increases exponentially and follows a somewhat complicated logarithmic formula which is unnecessary here. A rough rule of thumb for body part thicknesses in general is that for every 4 centimeters of additional thickness, the attenuation of the x-ray beam is doubled, so that the penetration of x-rays through to the film is cut in half. A body part that is 4 centimeters thicker than some other part will absorb about twice as much of the x-ray beam, and the radiographic image will turn out about one-half as dark in this area.

Suppose that tissue A has an attenuation factor of 40 percent, and tissue B has a factor of 10 percent. The subject contrast between tissues A and B is $40/10 = 4.0$. Now, let tissue B increase in thickness by 4 centimeters. This would double its attenuation factor from 10 percent to 20 percent. The subject contrast will now be $40/20 = 2.0$. Clearly in this case, with tissue B increasing in thickness, the *subject contrast has been reduced from 4.0 to 2.0.* On the other hand, let tissue A increase in thickness by 4 centimeters, thus doubling its attenuation factor from 40 percent to 80 percent. With tissue B at its original 10 percent attenuation, the ratio between the two tissues will now be $80/10 = 8.0$, and *subject contrast has increased from 4.0 to 8.0.* Hence, changes in tissue thickness may cause the subject contrast to either increase or decrease, depending on which tissue has changed.

TISSUE DENSITY

The physical density of a substance refers to the amount of physical mass that is concentrated into a given volume of space, such as grams per cubic centimeter. In the patient, the physical density may be considered as the concentration of atoms or molecules of a tissue. At higher tissue densities, there are more atoms or molecules packed into a given space. At lower densities, atoms or molecules are less concentrated and there is more space between them.

Clearly, if the number of atoms in a particular space is doubled, there will be twice as high a probability that an x-ray photon passing through will actually hit one of these atoms. If the tissue density is cut in half, the likelihood of attenuation of x-rays is cut in half. This probability applies equally to both Compton and photoelectric interactions. Therefore, it may be said that the occurrence of all interactions is *directly proportional* to the physical density of the tissue through which the x-rays are passing.

Visible radiographic contrast will occur between two tissues in the image only if they are *extremely* different in physical density, simply because the one tissue will absorb much more radiation altogether and leave a lighter, less exposed area on the radiograph. For example, air in the lungs is a gas and therefore has an *extremely low density* when compared to soft tissue. Soft tissue has a physical density roughly equal to that of liquid water. The density ratio of soft tissue to air is roughly 1000 to 1. Since the soft tissue will absorb 1000 times more radiation than the air, an extreme difference, visible image contrast results between the lungs and the heart on a chest radiograph.

Three types of body tissues may be distinguished from each other on a radiograph primarily because of the effect of tissue density: soft tissues (muscles and glands), fat, and gasses such as air in the lungs. Soft tissues absorb more x-rays than fat or gas

and result in the lighter shades of gray on the image, with fat appearing slightly darker and gas appearing the darkest.

Much radiography, however, involves the visualization of bones or of contrast agents. Bones, metals and contrast agents are not dramatically different from soft tissue in their physical densities. The reason these materials appear with contrast on a radiographic image is because of their high atomic numbers (larger atomic "size"), rather than because of differences in physical density.

TISSUE ATOMIC NUMBER

Most radiographic procedures fall in the categories of skeletal procedures and artificial contrast procedures. Soft tissues cannot be radiographically distinguished from each other without some form of intervention to artificially provide subject contrast. Contrast agents—substances usually based on the iodine atom or the barium atom—are introduced into cavities within organs or tissues where possible in order to provide an image of them.

Contrast agents, bone, and metallic objects are visible on a radiograph primarily because of the difference between their atomic numbers, that is, how "large" their atoms are on average. This is why iodine (atomic number 53) and barium (atomic number 56) are so effective at absorbing x-rays. Barium, for example, not only has 56 positively-charged protons in its nucleus, but it normally also has 56 electrons in its orbital shells. Interestingly, barium and other atoms with high atomic numbers are actually not significantly larger in their overall *diameter* than hydrogen with its atomic number of 1. Rather, as the atomic nucleus of atoms becomes larger and larger, the additional positive charge of all the protons "pulls" the electron shells in closer and closer to the nucleus. So, atoms with more shells actually have them "packed" in tighter and closer to the nucleus. This also means that all of the electrons within these shells are now packed more tightly into the small volume of space which the atom occupies. This *concentration* of the electrons within the space of the atom's diameter is referred to as *electron density*.

Hence, "larger" atoms are not spatially larger in actual size, but rather they are more *dense* with electrons. The likelihood, then, that a particular x-ray photon will be absorbed by one of these electron-packed atoms is greatly enhanced for elements with high atomic numbers. A particular tissue is comprised of several different types of atoms combined into molecules. Thus, the atomic number of a tissue must be expressed as an average, which takes into account the number of each different type of atom within these molecules. For example, the average atomic number of soft tissue, mostly comprised of water, is 7.4. (Water is composed of two atoms of hydrogen with an atomic number of 1, and one atom of oxygen with an atomic number of 8. The average atomic number, then, must fall between 1 and 8. It averages closer to 8 because the oxygen has a much greater effect than the two very small hydrogen atoms.)

To summarize, there are *two* aspects of tissue which determine its ability to attenuate the x-ray beam: The *physical density* of the tissue, which is the number of atoms concentrated into a volume of space, and the *average atomic number* for the tissue, which relates to the concentration of electrons within each atom. Bone, metallic objects, and contrast agents are demonstrated on radiographs primarily because of the *atomic numbers* being different from soft tissue. Gasses such as air, and fat, show up primarily because of extreme differences in their physical *density* when compared to soft tissue.

X-RAY BEAM ENERGY (kVp)

Changes in the energy levels of the x-ray beam, controlled primarily by the selected kilovoltage, dramatically alter the penetration characteristics of the x-rays. As illustrated in the last chapter, a high-kVp x-ray beam penetrates more different types of tissues and records them on the image as varying shades of gray density. As the number of shades of gray within the image increases, the difference between these densities becomes less. Gray scale is increased, and correspondingly, contrast is decreased. These effects are again due to the penetration of the beam versus the overall attenuation factor, and will hold true regardless of the particular prevalence of the photoelectric effect or the Compton effect.

However, there are implications for the relative prevalence of these two interactions as we study image contrast. Figure 4-6 is a graph showing the prevalence of the photoelectric interactions and the Compton interactions occurring in different types of tissue at increasing levels of kVp. As you examine this graph, you will note that the photoelectric curves plummet quickly toward zero at higher kVp levels, but the number of Compton interactions occurring only decreases slightly. Since higher kVp levels result in more penetration of the x-ray beam through the body, there are less interactions of all kinds at higher kVp's. But, since the photoelectrics are so much more quickly lost, *the Compton interaction becomes the more prevalent interaction at higher kVp levels.*

The photoelectric effect only occurs at discrete energy levels where the kilovoltage of the incoming photons is slightly higher than the binding energies with

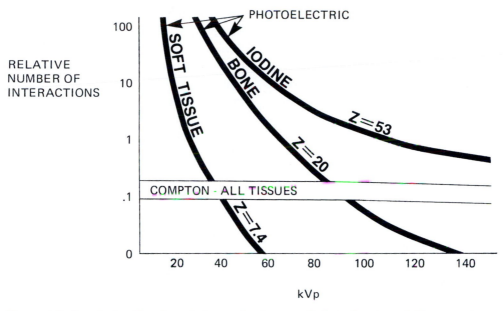

Figure 4-6. Graph showing the *relative* predominance of photoelectric and Compton interactions at increasing kVp levels. All interactions decrease in number at higher energies, as more of the x-ray beam penetrates through. However, photoelectrics quickly decrease to zero, especially in soft tissue, leaving Compton as the predominant interaction at high kvps. Also note that photoelectric interactions occur in much greater numbers in higher atomic number tissues such as bone, whereas Compton interactions occur at about the same rate for all tissues.

which the nucleus holds orbital electrons in their shells. This means that changes in kVp will have a dramatic effect upon the occurrence of photoelectric interactions.

As the kVp is increased to exceed those binding energies by large amounts, the occurrence of photoelectric interactions drops precipitously to zero. The photoelectric effect only occurs in the inner shells of the atom which are close enough to the nucleus to have significant binding energies. The use of atoms with larger nuclei and higher atomic numbers will raise the binding energies of these inner shells. When binding energies are increased enough to more closely match the particular kVp being used, without exceeding it, more photoelectric interactions will occur. Note that at 40 kVp, many more photoelectric interactions occur in bone tissue (having an average atomic number of about 20) than do in soft tissue (with an average atomic number of 7.4). For a given tissue, however, photoelectric interactions drop off rapidly as the kVp is increased. Thus, *the greatest number of photoelectric interactions will be achieved when the kVp is low and the tissue atomic number is high.*

Compton interactions occur only in the outer shells of an atom. Because these shells are far from the nucleus and have so little binding energy, their electrons are not selective in absorbing x-ray photons. Changes in atomic number do not affect these outer shells much. Furthermore, in the Compton interaction, only a portion of the photon energy is absorbed by the orbital electron, so that a variety of photon energy levels can result in this interaction taking place. Since binding energies are not significant, since the electrons are not selective, and since any portion of the photon energy can be absorbed, the occurrence of Compton interactions is not affected much by changing atomic numbers of tissues; nor is it affected much by changes in kVp. Specifically, higher kVp levels will penetrate the patient more and less Compton interactions will occur, but this reduction is very slight compared to the reduction of the photoelectric effect (Fig. 4-6). *Compton interactions may be considered as almost constant, regardless of atomic number or kVp.*

Now consider what happens within soft tissue when the kVp is increased from 40 to 80 kVp. By the graph, in soft tissue at 40 kVp, the lines for photoelectric and Compton interactions cross over each other: There are roughly equal numbers of photoelectric and Compton interactions taking place. About one-half of all interactions occurring within the patient are photoelectrics, which completely absorb x-rays and leave the image on the film relatively "white." At 80 kVp, there are *no photoelectric interactions* occurring within soft tissue. No portion of the image under this tissue will appear "white." The image of the soft tissue at 80 kVp is being created only by penetrating x-rays and by Compton scattered x-rays. The penetrating x-rays provide blacks and grays in the image, while the Compton scattered photons further gray the image. The only interactions occurring are "gray-producing interactions," and the soft tissues at this kVp can only be depicted as dark densities. Note, however, that the *bone* at 80 kVp *will* have "whites" in its image, because there are still plenty of photoelectrics occurring in the bone at this energy. Bone will show up well at 80 kVp, with good image contrast, whereas soft tissue will not.

Let us now increase the kVp all the way to 120, perhaps for a solid-column barium study, and see what fate awaits the bone image at this very high kVp: At 120 kVp,

the photoelectric interactions even within bone have nearly disappeared. The bone densities in the image now consist of mostly penetrating x-rays and scattered x-rays. This is why bones appear so poorly on barium studies. The barium itself follows a curve on the graph similar to the iodine curve, and still produces plenty of photoelectric interactions even at this very high kVp.

COMPTON SCATTER RADIATION

The key to understanding the effect of Compton scattered radiation upon image contrast is that *scattered radiation is random in its distribution, and therefore adds a roughly equal density to all areas of the image.* Figure 3-13 in the preceding chapter shows how scattered radiation is emitted in all directions from the patient. The chance that a particular scattered x-ray will strike the film where a bone image should be is equal to the chance that it will strike the film where a soft tissue image should be. Thus, as shown in Figure 3-14, the entire image is fogged with a "blanket density."

By assigning a value to this blanket fog density, it is easy to demonstrate numerically how scattered radiation reduces image contrast. Suppose a simple image is composed of an area of bone that measures a density of 1.0 on the densitometer, surrounded by a soft tissue area of darker density which measures 2.0 on the densitometer. The contrast of this simple image is found by the *ratio* of the two densities, 2/1 = 2.0.

Now, suppose that scatter radiation lays down a "blanket" of fog across the entire film, and that the fog density, if measured separately, would have a value of 0.5 on the densitometer. A fog density of 0.5 has been added to all tissue densities in the image. The density of the bone area now measures 1.5, and the density of the soft tissue area now measures 2.5. The contrast of this image is found by the ratio 2.5/1.5 = 1.67. Contrast has been reduced from the original 2.0 to 1.67 as a result of fog. There is less obvious difference between the bone and the soft tissue areas, because of the addition of the fog density to both. Scatter radiation and the fog it produces are always destructive to the image.

X-RAY BEAM INTENSITY

The following chapters proceed to analyze the effect of each radiographic variable upon image contrast. It will be of immense help to understand that anything which simply alters the overall *intensity* of x-ray beam, the *quantity* of radiation directed at the film, will generally *not* affect image contrast, unless the change were to also alter one of the variables discussed in this chapter. Two examples are changing mAs and changing source-image receptor distance (SID). If the mAs is cut to one-half the original, there will be one-half as many x-rays entering the surface of the patient, one-half as many photoelectric interactions will occur, one-half as many Compton interactions will occur, and one-half as many x-rays will penetrate through to the film. In like fashion, if the x-ray tube is moved closer to the film such that the concentration of radiation striking the patient is doubled, photoelectric interactions will double in number, Compton also, and the number of penetrating x-rays will also be doubled. As long as the *percentage of penetration* or the *ratio of attenuation* is unchanged, image contrast will not be affected.

Remember from the previous chapter, as illustrated in Figure 3-7, that an image can certainly be twice as dark or twice as light overall, yet maintain the same contrast, which is the *ratio* between the densities. This is what happens when beam intensity alone is changed. The mere quantity of radiation is not a controlling factor for image contrast, within the ranges of diagnostic practice.

SUMMARY

1. The *photoelectric* interaction, because of its total absorption of x-rays, produces necessary *contrast* in the image.
2. The *Compton* interaction is responsible for 99 percent of the *fog* in the image and must be controlled.
3. *Scatter* is that secondary radiation which has significantly changed *direction* from that of the primary beam. It arises from both Compton and Thompson interactions.
4. *Subject Contrast* is produced by the differential absorption of tissues, and is measured as the *ratio* of the attenuation factors for two adjacent tissues.
5. *Subject Contrast* is affected by tissue thickness, the physical density of tissue, the average atomic number of tissue, and the kVp of the x-ray beam. It is not directly affected by changes in beam intensity.
6. As *kilovoltage* is increased, photoelectric interactions in a tissue drop off rapidly in number, while Compton interactions only decrease slightly. *Contrast* in an image is lost when there is a loss of *photoelectric interactions.*
7. When *atomic number* is increased by using positive contrast agents, the number of *photoelectric* interactions rises sharply, while Compton interactions remain at about the same level, thus

restoring high image *contrast.*

8. Against a background of soft tissue, *subject contrast* is produced for metals, contrast agents and bone primarily because of their *atomic number.* Air in the lungs and fat tissue are made visible primarily because of extreme differences in their *physical density,* when compared to soft tissue.

9. Since *scatter radiation* from the Compton interaction is randomly distributed, it adds a fog density equally to all areas of the image. This added density diminishes the ratio between these densities and thus reduces contrast.

REVIEW QUESTIONS

1. What are two other names for the Compton interaction:

2. Draw a sketch of the Compton interaction, and label all parts.

3. A photon is completely absorbed by an inner-shell orbital electron in the patient, and the electron ejects from its orbit. Name this interaction:

4. Define scatter radiation:

5. What effect does increasing the x-ray beam energy (kVp) have on the *total* number of all interactions within the patient?

6. What effect does increasing the x-ray beam energy (kVp) have on the *proportion* of Compton scatter interactions compared to photoelectric interactions?

7. A photon with *much* more energy than the electron binding energies of the tissue through which it passes is most likely to undergo what type of interaction.

8. A photon with just *slightly* more energy than the electron than the electron binding energies of the tissue through which it passes is most likely to under-

go what type of interaction?

9. Roughly how much of the radiation striking the film is secondary radiation?

10. On a radiograph, bone shows up against a background of soft tissue *mostly* because of what difference in its molecules?

11. If barium causes just as many Compton scatter interactions as normal fluids in the stomach, why does it show up so white on radiographs?

12. List the end product(s) of the Compton interaction:

13. Which two interactions within the patient ionize atoms?

14. Which two interactions within the patient result in scatter radiation?

15. Which interaction contributes most to image contrast?

16. Most image fog is caused by which interaction?

17. In bone, which interaction is more prevalent at very low kVp levels?

18. How much thicker does the anatomical part need to be in order to absorb twice as much of the x-ray beam?

Part II

VISIBILITY FACTORS

Chapter 5

MILLIAMPERE-SECONDS

MILLIAMPERAGE, abbreviated *mA*, is a measure of the quantity of electrical current flowing through a circuit. It is actually a rate representing the number of electrons passing through a wire in the circuit per second. The milliamperage control on an x-ray machine console is actually the *rheostat* in the filament circuit and it controls the *intensity* of the electron flow rate. Higher milliamperage settings send more electrons through the x-ray tube filament per second, heating it to a greater temperature each time the *rotor* switch is depressed. Because of the high temperature of the filament, more electrons are *boiled off* by thermionic emission (as discussed in Chapter 1).

Thus, at higher mA settings, more electrons are released from the filament and made available to accelerate across the x-ray tube and strike the anode. The number of x-rays ultimately produced in the x-ray beam is directly proportional to the number of electrons striking the anode. Therefore, the intensity rate of the x-ray beam is directly proportional to the mA set at the console. Double the mA station, and the flow of x-rays is twice as much per second.

Exposure time, abbreviated *s* for *seconds*, is simply the amount of time over which the beam is activated and exposure is occurring. Since mA is a rate, the mA multiplied by the exposure time *s* will give an indication of the total intensity of the entire x-ray exposure made. In a similar way, the rate of speed in miles-per-hour (MPH) multiplied by the hours of travel will indicate the total number of miles covered on a road trip: MPH x hrs = total miles. Since milliamperage is actually the flow rate of electricity, multiplying the mA by the exposure time will yield the total quantity of electricity that was used during an x-ray exposure. This total quantity is referred to in units of *mAs*, commonly pronounced *"mass."* The unit name is indicative of the mathematical formula: *mA* x *s* = *mAs*. Since the total number of x-rays striking the film during an exposure is directly controlled by the total amount of electricity used in producing the exposure, we may say that *mAs controls the total quantity of x-rays used during an exposure.*

EFFECT ON X-RAY BEAM SPECTRUM

As described in Chapter 1, an x-ray beam is heterogeneous, having many different energy levels in it, and the spectrum of the beam may be graphed by plotting the number of x-rays produced at each energy level. Figure 5-1 shows how a change in milliamperage or exposure time affects the x-ray beam spectrum, changing the intensity at each energy level by an equal proportion, but not affecting the

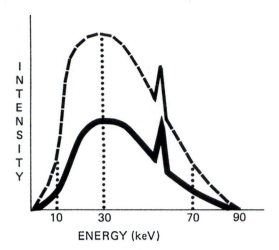

Figure 5-1. Graph demonstrating the effect of doubling the mAs on the x-ray beam spectrum. The number of photons produced at *every* keV level is doubled. Therefore, the minimum, average and peak energies remain the same.

peak, minimum or average energies. The solid curve represents the original x-ray beam, and the dashed curve depicts the new beam spectrum if the mAs were doubled.

If the *mA* is doubled, the exposure *rate* is doubled, and twice as many x-rays will be produced from the x-ray tube during the time the exposure occurs. If the mA is left unchanged, but the exposure time is doubled, once again there will be twice as many x-rays produced from the total expo-

sure. In either case, the *height* of the x-ray beam spectrum curve as shown in Figure 5-1 will double. The total area under the dashed line represents the total number of x-rays produced, and this area has indeed doubled when compared to the spectrum for the original beam.

Note in Figure 5-1 that the number of x-rays having just 10 kilovolts of energy has doubled; the number of x-rays produced at the average energy, 30 kV, has also doubled; there are also twice as many x-rays produced at 70 kV of energy. When the total *mAs* is doubled, the number of x-rays produced *at all energies* doubles. This means that the minimum, peak, and average energies of the beam (measured left to right on the spectrum) will be unchanged. For example, in Figure 5-1 the *average* energy of the original beam (solid line) is 30 kV. When the intensity of the new beam is doubled (dashed line), the average energy is still 30 kV. The *quantity* of the x-ray beam has increased, but the *quality* has not: The beam has the same penetrating characteristics because it has the same energy characteristics. The end result of doubling this intensity or quantity of the beam will be a radiographic image that is twice as dark, but other characteristics of the image, such as contrast, will not necessarily be affected.

RECIPROCITY LAW

The milliampere-seconds factor, indicated by the symbol *mAs*, directly controls radiographic image density when all other factors are constant. It is the product of the *milliamperage* (mA) and the duration of the exposure time in *seconds* (s). It is assumed that either factor, mA or s, may be changed at will to conform to required radiographic exposures as long as their product—*mAs*—remains the same. For example, approxi-

mately the same radiographic density will be obtained whether 50 mA is used for 0.1 second or 10 mA for 0.5 second, as long as their product comes to 5 mAs.

An important concept advanced by Bunsen and Roscoe in 1875 states that the reaction of a photographic emulsion to light is equal to the product of the intensity of the light and the duration of exposure. This is known as the *reciprocity law*. It implies that exposure rate (mA) may be exchanged with exposure time and still get the same film exposure. In radiography, reciprocity holds strictly true for direct exposure of the film to x-rays; however, when intensifying screens are used, the reciprocity law is not completely valid. This is because in order to chemically convert a silver bromide crystal into a developable grain, only one x-ray photon is required, but for light photons from an intensifying screen, more than one photon is required.

Failure of the reciprocity law may be observed during screen radiography when extremely short exposures (less than 0.05 second) with a high mA or extremely long exposures and a very low mA are used. Under these exposure conditions, even though the total product of the *mAs* may be the same, the resulting image densities using different mA and time combinations may not be consistent. Specifically, the image density will fall slightly short of the expected darkness. Fortunately, reciprocity law failure is seldom encountered in modern radiography and has been largely compensated for by the characteristics of modern x-ray film emulsion. Therefore, the total *mAs* value may be considered reliable for use as an exposure factor in general radiography.

In radiography, the density produced on the film will be directly proportional to the total exposure received by the film. The intensity of the total exposure is controlled by the total mAs. Therefore, *the overall radiographic density of an image will be directly proportional to the mAs used.*

CONTROL OF DENSITY

Milliampere-seconds is the primary electrical control over image density, because within normal ranges it affects *only* image density. If *either* the mA or the exposure time is doubled, the resulting image density will double. Since the total image density is a function of the total mAs, it may be said that mA and exposure time are inversely related *to each other* when maintaining a certain level of image density. That is, if the mA were doubled, the exposure time should be cut in half in order to maintain the original density. These relationships are important and are illustrated by the follow set of experiments.

EXPERIMENT:
TIME–DENSITY RELATION

Two series of radiographs of the hand, Figure 5-2, were taken employing 35 kVp for the first set and 50 kVp for the second set. After the first exposure was made for each set, the exposure time was doubled for each subsequent exposure. All other factors were kept constant. The total mAs resulting from each increase in exposure time is marked on each film. For Series A, the top row of images, note that at this low kilovoltage of 35 kVp, sufficient exposure through the bones of the hand is never achieved and details within the bones are never satisfactorily visualized. One can observe, nonetheless, that the *background* density of these radiographs visually doubles with each doubling of the exposure time.

In series B, the bottom row, 50 kVp was used providing good penetration of radiation through the bones of the hand. Note that in this case, the density of the anatomy itself, the actual bones and soft tissues of the hand, clearly doubles in darkness with each doubling of the exposure time. Of all

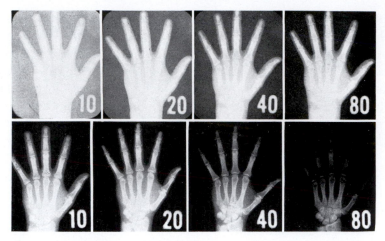

Figure 5-2. Demonstration of the effect of exposure time on radiographic density when an absorber (hand) is used (*Top*) using 35 kVp, and (*Bottom*) using 50 kVp. The respective total mAs values are noted on each radiograph.

these images, the most satisfactory is that taken at 50 kVp (bottom row) and employing 40 mAs. This image provides the greatest amount of bony detail. When all other factors but exposure time are constant, the quantity of x-rays emitted by the x-ray tube increases in direct proportion to the time of exposure.

EXPERIMENT: mA–DENSITY RELATION

Three radiographs of the hand were taken using 10, 50 and 100 mA respectively, while maintaining all other factors equal, Figure 5-3. The radiographic effect is similar to the influence of exposure time on image density. Radiograph #2 shows five times the density of radiograph #1 as expected for a proportional relationship. Radiograph #3 is severely overexposed, because 10 times the original mA was used. The most satisfactory radiograph is #2 taken at 50 mA. When all other factors but mA are constant, the quantify of x-rays emitted by the x-ray tube increases in direct proportion to the mA station set at the console.

EXPERIMENT: mA–TIME RELATION

Three radiographs of the hand, shown in Figure 5-4, were taken using the following techniques:

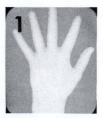
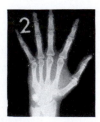
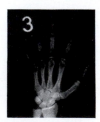

Figure 5-3. Demonstration of influence of mA on radiographic density with absorber (hand). The respective exposures are (1) 10 mA, (2) 50 mA, and (3) 100 mA.

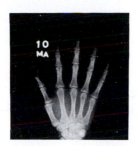 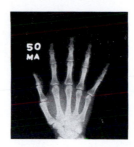 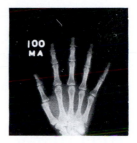

Figure 5-4. Demonstration of the compensatory (inverse) relationship between mA and exposure time on radiographic density. Time was adjusted downward in inverse proportion to the mA increases which are indicated on each radiograph, to maintain equal total mAs.

Exposure No	mA	Exp. Time	Total mAs
1	10	5 sec.	50
2	50	1 sec.	50
3	100	0.5 sec.	50

Note that as the mA stations were increased, the exposure times were reduced by an inversely proportionate amount, such that the total mAs values were all equalized at 50 mAs. The resulting densities of the hand image were all approximately equal. The original radiograph taken at 10 mA demonstrates a good density, which was maintained in the subsequent exposures. With respect to a given density level in the image, the mA and exposure time settings are inversely proportional to each other.

ARITHMETICAL RELATIONS

Mathematically, the *inversely proportional* relationship between mA and the time of exposure may be expressed by the formula:

$$\frac{mA_o}{mA_n} = \frac{Time_n}{Time_o}$$

where *o* is the original technique and *n* is the new technique. If one cross-multiplies this formula, one can see that it is just another way of stating that

Original mA x Original s = New mA x New s

or

Original *mAs* = New *mAs*

Example 1. Assume that 10 mA and an exposure time of 0.5 sec. was employed in making a radiograph. It is desired to decrease the exposure time to 0.05 sec. What milliamperage would be needed to assure comparable density?

Solution:
$$\frac{10}{X} = \frac{0.05}{0.5}$$

$$X(0.05) = 10(0.5)$$

$$X = \frac{10(0.5)}{0.05} = \frac{5}{0.05} = 100 \text{ mA } answer$$

Example 2: Assume that 500 mA and exposure time of 0.5 sec. was employed in making a radiograph. It is desired to decrease the milliamperage to 100 mA. What exposure time would be needed to obtain a comparable density?

Solution: $$\frac{500}{100} = \frac{X}{0.5}$$

$$X(100) = 500(0.5)$$

$$X = \frac{500(0.5)}{100} = \frac{250}{100} = 2.5 \text{ seconds } \textit{answer}$$

CALCULATING mAs VALUES

Some older x-ray machines may list the exposure times available in fractional form (i.e., 1/5 sec., 1/20 sec.). In computing mAs values, it is best to form a habit of employing decimal exposure times as are found on most modern equipment. To find the decimal equivalent of any fraction or ratio, simply divide the *numerator*, the number above the line, *by the denominator*, the lower number. For 1/5 second, just divide 1 by 5, yielding the decimal value 0.2. The total mAs value is determined by multiplying the mA station and the exposure time.

Table 5-1 may be very useful as a quick reference in determining mAs values when the mA and the exposure time to be used are known. To use this table, find the exposure to be employed in the left-hand vertical column; then, in the horizontal row at the top of the table, find the mA station to be used. The resulting mAs value is found where this column and row of the table meet.

Example 1: An exposure of 1/30 second is used with the 100 mA station. What is the mAs value? Find 1/30 second in the left-hand vertical column of the table, then locate 100 in the horizontal row at the top of the table. The row for 1/30 second intersects the column for 100 at the mAs value 3.33. This technique produces 3.33 mAs.

Example 2: An exposure of 0.07 second is used with the 50 mA station. What is the mAs value? Find 0.07 second in the left-hand vertical column of the table, then locate 50 in the horizontal row at the top of

the table. The corresponding row and column intersect at the mAs value 3.5. This technique produces 3.5 mAs.

WORKING WITH DECIMAL TIMERS

Radiographers must often adjust techniques using *mental math* rather than with pencil, paper, or calculator. On x-ray machines, most mA stations are in multiples of 100. On exposure timers, the most used decimal times frequently have two digits after the decimal point, that is, they are rounded to "hundredths" (e.g., 0.35, 0.02). This provides an easy starting point for practicing *mental* decimal conversions. To figure the total mAs, get into the habit of moving the decimal point on the exposure timer *two places to the right,* in your mind– then *ignore the two zeros on the mA station while multiplying.* You are simply cancelling out hundreds with hundredths.

For example, find the total mAs for

300 mA at 0.05 seconds

Moving the decimal in the timer two places to the right, you have 5. Ignoring the two zeros in the mA, you have 3. This is simply 3 times 5, or 15 mAs.

Think of 300 mA at 0.08 seconds as simply 3 times 8 for 24 mAs. And, 100 mA at 0.025 seconds is 1 times 2.5, or 2.5 mAs.

If there are three digits after the decimal, as in 0.008 seconds, you can use the same method but will be dealing with a decimal number when multiplying. For example, 200 mA at 0.008 seconds should be though of as 2 times 0.8 for a total of 1.6 mAs. If there is only one digit behind the decimal point, such as in 0.4 seconds, again, move the decimal two places to the right, in this case adding a zero to the number so that you would consider 0.4 as 40. Hence, 200 mA at 0.4 seconds will be thought of as 2

Table 5-1
MILLIAMPERE-SECONDS (mAs)

		Milliamperes							
Time Decimals	*Time Fractions*	*25*	*50*	*100*	*200*	*300*	*400*	*500*	*600*
0.0083	$1/120$	0.21	0.42	0.83	1.67	2.5	3.33	4.17	5.
0.007	—	0.18	0.35	0.7	1.4	2.1	2.8	3.5	4.2
0.01	$1/100$	0.25	0.5	1.	2.	3.	4.	5.	6.
0.0125	$1/80$	0.31	0.63	1.25	2.5	3.63	5.	6.25	7.5
0.0167	$1/60$	0.42	0.83	1.67	3.33	5.	6.25	8.33	10.
0.02	$1/50$	0.5	1.	2.	4.	6.	8.	10.	12.
0.025	$1//40$	0.62	1.25	2.5	5.	7.5	10.	12.5	15.
0.033	$1/30$	0.83	1.67	3.33	6.67	10.	13.33	16.67	20.
0.035	—	0.88	1.75	3.5	7.	10.5	14.	17.5	21.
0.05	$1/20$	1.25	2.5	5.	10.	15.	20.	25.	30.
0.067	$1/15$	1.67	3.33	6.66	13.33	20.	26.67	33.33	40.
0.07	—	1.75	3.5	7.	14.	21.	28.	35.	42.
0.083	$1/12$	2.08	4.16	8.33	16.67	25.	33.33	41.67	50.
0.1	$1/10$	2.5	5.	10.	20.	30.	40.	50.	60.
0.125	$1/8$	3.13	6.25	12.5	25.	37.5	50.	62.5	75.
0.133	$2/15$	3.33	6.67	13.33	26.67	40.	53.33	66.67	80.
0.15	$3/20$	3.75	7.5	15.	30.	45.	60.	75.	90.
0.167	$1/6$	4.17	8.33	16.7	33.33	50.	66.67	83.33	100.
0.2	$1/5$	5.	10.	20.	40.	60.	80.	100.	120.
0.25	$1/4$	6.25	12.5	25.	50.	75.	100.	125.	150.
0.3	$3/10$	7.5	15.	30.	60.	90.	120.	150.	180.
0.35	—	8.75	17.5	35.	70.	105.	140.	175.	210.
0.4	$2/5$	10.	20.	40.	80.	120.	160.	200.	240.
0.5	$1/2$	12.5	25.	50.	100.	150.	200.	250.	300.
0.7	—	17.5	35.	70.	140.	210.	280.	350.	420.
0.75	$3/4$	18.75	37.5	75.	150.	225.	300.	375.	450.

times 40 for a total of 80 mAs. Think of 100 mA at 0.2 seconds as 1 times 20, and 500 at 0.8 as 5 times 80.

Do the following exercise, calculating the total mAs values *mentally*. When completed, check your answers from the Appendix.

EXERCISE #1

mA x *time* = *mAs*

1. 100 @ .05 =
2. 100 @ .8 =
3. 200 @ .02 =
4. 200 @ .125 =

5. 200 @ .3   =
6. 300 @ .7   =
7. 300 @ .04   =
8. 300 @ .025 =
9. 400 @ .04   =
10. 400 @ .016 =
11. 400 @ .33   =
12. 500 @ .03   =
13. 500 @ .7   =
14. 600 @ .25   =
15. 600 @ .008 =

WORKING WITH
MILLISECOND TIMERS

Modern radiographic equipment with a high-capacity generator may use a millisecond timer. As with decimals and fractions, the mathematics involved is simple, yet a little practice is very helpful in developing the required skill. To convert a millisecond exposure time into a decimal time, simply move the decimal three places to the *left* and delete any zeros at the end of the number. For example, the decimal time for 700 milliseconds is 0.700 = 0.7 seconds, and 350 milliseconds is 0.350 = 0.35 seconds.

If the millisecond time has only one or two digits, zeros must be added in front of it (to the left of it) as the decimal point is shifted to the left. For example, the decimal time for 50 milliseconds is 0.05 seconds—one zero must be added before the "5" as the decimal point shifts to the left. The decimal time for 25 milliseconds is 0.025 seconds. What is the decimal time for 4 milliseconds? Shifting the decimal point three places to the left and adding two zeros in front of the "4," the answer is 0.004 seconds.

When converting decimal times into milliseconds, the decimal is moved three places to the *right*, adding zeros as required. Thus, 0.8 seconds is 0800. = 800 milliseconds. Two zeros were added as the decimal

was shifted to the right. What is 0.15 seconds in milliseconds? Moving the decimal to the right three places and adding one zero, the answer is 0150. = 150 milliseconds. A decimal time of 0.135 seconds is 135 milliseconds.

Complete the following brief exercise *mentally*, without paper or calculator. Then check your answers in the Appendix.

EXERCISE #2

Decimal = Milliseconds

1. 0.75   =
2. 0.3   =
3. 0.125 =
4. 0.04   =
5. 0.083 =
6. 0.0333 =
7. 0.005 =
8. 0.0012 =

Milliseconds = Decimal

9.   200 =
10. 167 =
11. 250 =
12. 35   =
13. 70   =
14. 15   =
15. 8   =
16. 1200 =

When calculating mAs conversions with millisecond times, you may move the decimal point on the *mA* to the left three places and multiply, but it is often easier to move the decimal for the *exposure time* three places to the left and multiply the mA by this number. In other words, it is easier to convert the millisecond time into a decimal time, as we have just practiced in Exercise #2, then multiply the mA by that decimal time. Now try the following mAs calculations, finding the total mAs mentally. These problems are identical in format to

Exercise #1, but they use millisecond times instead of decimal times. Check your answers from the Appendix.

EXERCISE #3

$$mA \times time = mAs$$

1. 50 @ 50 ms   =
2. 100 @ 500 ms =
3. 100 @ 35 ms   =
4. 100 @ 8 ms   =
5. 200 @ 200 ms =
6. 200 @ 125 ms =
7. 300 @ 33 ms   =
8. 300 @ 6 ms   =
9. 400 @ 250 ms =
10. 400 @ 80 ms   =
11. 500 @ 5 ms   =
12. 600 @ 150 ms =

WORKING WITH FRACTIONAL TIMERS

Exposure timers reading in fractions, common on older equipment, are somewhat more difficult than decimals to work mentally, yet they tend to follow patterns and can be learned with a little practice. Particular patterns of number pairs always go together, for example, 2's and 5's go together since $1/2 = 0.5$ and $1/5 = 0.2$. Such number pairs are found at the 100 and 300 mA stations: At the 100 mA station, the following pairs of numbers always go together:

3 and 33
4 and 25
5 and 2
6 and 16
7 and 15
8 and 12

For example, 100 mA at 1/8 second is approximately 12 mAs (12.5), and 100 mA

at 1/12 is approximately 3 mAs (8.33). At the 300 mA station, the following pairs are found:

5 and 6
15 and 20
12 and 25

For example, 300 mA at 1/15 second is 20 mAs, while 300 mA at 1/20 second is 15 mAs. For the 50 mA and 200 mA stations, use the numbers listed above for the 100 mA station but simply cut the results in half or double them respectively. Likewise, multiply these results by 4 for the 400 station, by 5 for 500 mA, and so on. Try Exercise #4 below, completing all the calculations *mentally*, then check your answers in the Appendix.

EXERCISE #4

$$mA \times time = mAs$$

1. 100 @ 1/20 s =
2. 100 @ 1/8 s =
3. 100 @ 1/120 s =
4. 100 @ 1/6 s =
5.   50 @ 1/20 s =
6. 200 @ 1/5 s =
7. 200 @ 1/40 s =
8.   50 @ 1/30 s =
9. 300 @ 1/60 s =
10. 300 @ 1/15 s =
11. 300 @ 1/25 s =
12. 600 @ 1/5 s =
13. 400 @ 1/8 s =
14. 500 @ 1/15 s =

Complex Fractions

Complex fractions involve numerators other than "1" on top, such as 2/5 or 7/20. You must convert them in two steps, dividing the bottom denominator into the mA station first, then thinking of the top number as "sets." For example, to solve 200 mA at 2/5 second, first, ignore the top numerator of the fraction, considering it as a "one"–in other words, find 1/5 of 200. When you have this, multiply it by the top of the fraction thinking in "sets," as follows:

>200 mA @ 2/5 sec. =
>1/5 of 200 = 40
>2 SETS of 40 = 80 mAs *answer*

Using 200 mA at 7/20 second yields 7 *sets of 10* or 70 mAs. 300 mA at 3/15 second results in *3 sets of 20* or 60 mAs. Using this approach, solve the problems in Exercise 5 below mentally, then check your answers in the Appendix.

EXERCISE #5

$$mA \times time = mAs$$

1. 100 @ 2/15 s =
2. 100 @ 3/20 s =
3. 200 @ 3/5 s =
4. 200 @ 7/20 s =
5. 400 @ 2/5 s =
6. 300 @ 3/20 s =

FINDING mA AND TIME COMBINATION FOR A DESIRED mAs

Probably the most common mathematics problem a radiographer faces every day is that of having a desired total mAs in mind, and trying to mentally determine an mA–time combination that will yield that total. If there is a *mAs Table* available, such as the one presented in Table 5-1, you can simply scan downward and to the right for a mAs value close to the mAs desired, and read the table "backwards" by following the column upward to find the mA station, and following the row to the left to find the exposure time. Naturally, there are several combinations to obtain the same total mAs, and if you wish to extend the exposure time for a breathing technique, or to minimize it in order to reduce motion, the first combination you find on the table may not be adequate. In this case, go back to the total mAs where you started, and scan diagonally upward and to the right, or downward and to the left. You will find that the same total mAs value (or others close to it) repeats itself with various combinations of mA and exposure time.

Such conversion charts are not always available, and it is an important skill for the radiographer to develop an ability to also be able to make such calculations mentally. In this case, you must first determine what mA station the desired total mAs would divide into easily. With a little practice, the correct time fraction will then come to mind.

One unique thing about fractions (which you will not find with decimals) is that some of the answers can only be found in "complex fractions," which have a number other than "1" as their numerator, such as 2/5 or 3/20. To solve these, you must learn to think in "sets," such as using two sets of 20 mAs to obtain 40 mAs.

Example: It is desired to obtain 80 mAs, using the 200 mA station. Since 80 does not divide *evenly* into 200, no usable fraction with a numerator of "1" on top can be found. However, if you learn to recognize *80 as two sets of 40*, you can find the usable time as follows:

First, *divide 40 mAs into 200 mA = 5*

5 will be the denominator of your fraction time

(That is, 40 mAs would be obtained at 1/5 sec.)

Now, simply go back and *take two sets of 1/5, by changing the numerator to 2*

The answer is 2/5 second

80 mAs = 200 mA at 2/5 second

80 mAs = 2 sets of 40 mAs

The following exercise will provide practice in finding such fractional times. For each total mAs listed, express it as so many sets of a smaller number which will easily divide into a typical mA station. Some of the calculations may have more than one workable answer, yet you should *reduce* any fractions as far as possible. For example:

120 mAs may be expressed as ___ sets of ___?

If you use *6 sets of 20*, this ratio could be further reduced to *3 sets of 40*, which is a better answer.

Another good answer for this problem would be *2 sets of 60*, since, again, this number of sets could not be further reduced.

Note that *sets of 40 will be easily divisible into the 200 mA station*, while *sets of 60 would be easily divisible into the 300 mA station.*

This may sound complicated at first, but try the exercise below, and you will find it is not as difficult as expected. When completed, check your answers from the Appendix.

EXERCISE #6

1. 80 mAs can be expressed as __ sets of __.
2. 45 mAs can be expressed as __ sets of __.
3. 66 mAs can be expressed as __ sets of __.
4. 75 mAs can be expressed as __ sets of __.
5. 180 mAs can be expressed as __ sets of __.
6. 120 mAs can be expressed as __ sets of __.
7. 160 mAs can be expressed as __ sets of __.
8. 240 mAs can be expressed as __ sets of __.
9. 90 mAs can be expressed as __ sets of __.
10. 320 mAs can be expressed as __ sets of __.

In the following two exercises, the total mAs desired is given along with a suggested mA station. For each one, determine which exposure time to use to obtain the total mAs value. On the first exercise the answers must be given as fractions, and on the second exercise the answers must be in decimals. Do the exercise *mentally*, then check your answers from the Appendix.

EXERCISE #7:

Answers must be in *fractions*:

Total mAs = mA x seconds

1. 2.5 mAs = 100 mA x
2. 7 mAs = 100 mA x
3. 3.3 mAs = 100 mA x
4. 1.7 mAs = 100 mA x
5. 1.25 mAs = 100 mA x
6. 0.8 mAs = 100 mA x
7. 2.5 mAs = 50 mA x
8. 40 mAs = 200 mA x
9. 5 mAs = 200 mA x
10. 14 mAs = 200 mA x
11. 20 mAs = 300 mA x
12. 2.5 mAs = 300 mA x
13. 45 mAs = 300 mA x
14. 240 mAs = 300 mA x
15. 240 mAs = 400 mA x

EXERCISE #8:

Answers must be in decimals:

Total mAs = mA × seconds

1. 2.5 mAs = 100 mA ×
2. 7 mAs = 100 mA ×
3. 3.3 mAs = 100 mA ×
4. 1.7 mAs = 100 mA ×
5. 40 mAs = 100 mA ×
6. 1.25 mAs = 50 mA ×
7. 25 mAs = 200 mA ×
8. 5 mAs = 200 mA ×
9. 2.5 mAs = 200 mA ×
10. 14 mAs = 200 mA ×
11. 50 mAs = 300 mA ×
12. 6 mAs = 300 mA ×
13. 21 mAs = 300 mA ×
14. 180 mAs = 300 mA ×
15. 240 mAs = 400 mA ×

VISIBLE DENSITY CHANGE

Generally, the most common cause of repeated exposures is improper density– the radiograph turns out too light or too dark. A repeated exposure doubles the radiation dose to the patient in order to obtain a particular view. It seems unconscionable that a third exposure might be necessitated, thus tripling the patient dose, because the radiographer did not accurately assess the needed technique correction the first time. Every radiographer should have developed the fundamental skill to confidently determine how much a technique must be increased or decreased by observing the original radiograph. An exercise to help develop this skill is found in Chapter 24.

By far, the most common error in making such technique adjustments for improperly exposed radiographs is to *not make a big enough change.* For example, to compensate for a light radiograph, it is somewhat common to "go up one step in time." In most cases, this is a foolhardy notion, since the resulting radiograph may not appear obviously darker than the original, and another repeat could easily result. This is demonstrated in Figure 5-5 using manual techniques with the actual mAs listed: Note that in this case a 25 percent increase in exposure did *not* result in an obviously darker radiograph. The 47 percent increase

in mAs did result in a darker film.

This is not to say that a 25 percent change in mAs is *never* visible, but for most daily procedures, it is not worth risking this type of increase and the additional repeat it may lead to. What is needed is a good rule of thumb for minimum technique corrections, to ensure that the change will be substantial enough to make a difference. A traditional rule of thumb was to always adjust technique (mAs) by at least one-third. The advent of rare earth screens has indeed lowered this amount slightly, but not as dramatically as some authors have suggested. (If this type of experiment is performed in the lab using a step-wedge penetrometer, results as low as 17 percent may be obtained; such results must *not* be translated into clinical practice for two very important reasons: First, the step-wedge is made of homogeneous material, whereas the human body is composed of heterogeneous tissues forming thousands of trabecular densities, so that greater changes are required before they become obvious in the image. Second, the step-wedge is small in thickness and produces very little scatter radiation, whereas the human body can produce large amounts of scatter. This also obscures density changes so that they are less obvious. The rule of thumb we seek must address practical clinical results on

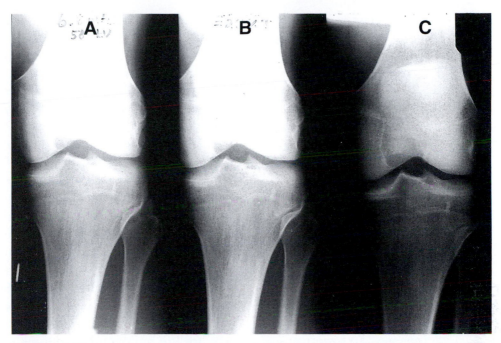

Figure 5-5. Demonstration of minimum mAs adjustment to cause a visible change in image density for knee radiographs. Radiograph B shows a 25% increase in mAs from the previous Radiograph A: Note that the density of B is *not visibly darker than A.* Radiograph C shows a 47% increase in mAs, which does result in an obviously darker image. Factors = 58kVp, A = 6.8 mAs, B = 8.5 mAs, C = 10 mAs.

real patients.)

In practice, as illustrated in Figure 5-5, a 25 percent increase is usually not visible. A 25 percent *decrease* in technique usually is just visible, as shown in Figure 28-2 in Chapter 28 demonstrating the effects of changing the density knob setting for automatic exposure control. The 25 percent *decrease* results in an exposure that is **3/4** of the original mAs. The new exposure ratio is 3/4. The opposite of this change, that is, a corresponding *increase* in technique, is actually **4/3** (3/4 inverted). If technique must be reduced to 3/4 to be visibly lighter, it would be expected that an increase to 4/3 would be needed to be visibly darker. Expressed as a percentage, 4/3 of the original technique is a 33 percent increase or an increase of 1/3; this is in keeping with the traditional rule of thumb.

Suppose that the radiologist asks for a repeated exposure in order to darken the image, and the technologist makes this correction by increasing "one step in time." There are two inherent problems with this approach: First, it is not always specific, since the actual percentage of change achieved by the "next step" on the exposure timer depends upon the particular format the manufacturer of the x-ray equipment has used, and these formats vary. The "next step in time" on one machine might be a 25 percent increase, whereas on another brand of equipment it might be as much as a 50 percent increase. Second, and most importantly, "steps" on the exposure timer may fall below the one-third increase required for a visibly darker image.

As an example, suppose that a combination of 300 mA and 0.2 (1/5) second resulted in a light radiograph. This is 60 mAs total. The next step in time on many machines is 0.25 (1/4) second. An increase of "one step" to 300 mA at 0.25 second would yield 75 mAs total. This change from 60 to 75 mAs only represents a 25 percent increase, well below the rule of thumb. It is likely that the repeated radiograph would *not be distinguishably darker* than the original, and this may lead to yet a third exposure to the patient.

The rule of thumb for minimum technique corrections is affected by the response of the image receptor system, but is not brought about by it. The need for such a rule is simply based upon the limitations of the *human eye* in distinguishing subtle density differences. It is important to note that the discussion thus far has dealt only with *minimum* visible changes, not with *recommended* changes. **In practice**, one is not trying to produce a change in technique that is *barely* distinguishable from the previous image, but rather a change that is visibly *obvious*. The older rule of thumb, "reduce technique by at least 1/3 or increase it by at least 1/2," is still quite functional as a *recommendation for daily practice*. Note that these are again mathematically opposite to each other: An increase by 1/2 or 50 percent yields an overall ratio that is 3/2 the original. A decrease of 1/3 or 33 percent yields an overall ratio that is 2/3

the original. These are exactly inverted ratios, 3/2 and 2/3.

Thus, the practical, workable rule of thumb for adjusting image density in modern radiography is still: ***Always increase technique by at least one-half, always decrease technique by at least a third***.

When using automatic exposure control or "phototiming," the most common selections for increasing technique are +25%, +50%, and 75%; Given these choices, as shown in Figure 5-5, it is almost always wiser to select the +50% in order to darken up an image, thus increasing technique by 1/2.

Another general rule of thumb has proven valuable when correcting for *serious* underexposures and overexposures: It is useful for the radiographer to think of substantial technique corrections in factors of 2. Most serious underexposures can be corrected by doubling the initial mAs. In the case of serious overexposures, cutting the mAs to one-half the initial value will usually suffice. There are certainly situations that require more dramatic alterations, and the density correction exercise in Chapter 24 addresses these. But, this "factor of 2" concept is workable in perhaps 80 percent of the circumstances when a radiograph turns out much too light or very dark.

UNDEREXPOSURE AND QUANTUM MOTTLE

During a light rain shower, you can see the individual raindrops on a sidewalk. If you count the raindrops on each square of cement, you can see that they are not evenly distributed: more raindrops fall in some areas than in others. It is a random phenomenon, a matter of statistical probability, which squares of cement will be exposed to more raindrops. When a very *heavy* rainfall comes, the same uneven dis-

tribution of raindrops is still there, but you can no longer tell, because the sidewalk is now saturated with water and there are no dry spots between the drops.

The x-ray beam is a *shower* of x-rays which have a random distribution just like a rain shower. When very low mAs values are used, there are few photons striking the film and one can see the uneven distribution of the densities resulting. The radiograph appears *grainy*–that is, very small blotches of density are seen across the film when examined up close. These blotches are referred to as *quantum mottle*, a mottled appearance of the image caused by the *quanta* or photons in the x-ray beam. Vis-ible mottling of the image indicates that an insufficient amount of x-rays have reached the film, most commonly because insuffi-cient mAs values were used for the expo-sure. To correct it, the intensity of the beam must be increased by increasing mAs.

EFFECT ON CONTRAST

Radiographic contrast is determined by the *ratio* of penetrating x-rays between dif-ferent types of tissues within the patient. As shown on the beam spectrum graph in Figure 5-1, changes in mAs control the total number of photons produced but do *not* change the proportion of photons at one energy level to those at another energy level. For example, the number of photons having 35 keV may be doubled, but the number of photons having 70 keV are also doubled, so that their proportion to each other remains the same. Milliampere-sec-onds cannot have any effect upon the *types* of interactions taking place, only upon the total number of all interactions.

For example, doubling the mAs will have the following effects: Twice as many x-ray photons will enter the surface of the patient. In soft tissue, twice as many photo-electric interactions will occur and twice as many Compton scatter interactions will occur, so that the overall absorption of x-rays has doubled. *However, there will also be twice as many photons penetrating completely through the soft tissue without interacting.* Everything doubles, including the number of penetrating rays. Therefore, the *ratio* of penetration to absorption in the soft tissue is unchanged–this tissue still has the same subject contrast characteristics. The same is true for bone tissue: Twice as many x-rays are absorbed, but twice as many penetrate through as well, so that the penetration/absorption *ratio* is unchanged and the bone still possesses its characteristic subject con-trast.

As illustrated in Chapter 4, image con-trast will not change as long as the absorp-tion ratios between the tissues is unchanged. Let us assume that, originally, the absorption ratio for the soft tissue was 90 percent, and that the ratio for the bone was 70 percent. Doubling the quantity of x-rays entering the patient does not change these ratios. Thus, the contrast between the bone and the soft tissue will still be 9/7. Contrast is unchanged.

Figure 3-7 in Chapter 3 shows that a radiograph can be twice as dark overall, and yet still possess the same contrast. Figure 5-2, just a few pages back, demon-strates the same concept if you observe the two middle radiographs on the bottom row, using 20 mAs and 40 mAs respective-ly. The soft tissue may appear twice as dark, but as long as the bone *also* appears twice as dark, the ratio of density difference *between* the bone and the soft tissue will still be equal. (Note that in evaluating image contrast, the *background* density must be ignored–comparisons should only be made between between the different tissue areas *within the anatomy*, in this case, the soft tissue density versus the bone density.) For practical purposes, *mAs should not be considered as a variable affecting contrast.*

Now, if *extreme* changes in mAs are made, an exception occurs which also can be seen in Figure 5-2 by observing the two extreme ends of this series of radiographs: On the one hand, if there is just insufficient exposure to the film to produce any reasonable density, all tissues, both bone and soft tissue, will appear nearly blank white, and the contrast between them is lost. On the other hand, if extreme amounts of mAs are used so that the film is grossly overexposed, the soft tissue areas will have reached the maximum density the film can produce—"pitch black," while the bone areas will continue to darken, and contrast will diminish. These are both exceptional cases: Note that in Figure 5-2, the difference in mAs to illustrate these effects was *8 fold*, while in daily practice, changing technique by 8 times would be unheard of. The *mAs should never be considered as a controlling factor over image contrast* when used in diagnostic ranges.

EXPOSURE TIME AND MOTION

Long exposure times are not the direct cause of motion—it is the patient who moves. But in chest radiography, for example, the movement of the heart is unavoidable, and can only be eliminated from the radiographic image by the use of very short exposure times, effectively "freezing" the motion. In a similar way, sports photographers must use extremely short exposure times to "freeze" the motion of athletes or speeding cars. Besides heart motion, the longer the exposure time used, the greater the chance for peristaltic motion in the stomach or intestines, and the greater the possibility that the patient might breath or move.

Therefore, exposure time is generally considered to be a *contributing factor* for motion during radiographic exposures. Motion is the greatest enemy to sharpness of recorded detail in the image. Shorter exposure times cannot *guarantee* that motion will not occur any more than longer exposures guarantee that it *will* in every case. Yet, since heart and peristaltic motion are beyond the control of the radiographer, *it is generally assumed that the shorter the exposure time, the sharper the recorded detail in the image.*

EFFECTS ON OTHER IMAGE QUALITIES

Milliamperage and exposure time have no direct effect upon magnification or distortion of the radiographic image. Magnification and distortion are *geometrical* in nature and depend upon the geometry of the beam, whereas mA and exposure time are essentially *electrical* factors, unrelated to beam geometry.

SUMMARY

1. Milliamperage is an electrical factor controlling the *rate* of x-ray emission from the x-ray tube.
2. Milliampere-seconds (*mAs*) multiplies this rate by the exposure time to represent the total amount of electricity employed during an exposure. It controls the *total exposure* intensity to the film.
3. Milliampere-seconds is the primary

control for image *density*. This is for two reasons: First, density is *directly proportional* to the mAs, and second, mAs has no direct effect upon the other image qualities, within practical ranges.

4. For a given mAs value, mA and exposure time are *inversely related* to each other. A higher mA and a shorter time can be used, as long as the total mAs is equal, to achieve a certain image density.

5. When correcting mAs for and improperly exposed radiograph, *decrease by at least 1/3 or increase by at least 1/2 to produce a visible change in the density*. For serious corrections, generally change mAs by a factor of 2.

6. Insufficient mAs can lead to visible *quantum mottle* in the image.

REVIEW QUESTIONS

Calculate the following total mAs values from the given mA and time combination:

$$mA \times time = mAs$$

1. 100 @ .125 sec =
2. 200 @ .035 sec =
3. 300 @ .006 sec =
4. 400 @ .007 sec =
5. 500 @ .125 sec =
6. 50 @ 300 ms =
7. 200 @ 35 ms =
8. 300 @ 25 ms =
9. 600 @ 12 ms =
10. 100 @ 2/5 sec =
11. 200 @ 4/5 sec =
12. 300 @ 4/5 sec =
13. 400 @ 3/20 sec =

Give the *fractional* exposure times that must be used to complete the following quotations:

$$Total\ mAs = mA \times seconds$$

14. 40 mAs = 100 mA ×
15. 120 mAs = 200 mA ×
16. 6 mAs = 300 mA ×
17. 180 mAs = 300 mA ×
18. 80 mAs = 400 mA ×

Give the *decimal* exposure times that must be used to complete the following equations:

$$Total\ mAs = mA \times seconds$$

19. 16 mAs = 100 mA ×
20. 2.5 mAs = 50 mA ×
21. 120 mAs = 200 mA ×
22. 75 mAs = 300 mA ×
23. 80 mAs = 400 mA ×

24. Failure of the reciprocity law implies that mAs values may not always be exactly proportional to image density when using _____.
25. What electrical factor controls the rate of the x-rays coming from the tube?
26. In controlling image density, why it is important to talk of total mAs rather than just mA or time separately?
27. Give two reasons why mAs should be considered as the *primary* control for image density.
28. In maintaining a given density, mA and time are _____ related to each other.
29. The fraction 1/8 second is equal to which decimal time.
30. 80 milliseconds is _____ second in decimal time.
31. In normal ranges, changing the mAs does not affect image contrast because

the number of incoming photons does not alter the _____ -contrast of the tissues.

32. What would be a good practical reason for using low mA and a long exposure time to achieve a particular total mAs?

33. In practice, when repeating a radiograph that was too dark, always decrease the mAs by at least _____ to *ensure* a visible difference.

34. In practice, when repeating a radiograph that was too light, always increase the mAs by at least _____ to *ensure* a visible difference.

35. When repeating a radiograph that was *much* too dark or *much* too light, always change the mAs by at least a factor of _____.

36. What technique error can cause the uneven distribution of x-rays within the beam to show up as a "grainy" appearance on the radiograph?

Chapter 6

KILOVOLTAGE-PEAK

KILOVOLTAGE, abbreviated keV or kV, is a measure of the electrical force or *pressure* behind a current of electricity, which causes it to flow. In the x-ray machine, the kilovoltage control is actually the *autotransformer* in the high-voltage circuit. Whenever a potential difference exists between two points in a conductor, one end having a relative negative charge and the other end a relative positive charge, a current of electrons will flow through the conductor toward the positive charge. The greater the difference is in the electrical charge or potential, the more *pressure* is exerted on the current to flow, and the more kilovoltage will be measured. Recall from the last chapter that *mAs* actually measures the quantity of electricity flowing through a wire. Kilovoltage measures the *quality* of the electricity, that is, its *energy level.*

Due to the rotation of the magnetic fields in a generator that produces electricity, the actual kilovoltage of the current supplied to a typical x-ray machine varies up and down in a sine-wave pattern, rising to a peak and then falling back to zero repeatedly. Since the kilovoltage is constantly changing, it must be measured in terms of either an average value or as a peak value attained during this cycle (Fig. 6-1), hence the use of the term *kilovoltage-peak,* or *kVp.*

EFFECT ON X-RAY BEAM SPECTRUM

The kVp meters on the console of a typical x-ray machine read in *peak* kilovoltage, but it is important to remember that this reading indicates the energy of only a very small portion of the current. Most of the current has much less than the peak energy. The x-rays produced cannot possibly have more energy than the electrons that produced them. Only a few x-rays in the beam will actually have the *peak* energy. The *average* energy of the x-rays in the beam is about *1/3 of the peak energy.*

The characteristic curve of the spectrum of energies in an x-ray beam plots the kV energy levels against the number of x-rays produced at each kV, i.e., the intensity at each kV level, as shown in Figure 6-2. Note that the greatest number of x-rays for an 80-kVp beam occurs at about 27 keV (1/3 of the peak). When kVp is increased to 90, as shown by the dotted curve, the *average* energy of the beam increases to 30. In addition, the shifting of the right half of the curve toward the right results in a larger total area under the curve; this indicates that the total number of x-rays produced has also increased.

When the kilovoltage applied across the x-ray tube is increased, the electrons emitted from the filament accelerate to a greater speed before reaching the anode. Since they each have higher energy, these

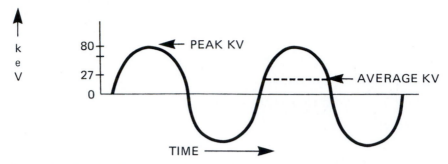

Figure 6-1. Graph of sine wave showing the changing kilovoltage during normal electrical cycles. Kilovoltage must be measured as a peak value or as an average value. For single-phase equipment, the *average* kilovoltage is about one-third of the *peak* kilovoltage.

electrons are capable of losing more energy when they interact with atoms in the anode. X-rays with higher energies will be produced. Not *all* of the additional x-rays produced will have higher energies than those originally in the beam, but many will, and so the average energy of the beam will increase (Fig. 6-2).

At the same time, electrons traveling at higher speeds are likely to undergo *more* interactions with atoms in the anode before they are completely stopped. Each interaction results in the production of an x-ray.

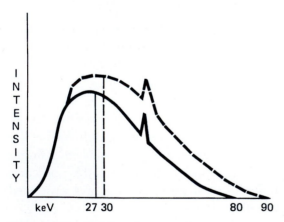

Figure 6-2. Graph of x-ray beam spectrum changes resulting from an increase in kVp. The peak and average energies of the beam increase, while the minimum energy remains the same. Also, the total number of x-rays emitted from the x-ray tube increases by 25% to 40%.

With more interactions occurring, more x-rays will be produced at higher kVp settings. Reviewing the *bremsstrahlung* interaction in Chapter 1, you can surmise that, since an electron is only *partially* slowed down from this interaction, the electron may undergo *several* bremsstrahlung interactions before losing all of its speed energy. This means that one single electron can produce several x-rays, one from each interaction. At higher kilovoltage, the electrons enter the anode material at higher speeds, and can undergo more interactions before losing all their energy. As shown in Figure 6-2, more x-rays will be produced resulting in a *higher* spectral curve graphed, as well as an increased area under this curve. To summarize, *at higher kVp levels,* **both** *the quality and the quantity the x-rays emitted by the tube are increased.*

With higher kVp, even though more x-rays are produced at *all* energy levels, those with low energies will be absorbed by filtration. The *minimum* energy of the beam is denoted in Figure 6-2 as the point to the left at which the curve is cut toward zero. This *left* portion of the spectrum curve is unchanged. The minimum energy the x-ray beam is controlled by filtration, not by kVp.

An x-ray beam with higher energy will

be capable of *penetrating* through more different types of tissue. As discussed in Chapter 4, such a change in penetration will affect the gray scale, and consequently also the contrast, on the finished radiographic image. Higher kVp levels also result in more x-rays being initially produced, and with higher penetration power, these are more likely to reach the film, darkening the overall density of the image. Therefore, changes in kVp have profound effects on *both contrast and density* in the final image.

CONTROL OF CONTRAST

Subject contrast, the difference in intensity between one portion of the remnant x-ray beam and another, is completely essential for a radiographic image to be produced. Three situations, all of which can be related to kVp, can prevent this production of subject contrast in the image. In the first case, insufficient penetration of the x-ray beam through the tissues leads to a failure to record each different tissue density on the radiograph. Two underpenetrated areas will both be recorded as blank white, so that there can be no distinction between them. In the second case, alteration of the directions of the remnant x-rays by scattering interactions within the patient leads to a crossing over of exposure intensities, so that there is less distinction between them. In the third case, extreme overexposure of the film leads to all areas reaching a level of pitch-black density, so that there can be little or no distinction between them.

PENETRATION AND GRAY SCALE

The most important function of kVp is to provide penetration of the x-ray beam through the patient's tissues. At higher levels of kVp, the penetrating ability of the x-rays is increased. Therefore, *more* different types of body tissues may be penetrated and recorded on the radiograph as a representative density. As greater numbers of different tissues are recorded on the radiograph, more different gray shades will be present in the image. Gray scale increases. Penetration is a primary controlling factor over image gray scale.

Let us examine this relationship more closely by considering low, medium, and high kVp levels one at a time: If kVp is so low that there is insufficient penetration, virtually all tissues are recorded as a light or "white" density on the image, and by definition, there is little contrast. As kVp is gradually increased, tissues with lower atomic numbers are recorded as gray shades, while bones, barium, iodine, and other tissues with higher atomic numbers are still "white." Differential absorption, due to *subject contrast* or *tissue contrast*, is now established. Gray scale can now be measured in the image (simply by counting the number of different densities), but this scale is too short, with only a few different shades of light gray and white present. Continuing to still higher energies, bones and similar tissues become penetrated and are recorded as light grays, while other tissues are seen as medium and dark grays. Gray scale increases. Eventually, if the kVp is high enough, even barium and iodine will be penetrated enough to be recorded as a light gray rather than a blank white (which possesses no radiographic information.)

By increasing kVp, more and more different types of tissue are recorded on the image, more different shades of gray are produced, and gray scale is gradually lengthened. Since this represents more information, it is usually *desirable* to have such long gray scale in the image.

As discussed in Chapter 3, gray scale is the opposite of image contrast, and when there are many more different shades of gray present in the image, the result is that there is less difference from one gray shade to the next. Hence, contrast is reduced.

This implies that *even when fogging of the image from scatter radiation is eliminated, changes in kVp will still have a considerable effect upon image contrast by virtue of their effect on beam penetration. Higher kVp levels will increase image gray scale, thus reducing image contrast.* For example, the hand is such a thin anatomical part that it produces practically no scatter radiation during an expo-

sure. Nonetheless, even though scatter is negligible, increasing the kVp on a hand exposure will *still* reduce the contrast of the image, because of the effect of increased penetration in lengthening gray scale. This is also true for chest radiography where very little scatter radiation is produced within the lung fields. Contrast will still diminish at higher kVp levels.

Demonstration No. 1

The influence of kilovoltage on gray scale can be demonstrated by a series of radiographs of a dry skull (Fig. 6-3). The absence of the soft tissues of the brain and face in this specimen eliminates most of the scatter radiation that might have been produced. These images, therefore, may be considered essentially free of scatter fog.

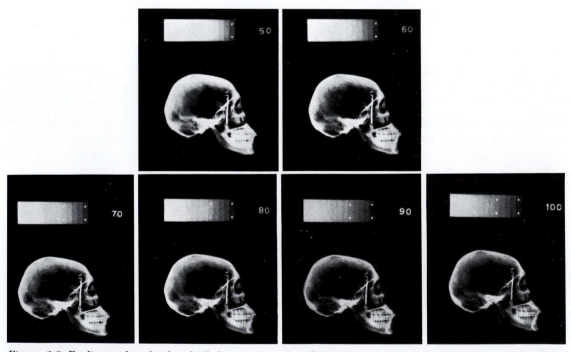

Figure 6-3. Radiographs of a dry skull demonstrate that the increased *penetration* obtained at higher kilovoltages leads to lengthened image gray scale. Note that with no soft tissue present, scatter is negligible. Therefore, this effect is entirely due to increased penetration of various tissues. The kVp used is shown on each image.

The radiographs were exposed in 10 kVp increments from 50 to 100 kVp. The density effect of each kilovoltage was offset by compensating mAs. A step wedge was included in each image as a "control" in order to determine the exact mAs compensations needed to maintain density. This procedure made it possible to demonstrate the gray scale characteristics produced at each kVp level.

Note that in the 50-kVp image, very high densities (blacks) are apparent, yet there are also areas in which no details are exhibited because of insufficient penetration through bone. As the kVp is advanced, details in the jaws, pars petrosae, and superior portions of the cranial vault begin to appear. At 90 and 100 kVp, all structures are thoroughly penetrated and all radiographic details are visible. In comparing the 50-kVp and the 100-kVp radiographs, a clear difference in "brightness" in the image is manifest. The lower kVp image attracts the eye at once because of its brilliance. Yet, many details of the anatomy are absent. At 100 kVp, there is a more uniform distribution of densities over the entire image. This radiograph appears less "bright," but upon close examination an abundance of details within the anatomy are apparent. This is essential for diagnostic purposes. The 50-kVp radiograph represents short gray scale, the 100-kVp image possesses long gray scale. The former is to be avoided and the latter attained.

Demonstration No. 2

The chest is a unique area of the body to radiograph, in that the air contained within the lungs is a gas with such low physical density that very few scatter-producing interactions occur. This effect is so substantial that chest radiographs of *small and average patients* may be considered to be virtually scatter-free. In this demonstration, radiographs were taken of a real patient of average thickness (22 cm). Four exposures were made at 50, 60, 80, and 100 kVp respectively (Fig. 6-4). Adjustments were made in mAs to maintain the density of the right upper lobe of the lung. (The respective mAs values were 20, 8.33, 3.33, and 1.66.) With each successive rise in kilovoltage, details of heavier and more dense tissue structures, especially notable in the mediastinum, gradually made their appearance, indicating gradual penetration by the shorter wavelength x-rays.

These radiographs were taken with no grid. The 80-kVp radiograph demonstrates all essential thoracic detail. At 100 kVp, without a grid, gray scale actually becomes somewhat excessive and the distinction between some of the vessels around the heart becomes lessened against the background of the lung field. Note that the 50-kVp radiograph with its very short scale has the least presentation of diagnostic information and anatomical details. As kilovoltage increases, gray scale is lengthened and more densities become visible—up to a certain point. Above this level, gray scale can become too long, and the necessary contrast to distinguish between adjacent densities is lost.

INFLUENCE OF SCATTER FOG

As explained in Chapter 4, a higher-energy x-ray beam results in a drastic loss of photoelectric interactions, leaving high *proportions* of Compton interactions, which result in scattered x-rays. Although Thompson interactions also emit x-rays in random directions, Compton interactions account for over 99 percent of all scattered x-rays reaching the film. Any radiation emitted as a result of interactions within the patient's body is considered as *secondary* radiation. Not all secondary radiation is significantly scattered. A small amount may be emitted in very nearly the direction of the original x-ray which caused the interaction and therefore will still be carrying an image.

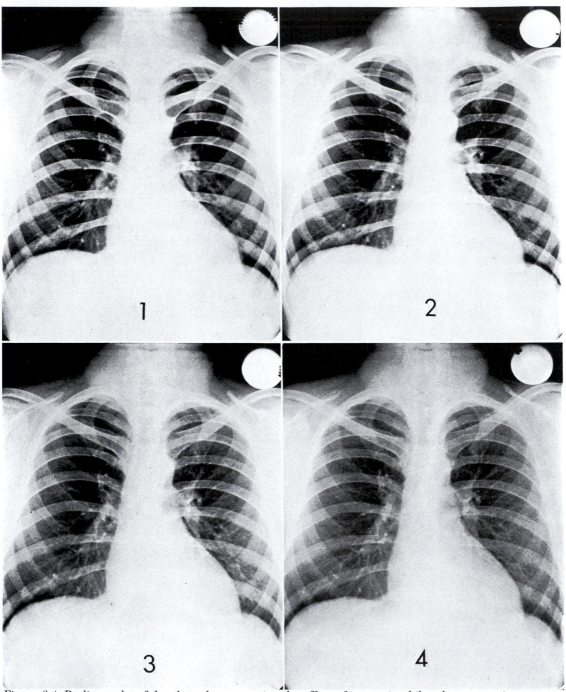

Figure 6-4. Radiographs of the chest demonstrating the effect of increasing kilovoltage upon image contrast and gray scale. Radiograph No. 1 was taken at 50 kVp, No. 2 at 60 kVp, No. 3 at 80 kVp, and No. 4 at 100 kVp.

An image cannot exist without *subject contrast*, the difference in radiation intensity between two areas within the remnant beam exiting the patient. The area under a bone, for example, would have much less intensity left than the area under soft tissues, since the bone attenuates more of the original beam. It may, therefore, be said that the remnant beam *carries* an image or a *signal*. The subject contrast carried by the remnant beam is directly responsible for the image contrast on the finished radiograph. Most of the secondary radiation resulting from Compton interactions is scattered in random directions. Subject contrast can only exist in the remnant beam while the x-rays are travelling in straight lines. When scattered rays cross over from one area into another within the remnant beam, these rays no longer carry organized image information, but only cause an overall blackening of the film, a general increase in image density (Fig. 6-5). Scattered radiation cannot carry the contrast differences required for an image to exist.

Fog as Noise

Since scatter radiation cannot carry any useful signal, it contributes nothing of value to the radiographic image. It can only be destructive, veiling over the useful image with a nebulous layer of density called *fog*. This fog obscures image details, reducing their visibility.

Any useless density recorded on an image which obscures the desired image is considered a form of *noise*. A certain degree of noise is present in any image. The visibility of the image is enhanced by keeping this noise level low in proportion to the useful signal. It should be recalled that in radiography, the useful signal is produced primarily by the occurrence of photoelectric interactions within the patient, which result in subject contrast in the remnant x-ray beam. At high levels of kVp, these photoelectric interactions are rapidly lost, while much of the scatter interactions remain. This remaining noise then comprises a much larger *proportion* of the total information reaching the film. The fogging effect of the scatter radiation becomes visible in the image.

In addition to these differences in the proportions of interactions, two other effects of high-beam energy levels upon scatter radiation must be remembered: First, at higher kVp levels the scattered radiation produced will also have higher ener-

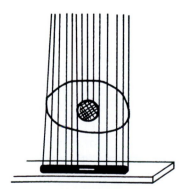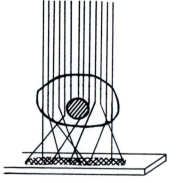

Figure 6-5. Diagram showing how subject contrast is lost in the remnant beam by scattered x-rays randomly crossing over image boundaries and fogging the film.

gies, making it more likely to penetrate out of the body and reach the film. Second, the higher the energy of the scattered radiation, the more it tends to be emitted in a forward direction, rather than backward or sideways, so that more of it actually strikes the film. Together, these two effects more than compensate for the slight reduction in Compton interactions that are actually occurring within the patient, graphed in Figure 4-6. *The result is that the **net** amount of scatter radiation reaching the image receptor or film is gradually increased at higher energy levels.*

To summarize, at higher kVp's, even though fewer Compton interactions are actually occurring within the patient, a higher *percentage* or *proportion* of those that are produced penetrate out of the patient in a more forward direction and strike the film. The *net* result is that *more fog is produced in the image.*

High kVp techniques, then, result in low contrast images for three important reasons:

1. Increased penetration of the primary beam through various tissues lengthens the image gray scale.

2. Photoelectric interactions are rapidly lost, leaving a high Compton-to-photoelectric ratio: In the image, "white" densities are lost, leaving fog more apparent in the image.

3. Scatter radiation produced by the Compton interaction is both more energetic and scatters in a more forward direction, so that an increased amount of scatter *reaching the film* produces more fog in the image.

Fog darkens the relatively light areas of the image, while those areas which are already pitch black cannot become visibly any darker. The diffuse exposure of all of the various areas of the image to fog results in less difference between these densities. Contrast is reduced.

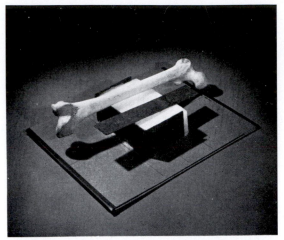

Figure 6-6. Photograph of paraffin emitter and associated objects used to illustrate the influence of kilovoltage on the production of scatter radiation in Figure 6-7.

Increased scatter radiation reaching the film constitutes a second mechanism by which image contrast is reduced when higher kVp's are employed. The first mechanism, increased penetration and gray scale, is considered generally desirable. The second, scatter fogging, is never desirable. The task of the radiographer is achieve good penetration and gray scale while controlling the effects of this scatter. Other means, such as the use of grids, provide this control over scatter radiation and make it possible to use high kVp levels on large body parts.

Demonstration

The influence of kilovoltage on the proportion of scatter radiation and its fogging effect on the image is illustrated by a series of radiographs shown in Figure 6-7. The arrangement of a paraffin block to be used as the emitter of scatter radiation, a dried femur, a slab of 1/8-inch lead and a lead sheet barrier is shown in Figure 6-6. The dried femur and lead produce such small quantities of scatter radiation that neither can be considered an effective emitter. A sheet of 1/8-inch lead when wrapped around the emitter on three sides serves as a barrier to the scatter radiation that would reach the film on one side of the exposure. Radiographs A-D in Figure 6-7 were made with the bone and lead sheet placed on *top* of the paraffin scatter emitter, thereby creating a 2.5-inch OID for these objects. The lead strip and femur were permitted to project over the lead barrier on both sides of the paraffin block as shown in Figure 6-7. These radiographs were made with a constant mAs of 40. The kVp employed for radiograph A was 40; B, 60; C, 80; and D, 100.

Note in Figure 6-7 that as kVp increases and all other factors remain constant: (1) radiographic density and fog increase in the presence of an emitter of scatter radiation, and (2) full penetration through the bone itself is effected at 60 kVp. In each radiograph, there are six numbered areas that should be observed as the kVp is increased:

Area 1 is that portion of the image of the femur that is covered by the image of the paraffin scatter emitter. As the kVp increases, the density of this area increases. It is affected by both the increasing penetration of the radiation *and* by the increasing scatter radiation emitted by the paraffin block. The ease with which details are visualized in this area is greatly diminished in the 100-kVp film (D) due to scatter radiation. (Note that there are virtually no details present in the 40-kVp image (A) due to insufficient penetration.)

Area 2 is that portion of the image of the femur that projects over and *beyond* the lead barrier. Since the lead prevents scatter radiation from affecting this portion of the image, the increased density is solely due to the increase penetration achieved at a higher kVp. As with *Area 1*, this portion was not penetrated at the low 40 kVp setting (A). At 100 kVp (D) *Area 2* is not fogged, yet it is *overexposed* by the amount of remnant radiation reaching the film to the point where details in the inner bone marrow are too dark and lost to the image.

Area 3 is that portion of the image of the lead strip covered by the image of the paraffin scatter emitter. Because the object-film distance is 2.5 inches, scatter radiation undercuts the lead strip and this area of the image becomes fogged. One can readily see the graduated increase in fog as the kilovoltage is increased in increments. Because the lead strip is not penetrated by the primary beam, the silver deposits in this image area may be entirely attributed to exposure by secondary scatter radiation.

Area 4 is that portion of the image of the lead strip that extends beyond the lead barrier. No appreciable change in density occurs in this image area because no primary radiation penetrates through the lead and no scatter radiation penetrates from the paraffin block through the lead barrier.

Area 5 that *unshielded* portion of the femur to the side of the scatter emitter. Details in the femur nearest the emitter become somewhat fogged, but this effect diminishes as the bone becomes more remote from the paraffin block. Here, the inverse square law is demonstrated to apply to scatter radiation, as the fog diminishes away from the source of scatter radiation.

Area 6 is that portion of the image representing the lead strip that projects over and beyond the unshielded side of the emitter. The diminution of fog by undercutting as the strip becomes more remote is shown. The condition is similar to that in *Area 5* except that details are not present in the image area.

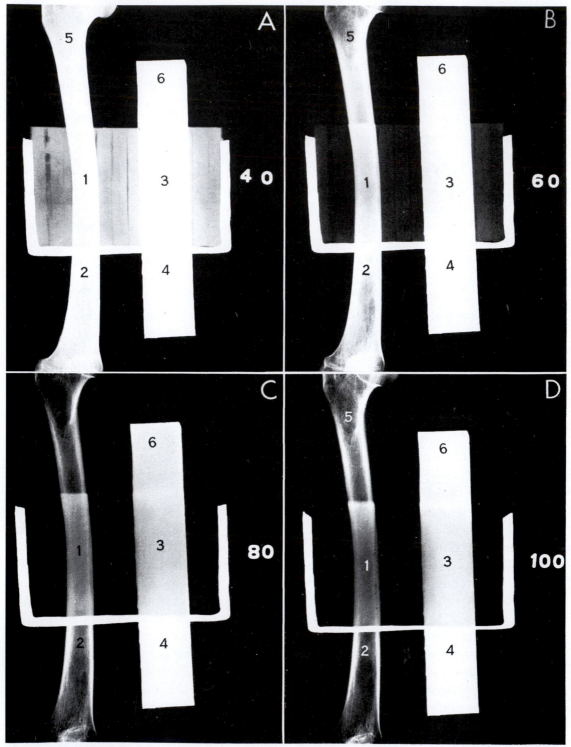

Figure 6-7. Radiographs of paraffin emitter and associated objects. Kilovoltages are noted on each radiograph. Note the presence of scatter fog (from the paraffin) in areas 1 and 3 at high kVp levels.

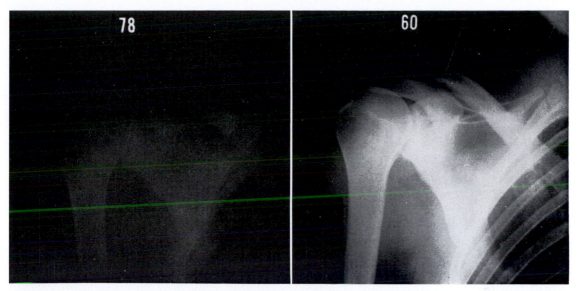

Figure 6-8. Non-grid radiographs of the shoulder showing effect of kVp overexposure. Kilovoltage used is noted on each radiograph. Note the fog on the 78 kVp image.

OVEREXPOSURE BY KILOVOLTAGE

The real function of beam penetration, controlled by kVp, is to leave a sufficient intensity of x-rays in the remnant beam to expose the film and thus produce an image. It is possible to extend the penetration capacity of the beam to such an extreme level that a great majority of the x-rays penetrate through every type of tissue in the patient. For example, the use of 120 kVp for any procedure other than chest radiography or barium studies will result in an overexposed image. At this high level, even the bones are unable to attenuate more than a few of the x-rays. With excessive amounts of x-rays exposing the film, light areas in the image will turn dark gray, while pitch-black areas will remain pitch-black (having used up all of the silver available in the film). Radiographic contrast will be lost, as the image will have no more light areas present. This is demonstrated in Figure 6-8.

CONTROL OF DENSITY

The single most essential quality of the x-ray beam is its *penetration*, the ability to pass through an object and reach the image receptor to expose it. Without penetration, there can be no production of densities on the film. Penetration is the opposite of attenuation. Seventy-five to 80 percent of the typical diagnostic x-ray beam is attenuated within the patient, so the average remnant beam has about 20 percent of the intensity of the original primary beam. It may be said that the penetration of the typical x-ray beam is about 20 percent or 1/5. Penetration is characteristic of the energy level or quality of the x-ray beam and is therefore controlled by kVp. The higher the kVp, the higher the penetration of the beam.

Greater penetration through an object results in higher intensity levels of the radiation reaching the film, which increases film exposure and image density. Although kVp is a controlling factor for image contrast, it will also affect image density each time it is altered. This consideration must be kept in mind each time the radiographer manipulates electrical technique factors.

Since x-ray energies are inversely related to their wavelengths, it may also be said that x-ray wavelength controls penetration, affecting film exposure and image density.

Long Wavelength, Low kVp Exposure

Reference to Figure 6-9 will serve to explain theoretically the penetration and absorption of x-rays. In diagram *A*, a low kVp is employed, producing long wavelength x-rays. These long wavelength rays are shown to penetrate various distances within the object, but none emerge to expose the film. In reality one or two of these would make it through to the film, but this number would be so small that no satisfactory density will be produced in the image regardless of the extent of the exposure time used; This is demonstrated in the accompanying radiograph *E*. Figure *B* shows that when the *number* of long wavelength x-rays produced is increased by using more mAs, these are also absorbed and still fail to reach the image receptor. The accompanying radiograph *F* was made employing the same kilovoltage and wavelength as in *A*, but with a very long exposure time and a resulting higher mAs. A satisfactory image is still not obtained. Even though the background density shows the effect of the increased exposure, the long wavelengths of these x-rays are insufficient to penetrate the bones and thicker portions of the hand. Except in the very thinnest anatomical areas, the tips of the fingers, there is not appreciable gain in image details.

Short Wavelength Exposure

Figure 6-9 goes on to show that when the wavelength is shortened by increasing kVp, as in *C*, even though low mAs is used and few x-rays directed toward the object, penetration through the object easily takes place. The emergent remnant radiation is sufficient to produce radiographic density in the image. In the accompanying radiograph *G*, note that there are some details visible in various portions of the bones of the hand, yet in those *thicker* portions of the hand, the weak densities produced indicate an insufficient *quantity* of exposure. The radiation may now be considered *qualitatively* correct and penetration of the hand is attained, yet the *number* of x-rays reaching the image receptor is still too small to produce a completely satisfactory image. With the same kilovoltage and an increase in mAs, shown in *D*, a satisfactory image showing details throughout the bones of the hand is attained in the accompanying radiograph *H*.

Demonstration No. 1

A series of four PA radiographs of the hand were made employing kVP increases in increments of 10. All other factors were maintained equal and mAs was not changed. As shown in Figure 6-10, the overall density of each image increases with the kVp. The darker images are obtained due to the greater tissue penetration that is coincident with shorter wavelengths of radiation. In this range, the density of each image has roughly doubled from the previous one due to a 10-kVp increase.

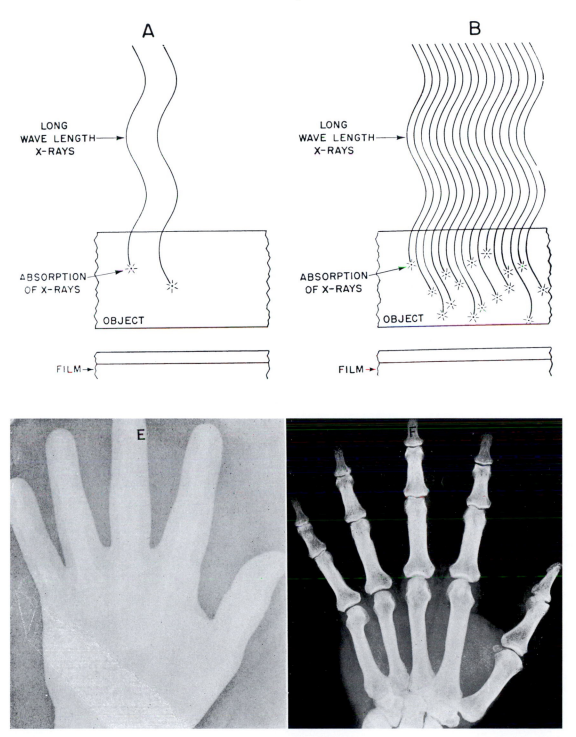

Figure 6-9. Illustrations of the relationship between beam penetration and radiographic density. (A) and (B) effects of long wave length (low energy) radiation, (C) and (D) effects of short wave length (high energy) radiation. Radiographs of the hand (E) through (H) that simulate the theoretical conditions shown above.

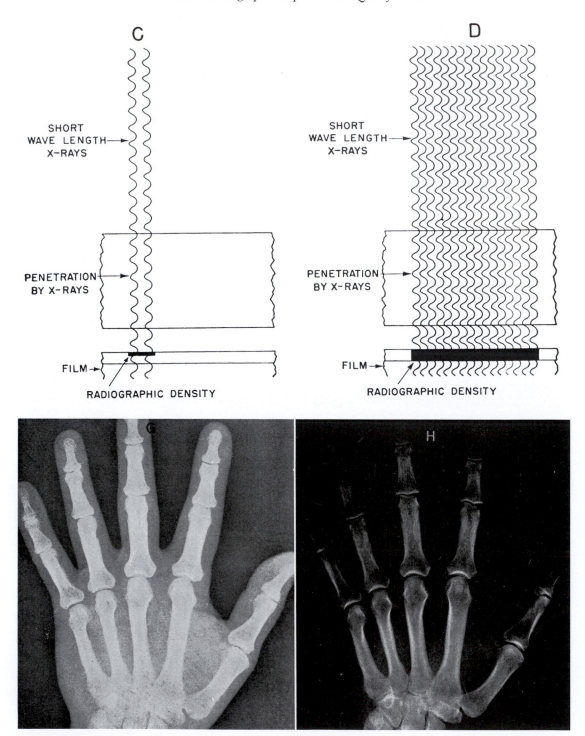

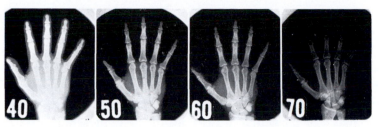

Figure 6-10. Demonstration of kVp-density relation. Kilovoltages are noted on each radiograph. Note the dramatic change in density caused by a 10 kVp adjustment.

Demonstration No. 2

In medical radiography it can also be shown in a series of PA chest radiographs, Figure 6-11, that as the kilovoltage advances, radiograph density and gray scale increase. For this series of radiographs, the kVp was increased in increments of 10, with a range of 60 to 100 kVp, all other factors being kept constant. No grid was used, so that any scatter fogging might become apparent. Since the lungs are full of air, very little scatter fog is produced. The increasing gray scale can thus be attributed primarily to enhanced penetration. However, at 100 kVp, overexposure occurs, and scatter fogging becomes apparent. The ideal kilovoltage in this particular case would be 90 kVp.

SUFFICIENT PENETRATION

X-ray film requires a certain minimum exposure in order for the silver crystals to be developed into black metallic silver deposits and produce image density. It

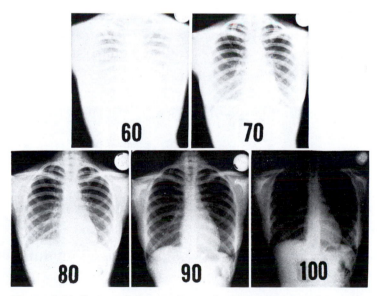

Figure 6-11. Series of chest radiographs demonstrating that as the kilovoltage advances and all other factors are constant, density increases dramatically. Kilovoltages used are noted.

actually takes several x-ray photons, not just one, to sensitize a silver crystal enough that it will be successfully developed into black metallic silver during processing. Suppose that the kVp set results in 10 percent penetration through the patient. Suppose further that the particular x-ray film being used requires at least 200 photons striking each square millimeter of the emulsion in order to develop a visible density there. If a setting of 100 mAs were to result in 10 photons striking each square millimeter, then an increase to 200 mAs would produce 20 photons striking the same area; at 500 mAs there would be 50; at 1000 mAs (about the limit of most x-ray equipment), there would still be only about 100 photons striking each square millimeter. Since this film requires 200 to produce a visible density, this level of exposure will still be insufficient. When penetration is insufficient, it cannot be realistically compensated for by more intensity. For practical purposes, no amount of output from the x-ray tube will ever compensate when there is inadequate energy in the x-ray beam. From a technique standpoint, this means that *no amount of mAs will ever compensate for insufficient kVp.*

Excessive mAs values are dangerous to the patient and are never justified in medical radiography. All general medical radiography can be adequately performed within the range of 50 to 120 kVp. It is well to remember that when a kilovoltage is to be assigned to a given projection, one must think of it in relation to *tissue penetration,* and whether the radiation will penetrate the part and provide remnant radiation of a quality and quantity that will produce a satisfactory image. The following example illustrates the futility of employing inadequate kilovoltage.

Demonstration No. 1

A series of direct exposure PA radiographs of the hand were made to determine the mAs value that would produce a translucent image of all structures in the hand (Fig. 6-12). The kilovoltage employed was 30 kVp. The first radiograph was made using 45 mAs, and for each succeeding exposure, the mAs was doubled in an attempt to produce a dark enough image density. Even in radiograph *E* with a final mAs value of 720, the image is still unsatisfactory: Note that still no details are visible within the bones of the hand. The lack of penetrating power renders the remnant

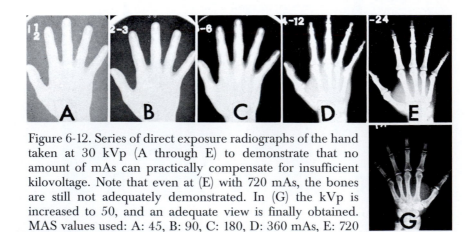

Figure 6-12. Series of direct exposure radiographs of the hand taken at 30 kVp (A through E) to demonstrate that no amount of mAs can practically compensate for insufficient kilovoltage. Note that even at (E) with 720 mAs, the bones are still not adequately demonstrated. In (G) the kVp is increased to 50, and an adequate view is finally obtained. MAS values used: A: 45, B: 90, C: 180, D: 360 mAs, E: 720 mAs, (G) was taken at 50 kVp and 50 mAs.

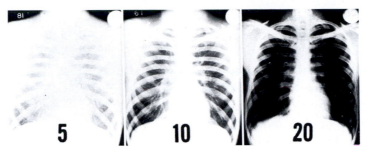

Figure 6-13. Screen exposures of the chest taken at an insufficient 50 kVp. Respective mAs values are shown on each radiograph. Note that after two doublings of the mAs, the heart and mediastinum are still not penetrated.

beam insufficient, no matter how much the mAs is increased, making the objective entirely hopeless.

For comparison, radiograph *G* was taken exposing the same hand with 50 kVp and 50 mAs, and a diagnostic image was obtained at this kilovoltage level. This radiograph provides an image in which *all* of the densities are translucent and details throughout the entire image were clearly recorded, when a relatively short exposure time was employed. The excessive mAs values used in *C* through *E* represent excessive and unnecessary exposure to the patient, which becomes a critical issue in other body areas where more sensitive organs would be exposed. The key to avoiding this type of malpractice is to always ensure sufficient kVp for full penetration.

Demonstration No. 2

A second example of this principle is demonstrated in Figure 6-13, where only 50 kVp was employed on a chest radiograph. It should be recalled that chest radiography is largely performed for examination of the heart size and condition, not only for the lung fields. Adequate penetration on a chest radiograph is determined by the rule of thumb that some details of the spine should be visible through the heart tissue. In this example, 50 kVp was insufficient to penetrate the heart tissue, even after the mAs was doubled twice. Note that although the lung areas are shown somewhat upon the first doubling of the mAs, and were completely overexposed upon the second redoubling, the heart area is still underpenetrated and inadequate for diagnosis.

OPTIMUM kVp

A certain optimum kVp is required to expose the x-ray film properly. As discussed in the first chapter, whether a given photon with a certain energy level will be attenuated or not by an atom depends upon the atomic number of the atom, i.e., how many electrons it has. The penetration level required for an x-ray beam to make it through a particular body part is determined by the *proportions* of the various atomic numbers present in the tissues that make up that body part. When exposing a lateral lumbar spine, for example, roughly 90 percent of the tissue being penetrated is soft tissue, with an atomic number averaging about that of water, and only 10 percent is bone. But, when exposing a lateral projection of the lumbosacral joint at L5-S1, the overlying iliac bones of the pelvis are added to the sacrum and spine so that roughly 20 percent of the tissue being penetrated is now bone, and only 80 percent soft tissue. With a higher *ratio* of bone, which has a much higher atomic number than soft tissue, increased penetration is needed.

Similarly, filling the stomach with barium causes as much as 25-50 percent of the substance being penetrated by the x-ray beam to have the atomic number of barium. Thus, the average atomic number of the abdomen in that area is increased. In such procedures, the tissue of interest (the bone or the barium) must be penetrated by the x-ray beam so that the radiologist can see *through* it to the other side of the organ. If it is not penetrated, the image will be blank white where the barium or bone is, and the only information the radiologist can discern is the information at the *edges* of the organ, only about 10 percent of the information he needs to see. It is like looking at a silhouette of the organ, where you cannot discern anything within the shadow, but only the edges. Figure 6-14 demonstrates this "silhouette" condition in an image of the barium-filled stomach. Adequate kVp is essential to the visibility of information in the image.

Once sufficient penetration of the body part is achieved such that image gray scale is lengthened to that level at which maximum details are visible in the image, further increases in kVp result only in unnecessary scatter radiation being produced. This slightly fogs the image, with no further gain in other image qualities. So, rather than striving for *maximum* or *minimum* kVp, the ideal practice is to find the *optimum* kVp level for each body part. Optimum kVp may be defined as the min-

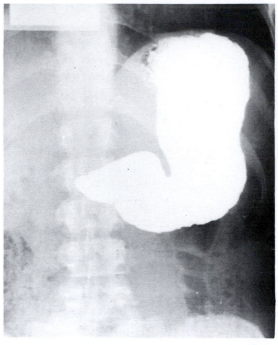

Figure 6-14. Radiograph of barium-filled stomach taken with 80 kVp. Note that with inadequate penetration through the barium, the only details visible in the stomach are those at the very edge of the barium bolus. Such a silhouette image is of little diagnostic value.

imum kVp which still provides fully adequate penetration of the body part and sufficient gray scale.

Optimum kVp does *not* vary from machine to machine, between different machine phases, different image receptor systems, or even different sizes of patients. It is based primarily upon the relative proportions of the types of tissues that are normally present in the particular body part, with average part thickness being a secondary consideration. As in the example previously mentioned, a male patient may measure precisely the same thickness for a lateral lumbar spine projection and for a lateral projection of the lumbosacral joint at L5-S1; yet, kVp must be substantially increased for the lateral lumbosacaral joint when compared to the lateral L-spine.

(Most radiographers increase by 10 kVp between these two views.) This is because of the higher *ratio* of bone within the pelvic area when compared to the waist.

Optimum kVp is determined by the *tissue composition* of the body part as much as by its thickness. Accordingly, when iodine or barium contrast agents are introduced into the body, this tissue composition has been changed; the optimum kVp is determined by the characteristics of that iodine or barium in absorbing x-rays rather than the simple thickness of the body part being examined. Most authors place the optimum kVp for penetrating iodine-based contrast agents in the range of 70-76 kVp. For solid-column barium studies in the abdomen, the convention is to use 116-120 kVp. For air contrast/barium studies and for barium coating within the esophagus, most radiographers use 90-94 kVp. Table 6-1 is a listing of optimum kVp's commonly used, and should be committed to memory, as it will apply to most situations.

Table 6-1

OPTIMUM KVP FOR
DIFFERENT PROCEDURES

Procedure	Optimum kVp
Hand/Wrist	54
Elbow/ Foot	60-62
Ankle	64
Knee	70
Femur/Shoulder/Sinus/Ribs	74-76
Cervical/Thoracic Spine (all views)	74-76
General Torso Anatomy (Pelvis, Abdomen, Lumbar Spine)	76-80
All Iodine Procedures (IVP, cystogram, etc.)	70-76
Non-Grid Chest	80
Air Contrast/Barium Studies	90-94
Esophagram	90
Solid-Column Barium Studies	116-120
Grid Chest	110-120

*NOTE: Unlisted procedures may be extrapolated with fair accuracy by splitting the difference between the two adjacent anatomical parts listed. For example, the humerus would be half-way between the elbow and the shoulder, yielding about 66kVp. Tangential or partial types of skull procedures, such as the mandible, would be about equal to the cervical spine at 70 kVp. Most techniques ever needed can be derived from this basic list.

THE 15 PERCENT RULE

The relationship between kVp and image density is not a linear, proportionate one. Some radiographic physics textbooks present a formula relating kVp to x-ray tube output, which states that the intensity of x-rays emitted from the tube is proportional to the *square* of the kVp. In other words, the relationship is an *exponential* one rather than a linear one. Even so, this formula applies only to intensity of *primary* radiation emitted at the x-ray tube, *not the end result density at the film.* To determine this final result, one must also take into account the effects of *increased penetration,* and the condition and intensity of the *remnant* beam after attenuating interactions in the body has taken place. This is an entirely different question than the initial beam output at the x-ray tube.

In practice, the radiographer needs a rule of thumb relating changes in the kVp setting to the end result in image density. Objective experience has provided enough empirical evidence to establish a very simple rule of thumb for this purpose: *The 15 percent rule.* While not perfectly accurate from a mathematical standpoint, the 15 percent rule is very workable in practice, and provides an easily remembered formula that can be readily applied to most situations for diagnostic radiography.

The 15 percent rule states that: *A 15 percent change in kVp will result in a change in image density by a factor of 2.* If kVp is increased 15 percent, the radiographic density will roughly double. If it is decreased by 15 percent, the image density will be roughly cut to one-half the original. Students should memorize and practice applying this rule in all of the various ranges of kVp, because it is of eminent use and value in daily practice.

The 15 percent rule works for *two* reasons: As described at the beginning of this chapter, an increase in kVp results in *both* higher radiation output and higher beam energy. With a higher average energy in the x-ray beam, a much greater percentage of x-rays incident upon the body make it through to the film. When this effect is added to the increase in the original beam intensity from the tube, the *total amount of remnant radiation* reaching the film is increased by nearly 2 times, or 100 percent. The resulting image density will be twice as dark.

There is a physics formula which approximates the 15 percent rule for density. It is

$$\frac{(kVp_2)^4}{(kVp_1)^4} = \frac{D_2}{D_1}$$

Rephrased in common English, this formula states that the density will change according to the fourth power of the kVp change. In effect, it is the 15 percent rule stated algebraically, and it results in similar answers. In daily practice, however, radiographers need a rule of thumb that can be quickly calculated *mentally.* The 15 percent rule is perfectly adaptable for this purpose.

Students and technologists often hear the phrase, "go up or down 10 kVp." While the approach is functional in many situations for doubling image density or cutting it to one-half, it is not as accurate an approach as the proper calculation using a *percentage* change applied to the initial kVp. In fact, the saying originates from the fact that the average kVp for all the various diagnostic procedures turns out to be about 70 kVp, and 15 percent of 70 is 10.5. One must beware particularly of very high and very low kVp ranges if the "10 kVp" notion is used; take, for example, a chest radiograph taken at 100 kVp: A 10-kVp increase in this range will not be nearly adequate to double image density—the proper adjustment would be 15 percent of 100, or 15 kVp. On the other hand, in the range of 40-50 kVp, only a 6 kVp adjustment is required to double image density.

To find 15 percent of any number mentally, simply take 10 percent of it and then add one-half that much again. Thus, 15 percent of 80 would be 8 plus one-half of 8 for a total of 12 kVp. In the range of 80-90 kVp, a 12-kVp change is required to cause a doubling effect on the image. Examine the three pairs of techniques presented in Table 6-2. Using the 15 percent rule, you should be able to surmise that each of these pairs consists of two roughly equivalent techniques in terms of the radiographic density that will be produced.

It is also important to remember, in solving density problems, that the 15 percent rule must be applied *in steps* for accuracy. For example, suppose it is desired to cut the mAs to 1/4 the original value and maintain density by adjusting kVp. First, one should think in terms of doubling or halving the mAs in steps. This way, 1/4 the original mAs represents two steps of cutting in half. To compensate, the kVp must be changed in such a way as to effectively double the image density two times, or in two steps. To do this, one cannot simply

Table 6-2
EQUIVALENT TOTAL TECHNIQUES

The 15 percent rule applied, each of the pairs of techniques below consists of two equivalent techniques in terms of the density that will be produced on the finished film.

A	B	C
60 mAs at 40 kVp	25 mAs at 92 kVp	15 mAs at 110 kVp
30 mAs at 46 kVp	50 mAs at 80 kVp	7 mAs at 126 kVp

double the 15 percent rule and add 30 percent of the original kVp; rather, one step of 15 percent must be applied, and then an additional 15 percent added *to that result*: If the original kVp were 80, first add 15 percent of 80 = 12 to get 92 kVp, then calculate 15 percent *of 92* which is about 14, and add that to 92 for a total of 106 kVp. The 15 percent rule is very helpful indeed if one learns to always think in terms of steps of doubling or halving the density.

Demonstration

The series of radiographs of the PA chest in Figure 6-15 demonstrate a typical exam-

ple of the 15 percent rule applied. Radiographs *A-C* were made with 80 kVp, 92 kVp and 106 kVp, respectively with only slight reductions in mAs, resulting in the expected darker overall densities. Radiographs *D-F* were made with the very same kVp values, representing an increase of 15 percent each time, but the mAs values were cut to one-half each time *(D = 6.66 mAs, E = 3.3 mAs, and F = 1.7 mAs)*. When the 15 percent kVp increases were compensated with changes in mAs by a factor of 2, halving the mAs each time, the overexposures seen in *A-C* were precisely corrected and the overall density is seen to be clearly maintained close to the original. By using

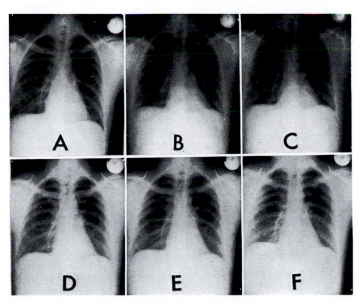

Figure 6-15. Series of screen radiographs of the PA chest showing examples of the effects of overexposure (A-C) and correct exposure (D-F) when using the 15 percent rule.

this rule of thumb, more consistency in producing desirable images may be attained.

APPLYING THE 15 PERCENT RULE

The ability to make 15 percent adjustments mentally should be second-nature to the radiographer. It is not very difficult to develop this ability, but it does require some practice. To find 15 percent mentally, think of the operation as taking 10 percent first, then adding half as much again. For example, to find 15 percent of 60 kVp:

> 10% of 60 = 6
> 1/2 of 6 = 3
> 6 + 3 = 9
> *Solution:* 15% of 60 kVp is 9 kVp

This number is added to the original kVp in order to double the image density, it is subtracted in order to obtain one-half of the original image density. In the above example, using 60 kVp as a starting point, what new total kVp would result in twice as dark an image? The answer is 69 kVp. This is also the answer to the question, what new kVp would *compensate* for cutting the mAs value in half? Suppose that using 60 kVp a radiograph turned out twice too dark. It is desired to reduce this density to one-half the original, using kVp. What should be the new total kVp? The answer is 60 - 9 = 51 kVp.

> 15% of 80 kVp would be 8 + 4 = 12.
> 15% of 120 kVp would be 12 + 6 = 18.

You should also become comfortable applying the 15 percent rule both in sequential steps and in portions, as follows.

Applying the Rule in Steps

Sometimes the desired adjustment in image density is much greater than a dou-

bling or halving. Suppose a radiograph has turned out extremely light due to under-penetration, and the density needs to be increased four-fold. Always translate the desired changes into terms of doublings or halvings (factors of two), and you can apply the rule. To produce an image four times darker, think of this change as two doublings. To obtain two doublings, increase the kVp by 15 percent *in two steps.*

A practical example can be found by comparing a routine abdomen technique to a solid column (not air contrast) barium technique, such as for a barium enema or upper GI series. A typical technique for an AP projection of the abdomen might be approximately 20 mAs at 80 kVp. The following calculation allows adequate penetration of the barium-filled stomach while maintaining overall image density:

20 mAs at 80 kV	Routine AP Abdomen
10 mAs at 92 kVp	First step increase of 15% in kVp, (12 kVp) accompanied by halving the mAs to maintain the original density
5 mAs at 106 kVp	Second step increase of 15% in kVp, (14 kVp) accompanied by another halving of the mAs

This technique of 106 kVp at about 5 mAs is a practical technique for a solid column barium procedure, providing good penetration through the barium. (For an air contrast procedure with barium, simply reduce 10 to 15 kVp, but this time leaving the mAs at 5, for a result of 5 mAs at about 90 kVp.)

Applying the Rule in Portions

Suppose that it is desired to increase the density only by $1\frac{1}{2}$ times the original, that is, half-way to doubling. Since a 15 percent increase in kVp will double the density, one-half of 15 percent should bring the density up to this level. In other words, to increase the density 50 percent, increase the kVp by one-half of 15 percent. For example, suppose a radiograph taken at 80 kVp comes out too light, but it is estimated that a complete doubling of the technique would be too much. For a 50 percent increase in density:

15% of 80 kVp = 12	Find 15% of the kVp
1/2 of 12 = 6	Take 1/2 of that amount
80 + 6 = 86	Add this number to the original

Solution: 86 kVp will increase the image density by about 50%

In reducing technique, keep in mind that cutting the density to one-half the original represents a percentage reduction to 50 percent. Suppose that it is desired to reduce the density, but not all the way to one-half. A reduction to 75 percent, or three-fourths, of the original density may be thought of as reducing it *half-way to one-half.* Again, find one-half of 15 percent, but this time the result will be subtracted. In the above example using a starting point of 80 kVp, the answer would be to reduce the kVp by one-half of 15 percent, subtracting 6 kVp from 80. A reduction to 74 kVp will reduce the original density to about three-fourths.

Complete the following exercise applying the 15 percent rule. The later problems will require application of the rule in steps or in portions. After completing it, check your answers in the Appendix. Be sure to do all of these *mentally* to benefit most from the exercise.

EXERCISE #9

1. What is 5 percent of 80?
2. What is 5 percent of 50?
3. What is 15 percent of 70?
4. What is 15 percent of 110?
5. What is *one-half* of 15 percent of 80?
6. What is *one-half* of 15 percent of 120?
7. Staring at 120 kVp, what new kVp would result in a density one-half as dark as the original?
8. Staring at 60 kVp, what new kVp would result in a density 50% darker than (1½ times) the original?
9. Staring at 80 kVp, what new kVp would result in a density 1/4 as dark as the original?

In the following problems, fill in the kVp that would maintain *equal* density upon changing from the original technique, listed first:

10. 400 mA 1/20 sec. 90 kVp
    300 mA 1/60 sec. ___ kVp
11. 50 mA 1/60 sec. 50 kVp
    400 mA 1/120 sec. ___kVp
12. 300 mA 1/30 sec. 120 kVp
    400 mA 1/10 sec. ___ kVp
13. 300 mA 1/20 sec. 70 kVp
    150 mA 3/20 sec. ___ kVp

The 15 percent rule for kVp is useful not only for practical adjustments on a daily basis but for the development of accurate technique charts as well. Table 6-3 was developed using the 15 percent rule to derive mAs conversions to compensate for changes in kVp across the diagnostic ranges.

By the use of mAs multiplying factors, approximate mAs values may be obtained for changes in the kVp range of 50 to 100 in increments of five.

Some mAs values derived from this table may require the use of a time value that is not within the practical scope of the timer. It is then necessary to employ the *nearest* practical value. In most instances, these approximations will be so close that the difference is not visibly recognizable. Due to variations in x-ray equipment and generators, no table can be expected to

Table 6-3
mAs MULTIPLYING FACTORS FOR USE WHEN KILOVOLTAGE IS CHANGED (SCREEN EXPOSURES ONLY)

Old kVp	New Kilovoltage mAs Multiplying Factor													Old kVp
40	1.	.4	.23	.15	.11	.08	.064	.05	.04	.032	.025	.02	.017	40
45	2.5	1.	.52	.3	.22	.16	.12	.1	.076	.06	.05	.04	.032	45
50	4.	1.7	1.	.68	.5	.35	.27	.21	.16	.13	.1	.08	.066	50
55	8.	2.5	1.5	1.	.74	.56	.43	.35	.28	.22	.18	.15	.12	55
60	10.	4.	2.3	1.5	1.	.78	.6	.46	.37	.3	.25	.2	.17	60
65	12.	5.	3.	2.	1.4	1.	.8	.62	.5	.4	.32	.26	.21	65
70	16.	7.	4.2	2.6	2.	1.4	1.	.8	.6	.5	.39	.31	.25	70
75	20.	9.	5.4	3.5	2.5	1.8	1.3	1.	.76	.6	.47	.38	.3	75
80	24.	11.	6.6	4.5	3.2	2.3	1.7	1.3	1.	.8	.6	.47	.37	80
85	28.	13.	8.	5.4	4.	2.9	2.2	1.7	1.3	1.	.8	.64	.5	85
90	34.	15.	9.	6.2	4.5	3.4	2.6	2.	1.6	1.25	1.	.8	.64	90
95	48.	18.	11.	7.8	5.6	4.2	3.2	2.5	2.	1.6	1.3	1.	.8	95
100	60.	22.	13.	9.	6.8	5.	3.8	3.	2.4	1.9	1.5	1.2	1.	100
	40	45	50	55	60	65	70	75	80	85	90	95	100	

apply accurately to all situations, but this table can provide a very close guide to an anticipated value.

It is important to remember that when kilovoltage is employed to change radiographic density, radiographic contrast and the quantity of scatter radiation produced also change.

Example: Assume that 55 kVp and 10 mAs were used in obtaining a PA view of the chest. It is desired to penetrate the chest more thoroughly and to lengthen the gray scale so that more structural details can be visualized. A new kVp of 80 is selected for this purpose. What mAs value should be employed at this new kVp to maintain overall image density? Consulting Table 6-3, locate the original kVp value of 55 in the left-hand column. Pass the finger horizontally across the chart to the column for 80 kVp, indicated at the bottom of the table. The mAs multiplying factor is 0.28. Multiply the original mAs of 10 by 0.28. The new compensated mAs should be set at 2.8.

Demonstration

A series of radiographs of the PA chest with a range of 40 to 100 kVp as shown in Figure 6-16. The mAs was adjusted to compensate for the increasing kVp with the assistance of Table 6-3. Using the upper right pulmonary area as a guide, the overall densities of this series are seen to be maintained relatively equal.

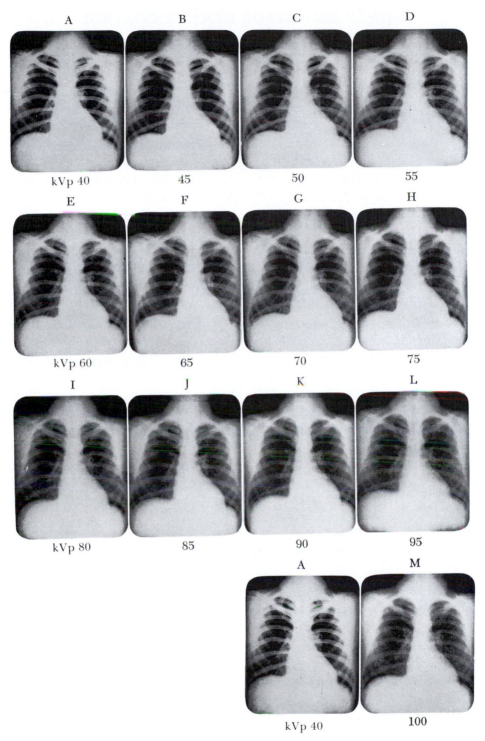

Figure 6-16. Series of screen radiographs of the chest in which the mAs was decreased, using the 15 percent rule, in compensation for increasing kVp. The kilovoltages are shown under the radiographs. Note that the gray scale becomes longer with higher kVp, but the overall density is maintained. MAS factors used: A: 70, B: 40, C: 20, D: 10, E: 8.3, F: 6.3, G: 5, H: 4.12, I: 3.3, J: 2.15, K: 2, L: 1.6, M: 1.6.

Kvp VERSUS mAs FOR DENSITY CONTROL

In the previous chapter, it was learned that excessive amounts of mAs will overexpose the x-ray film, and that overexposure is not the same thing as fogging the film with scatter radiation. When excessive levels of kVp are used, fog becomes visible. The film may also be overexposed, because the increase in penetration of the beam through the patient makes the remnant beam more intense, just as if mAs had been increased. Therefore, *excessive kVp levels both overexpose and fog the radiograph, while excessive amounts of mAs merely overexpose it.*

It is generally *not* recommended that kVp be used as a control for radiographic density. Since mAs is directly proportional to density, it is predictable and easy to work with. Furthermore, mAs has no effect upon other image qualities such as contrast. Kilovoltage cannot be changed without affecting *both* density and contrast. The proper use of kVp is in controlling penetration and radiographic contrast. When the proper level of contrast is achieved for the particular body part, then mAs should be used to adjust density for different sizes of patients.

Different optimum kVp levels must be used for procedures involving different anatomy. But, *within a given procedure, it is important that the radiologist be provided with the same type of contrast from one view to the next.* Significant changes in contrast and gray scale between, say, a PA skull and a lateral skull in the same series, can hinder the radiologist's ability to diagnose the patient's condition, because some detail which is visible on the one radiograph may be obscured on the other. There is some flexibility afforded by the fact that it takes a somewhat drastic change in kVp to really cause such an effect. This flexibility is on the order of plus or minus 10 percent. There are also a few clear exceptions to this rule, such as the lateral projection of the L5-S1 "spot," which requires a 10-kVp increase over the lateral projection of the L-spine. Nonetheless, it may be said that generally, *within a given procedural series, kVp should be kept fairly stable while mAs is normally adjusted for different views. This will ensure a set of images which have both proper density and consistent contrast characteristics.*

VISIBLE DENSITY CHANGE

As discussed in Chapter 5, the human eye cannot discern any change in radiographic density of less than about 30 percent. There are occasions when the radiographer may wish to make a density change of this magnitude, 30-40 percent, but the next available exposure time on the timer knob is an increment of 50 or even 67 percent, too much for what is desired. In such a situation, the use of kVp to make this small density adjustment can be justified.

Based upon the 15 percent rule for the kVp density relation, recall that a 15 per-

cent increase in kVp would double the image density, or increase that density by 100 percent. It may be extrapolated, then, that approximately one-third of that kVp change, or a 5 percent increase, would result in a density change one-third of the way to 100 percent, or about a 33 percent increase in density. This closely matches the 30 percent rule of thumb for visible density change. One-third of the 15 percent rule represents a change in kVp of 5 percent. It may be confidently stated, then, that *a 5 percent change in kVp is the minimum change that*

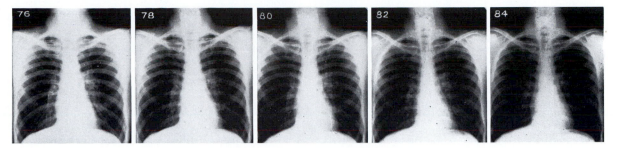

Figure 6-17. Screen exposures of the chest to demonstrate the negligible density effect with small changes in kilovoltage. The respective kVp used for each radiograph is noted.

will lead to a visible difference in the image.

A quick calculation of 5 percent in the various ranges of diagnostic kVp's will reveal that the common practice of changing 2 kVp to control image density is a superstitious practice. Even in the lower ranges of kVp (50 to 80), the 5 percent rule implies that kVp would have to be changed by at least **4** to make a visible change in the image. In ranges above the 80's, a change of at least **6** kVp would be required to make a visible difference.

Demonstration

The above facts may be illustrated by a series of PA views of the chest shown in Figure 6-17. Exposures were made employing a range of 76 to 84 kVp in 2-kVp steps. All other factors were kept constant. Comparison of the densities in the first two radiographs, 76 kVp and 78 kVp, shows no visible difference in the darkness of the images. The same holds true when comparing the 80-kVp radiograph to the 82-kVp image. Some distinction can be made between those images that have a difference in exposure of 4 kVp. A very noticeable difference exists between the 76-kVp and the 84-kVp radiographs. Hence, there is no advantage to be derived by changing kVp in any increment less than 4 in these ranges.

EFFECTS ON OTHER QUALITIES

Note that kVp affects *all* of the *visibility* functions in an image: An increase in kVp causes the density to increase, the noise (in the form of fog) to increase slightly, and the contrast to diminish. Kilovoltage does *not* affect any of the geometrical *recognizability* functions in the image.

Kilovoltage is an electrical factor, just as is mA, and has no bearing upon projection geometry in the x-ray beam. This means kVp cannot possibly have any effect upon the recognizability characteristics of the final image, which are all based upon beam geometry. Sharpness of recorded detail, magnification of the image, and shape distortion are not affected directly by kVp in any way.

EXPOSURE LATITUDE

When a body part is radiographed, the absorption properties of the tissues are largely unpredictable. Naturally, the question arises as to how great an error can be made in the exposure factors without degrading the image to a noticeable degree. The term, "correct exposure" does not imply that there is one single set of exposure factors that will produce the best diagnostic image, but rather that, depending on the kilovoltage used, there is a range of different exposures that can be employed to yield radiographs diagnostically acceptable to the radiologist. This phenomenon is linked to the concept of *exposure latitude.*

Exposure Latitude

Exposure latitude may be defined as the *range* between the minimum and the maximum exposures that will produce an acceptable scale of densities for diagnostic purposes. In other words, it is the *margin for error* in setting a proper technique. As previously demonstrated, the scale of image densities is determined by the kilovoltage

applied. Hence, exposure latitude varies with the kilovoltage employed.

Wide Exposure Latitude

When high kilovoltage values are used, the exposure latitude is wide because long scale is produced in the image which can compensate at times for wide errors in mAs. The large number of densities produced by using more penetrating radiation serves to retain image details even to the extremes of tissue thickness; that is, details in the *thin and thick* portions of the anatomy may be shown.

Example: A demonstration of wide exposure latitude using 80 kVp and an 8:1 grid is shown in Figure 6-18. A series of lateral exposures of a 10-cm knee were made employing mAs values of: (1) 12.5, (2) 25, (3) 37.5, (4) 50, (5) 75, (6) 100, and (7) 125. Radiographs Nos. 1 and 2 may be considered as underexposed. Radiograph No. 7 is overexposed. Radiographs Nos. 3 to 6 may be considered to possess diagnostic densities and the exposure latitude is 37.5 to 100

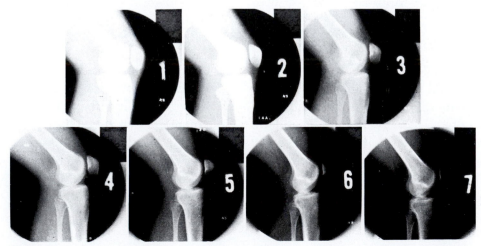

Figure 6-18. Series of lateral views of the knee to demonstrate exposure latitude. The range between 37.5 and 100 mAs (Nos. 3-6) may be considered the exposure latitude in this case.

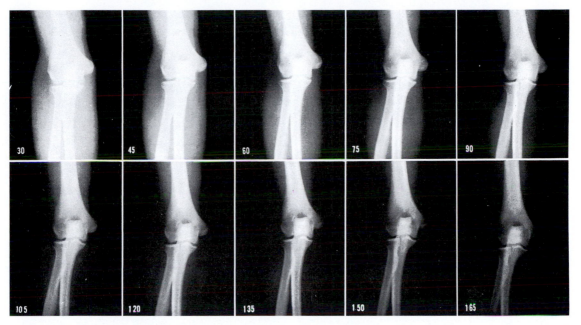

Figure 6-19. Radiographs of the elbow demonstrating exposure latitude. The range between 90 and 135 mAs may be considered the exposure latitude in this case.

mAs. Between these values lies the range of diagnostic exposures, 62.5 mAs in width.

Narrow Exposure Latitude

Exposure latitude is usually narrow when short scale prevails, as produced at lower kilovoltages. The small number of usable densities present in the image requires that the exposure be more nearly correct to obtain densities that are representative of the thinnest or the thickest portions of the part. The gray scale, however, is seldom such that all desired tissues are shown in the same image. Also, the mAs values required are usually so great as to be impractical in application.

Example: In a series of radiographs of the elbow (Fig. 6-19), 60 kVp was considered to be the optimum kilovoltage. The mAs was varied in steps of 15 mAs from 30 to 165. The exposure latitude in this series may be considered to be between 90 and 135 mAs, a range of 45 mAs in width. The

selection of this range was based upon the fact that visualization of all required details was attained in the images although they possessed varying degrees of density. Selection of the optimum density may easily be made by choosing three adjacent radiographs in the series that approach nearest to the required density—90, 105, and 120 mAs. A desirable density may be considered as produced by 105 mAs.

In review, the 80 kVp used for the knee radiographs in Figure 6-18 yielded an exposure latitude ranging across 62.5 mAs, while the 60 kVp series used for the elbow in Figure 6-19 yielded a latitude range of only 45 mAs. When the kVp is so low that adequate penetration is not achieved, as in Figure 6-12A-G, no amount of mAs will produce an acceptable density level and it may be said that the exposure latitude approaches zero. *The longer gray scales achieved at high kVp levels allow a greater margin of error or exposure latitude. When the gray scale is short, (for instance, at lower kVp levels),*

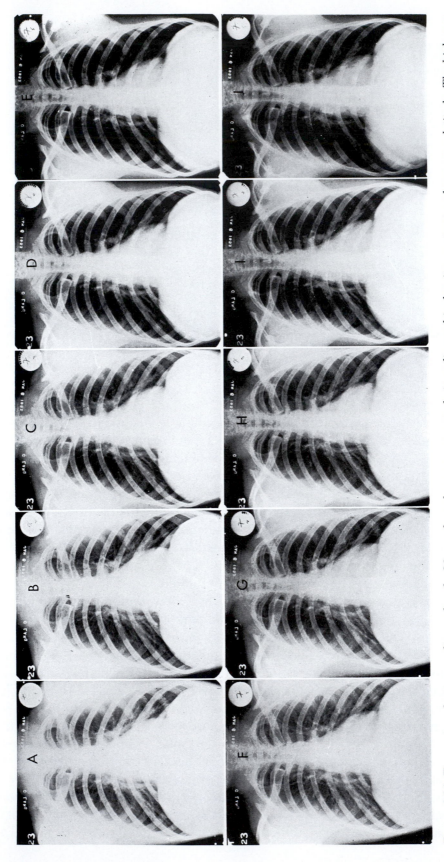

Figure 6-20. Two series of screen radiographs of a 23-cm chest that serve as a study in radiographic density, contrast and exposure latitude. The high contrast series A to E, taken at 50 kVp, demonstrates narrow exposure latitude. The low contrast series F to J, taken at 80 kVp, demonstrates wide exposure latitude.

exposure latitude is also very narrow and there is little margin for error.

CONTRAST VERSUS EXPOSURE LATITUDE

The close relationship between contrast and exposure latitude may be observed by a study of Figure 6-20. This relationship obviously is dependent upon the factor of kilovoltage.

Example: In Figure 6-20, radiographs *A-E* were produced with 50 kVp at mAs values of (A) 7.5, (B) 10, (C) 13.3, (D) 20, (E) 30. Radiographs *F-J* were made with 80 kVp and mAs values of (F) 2.5, (G) 3.3, (H) 4.16, (I) 5, and (J) 6.6.

For radiographs *A-E,* note that as the mAs increased, the overall density of the image increased. *D* and *E* contain areas where the opaque silver deposits are dark enough to obscure some details. In radiograph *A,* the contrast differences were so great that many of the finer details have been lost due to a lack of tissue penetration. This is a condition typical of high contrast. The exposure latitude was constricted to radiographs *B* and *C,* which is too narrow a range for good chest radiography.

Overall image densities also increased in radiographs *F-J,* yet all silver deposits are translucent even in *J* which exhibits some overexposure. Note that radiograph *F* demonstrates details that are completely absent in *A.* All essential details are recorded with varying levels of overall density in radiographs *F-I,* which is typical of low-contrast images. In radiograph *J* some details are obscured because of overexposure. The correct exposure may be considered as represented in radiograph *G.* The exposure latitude is wide, represented by radiographs *F-I.*

These examples demonstrate that when high contrast prevails, the resulting narrow exposure latitude prevents the rendition of a large number of different overall densities for diagnostic use. A radiographer operating with optimum kilovoltage technique is more likely to produce greater uniformity of radiographic results than one who uses low kilovoltage techniques. In fact, the latitude available at higher kVp levels is the very factor that permits consistency of results when employing a fixed kilovoltage approach to technique. A general rule may be stated: *Anything which leads to longer gray scale will also result in wider exposure latitude.*

USE OF HIGHER KILOVOLTAGES

The use of higher kilovoltages provides greater exposure efficiency in radiography for the following reasons:

1. Anatomical details in all tissue thicknesses are rendered as translucent densities. The relative absorption properties between bone and flesh are reduced making possible visualization of more structural details. At lower kilovoltages, bone detail often tends to obscure details of soft tissues that lie behind the bone. Complete penetration of bone by higher kilovoltages reveals soft tissue details that are often not visible at lower kilovoltages. The greater penetration afforded by higher kilovoltage radiation makes possible the rendition of a greater number of anatomical details then when lower kilovoltages are employed.

2. When high kilovoltages are employed *in combination with lower mAs values,* the radiation dose to the patient is reduced because the body absorbs less radiation. More radiation can, therefore, reach the film to expose it, and exposure can be reduced.

3. Heat production in the x-ray tube is reduced because smaller energy loads (mAs) can be employed, thereby increas-

ing x-ray tube life. As the kVp increases, x-ray tube efficiency increases. More radiation is produced per watt of electrical power consumed. Correct exposures may therefore be produced with less heat generated in the tube, and the tube will last longer.

4. Greater exposure latitude may be secured. As the kilovoltage increases, exposure latitude increases because of the reduced absorption of body tissues created by virtue of the complete penetration. Details become visible in tissues of wide density and thickness. There is a greater margin for error in selecting an acceptable mAs value; thus, the chances of having to repeat exposures to the patient are improved.

SUMMARY

1. Increasing kilovoltage increases beam *penetration* through the patient. This is essential to image production.
2. No amount of mAs can ever compensate for a kVp level that is *inadequate* to penetrate the anatomy.
3. Kilovoltage is a primary electrical control for image *gray scale.* Higher kVp levels penetrated more types of anatomy to expose the film, so that there are more gray shades and fewer unexposed blank areas in the image.
4. Kilovoltage is the primary electrical control for image *contrast.* Higher kVp levels reduce image contrast for three reasons: (1) Gray scale (which opposes contrast) is increased through enhanced tissue penetration; (2) Photoelectric interactions are lost, so that the remaining scatter interactions comprise a greater proportion of all interactions occurring; and (3) that scatter radiation produced is more energetic and emitted in a more forward direction, causing increased fog in the image. With lengthened gray scale, fewer photoelectric interactions, and increased fog, image contrast will decrease.
5. *Scatter radiation fogs* the image with a useless veil of density. Thus, increasing kVp increases the proportion of *noise* in the image.
6. Increasing kilovoltage increases image *density* dramatically. However, because kVp also affects contrast, it should not generally be used to control density. Density changes caused by kVp must be compensated for by adjusting mAs.
7. A *15 percent* change in kVp changes image density by roughly a factor of 2, doubling or cutting the density to one-half the original.
8. A 5 percent change in kVp (4-6 kVp in most ranges) is the required minimum to cause a visible *density change* in the image.
9. *Optimum kVp* is the minimum level required to sufficiently penetrate *all* of the tissues within a body part, based upon the relative proportions of bone or air to soft tissue within the part.
10. Increasing kVp increases the *exposure latitude*, so that there is a greater margin for error in selecting mAs values. *Anything* which increases image gray scale also increases exposure latitude.
11. Kilovoltage has no effect upon sharpness of detail, magnification, or distortion because it has no relationship to beam projection geometry.

REVIEW QUESTIONS

1. What, in one word, is the single most important function of kVp?
2. Explain the *three* reasons why higher kVp levels reduce contrast in the image:
3. Define *optimum* kVp:
4. A chest radiograph demonstrates that the spine is not at all visible through the heart. Why would increasing the mAs to darken up the film *not* solve this problem?
5. Why is kVp not generally recommended as a density control?
6. Radiographs with long gray scale also allow more exposure latitude. What does this mean in setting techniques?
7. A technique of 100 mA, 1/2 second, and 90 kVp results in a radiograph of the abdomen which is fogged and *also* has motion on it. Using the 15 percent rule, list a new technique that will solve *both* of these problems without changing the overall density of the original:

_____   _____   _____
mA   Time   kVp

8. What is the minimum visible density change rule-of-thumb for kVp?
9. Assume that a good abdomen technique for a particular machine is 40 mAs at 80 kVp. Adding barium in the colon for a barium enema requires the same *overall* technique, but much more penetration. If the mAs is adjusted from 40 down to 5 mAs for the BE, what must your new kVp be?
10. If scatter radiation has changed direction, why doesn't it reduce the sharpness of recorded detail in the image?
11. A graph of the x-ray beam spectrum change caused by a decrease in kVp from 100 to 70 would show an (increase or decrease) in the number of x-rays at each of the following energies:
    15 keV:
    55 keV:
    70 keV:
12. If you reduced kVp by *three steps* of 15 percent each, even though you doubled the mAs three times, the radiograph may still turn out light because of:
13. Even if higher kVp levels did not increase fog on the radiograph, they would still result in less contrast and longer gray scale because of:
14. The *average* energy of an 80 kVp x-ray beam is about:
15. Why can't increasing mAs compensate for a below-optimum kVp?
16. Sketch a curve in the graph below showing the change in the shape and position of the x-ray beam spectrum caused by an increase in the kVp from 60 to 100:

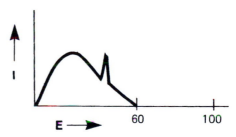

17. Higher kVp levels reduce image contrast because gray scale is _____, photoelectric interactions are _____, and fog is _____ (increase or decreased).
18. What electronic device in the x-ray machine is controlled by the kVp settings at the console?
19. Even though less scatter is actually produced within the patient at higher kVp levels, why does *more* scatter reach the x-ray film?

Chapter 7

MACHINE PHASE AND RECTIFICATION

IN ATTEMPTING TO INCREASE the efficiency of electrical generators, a design was developed that spins three coils of wire, rather than a single coil, within a magnetic field. This new type of generator resulted in overlapping pulses of electricity being produced (Fig. 7-1). Previously, x-ray machines using a single coil generator would produce individual "bursts" of x-rays emitted from the x-ray tube, one for each pulse of electricity. By *overlapping* electrical pulses, this new generator prevented the voltage from ever dropping all the way to zero, as the next rising pulse would boost the voltage back up before the current pulse ended, as shown in Figure 7-1. X-ray machines using this new device emitted x-rays *continuously* instead of in pulses. The *rate* of emission of x-rays from the x-ray tube was thus enhanced.

Radiographic machines using the overlapping pulses of a three-coil generator came to be known as *three-phase* machines, and those with a single coil as *single-phase* machines. In a single-phase machine, one electrical cycle consists of *two* pulses of electricity. A three-phase machine multiplies this number to *six* pulses in each cycle. It was later found that, by using additional coils of wire in the *transformer* of an x-ray machine, the number of overlapping pulses of electricity could be doubled again, for a total of *twelve* pulses per cycle. In this way, x-ray output was increased slightly over the three-phase, six-pulse machine.

The Greek letter *phi* (Φ) is used to abbreviate the machine phase and is often followed by a superscript number indicating the number of pulses of electricity pass-

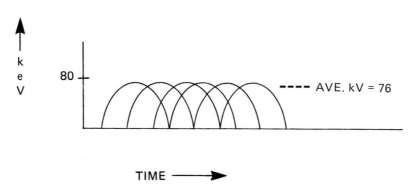

Figure 7-1. Diagram illustrating the overlapping of electrical pulses used in three-phase equipment to obtain continuous current and, consequently, continuous x-ray output. Also, note the ripple effect showing how three-phase equipment attains a much higher *average* keV than single-phase equipment operating at the same kVp.

ing through the x-ray tube during each electrical cycle. The abbreviation $1\Phi^2$ indicates the usual two pulses of electricity produced for each cycle of a single-phase machine. Three-phase machines are abbreviated $3\Phi^6$ or $3\Phi^{12}$ to indicate whether they are six-pulse or twelve-pulse machines.

In terms of radiographic technique, all three-phase machines are generally considered to be about twice as "hot" as single-phase machines. That is, if the same technique settings are used, any three-phase machine will produce a radiograph roughly twice as dark as a single-phase machine. Although a $3\Phi^{12}$ machine is slightly more efficient than a $3\Phi^6$ machine, the difference is not enough to be of concern in setting techniques. (Recall that a 30 percent difference would be required for a visible density change, and the difference between a 6-pulse and a 12-pulse machine is on the order of 6 or 7 percent.) The $3\Phi^{12}$ machine still produces radiographs approximately twice as dark as a single-phase unit. Whether $3\Phi^6$ or $3\Phi^{12}$, about one-half of the mAs is required for a three-phase unit to produce a desired density when compared to a single-phase machine.

HIGH-FREQUENCY GENERATORS

An increasingly popular type of x-ray machine generator is variously referred to as the *high-frequency, medium-frequency,* or *near-constant potential* generator (HFG, MFG, or CPG respectively). The popularity of this type of generator is understandable, since it can be plugged into any standard electrical outlet, is very small in size, and has about the same efficiency as a $3\Phi^{12}$ generator.

Details of high-frequency circuitry are beyond the scope of this text. Basically, a series of AC and DC electricity converters and a "DC chopper" are used to produce an extremely high-frequency electrical current that is supplied to the x-ray tube. The frequency of a single-phase unit is 60 cycles (120 pulses) of electricity per second, that of $3\Phi^6$ equipment is 180 cycles per second (3 times the single-phase), and that of $3\Phi^{12}$ equipment is 360 cycles per second. These newer generators produce an astonishing 60,000 cycles per second (for medium-frequency) to 100,000 cycles per second (for high-frequency). This means that the x-ray tube is receiving up to 200,000 overlapping pulses of electricity each second, and that the voltage fluctuation is much less than one percent (Fig. 7-2). A high-frequency machine is slightly more efficient than a 3Φ machine. This is for two reasons: First, the higher-frequency generator produces more x-rays per second (more mR/mAs) due to the more constant overlapping of electrical pulses. Second, the *average* energy of the high-frequency electrical current never falls more than a fraction of a percent below the kVp set at the console, as shown in Figure 7-2. The main advantages of high-frequency equipment over 3Φ equipment have to do with its smaller size and convenience.

The end result of all this technology is that image density is roughly doubled when compared to single-phase equipment operated at the same mAs values. Therefore, *high-frequency generators require about one-half the mAs used by single-phase equipment to obtain similar image density. Techniques for high-frequency generators are roughly equivalent to those for 3Φ equipment.*

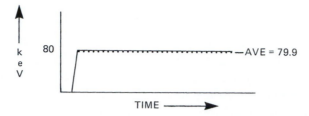

Figure 7-2. Graph illustrating the electrical pulse wave form for high-frequency generators and "constant potential" generators. Output is constant and the average keV is nearly 100% of the kVp set at the console.

EFFECT ON THE X-RAY BEAM SPECTRUM

Three-phase and high-frequency equipment are much more efficient (about twice as much) as single-phase equipment in producing a desired density on the radiograph. This is for two reasons:

X-RAY QUANTITY

Note in Figure 7-1 that by overlapping electrical pulses, two additional pulses of x-rays are begun before the first pulse returns to zero. In addition, note that the *valleys* between the pulses of the original current (where it returns to zero) are now filled with overlapping pulses of electrical current, so that current is continuous across the x-ray tube and never falls to zero. In this manner, the total quantity of current flowing across the x-ray tube per second is increased substantially. In the case of this three-phase, six-pulse machine, the rate of x-ray output from the tube (the *effective mA*) is increased over the single-phase machine. The high-frequency machine overlaps thousands of such pulses for the same effect (Fig. 7-2). A graph of the resulting x-ray beam spectrum is presented in Figure 7-3, where it will be noted that the total number of x-rays generated, represented by the height of the dotted curve, has increased substantially.

X-RAY QUALITY

Overlapping the pulses results in a voltage wave form which never falls to zero but *ripples* not far below the peak voltage level which was set at the console (Fig. 7-2). Compare the *average* energy of the electrical current produced by a three-phase machine in Figure 7-1 to that produced by a single-phase machine as shown in Figure 6-2 in Chapter 6. Now compare the further increase in *average* energy for a high-fre-

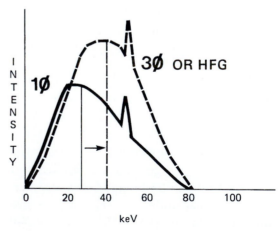

Figure 7-3. Graph of the x-ray beam spectra for single-phase and three-phase equipment. The three-phase machine shows a shift in average energy to higher levels (to the right) as well as an increased quantity of x-rays emitted per second (the height of the curve).

quency current in Figure 7-2 to the three-phase current in Figure 7-1. This *ripple effect* raises the average energy of the x-ray beam, even though the *peak* energy remains the same. With a higher average voltage, the x-ray beam will be more penetrating. The intensity of the remnant beam exiting the patient is thus increased even more, due to a higher percentage of beam penetration through the patient.

Figure 7-3 illustrates the effect of this change in average energy upon the graph of the x-ray beam spectrum when comparing a single-phase machine to a higher-power generator, either 3Φ or HFG, when both were set at 80 kVp: Even though the kVp in the graph is still indicated as 80, note that the shape of the curve has changed shifting the *average kV* to the right. This dotted curve represents a more penetrating beam of x-rays, even though the peak kV has not changed. It is due to the improved *efficiency* provided by higher-frequency generators.

To summarize, the dotted curve in Figure 7-3 implies that the beam has been changed in two ways—the additional height and area under the curve shows that more x-rays are actually being produced per second, while the shift in the mid-point of the curve to the right indicates that the average energy of the x-ray beam has also increased, providing additional penetration. To place a figure on each of these effects in regard to the final image density produced, it may be said that the increased *quantity* of radiation produced provides a 70-80 percent increase in image density, while the improved *quality* of this x-ray beam, the increased *penetration* due to a higher average kilovoltage, provides an additional 20-30 percent increase in image density. Adding these two figures, 70-80 percent plus 20-30 percent, we can expect a resulting final density effect of about 100 percent. This is a doubling of the radiographic density.

EFFECT ON DENSITY

We have seen from the above that when the increase in beam quantity is added to the increase in beam quality, the result of 3Φ or HFG equipment is radiographic densities that are roughly double that for 1Φ equipment, when *using the same kVp and mAs values set at the console* (Fig. 7-4). This higher efficiency allows shorter exposure times, about one-half those for single-phase, to be employed for like procedures. For this reason, all pediatric procedures and other procedures where there is a high probability of motion problems should be done in a three-phase x-ray room or a high-frequency room.

When changing from a single-phase room to a three-phase or HFG room, techniques for the same anatomy may be adjusted by simply cutting the mAs values to about one-half. Conversely, techniques should be doubled when changing from a three-phase or HFG room to a single-phase room.

EFFECT ON CONTRAST

Because of the increased *average* kilovoltage level for the three-phase or high-frequency x-ray machine, beam penetration is increased. As described in the previous chapter, a higher penetration level means that more of the various anatomical tissues

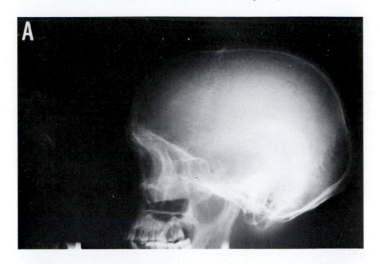

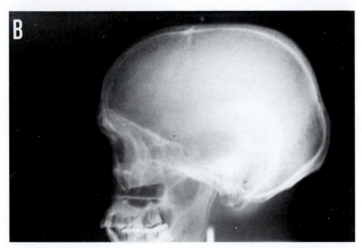

Figure 7-4. Radiographs of the lateral skull demonstrating the maintenance of density by cutting mAs values to one-half the original when changing from a single-phase machine to a three-phase machine. Factors: (A) 20 mAs, 76 kVp, single-phase; (B) 10 mAs, 76 kVp, three-phase.

will be radiolucent to the beam and recorded as gray shades on the radiograph, and gray scale will increase. Accordingly, contrast will usually be slightly lower for a three-phase or high-frequency machine than for a single-phase machine. Although this contrast loss may be measurable using a densitometer, it may not always be significant enough to detect visually.

The effect of a phase change on image contrast *is* visible in Figure 7-4, which compares two lateral skull views, one taken with a single-phase and one with a three-phase machine, while adjusting mAs to maintain equal density. Observe the densities in the area of the outer cranium: Note that in radiograph *A*, taken with a single-phase machine, the outer borders of the cranium are quite dark while the mid-portion of the cranium is relatively "white." This is high contrast. In radiograph *B*, the densities throughout the cranium are more balanced, presenting less contrast. This can also be seen in the area of the teeth, which are more "white and black" in radiograph *A*. Radiograph *A* possesses higher contrast, and radiograph *B* shows a decrease in contrast and a lengthening of the gray scale.

In conclusion, changing to a higher-phase x-ray machine results in an increase of the average beam energy which produces higher beam penetration through the part. This would be expected to lengthen gray scale and reduce contrast, and it does so, slightly. Nonetheless, because this reduction of contrast is not always visible, it is not a practical consideration in choosing machine phase. High-frequency equipment is purchased for its primarily for its electrical efficiency, and for the much shorter exposure times and control of motion that it allows.

EFFECT ON OTHER QUALITIES

As discussed above, three-phase or high-frequency equipment allows the use of much shorter exposure times. This reduces the *probability* of motion on the part of the patient and may therefore indirectly contribute to obtaining good sharpness of recorded detail. It should be considered, nonetheless, that this is only an indirect relationship; it is the motion itself, not the machine phase that is directly responsible for the resultant sharpness of detail. Thus, while the phase and frequency of the machine may considered as an indirect *con-tributing* factor for image sharpness, it must not be thought of as a *controlling* factor over image sharpness.

Sharpness of detail, magnification, and shape distortion in the image are all strictly geometrical factors and are directly controlled by beam projection geometry. Machine phase is an electrical factor which has nothing to do with beam geometry. The type of x-ray generator should not be considered to have any direct relationship with these *recognizability* functions in the image.

RECTIFICATION AND X-RAY GENERATORS

Not all x-ray equipment uses the fully rectified, pulsed electricity we have been discussing. Other variations include half-rectified units, capacitor discharge units and constant-potential generator units. These are all most frequently encountered in mobile radiography, discussed in Chapter 32.

Some older mobile units may still be in use which are *half-rectified*. This means that only every other pulse of electricity is allowed to reach the x-ray tube. Whereas a fully-rectified single-phase machine produces *two* bursts of x-rays with each cycle of electricity, a half-rectified machine will produce only *one* burst of x-rays with each electrical cycle. Its output is *one-half* that of a single-phase unit, and about *one-fourth* that of a three-phase machine. To compensate technique when using half-rectified equipment, all mAs values must be *doubled* from single-phase techniques in order to produce adequate radiographic density.

Capacitor-discharge units do not use pulses of electricity at all. Rather, they store up a preset electrical charge on a capacitor (somewhat like a battery) as described in Chapter 32. This charge is predetermined by the mAs set at the console. When the charging button is depressed, this amount of electrical charge is allowed to run from the incoming electrical line into the capacitor, where it is stored. After charging, the exposure button is activated, releasing this stored charge of electrons which rushes to and across the x-ray tube creating a single long burst of x-rays. For technique purposes, *the output of a capacitor-discharge unit is considered to be roughly equivalent to that of a single-phase unit.* The mAs values used would then be about double those for three-phase equipment, and double those used for battery-operated constant-potential units.

BATTERY-OPERATED MOBILE UNITS

Most modern "portable" or mobile x-ray units use a bank of powerful batteries as the power source for exposures. Such a machine is charge up between uses by plugging it into a wall outlet. Electrical charge from the incoming line is stored in the batteries and later used for both driving the mobile unit and making exposures. It is essential to keep these machines properly charged between uses, or the full mAs and kVp values set by the technologist may not be attained during exposure, resulting in light radiographs.

The batteries supply a direct (one-way) current. This electrical current is changed into alternating current in order to allow for manipulation and control at the console: Transforming electricity can only be done by *moving magnetic fields* which, in turn, can only be produced by *alternating* current which is constantly changing speed and direction. After the kVp is selected and the current is transformed to the desired level, the current is changed *back* into direct current before it reaches the x-ray tube so that it will always pass correctly from the filament to the anode. Direct current does not come in pulses, but is normally a steady flow of electricity. It has no voltage fluctuation like single-phase and three-phase generators produce (Figs. 6-1 & 7-1). In a battery-powered unit, because the current was transformed temporarily into AC and then back into DC, a very slight voltage fluctuation remains. But, this fluctuation is much less than a three-phase machine produces, and so slight that the final current is considered for all practical purposes to be "straight DC" current rather than pulsed DC (Fig. 7-2).

The importance of this waveform is that the average kilovoltage is essentially *equal* to the peak kilovoltage set at the console. It will be recalled that, with single-phase generation, the average kV produced is about one-third of the peak kV set (Fig. 6-1). With three-phase equipment, the average kV falls between 93 percent and 98 percent of the peak kV, depending on whether it is a 6-pulse or 12-pulse machine. With battery-powered mobile units, however, the average kV is virtually 100 percent of the peak kV set at the console (Fig. 7-2).

This explains why, in practice, lower kVp settings are frequently used on mobile equipment than on stationary x-ray machines in the x-ray department. For example, 76-80 kVp is typical for a *nongrid* chest projection in a standard x-ray room, such as an AP chest taken in a wheelchair. Yet, "portable" chest x-rays taken with a battery-powered mobile unit and *nongrid* are often done at 68-72 kVp, about 6-8 kVp less. This can be done because the *average* kV on the mobile unit is a higher percentage of the set kVp.

Lower mAs values may be used on these modern mobile machines for the same reasons. Battery-powered units are more efficient than three-phase or single-phase machines, both in terms of effective mA and average kVp. A rough rule of thumb is that *battery-powered mobile units require about six kVp less than three-phase, six-pulse machines.*

SUMMARY

1. Three-phase x-ray machines are twice as effective in producing radiographic *density* as single-phase machines. This is due to (1) more x-ray output per mA, and (2) increased average beam energy, resulting in higher penetration.
2. When changing from a single-phase room to a three-phase room, all *techniques* may be adjusted by cutting mAs to one-half, and vice versa.
3. Three-phase machines cause a slight decrease in the image *contrast* because of their higher average kV. Visually, however, this change is not always noticeable.
4. Phase has no direct relation to the recognizability functions of sharpness, magnification, or distortion. However, the probability of motion with pediatric or problem patients can be reduced by using three-phase equipment, since shorter times can be used. It may be said then that higher-phase machines

indirectly contribute to improved sharpness of recorded detail.
5. Machines that are not fully *rectified* provide only one-half the x-ray output per mA when compared to a fully-rectified single-phase unit. Compared to single-phase, techniques must be doubled when using these units.
6. *Capacitor-discharge* mobile units are roughly equivalent to single-phase equipment, requiring twice the mAs than a three-phase or constant-potential machine.
7. *Battery-operated mobile units* are slightly more efficient than three-phase equipment, requiring about 6 kVp less to produce equal radiographic density.
8. *High-frequency generators* require about the same techniques as three-phase equipment to produce equal image density, and one-half the techniques needed for single-phase equipment.

REVIEW QUESTIONS

1. Compared to a single-phase machine, a three-phase machine will produce an x-ray beam spectrum showing the same minimum energy, and the same peak energy, but increased _____ energy.
2. What factor would you change and by how much, for a given procedure, when changing from a three-phase machine to a single-phase machine.
3. Explain the *two* reasons why the total density effect of the different phases of machines is different:
4. Why does a half-rectified mobile x-ray unit produce lighter radiographs than a fully-rectified unit using identical techniques?
5. When changing from a three-phase machine to a capacitor-discharge mobile unit, adjust the mAs values to _____ the original.
6. When changing from a single-phase machine to a high-frequency generator unit, adjust the mAs values to _____ the original.
7. For three phase-six-pulse, three phase-twelve-pulse, and high frequency units, mAs values are approximately _____.
8. A battery-powered constant potential mobile unit will require _____ (more, less, or equal) technique when compared to a three phase-six-pulse unit.
9. The effect whereby the waveform for

the electricity passing through the x-ray tube of a 3-phase machine never drops very far below the *peak* kV before it is pushed up again is called:

10. Which type of x-ray machine produces the highest average kV:

Chapter 8

BEAM FILTRATION

WHEN ANY MATERIAL such as a sheet of aluminum is placed in the x-ray beam at the portal of the x-ray tube, both the quantity and the quality of the emergent radiation is altered. The effect of aluminum filtration is to screen out the non-penetrating, low-energy radiation that is not needed for routine radiography and which may be hazardous to the patient. The quantity of x-rays in the beam is reduced, but the quality of the x-ray beam is increased, because the removal of low-energy photons will lead to an increase in the *average* energy of the photons in the beam.

Imagine a graduating class of 100 high school seniors, for whom we want to determine the average height. We measure how tall each one is, divide by 100 and report the average to be 5 feet, 4 inches. Now remove the *shortest* 20 individuals and repeat the calculations. There are fewer individuals left in our study, only 80, but the average *height* has *increased* to perhaps 5 feet 8 inches. This is precisely what filtration does in the x-ray beam: The intensity of the beam is lessened because there are fewer x-rays remaining; nonetheless, their *average kilovoltage*, and consequently their *average penetration power* has been increased. A higher percentage of these 80 will penetrate through the patient to the image receptor. This is frequently referred to as "hardening the beam." A more penetrating beam is a "harder" beam of x-rays. Figure 8-1 is a graph of the x-ray beam spectrum

showing how the elimination of the low-energy x-rays results in an *increase* in the average energy of those x-rays remaining in the beam.

The total filtration within an x-ray beam can be divided into two categories: *Inherent* filtration and *added* filtration. *Inherent filtration* consists of the normal absorption of some of the x-rays by the glass of the x-ray tube itself, the oil in the tube housing, the beryllium window and the mirrors and plastic windows in the collimator through which the x-ray beam must pass. Inherent filtration includes all those devices which would be practically difficult or impossible to remove from the path of the beam. *Added filtration* is the additional thin slabs of

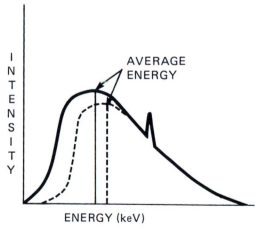

Figure 8-1. Graph showing the effect of increasing filtration on the x-ray beam spectrum. Minimum and average energy increase (shift to the right), but maximum energy does not Overall intensity (the height of the curves) is reduced.

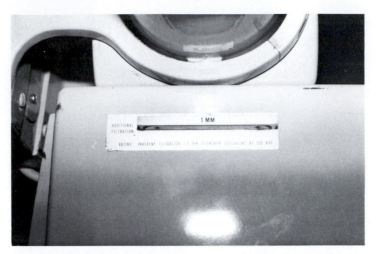

Figure 8-2. Photograph of the slot for added filtration on the side of a mobile unit collimator.

aluminum which may be installed within the collimator or between the tube and the collimator, and which is accessible enough to be easily removed or added. Figure 8-2 shows the slot in the side of a modern mobile x-ray machine collimator into which added filtration may be inserted.

In modern equipment, inherent filtration is normally equivalent in its cumulative absorption to 1-1.5 millimeters of aluminum. All equipment operating above 70 kVp must have a minimum total filtration of 2.5 mm of aluminum equivalency. Subtracting these two figures, it can be seen that the *added* thickness of aluminum slabs required will usually be between 1 and 1.5 mm. It is not unheard-of for a radiographer to remove aluminum slabs from the slot in the collimator, or from between the x-ray tube and the collimator in order to perform a mammogram or for some other reason, and then forget to replace the aluminum afterward. This practice poses a real risk of unnecessary high radiation dose to the patients and should be forbidden. There should always be slabs of aluminum present unless a certified radiation physicist has verified that adequate HVL is achieved

without the slabs. HVL will be discussed later in this chapter.

If the proper amount of filtration is not used, the low-energy x-rays, which are not penetrating, will nearly all be absorbed within the patient. They never reach the x-ray film and, therefore, make no contribution to image density. Hence, such low-energy x-rays only increase dose to the patient (especially skin dose), and for no beneficial purpose. Protective filtration reduces this unnecessary hazard to the patient. Under no circumstances should radiography be performed without proper aluminum filtration in the beam.

EFFECTS ON IMAGE QUALITIES

If the filtration were increased much beyond about 3.5 millimeters of aluminum equivalency, it would begin to visibly affect the radiographic density, since at such high levels it would begin to take out some of those useful x-rays that would otherwise have reached the film. In addition to this visible loss of density, there would also occur a slight increase in gray scale and a loss of image contrast, due to the fact that elimination of the lower energies in the beam spectrum leads to an increase in the *average* energy (Fig. 8-1). However, while this effect on contrast might be measurable using a densitometer, it is not significant enough to normally be visible.

Excessive filtration in the beam defeats the purpose of exposing the radiograph. When density losses become visible, they necessitate an increase in mAs to compensate. Such an increase in mAs simply reintroduces additional patient skin dose, which the filters were added to eliminate.

Therefore, an *optimum* level of protective filtration has been established to achieve the maximum level of protection for the patient *without* affecting the radiographic density. The requirement is 2.5 millimeters of aluminum equivalence for the total filtration in the beam. This amount eliminates the lowest-energy, most damaging x-rays in the beam—those which would *not* make it to the film anyway and therefore would have no radiographic value.

For practical purposes, protective filtration should not be considered a significant factor in *any* of the radiographic qualities, including density and contrast. For example, no increase in image density would be discernable when working with a real patient if the filtration was reduced from 2.5 mm to 1.5 mm of aluminum; this is because the additional low-energy x-rays released in the primary beam will virtually all be absorbed in the patient and never reach the film. Protective filtration only affects the image when it is increased to excessive amounts.

To summarize the effects of protective filtration, remember that although it alters the primary beam prior to reaching the patient, the *remnant* beam which exits the patient and reaches the film is not appreciably affected. In daily practice, protective filtration has no appreciable effect upon radiographic contrast or density. It also has no effect upon sharpness of recorded detail, magnification, or distortion in the image, since it does not alter the geometry (the distances, sizes and angles and alignment) of the projected x-ray beam.

COMPENSATING FILTRATION

There are occasions when it is difficult to balance densities in radiography of irregular anatomical areas. Regardless of attempted adjustments in mAs or kVp, the drastic change in thickness or density of the body part from one end to the other is so pronounced that one end of the image turns out too dark or the opposite end turns out too light. Examples include the AP foot, the AP T-spine, and the AP femur. However, if very thick, specially-shaped filters are employed to selectively absorb various portions of the x-ray beam *before* it reaches the patient, balanced image densities may be secured.

Absorption of the beam can be effected by placing a *compensating filter* such as a graduated aluminum wedge in the filter channel at the bottom of the collimator. The material is so shaped that the x-ray beam must pass through the larger amounts of absorbing material when directed toward the thinner anatomical portions. To cause a dramatic, visible reduction in image density these compensating filters must be quite thick, often thicker than 1 cm, when compared to protective filters which are slabs of only 1 or 2 mm. The material should be thin or omitted for that portion of the beam passing

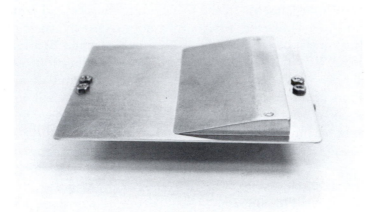

Figure 8-3. Photograph of a wedge filter which may be inserted in the collimator rails for anatomy of graduating thickness, such as AP views of the T-spine, foot, or femur.

toward the heavier, thicker parts of the anatomy.

Two of the most common types of compensating filters are the *wedge* filter (Fig.8-3) and the *trough* filter (Fig. 8-4). The wedge filter is particularly recommended for lengthwise use on AP thoracic spines and AP feet. The wedge can also be used lengthwise for AP femur projections, or crosswise for fetogram or pelvimetry views. The trough filter is used to obtain balanced densities in both the mediastinum and the lung field areas on one AP view of the chest. Thick trough filters have been designed to minimize breast dose on female patients for AP scoliosis projections, while allowing radiation through the central area to demonstrate the spine. Several types and shapes of of compensating filters are available and can be custom-made for special needs.

In most applications of compensating filters, techniques will need to be increased by 8 to 10 kVp. This is due to the fact that most techniques for uneven anatomy are selected to record the thinner portions of the anatomy. In these thinner areas, the thicker end of the filter will cancel out the effect of the 8-kVp increase, while the thinner end of the filter allows the increased technique through to darken the density in the areas of those thicker anatomical parts.

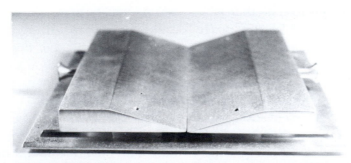

Figure 8-4. Photograph of a trough filter, used for the AP T-spine.

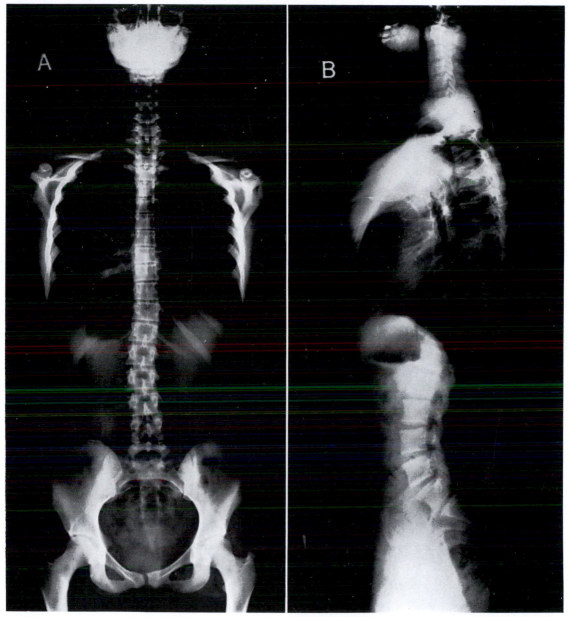

Figure 8-5. AP and lateral radiographs of the entire spine exposed with compensating filtration. Note the balanced densities along the spine.

The result is a proper density level across all anatomical areas in the image.

In radiography of the entire spine on a 14 x 36-inch film, a normal radiograph would exhibit high density in upper segment of the vertebral column, since the technique would have to be adjusted to suit the heavier lumbosacral portion of the spine. By constructing suitable compensating filters, both AP and lateral views of the entire vertebral column that exhibit balanced densities may be secured (Fig. 8-5). Custom-made filters can even be made to produce radiographs of the total body - two

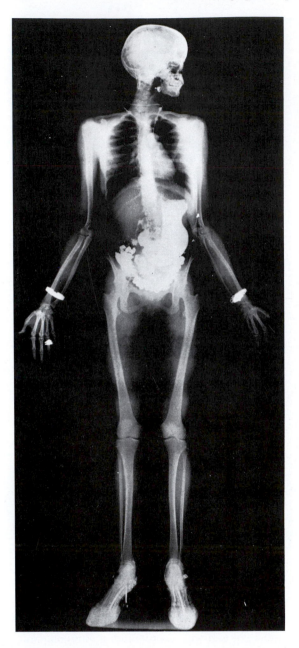

classic examples of these are demonstrated in the frontispiece of the book (inside cover) and in Figure 8-6. Such a practice is certainly *not* recommended in modern diagnosis, for a situation requiring demonstration of the entire body on a single exposure would never be justified, but these historical radiographs are dramatic in exhibiting just how effective compensating filtration can be.

Compensating filters are used to control image density alone. As with protective filtration, the addition of a compensating filter hardens the x-ray beam, increasing the average kV in those areas where the filter is thick. This would be expected to increase penetration, lengthen gray scale, and slightly reduce contrast in those areas of the image, but this effect is quantitatively negligible. Contrast changes in the image due to filtration are not normally noticeable, and certainly not a consideration in determining when to use a compensating filter. Compensating filters also have no direct effect on sharpness, magnification, or distortion. They are strictly used in density control.

Figure 8-6. Entire body radiograph of a living girl made with a compensating filter. The stomach and intestinal tract was filled with barium sulfate for their delineation.

X-RAY BEAM QUALITY AND HVL

The quality of the x-ray beam may be thought of as its *average energy*, or its overall ability for *penetration*. The average energy of the beam depends primarily upon two important factors: the kVp set at the console and the amount of total filtration in the beam. Increasing either one of these will pull up the average energy, making it more penetrating and of higher quality. Elevating the kVp raises average beam energy by *adding high-kV photons* to the beam; Adding filtration raises average beam energy by *eliminating low-kV photons* from the beam. Both "harden" the beam.

Since filtration also plays so vital a part, it is not customary or accurate to refer to the quality of an x-ray beam solely in terms of the kVp. A special unit, the *half-value layer*, directly measures beam quality by determining its actual penetration capability. The half-value layer, or *HVL*, is that amount of absorbing material required to reduce the intensity of the x-ray beam to one-half the original. Requirements for HVL and how it is determined are fully discussed in Chapter 30.

Any increase in inherent or added filtration, or any increase in kVp, will result in a higher HVL. Since all of these changes ultimately result in a more penetrating x-ray beam, it will take more absorber to attenuate one-half of that x-ray beam. The more penetrating the beam is, the higher the HVL. It may be said that beam penetration is *controlled* by filtration and kVp, but it is *measured* in HVL.

SUMMARY

1. Normal amounts of protective filtration are used only to reduce patient radiation *dose* and in practice have no appreciable effect on any aspect of the final radiographic image. Excessive amounts of filtration may result in a loss of image density, with no other significant change in the image.

2. Compensating filters are designed to reduce *density* in areas of thinner anatomical parts on the radiograph, and have no significant effect on other image qualities.

3. Most compensating filters require an increase in *technique* of 8 to 10 kVp.

4. Overall beam quality, based on its penetration ability, is measured in HVL units. This beam quality is affected by both the kVp set and the protective filtration present.

REVIEW QUESTIONS

1. In an 80 kV x-ray beam, a decrease in filtration would (increase, decrease, or not affect) the number of photons at the following energies:
   15 kVp:
   50 kVp:
   80 kVp:

2. List all of the image qualities which are noticeably affected when adding a thick compensating filter such as a wedge filter.

3. How much should you increase kVp when adding a thick wedge filter?

4. What is the minimum amount of protective filtration required on all x-ray machines capable of operating above 70 kVp? Be sure your answer is complete:

5. Give an example of a procedure on which you would use a wedge filter *and* explain why you would use it on *this* procedure.

6. Which image qualities would be noticeably changed when removing 0.5 mm of protective filtration from a beam that originally had 2.5 mm in it?

7. Define half-value layer:

8. Total protective filtration consists of which two subcategories of filtration:

9. For most x-ray machines, what range of *added* filtration thickness is required to meet standards:

10. What *two* factors determine the HVL or quality of the x-ray beam.

Chapter 9

FIELD SIZE LIMITATION

THE PURPOSES OF beam size limitation are twofold: (1) to reduce exposure to the patient and (2) to increase image contrast. The minimizing of patient exposure should be of paramount concern to every radiographer, and limiting the size of the x-ray beam is one of the most effective ways to do this. By controlling field size, organs with critical sensitivity to radiation such as the gonads, thyroid gland, and eye lens can be kept outside of the primary x-ray beam. The resulting reduction in dose to these organs can be as much as a hundred-fold. A variety of devices is available for this purpose.

COLLIMATION DEVICES

Devices commonly used to limit beam size include manual collimators and positive beam limitation (automatic) collimators installed on most modern equipment, cones, extension cylinders and aperture diaphragms (Fig. 9-1). The most effective of these devices in providing a sharp border on the x-ray field are those which cause the beam to pass through two apertures (openings) rather than one. The collimator and the extension cylinder (commonly misnamed a "cone") provide double apertures (Fig. 9-2). The modern collimator looks like a metal box connected to the x-ray tube, as shown in the previous Figure 8-2, with a plastic window in the bottom. Inside the collimator are two pairs of metal shutters and a series of gears and bands for moving them in tandem (Fig. 9-3). The extension cylinder (the middle device in Fig. 9-1) also provides for double apertures, since the radiation must make it through both the upper opening as it enters the cylinder and through the second opening at the bottom end.

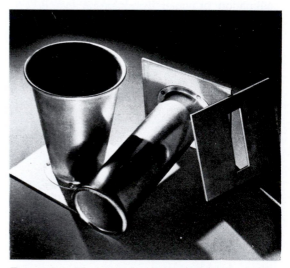

Figure 9-1. Photograph of cone, extension cylinder and aperture diaphragm, devices used to restrict field size.

The main purpose of the secondary aperture is actually to absorb *off-focus radiation*. Off-focus radiation is produced in the x-ray tube when a few of the high-speed electrons accelerating toward the anode veer off-track and strike the anode some-

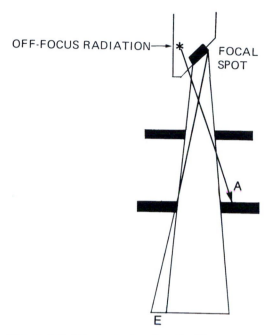

OFF-FOCUS RADIATION→ * FOCAL SPOT

A

E

Figure 9-2. Diagram showing double-aperture collimation provided by extension cylinders and automatic collimators. The second set of shutters, or the lower aperture, absorbs off-focus radiation (A) and provides a sharper field edge (E).

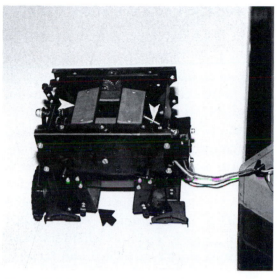

Figure 9-3. Photograph of collimator mechanism, showing upper set of shutters (horizontal white arrow) and lower set of shutters (black arrow). The screw for adjusting the angle of the field light mirror is demarcated by the vertical white arrow.

where other than at the focal spot. Remember that these electrons from the filament are being focused into a very tight, narrow beam as they approach the focal spot on the anode—some get too close to each other, having a "collision" in which their repulsive negative charge makes them ricochet off in random directions out of the focused beam. Where these off-focused electrons strike the anode, x-rays will be produced which are not part of the controlled beam of x-rays. Some of these off-focus x-rays will be emitted in directions that allow them to exit the window of the x-ray tube along with the primary beam, yet they will not be aligned with the rest of the beam. Figure 9-2 shows an off-focus x-ray (*A*) which has made it through the first set of collimator shutters along with the primary beam, but in a misaligned direction.

Off-focus x-rays are technically *primary* radiation (not secondary), but they travel in a crooked direction in relation to the rest of the beam, and are thus destructive to the final image. Off-focus x-rays must not be confused with secondary scattered radiation, which originates within the *patient* rather than in the x-ray tube. Nonetheless, they have similar effects upon the image, causing a random fog density which reduces image contrast. By placing a second set of lead shutters in the modern collimator (Fig. 9-3), many of these off-focus x-rays can be eliminated from the primary beam as it exits the collimator.

Since a secondary aperture is closer to the patient and film, it also provides a smaller projected field with sharper edges (Fig. 9-2). Sharper edges on the x-ray field itself, however, must not be confused with sharpness of the actual details of the image, which is *not* affected by field size limitation.

POSITIVE BEAM LIMITATION

From the mid-1970s to the mid-1990s, all new x-ray machines produced were required to have *positive beam limitation* or "automatic collimators." Most modern equipment provides *PBL*, but with an optional switch to override it when manual collimation is desired. For PBL, there are detectors connected to the film clamps in the Bucky tray which, when the clamps are closed on a cassette, measure the cassette size. This information is electronically relayed to the collimator, where the shutters are electrically activated and move to match the cassette size. This ensures that the field size will never be larger than the film/cassette size, and thus protects the patient from radiation exposure to unnecessary portions of the body.

Historically, automatic collimation turned out to be a curse as well as a blessing: There are many projections which should be taken with the field size collimated *smaller* than the film size. PBL inadvertently contributed to sloppy practice by radiographers who mistakenly thought they no longer needed to concern themselves with manual collimation at all, and stopped collimating smaller than the film when they should. Consequently, the *requirement* for PBL was rescinded. Although PBL is still installed on most x-ray machines and is valuable in controlling patient exposure, whenever a "coned-down" view is in order, the radiographer should override the PBL and manually collimate. Failure to do so results in unnecessary exposure to the patient and defeats the very purpose for which the collimator was invented.

OVERCOLLIMATION

The anatomy of interest must always be fully included within the x-ray field. Overzealous collimation can result in "clipping" essential anatomy of interest from the view and result in a repeated exposure. By so doing, one defeats the most important purpose of collimation—minimizing patient dose. In fact, a repeated exposure doubles the necessary dose for that view.

With experience, the student will come to appreciate that the edges of the actual x-ray beam are not always perfectly aligned with the edges of the projected light field. This is due to the fact that the light field is projected from a light bulb mounted in the side of the collimator and reflected downward from a mirror, while the x-ray beam itself passes through the mirror from above. The angle of the mirror can be adjusted by a lever inside the collimator (Fig. 9-3) and it is not uncommon for the light field to be projected as much as one-half inch off of the actual x-ray beam. In fact, each edge of the light field is only required to be within about one-half inch of the edges of the x-ray field.

With this in mind, a word to the wise would be to *always allow at least one-half inch of light beyond each edge of the anatomy of interest,* as long as it does not extend beyond the edge of the film. For example, when radiographing the hand, allow at least one-half inch of light beyond the fingertips and to each side of the hand shadow. This will ensure that the fingertips are not clipped off at the edges of the actual x-ray beam. Neglecting this guideline may result in unnecessary repeated exposures to the patient.

SCATTER RADIATION

Limitation of the size of the x-ray field is extremely important in the control of fog from scattered radiation. When an anatomical area is small, a field should be used that is small enough to include just the area of interest. In limiting the size of the x-ray beam, less tissue is irradiated within the patient, reducing patient dose. Further, the number of different areas within the patient and the table, as well as the number of different angles, from which any given point on the film may receive scattered photons, is reduced.

Figure 9-4 demonstrates this effect. With a wide beam, *A*, scattered radiation may be produced within a large volume of exposed tissue (dashed area). This scattered radiation emanates from various points within the body part, and can reach any point on the film from many different angles. Any one of these scattered rays could strike the small square area of interest on the film, fogging this area. (Scattered rays are in fact emitted in all directions, and can strike anywhere on the film, but for this demonstration in Figure 9-4, we shall consider a small chosen area of interest.) When the x-ray beam is collimated to a smaller size, *B*, scattered rays can only be produced in the smaller volume of exposed tissue represented by the solid lines. Also, there are fewer different angles from which this scat-

tered radiation may reach the indicated square on the film. The small square on the film will be more fogged with the wide beam *A* than with the narrower, collimated beam *B*.

It is important to remember that *scattered radiation is produced in and from tissue. Literally, the more tissue exposed, the more scatter produced.* Limiting the field size limits the volume of tissue exposed. Hence, it also limits the production of scatter fog in the final image.

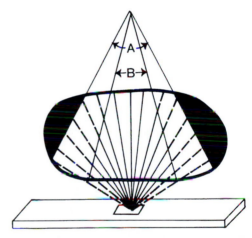

Figure 9-4. Diagram illustrating how smaller field sizes expose a lesser volume of tissue and a narrower range of angles (solid lines) from which scattered radiation can fog a given area on the film. This reduction in scatter decreases density and increases contrast.

EFFECT ON CONTRAST

In Chapter 4, we learned that for image contrast to be changed, the interactions of the x-ray beam must be considered *relative to each other*. We have established that less scatter is produced with narrower x-ray beams, but for this to result in any change in image contrast, we must also show that

photoelectric interactions and penetrating x-rays have *not* decreased by the same amount. If this were so, they would cancel out the effect of decreased scatter and overall image contrast would not change.

Figure 9-5 provides this demonstration, using diagrams of penetrating and absorbed portions of the primary x-ray beam. Once again, we focus on a small chosen area of the film. Note that the number of penetrating primary x-rays *striking the black square* is equal regardless of whether the collimated beam is wide, *A*, or narrow, *B*. In *A*, four x-rays reach the square and one, in the middle, is totally absorbed by photoelectric effect, leaving a small white spot in the middle of the square. In *B*, there are still four penetrating x-rays reaching this area. Furthermore, the white spot is unchanged in position and appearance. The *concentration* of penetrating and absorbed rays is not affected by the width of the overall x-ray beam.

The reason that penetrating and absorbed x-rays are *not* affected by beam size is that they are produced in the *x-ray tube* (not the patient). They follow straight, geometrically predictable paths which do not change, whether in tissue or outside the tissue, just because the location of the edges of the beam is altered (Fig. 9-5).

The reason that the amount of *scatter* radiation *is* affected by beam size is that scatter is produced in *tissue within the patient*, and since it is geometrically unpredictable and random in direction, it can reach the small square on the film from *anywhere* in the patient's body (Fig. 9-4).

If scatter radiation, produced by the

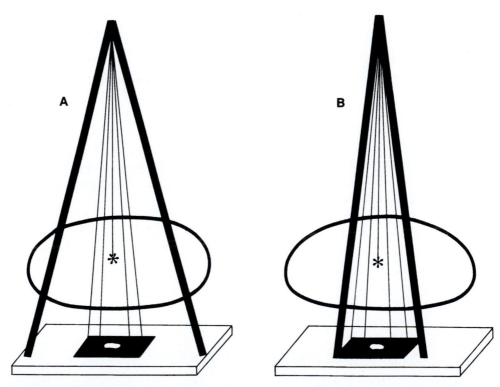

Figure 9-5. Diagram illustrating that field size does not affect the concentration of *primary* radiation nor the occurrence of the photoelectric effect (asterisk). Field size is indicated by bold lines. In (A), four x-rays reach the square area on the film, and one is absorbed by the photoelectric interaction, leaving a white spot on the radiograph. In (B), the edges of the light field are collimated in to obtain a smaller overall field. The square area on the film still receives four x-rays with a white spot in the middle. The effects of field size upon image density and contrast are *entirely* due to changes in the amount of scatter radiation produced within the body, not to any change in the intensity of the primary beam.

Compton interaction, decreases, while photoelectric interactions and penetrating x-rays remain unchanged, then the image contrast will change. The Compton/photoelectric ratio has decreased, and so has the Compton/penetration ratio. This means that visible fog in the image will decrease. With the reduction in fog, image contrast will improve.

It is worth noting that the effects of changing field size upon both density and contrast are limited to field sizes less than about 150 square inches, roughly equivalent to an 11 x 14 inch field. With field sizes larger than this, additional scatter radiation is produced at such a distance from our theoretical point (square) of fogging on the film that very few of these additional low-energy scattered rays reach that point and fog it. In other words, changing from an 11 x 14 inch field to a 14 x 17 inch field will not result in a *visible* change in image density or contrast. *Only when changing to or from field sizes less than 11 x 14 inches are these density and contrast effects noticed.*

EFFECT ON DENSITY

It may be said that the density for any particular area on a radiograph depends on the *concentration* of x-rays striking there. The more concentrated the radiation is, the greater will be the *total* number of x-rays striking within that area. Figures 9-4 and 9-5 illustrate the effects of changing field size on the concentration of radiation reaching a small square area on the film. In Figure 9-5, one can see that the same four primary x-rays reach the small square regardless of where the edges of the beam are located. The concentration of *primary* radiation is not affected by the size of the field. However, as shown in Figure 9-4, the concentration of *scattered radiation* in this small square area on the film *is changed* by the field size. When the field is collimated to a smaller area, a lesser volume of tissue is exposed and less scatter is produced. There are also fewer angles from which scatter produced in the patient may reach the small square. The amount of scatter rays striking this area is reduced.

In determining the *total* amount of radiation reaching the film, both the primary rays and the scattered rays must be considered. After all, fog density from scatter radiation, even though it is undesirable, *is* part of the total density produced in the image. Therefore, even though the concentration of *primary* x-rays is unaffected by field size, the loss of scattered rays results in a reduction in the *total* amount of radiation reaching the small square on the film. There will be less density in the image. The radiograph will turn out lighter.

This effect is true for all other small areas on the film, so that the overall density of the radiograph is likewise affected. Smaller field sizes result in lower overall density, because the reduction in scatter radiation leads to a reduction in the total amount of radiation reaching the film. With larger field sizes, overall density is increased, due to additional scatter radiation. These effects are illustrated in Figures 9-6 and 9-7.

To maintain image quality, the density effects of field size changes must be compensated for by adjusting technique. It is recommended that such adjustments be made using mAs rather than kVp. Frequently collimation is used for the express purpose of reducing image fog and enhancing contrast. Use of a higher kVp level to compensate would result in more

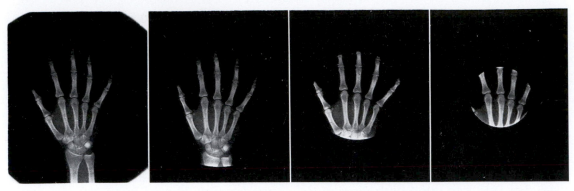

Figure 9-6. Series of radiographs of the hand to demonstrate the influence of the size of cones on the image. Note the enhancement of contrast and the loss of density with smaller cone sizes.

image fog, partially defeating this purpose. Since mAs compensation will not affect contrast, it will not cancel out the desired result, even partially. To maintain a given density, *collimation of the field size to a smaller area requires an increase in mAs from 35 to 50 percent* (and additional one-third to one-half the original mAs) depending on how extreme the change in field size is.

Changing from a 10 x 12 inch (24 x 30 cm) field to a typical cylinder on "cone" necessitates a 35 percent increase. For example, suppose that 30 mAs were used for a good view of the lumbar spine. The radiologist asks for a "coned-down" view of a few vertebrae. For this exposure, use 40 mAs, an increase of one-third. The most extreme change in field size would be encountered when changing from a 14 x 17

inch (35 x 43 cm) field to a cylinder, such as deriving a technique for a "coned-down" view of the gall bladder from a previous full abdomen view. In this case mAs must be increased by 50 percent or one-half. If the original abdomen were exposed using 40 mAs, increase to 60 mAs for the coned view.

Apparent exceptions to this rule can be attributed to other variables. For example, sinus radiographs are often "coned down" while a skull series is not, yet sinus techniques are usually somewhat *less* than skull techniques. In this case, the sinuses are air-filled cavities with fairly thin bones around them, very different tissue on average than the cranium, and much less technique is required for the sinus area. This required reduction is simply much greater than the effect from collimating affords in lightening

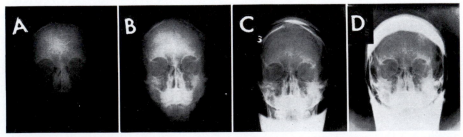

Figure 9-7. Series of radiographs of the PA sinuses which were all made using the same technique factors. (A) made without a cone, (B) made with a large cone, (C) and, (D) made with progressively smaller cones. Note the dramatic improvement of contrast and lesser density at smaller field sizes.

the image. Even though the smaller field size *does* lighten the image, additional reduction in technique is still needed here.

In the case of the coned-down view of the lumbosacral junction (L5-S1), technique must be increased much more than 50 percent as compared to the full lateral view, because, in addition to adjusting for coning down, additional penetration through the iliac bones is also required. Radiographers typically increase ten kVp from the full lateral technique for this view, equivalent to almost doubling the mAs. In the absence of other modifying conditions like these, the 35-50 percent rule of thumb may be applied with confidence to achieve consistent densities at different field sizes. As mentioned in the previous section, changing field size from 11 x 14 inches to 14 x 17 inches does not require any adjustment, simply because the added scatter radiation reaches a "saturation point" above 11 x 14 inches.

Example: The radiographs in Figure 9-6 were exposed using the same technique, but with progressively smaller field sizes. The presence of scatter fogging is apparent in the first of the series, causing an overall grayness and a loss of contrast. In Figure 9-7, the scattered radiation was mostly produced by the tabletop and cassette surrounding the anatomy of interest. As the field size is diminished, it can be clearly seen that the contrast is substantially enhanced. Further, the smaller field sizes demonstrate a significant loss of *density*. The mAs value should be increased by roughly one-third of the original to compensate for this density loss, assuming that the original density was desirable.

Ratio of Secondary to Primary Radiation

The ratio of secondary to primary radiation emitted by thin parts, such as the hand, is small, irrespective of the size of the field, because of the small amount of tissue irradiated. This does not hold true for the thicker and more dense structures. This fact is demonstrated in a series of radiographs of the frontal sinuses in Figure 9-7, wherein radiographs *A* to *C* were exposed with the same factors.

Radiograph *A* was made *without* a cone or cylinder; note the high image density that is largely attributable to fog generated by the neck and shoulder girdle. Radiograph *B* was made with a large cone and the fog is somewhat reduced because the tissue in the shoulder girdle has not been irradiated. Radiographs *C* and *D* were made with smaller cones and the fog density has been greatly reduced. The visibility of details is much improved because the small cone limits the *amount* of tissue exposed to radiation; hence, the quantity of secondary radiation is greatly diminished.

EFFECTS ON OTHER QUALITIES

While contrast increases and density decreases when employing smaller x-ray fields, sharpness of recorded detail, magnification, and distortion are unaffected. A common misconception is that scatter radiation affects the sharpness of recorded detail. This is false and is fully explained in Chapter 12. These recognizability functions involve the recording on the film of the edges of the anatomy of interest, all of which lies *within* the beam, and have nothing to do with where the *edges* of the beam might be, or in other words, how large the field size is.

CALCULATING FIELD SIZE COVERAGE

The total area of field size coverage is directly proportional to the square of the distance from the x-ray tube target to the film or image receptor. Any given side of a rectangular field, or the diameter of a circular field, is directly proportional to the SID. This relationship simply follows the laws of similar triangles, where the distances involved represent the height of the triangles and the sides or diameter of the fields represent the bases of the triangles, as illustrated in Figure 9-8. Where there are two apertures, as in collimators or extension cylinders, it is easiest to always use the diameter of the aperture *farthest away from the x-ray tube* as the base of the smaller triangle. This distance from the x-ray tube focal spot to that opening will be the height of the smaller triangle. Either of the two similar triangle formulae below may be used to arrive at a correct answer:

$$(1) \quad \frac{D1}{F1} = \frac{D2}{F2} \quad \text{or} \quad (2) \quad \frac{D1}{D2} = \frac{F1}{F2}$$

where *D1* is the distance from the x-ray tube focal spot to the aperture of the collimator or extension cylinder, *D2* is the distance from the focal spot to the film, *F1* is the size of the aperture opening, and *F2* is the field size at the film. These formulas are simple ratios and may be expressed in common English as follows:

(1) Distance 1 (collimator) is to Field size 1 (collimator) as Distance 2 (film) is to Field size 2 (film)

or

(2) Distance 1 (collimator) is to distance 2 (film) as Field size 1 (collimator) is to Field size 2 (film)

In practice, the radiographer should be able to make simple calculations of this type quickly *in his/her head*, since they are direct proportions. For example, if the distance to the film is twice the distance to the end of an extension cylinder, the round light field at the film will simply have twice the diameter of the end of the cylinder. For a rectangular field, the problem would have to be worked through twice, once for the length of the field, and once for its width.

Example: Collimator Coverage

Suppose that the indicators on an old collimator are not readable and the field light burned out. The bottom of the colli-

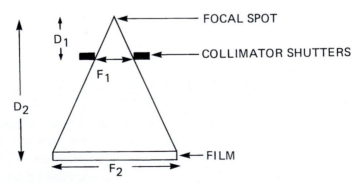

Figure 9-8. Diagram of similar triangle geometry formed by the x-ray beam. The field size is directly proportional to its distance from the focal spot.

mator is about 15 inches from the x-ray tube focal spot (which can be assumed to be 1-2 inches below the center of the cylindrical tube housing), and the SID being used is 45 inches. If the two pairs of shutters, which you can see through the collimator window, are three inches apart, what will be the length of the field at the film?

Solution using formula #1: $\dfrac{15}{3} = \dfrac{45}{X}$

$$X = \frac{3 \times 45}{15}$$

$$X = 9 \text{ inches}$$

This solution may be *mentally* found as follows: If the field size at the collimator is one-fifth the distance to the bottom of the collimator, the field size at the film will be one-fifth the distance to the film. One-fifth of 45 inches is 9 inches.

Example: Cone coverage

Suppose a new extension cylinder has been purchased. The bottom diameter of the cylinder is 4 inches, and the distance from the x-ray tube focal spot to that bottom rim is 10 inches. What is the diameter of the field coverage at an SID of 40 inches?

Solution using formula #1: $\dfrac{10}{40} = \dfrac{4}{X}$

$$X = \frac{4 \times 40}{10}$$

$$X = 16 \text{ inches}$$

This solution may be *mentally* found as follows: If the SID is 4 times the distance to the bottom of the collimator, then the field size at the film will be 4 times the field size at the collimator. Four times 4 inches is 16 inches.

A little practice will help the student become comfortable with these direct proportion ratios. Try Exercise 10 below, then check your answers from the Appendix.

EXERCISE #10

In the following exercises the "aperture" refers to the width of the bottom opening of a cone or extension cylinder or the bottom set of shutters in a collimator. Use the similar triangle proportions to fill in the missing size or distance:

	Distance from target (focal spot) to Source-Image Aperture	Field Size Receptor Distance	Size of Aperture	Field Size at Film
1.	10 inches	40 inches	6 inches	_____
2.	12 inches	36 inches	5 inches	_____
3.	20 inches	50 inches	4 inches	_____
4.	15 inches	60 inches	_____	16 inches
5.	18 inches	36 inches	_____	12 inches
6.	18 inches	45 inches	_____	25 inches
7.	15 inches	_____	5 inches	10 inches
8.	20 inches	_____	4 inches	12 inches
9.	_____	40 inches	6 inches	16 inches
10.	_____	72 inches	3 inches	12 inches

SUMMARY

1. X-ray field size must never be larger than necessary to include the anatomy of interest, or unnecessary patient *dose* will result as well as poor image quality.
2. Restriction of field size enhances image *contrast* by reducing the volume of exposed tissue available to produce scatter radiation.
3. Field size restriction reduces image *density*, which may need to be compensated for by increasing mAs up to 50 percent.
4. Field size has no relation to the *recognizability* functions in an image—sharpness of recorded detail, magnification, or distortion, because the penumbral geometry at the edges of the *image* are not changed.
5. Changes in field size are directly proportional to changes in the SID/SOD ratio when the *SOD* is considered to be the distance to the final aperture through which the x-ray beam passes.
6. Double-aperture collimators and extension cylinders reduce *off-focus radiation*.
7. Positive beam limitation, or *PBL*, should be overridden whenever a field size smaller than the film is appropriate.
8. Always allow one-half inch of field light beyond the anatomy of interest, unless it exceeds the film size.

REVIEW QUESTIONS

1. What are the two purposes of reducing field size?
2. Explain why reducing field size reduces image density:
3. The lower shutters in a collimator are 12 inches from the focal spot. If these shutters are opened to a 4-inch square, how big will the x-ray beam be at 42 inches from the focal spot?
4. The end of a 6-inch diameter extension cylinder is 15 inches from the focal spot. At what distance from the focal spot will you get a circular field with an 18-inch diameter?
5. To compensate image density for coming from a 14 x 17 inch field to a 5-inch square, by what percentage must you increase the mAs?
6. Why do collimators have two sets of shutters?
7. Even though collimation improves image quality, what is the *most* important reason to use it?
8. When should PBL collimator be overridden?
9. Always allow _____ -inch of field light beyond the anatomy of interest, unless it exceeds the film size.
10. Scatter radiation reaches a saturation level at field sizes above _____.
11. The more tissue exposed, the more _____ produced.

For the following sets of geometrical factors, fill in the blank:

	Distance from target (focal spot) to Aperture	Source-Image Receptor Distance	Size of Aperture	Field Size at Film
12.	12 inches	36 inches	4 inches	_____
13.	15 inches	60 inches	_____	12 inches
14.	12 inches	_____	5 inches	10 inches
15.	_____	40 inches	3 inches	12 inches

Chapter 10

PATIENT STATUS AND CONTRAST AGENTS

THE RELATIVE DIFFERENCES in the composition and thickness of tissue components exert a great influence on the radiation traversing it. This applies not alone to different parts of the same body, but also to the same parts of different bodies.

Absorption is intimately associated with the atomic number of the tissue elements being irradiated. Bone is less penetrable than the surrounding soft tissue. The pathologic and physiologic states of tissue are also important when considering absorption differences. Selection and alteration of exposure factors must be made with these facts in mind.

PHYSIQUE

No two human physiques are identical. Not only do they differ in their general family and racial physical characteristics, but individual parts vary widely in size, shape, and tissue density. Naturally, gradations between the types of physiques do occur.

In radiography, therefore, any x-ray exposure system should encompass all of the body deviations with sufficient latitude so that radiographs of diagnostic utility can be produced with some measure of standardization.

BODY HABITUS

The analysis of a living body for radiographic purposes requires its classification into one of four types, or more pertinently, *somatotypes*. Also, some discernment as to the physiology of the body should be made as well as an estimate as to the influence of disease or trauma on tissues. There are four general types of physique classified under the term habitus—hypersthenic, sthenic, hyposthenic, and asthenic.

The characteristics of each body type resolve into states wherein they can be generally separated from each other. Although it is not possible to strike much of an average in classification, by studying the extremes of each type, a definite understanding of the variables in physique that must be met in radiography can be achieved and exposure compromises effected.

Hypersthenic

The hypersthenic body type is characterized by softness and roundness throughout the various body regions. The tissues tend to be flabby with an excess of subcutaneous fat. The torso is barrel-like. The AP and lateral thicknesses are comparable. Abdominal and thoracic volume is predominant as compared to the head and extremities. The chest is relatively short and wide at the base. The neck is short and thick and the waistline is high. The vertebral column is relatively straight when viewed laterally and the back is well padded with fat.

This type tends to become obese and is often a victim of hypertension. Degenerative diseases of the heart, arteries, and kidneys are common to the type.

Sthenic

The sthenic type is strong and active. The joints and bones are large. The physique is heavy in muscle and bone and relatively rectangular in shape. The skin is thick with an abundance of underlying connective tissue. These persons are physically well-balanced.

The measurement of the torso is typically eight centimeters less in the AP than in the lateral dimension. The well-developed chest is larger than the abdomen. The trunk is long with the waist slender and low. The neck is long and the clavicles are heavy and predominant.

Asthenic

The asthenic type exhibits a sense of linearity and delicateness of body. The neck is long and slender and projects forward. Small bones and stringy muscles prevail. The thorax is long, flat and narrow. The ribs are thin and prominent and the shoulders narrow without muscle relief. The scapulae tend to protrude posteriorly. The trunk is short and the limbs long. The abdomen is flat and shallow in depth.

Hyposthenic

The hyposthenic body habitus is not as extreme a variation as the hypersthenic or asthenic. In body size, it lies somewhere between the sthenic and the asthenic types, but may be described as very thin. The primary distinction between the asthenic habitus and the hyposthenic habitus is not in size but in condition: While the asthenic patient is physically weak and emaciated due to pathological conditions, appears sickly, and is often advanced in age, the hyposthenic patient is young, active, and relatively strong but is definitely underweight for his height and extremely thin compared to the average.

In spite of their small size, hyposthenic patients have a body composition with muscle/fat tissue ratios similar to sthenic patients, and, therefore, technique may be adjusted (from average technique) entirely in accordance with their size without further considerations as to condition. A technique chart with small enough measurements represented on it may be followed.

The foregoing physical characteristics are, of course, the extreme variants of the four somatotypes. The body being an intermixture of all types may exhibit in a more or less dominant manner special characteristics of one or the other type. Knowing the general characteristics of the extremes makes the analysis of the patient a little easier for radiographic purposes.

BODY TISSUES

For medical radiography, body tissues may be divided roughly into two groups: those consisting largely of *organic* materials (soft tissue) and those containing organic materials impregnated with *inorganic* substances (bone). Organic tissues comprise the skin, fat, muscle, cartilage, tendon, nerve trunks, brain, blood vessels, visceral organs, etc., which all contain a large amount of fluid when compared to inorganic tissues. Organic tissues are composed of carbon, hydrogen, nitrogen, and oxygen, and they possess low x-ray absorption properties. Muscle tissue contains approximately 75 to 80 percent fluid; fat stores little fluid–about 20 percent. Pulmonary tissue, on the other hand, contains a large quantity of moisture-laden air in the living state.

Muscles, body fluids, connective tissues, and solid viscera have about the same degree of x-ray absorption as water, whereas fat and air-laden pulmonary tissue offer considerably less absorption. Females and young children have a higher percentage of body fat than adult males. Alteration in the fat content is probably the most important single variable, other than disease, that determines the water content of the body at any given period of life.

The normal adult bony and cartilaginous skeleton comprises approximately 20 percent of the total body weight. Living bone is a versatile tissue possessing an organic matrix (collagen) upon which mineral salts have been deposited. It furnishes the supporting framework of the body. It is soft in young persons and hard in the older. The minerals in bone are primarily calcium phosphate and calcium carbonate in a ratio of 2:1.

An infant's bones are seldom as well delineated radiographically as those of an adult because their mineral content is less. The radiographic appearance of bone is directly related to its mineral content. Normal adult bone possesses high x-ray absorption characteristics. The function of the bone marrow is to form blood. The *erythroblasts* and other blood-forming cells in the marrow naturally have a high repro-

ductive rate, thereby making the bone marrow one of the more radiation-sensitive organs of the body. Bone is in a constant state of building up and tearing down a little at a time. In growth, bone is built by erosion (by osteoclasts) of the inside of the bone (medulla) thereby enlarging the medullary cavity, while bone-forming cells (osteoblasts) build up the bone externally. Bone fractures are repaired by the laying down of a soft fibrous tissue called *callus* that largely originates in the periosteum and joins the ends of the fractured segments. The callus is replaced gradually with hard, new bone due to the action of the osteoblasts. The jagged edges that might interfere with function are smoothed away by the osteoclasts. The old, healed fracture presents the appearance of a "swollen" portion of the shaft of a bone, where it has been made both thicker and denser for future protection. This increased density and thickness at the sights of large calluses may require an increase in radiographic technique (kVp) to be fully penetrated.

Growth in the length of bones is quite different. In childhood, each bone contains a disk of cartilage called the *epiphyseal plate* at its ends. As growth takes place, this disk of cartilage extends itself and the part nearest the bone absorbs calcium to make new bone. In adulthood this cartilage is replaced completely by bone.

On average, human body fluids comprise about 62 percent of body weight. Bodies of the lean muscular type may contain approximately 70 percent fluids, whereas obese bodies may contain as little as 42 percent. Fluid content is a major factor in the generation of scatter radiation by the body tissues. Fluids exist in localized quantities in the urinary, gastrointestinal, biliary and circulatory systems, in joint spaces, glands, spinal cord, and ventricular spaces of the brain. If such structures are to be differentiated from surrounding soft tissues, they must be infused with or surrounded with some contrast agent that will provide the necessary x-ray absorption to produce subject contrast in the image.

EVALUATION OF THE PATIENT

The radiographer must continually train his or her eyes and mind in evaluating the patient for radiographic purposes. The body must be viewed as a physiological or pathological entity with varying degrees of hydration, nutrition, calcification, or disease. Evaluation should be based upon the patient's physique and clinical situation. The radiographer should be able after some clinical experience to recognize deviations from the normal or average, since these changes intimately affect the choice of exposure factors. A lean, well-trained athlete will likely require more radiation, more penetration, and produce more scatter radiation than another patient of the same size but differing condition.

INFLUENCE OF AGE

During the early months of a child's life, weight gain is rapid, doubling in the first six months and tripling at the end of a year. Thence the gain in weight and size is slower but steady until about the eighteenth year. Throughout life there is a constant flux in bone mineralization. During the growth period, bone formation is more rapid that resorption. During middle-age, bone formation and bone resorption is in balance. In later life, resorption exceeds bone growth and mineralization decreases. Lower kVp levels are required to avoid overpenetration of bone and excessive density on radiographs of elderly patients. There is also some *atrophy*, or loss of body water and minerals, from soft-tissue organs.

Pediatric techniques are often derived by modifying adult techniques according to the proportionate thicknesses of the anatomy. It is well to note the proportionate differences in the growth of various body parts throughout our physical development: The femur (thigh) represents the extreme in growth—it is over five times longer and thicker in an adult than in an infant. On the other hand, the human skull expands less than three times its original diameter from infancy. This means that the pediatric technique for a skull will be roughly one-third to one-half that of an adult skull technique, while the pediatric technique for a femur will be as little as one-fifth that of an adult.

ANTHROPOLOGICAL FACTORS

There are physical differences in the mass, density, and shape of various bones for different human races, which are often substantial enough to require adjustments in technique. This is particularly true for skull radiography. A workable rule-of-thumb cannot be stated for any particular anthropological group, for at least two reasons: there is too much variation within a racial group, and racial groups have become widely intermixed. However, an observant radiographer will recognize those patients whose skull appears to have greater bony mass than average, and *increase techniques by approximately one-third from the average mAs.*

There are three anthropological categories for skull shapes: *Mesocephalic* skulls are roundly oval in cross-section, with an angle of approximately 47 degrees between the mid-sagittal plane and the petrous pyramids. These represent an average so far as radiographic technique is concerned. *Dolichocephalic* skulls are extremely oval in cross-sectional shape, narrow side-to-side, and long front-to-back, with a petrous ridge angle of roughly 40 degrees. On such skulls, there will be a greater difference in the technique required when changing from the PA projection to the lateral projection, and the lateral projection may require somewhat less technique than the average skull. *Brachicephalic* skulls are very round in cross-sectional shape and broad, with a typical petrous ridge angle of about 54 degrees. These types of skulls frequently present a thicker bony mass in addition to their broader shape, and may require up to one-third more mAs for *all* views taken.

SOFT TISSUE–BONE RELATION

The proportion of bone to soft tissue is fairly static for a given anatomical part. If the part is naturally large, the probabilities are that the bone is large and has a proportionate amount of soft tissue covering it. The radiographer must judge whether the part is *naturally* small, average, or large. The aggregate of the tissues possesses a certain thickness-density ratio that influences the degree of x-ray absorption that will take place. This fact must be considered when determining the amount of penetration that is necessary. This penetration level dictates the minimum kVp required for each body part, regardless of variable thicknesses between patients. Table 6-1 in Chapter 6 lists the optimum kVp levels for each body part.

BODY THICKNESS

Human beings are dissimilar in their thickness characteristics. These tend to change in varying degrees during life and in health and disease. Despite these human differences, it is possible to establish certain pattern measurements for radiographic purposes that conform to what may be termed *average* thickness ranges. Such measurements can be standardized and are an important means toward standardization of radiographic exposure factors.

The type of calipers to be used for measuring different body parts is shown in Figure 10-1. *All measurements should be made along the course of the projected central ray.* Usually the nonmovable leg of the calipers is placed opposite the body entrance point for the central ray and the movable leg is closed until it just makes contact with the skin. The calipers should not be squeezed for tissue will be displaced and a true measurement will not be obtained.

Chest measurements should normally be made with the patient standing or sitting as they will be radiographed, under normal respiration. The thickness of the pectoral muscles must be included, therefore measurements should be taken at the level of the seventh thoracic vertebra where the central ray is directed. Generally, this is the area about one inch above the nipple-line.

For radiography of the abdomen, measurements are normally made with the patient supine and at rest. The nonmovable leg of the calipers is place in a horizontal plane next to the skin posteriorly; the mov-

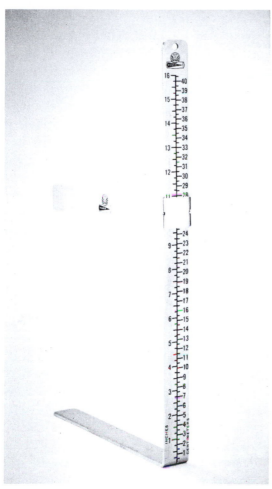

Figure 10-1. Photograph of calipers used for measurement of body parts.

the skin very tight. When gas or fluid are present, the radiographer should make allowances in setting the mAs factor. When the patient is standing or sitting erect, it should be recognized that abdominal organs will gravitate toward the pelvis, packing together and increasing the overall density and thickness to be penetrated. An increase in technique from average is usually required for upright abdominal and pelvic radiography.

Patient weight and patient height are not reliable indices of x-ray absorption and cannot be used as guides in formulating or standardizing radiographic exposures. Reliable techniques may be determined only by using the *measured part thickness* as a fundamental guide, with the patient's condition (and resulting alterations in tissue composition) taken into account by the radiographer.

THICKNESS RANGES

Statistically, the frequency with which adult patients conform to an average thickness range for a given projection is relatively high. Since the x-ray absorption properties of human tissues are *unpredictable*, some latitude in compensating for this fact can be made. Table 10-1 presents the data from thousands of accurate measurements of body part thicknesses that were made for various projections. The frequency with which various thicknesses appeared for each given projection was then tabulated. The higher thickness frequencies for each projection were then grouped into an *average thickness range*, to which could be applied a common set of exposure factors with the assurance that satisfactory radiographic quality would be obtained in more than 85 percent of cases.

The implications of Table 10-1 for radiographic technique are very significant

able arm is then closed so that it just touches the anterior wall of the abdomen. It is important *not* to simply place the nonmovable leg of the calipers on the tabletop, but rather to pull it up into contact with the patient's back. This way a true measurement will be obtained that does not include any air space in the gap behind the patient's lower back and the tabletop. Along with this measurement, the radiographer should gently palpate the abdomen to determine any condition of gas or fluid distention—a gas-filled abdomen feels unusually soft and malleable, whereas a fluid-distended abdomen feels hard and

Table 10-1

TABLE LISTING AVERAGE THICKNESS RANGES FOR VARIOUS PROJECTIONS AND THE FREQUENCY WITH WHICH THE ADULT PATIENT DIMENSIONS FALL INTO EACH AVERAGE RANGE

Region	AP	PA	LAT	Per Cent Frequency
Thumb, fingers, toes	1.5–4			99
Hand	3–5			99
			7–10	93
Wrist	3–6			99
			5–8	98
Forearm	6–8			94
			7–9	92
Elbow	6–8			96
			7–9	87
Arm	7–10			95
			7–10	94
Shoulder	12–16			79
Clavicle		13–17		82
Foot	6–8			92
			7–9	91
Ankle	8–10			86
			6–9	96
Leg	10–12			85
			9–11	89
Knee	10–13			92
			9–12	92
Thigh	14–17			77
			13–16	76
Hip	17–21			76
Cervical C1-3	12–14			77
Vertebrae C4-7	11–14			98
C1-7			10–13	90
Thoracic Vertebrae	20–24			76
			28–32	81
Lumbar Vertebrae	18–22			69
			27–32	77
Pelvis	19–23			78
Skull		18–21		96
			14–17	88
Sinuses Frontal		18–21		97
Maxillary		18–22		88
			13–17	96
Mandible			10–12	82
		20–25		82
Chest	OBL		27–32	84
	24–30			83

indeed. First, these statistics show that techniques can be usefully standardized, because a relatively high percentage of patients fall within the "average range" of thickness for most types of projections. Note that for most distal extremities, and skulls, more than 90 percent of all adult patients will conform to a single "average" technique. The lowest percentage in Table 10-1 is for the AP projection of the lumbar spine, at 69 percent. The AP lumbar spine may be considered equivalent to the AP abdomen projection. Therefore, it might be safely stated from this statistic, that even for abdominal radiography, two out of three patients will conform to a single "average" technique. *Radiographic technique can be confidently approached in a systematic way.*

Second, the radiography student can extrapolate average thicknesses to memorize from Table 10-1. These provide an essential starting point from which to derive techniques for various thicknesses of body parts. Note that, combining the figures for the chest, thoracic spine, lumbar spine, and pelvis, *average thicknesses for the adult torso in general may be stated as 22 centimeters (about 8 1/2 inches) in AP projection, and 30 centimeters (about 12 inches) in lateral projection.* You should memorize these two measurements so that technique adjustments can be made for various torso thicknesses.

Part thickness affects the absorption of x-ray photons in an exponential fashion, that is, small changes in thickness cause great changes in the absorption of photons. Radiographers must become adept at adjusting the mAs in exponential proportion to body thickness variations between patients. A very workable rule-of-thumb for this relationship is: *Every four centimeters of thickness affects image density by a factor of two.* A patient measuring 26 cm through the torso, then, would absorb twice as much radiation, and require twice the mAs to compensate, when compared to the average 22-cm patient. Failing to make this doubling of technique, the radiograph would turn out one-half as dark.

The corresponding rule-of-thumb for technique, then, is: *For every four centimeters of thickness, change the mAs by a factor of two.* Thus, an 18-cm patient would require one-half the mAs of the average 22-cm patient, and a 26-cm patient would require twice the mAs. This rule is not only useful on a daily basis but can also be applied effectively in developing technique charts to

standardize and control exposure to patients (Chapter 27).

Try the following brief exercise to practice the *four-centimeter rule*, then check your answers from the Appendix.

EXERCISE #11

For each of the following problems, list the actual mAs you would use based on the part thickness rule:

	Technique Chart		Actual Part	
Part	mAs	Thickness	Thickness	mAs Used
1. Elbow	5	6 cm	10 cm	_____
2. Femur	10	17 cm	13 cm	_____
3. UGI AP	7.5	20 cm	25 cm	_____
4. L-Spine AP	30	24 cm	16 cm	_____
5. Chest	10	22 cm	24 cm	_____

Scatter Radiation

The problem of scatter radiation fog increases in proportion to the thickness of the part. It has been found that the radiation emerging from a tissue thickness of 6 inches may assume a ratio of scatter radiation to primary radiation of 5 to 1, and with

greater thicknesses it may rise to 10 to 1.

Also, larger patients attenuate more of the primary x-ray photons and there is less useful exposure to the film. Radiographic density decreases, and, at the same time, since the ratio of scattered radiation to primary radiation has increased, radiographic contrast is reduced.

MOLECULAR COMPOSITION

Apart from the thickness of the part, the degree of absorption of x-rays in the patient is primarily determined by two molecular factors: (1) the average atomic number of the tissue, and (2) the average physical density of the tissue. Attenuation (absorption) of x-ray photons is affected by the atomic number of atoms through which they pass in an exponential way. Relatively small differences in atomic number between tissues will result in large differences in the penetration or absorption of the x-ray beam. Specifically, photon attenuation is roughly proportional to the cube

of the atomic number. For example, the average atomic number of bone is around 20 and that of soft tissue, which is mostly water, is about 7.4. Cubing each number yields 8000 and roughly 405, respectively. Now, by dividing 8000 by 400, it can be found that bone is approximately 20 times more effective in attenuating x-rays than is soft tissue by virtue of its larger atomic nuclei (calcium, phosphorus, etc.).

The physical density of the molecules in a particular tissue (how *tightly packed* they are) is directly proportional to x-ray absorption. Bone tissue is about twice as dense as soft tissue and will therefore absorb roughly twice as many x-ray photons by virtue of its density.

To find the *total* difference between bone and soft tissue in attenuating the x-ray beam, multiply the effect of atomic number (20 times) and the effect of physical density (2 times); overall, bone is 40 times more effective. That is, bone stops 40 x-rays for every x-ray stopped by soft tissue.

Comparing the exponential effect of atomic number with the proportional effect of physical tissue density, it can be clearly seen that the major molecular factor bearing upon the penetration of the x-ray beam is atomic number. This is further supported by the fact that atomic numbers in the human body vary much more than most tissue densities do. Most tissues are close to water density. This is why the stomach is not normally contrasty against the surrounding muscle tissue unless a contrast agent is added.

There are, however, two exceptions to the predominance of atomic number in producing subject contrast: lung tissue and fat tissue. In the exceptional case of the lungs, the density of the air with which they are insufflated is about 0.001, while the physical density of the surrounding soft tissues is about 1.0. This is a dramatic ratio of difference, 1000 to 1. On the other hand, the difference in atomic number in this case is very slight: air has an average atomic number of about 7.6, while soft tissue's atomic number is about 7.4. Clearly, the air is demonstrated on a radiographic image primarily due to an extreme difference in *physical density* rather than to the small difference in atomic number. Air in the lungs is demonstrated with contrast against the background of soft tissue primarily because of this extreme density difference.

Fat is also substantially less dense than other soft tissues. Fat is only about 20 percent fluid, while other soft tissues are as much as 80 percent fluid. This is enough difference for fat to show up slightly darker than surrounding muscles and organs on a radiograph. Careful scrutiny of the radiograph in Figure 10-2B demonstrates that the kidneys would not be distinctly visible against the background densities of muscles and other organs, if it were not for the fact that each kidney is encapsulated in a thick layer of fat which creates on a radiograph a darker density outlining each kidney. For differences in the physical density of tissues to produce visible subject contrast in the image, these differences in physical density must be very great.

There are basically only five types of materials visible on conventional radiographs: *gas, fat, fluid, bone,* and *metal.* All soft tissues are roughly of fluid density, equal to water radiographically. Barium and iodine compounds are, chemically, liquid metals. They show up very light on a radiograph for the same reason that a bullet or other solid metallic object would. Using soft tissue as a background, air and fat are demonstrated on a radiograph because of the *extreme* differences in their physical density. On the other hand, bones and metals including contrast agents are demonstrated primarily because of their different atomic numbers (larger atoms).

Generally, small deviations from the normal in tissue density or thickness can be ignored. Where a body part contains thick heavy bone surrounded by a large quantity of muscle and fat, as in the lumbar region, x-ray absorption differences become relatively wide (Fig. 10-2A). This is due mostly to differences in atomic number between bone and soft tissue. The image of the calcified body in Figure 10-2C provides easy visibility against the darker adjacent densities of its containing lung tissues because of their extremely low physical density. As a

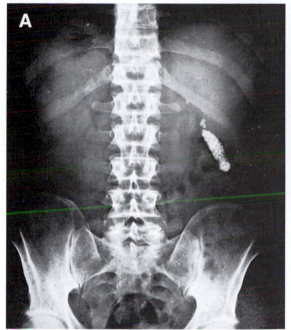

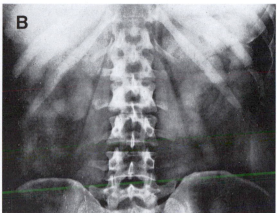

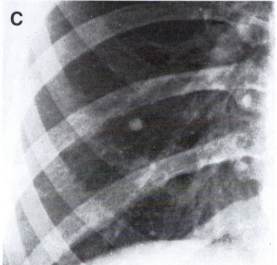

Figure 10-2. (A) Screen-grid radiograph of AP abodomen, showing wide absorption differences between tissues and contrast agent. (B) Screen-grid AP radiograph of kidney region that exhibits small differences in density between tissues of comparable physical density and atomic number. (C) Portion of PA chest radiograph showing a calcification of medium contrast against a background of pulmonary tissues.

rule, such parts provide little difficulty in recording even though large errors in exposure may be made.

In Figure 10-2B, the absorption differences between the kidney, liver and gall bladder are small and differentiation becomes difficult. These organs are all close in both their physical densities and their atomic numbers. A shorter gray scale (higher contrast) in the image would be helpful in better demonstrating these organs.

USE OF CONTRAST AGENTS

Contrast agents are employed to render high subject contrast in a viscus that normally has very low subject contrast. These agents comprise various nontoxic chemical preparations that have high absorption properties. They are either injected or ingested into the viscus before radiography if performed. Air is also very useful on occasion because of its very low x-ray absorption properties. The alimentary tract normally cannot be differentiated from surrounding soft tissues and it must be filled with a barium or iodine compound of high purity to be demonstrated (Fig. 10-3A). Study of the urinary tract function requires the injection of an iodine compound into the circulatory system, which will then be filtered out of the blood by the kidneys and passed along the ureters to the bladder. Study of the urinary tract can also be undertaken by inserting catheters into the ureters and injecting an iodinated agent in retrograde fashion up the ureters to the renal pelves (Fig. 10-3C). Air is often injected into the large intestine to augment the contrast properties of barium sulfate during a radiographic study of the colon (Fig. 10-3D). The gall bladder may be demonstrated (Fig. 10-3F) with the iodine digested from oral preparations.

Contrast agents may be categorized in several ways. The broadest division would be to distinguish between those agents which attenuate x-rays much *more* than soft tissue does, and those agents which attenuate much *less* of the x-ray beam than soft tissue, allowing the x-rays to penetrate through and reach the film. Contrast agents which attenuate x-rays, resulting in a light area on the radiograph, are called *positive* contrast agents. Positive contrast agents are normally fluids, and these may be further subdivided into injectables, ingestibles, and oily-viscous media. Contrast agents which allow more x-rays to penetrate through, resulting in a dark area on the radiograph, are referred to as *negative* contrast agents. Negative contrast agents are all gaseous. Common examples include normal room air which may be drawn up into a syringe or trapped in a bag, carbon dioxide, and nitrous oxide.

Although there are many types and brand names of positive contrast agents, each having different specific chemical formulae, they are all based on either the element *iodine* or the element *barium* bound into molecules with organic salts to make them nontoxic. These two elements are used on account of their very high atomic numbers. The viscosity, density or weight of these fluids has virtually nothing to do with their ability to attenuate x-rays. As discussed in the previous section, the atomic number (the *size* of the atoms used) is the single most significant control over x-ray absorption. The atomic number of iodine is 53 and that of barium 56. These atoms simply have lots of orbital electrons with which x-rays may "collide," 53 electrons and 56 electrons respectively, all packed into the small space of one atom. Since the absorption of x-rays is proportional to the cube of the atomic number, these elements in their pure form are *hundreds of times* more absorbing than soft tissue with its atomic number of 7.6. Iodine, for example, absorbs 531 times more x-rays than soft tissue. The content of iodine or barium in a typical contrast agent, however, is somewhat diluted by the other organic salts and water that make up the agent.

For maximum radiographic information, it is essential to be able to see *through* the bolus of a positive contrast agent. This means that the x-rays in the beam must be of sufficient energy to penetrate through the agent and record information on the film. Otherwise, the radiologist will only be able to observe the tangential edges of the bolus, that is, only a small portion of the outermost lining of the organ of interest (Fig. 6-14). The middle portions of the organ, filled with a thick bolus of contrast agent, will appear as a blank white density on the radiograph, with no information presented. In order for the beam to penetrate through the agent and record information on the film, a certain minimum kVp is required. As listed in Table 6-1, the *optimum kVp recommended for penetration of iodine is 76 - 80, that for a thick solid-column*

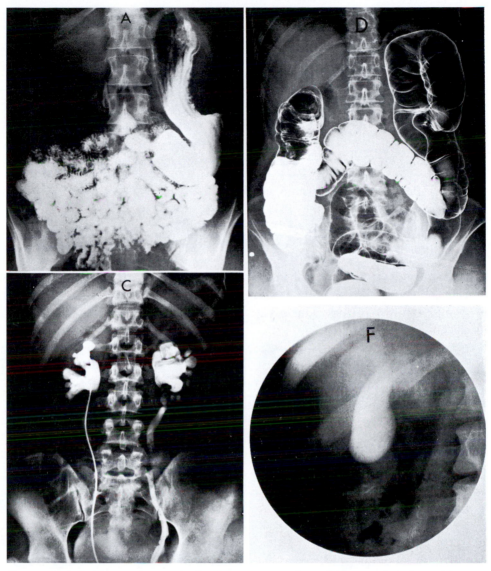

Figure 10-3. Radiographs in which contrast agents have been employed to delineate anatomic structures: (A) stomach and small intestine, (C) kidneys and ureters, (D) colon, and, (F) gall bladder.

of barium is 116-120 kVp, and for air-contrast barium studies about 90-94 kVp.

Negative contrast agents, which are always gases, do not present a significant difference in atomic number than soft tissue or water (Z# for air = 7.6, Z# for soft tissue = 7.4). Therefore, their ability to produce contrast in the image is not related to the ratio of photoelectric interactions to Compton interactions. Rather, because they have such an extreme difference in physical density (1/1000th that of soft tissue), *all* interactions, photoelectric and Compton, are so reduced that the majority of the x-rays in the beam penetrate through to darken the film.

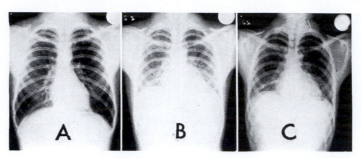

Figure 10-4. Screen radiographs of PA chest, (A) made upon inspiration, (B & C) upon expiration. All were taken at 80 kVp and the same distance; A and B: 2.5 mAs, C: 3.3 mAs.

INFLUENCE OF RESPIRATION

In radiography of the thorax, the influence of respiration on the overall image density should be recognized. The great permeability of air-containing tissues to x-rays presents no problem to radiographic exposure. But, when the patient is not cor-

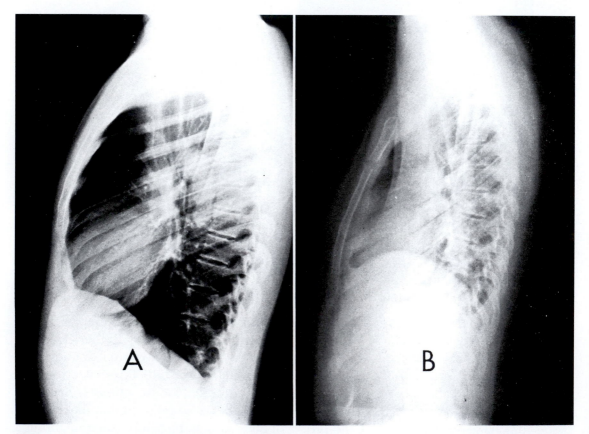

Figure 10-5. Screen radiographs of lateral chest demonstrating influence of respiration on density: (A) made at inspiration, (B) at expiration. Both were taken at 85 kVp and the same distance, A: 10 mAs, B: 13.3 mAs.

rectly instructed to take a large inspiration, confusing results may be obtained. If an exposure is made on expiration or on partial expiration, the resulting consolidation of pulmonary tissues will cause underexposure and a loss of radiographic density. Whenever an exposure to the lungs is made on expiration, an approximate increase of one-third in the mAs is necessary to maintain sufficient image density.

Example 1. These conditions may be illustrated by three radiographs of the PA chest in Figure 10-4. Radiograph *A* was exposed at full inspiration and radiograph *B* upon full expiration, using identical exposure factors. Note the overall loss of density in radiograph *B*. Radiograph *C* was

then made using an increase of one-third in the mAs. The position of the heart and diaphragms in *C* show it to be on expiration, but the increased mAs has restored the radiograph to a diagnostic density level.

Example 2. To demonstrate the appearance of the image obtained in both respiratory phases for lateral radiography of the chest, radiographs *A* and *B* in Figure 10-5 were obtained. Radiograph *B*, taken on expiration, also employed an increase in mAs of 33 percent to compensate for the consolidation of pulmonary tissues. In radiography of the chest, *the mAs should be increased by at least one-third when exposure is made on expiration.*

EFFECTS ON OTHER QUALITIES

The condition of the patient and the use of contrast media affect density and contrast, the visibility functions in the image. They do not, however, make details which are already visible any sharper, less magnified, or distorted. These geometrical functions are not directly affected by patient status. Nonetheless, there can be *indirect* relationships between patient status and the geometrical image qualities: first, large patient thicknesses *may* result in increased object-to-image receptor distance for some

particular parts of interest, such as the sternum, which are close to one side of the body. By changing the patient position from PA to AP or vice versa, this problem can be alleviated, thus preventing undue magnification and unsharpness. But, remember that it is the OID created by the position rather than the patient status which is directly responsible for these effects. Second, patient motion can destroy image sharpness. The effects of motion are discussed in Chapter 23.

SUMMARY

1. Average thickness ranges have been established which apply to more than 85 percent of all patients for all body parts. Standardized *technique charts* are therefore applicable to a high percentage of patients and should be regularly used by radiographers.

2. Although average techniques are faci-

litated by the use of standardized technique charts, each patient must be individually evaluated by the radiographer for fine *technique adjustments* based upon body habitus, condition including disease, gender, race, age, etc.

3. Hypersthenic and very large, muscular patients present a special problem with

reduced image *contrast* and loss of density, so that other technique factors must be manipulated to restore these image qualities to some degree.

4. Technique should be adjusted by a factor of two for every four centimeters change in body *thickness.*

5. The *five materials demonstrated on radiographs* are, from most radiopaque to most radiolucent: metals, bone, fluid, fat, and air.

6. *Subject contrast* between body tissues is primarily a function of average atomic number, because it has an exponential effect on the occurrence of photoelectric interactions. Two exceptions to this rule are the lungs and fat, where tissue density becomes the main factor.

7. *Positive contrast agents* work in producing high subject contrast because their high atomic numbers (large atoms) multiply the occurrence of photoelectric interactions, not because they are viscous, dense, or heavy.

8. *Negative contrast agents* produce subject contrast because of their extremely low physical density as gasses.

9. The penetration necessary for a body part depends upon the ratio of one tissue type to another, based primarily upon their atomic numbers. *Optimum kVp* levels have been established for each body part and for contrast media procedures.

10. *Expiration chests* require an increase in technique of at least one-third mAs.

11. Patient status and contrast agents have no direct relationship to the geometrical functions in the image–sharpness of recorded detail, magnification, and distortion.

12. The *average torso thicknesses* are 22 cm in AP projection and 30 cm in lateral projection.

13. Greater increases in technique are required for large muscular or fluid-distended patients than for fatty, obese patients of similar measurement.

REVIEW QUESTIONS

1. Define *hypersthenic.*
2. Define *asthenic.*
3. On which two types of body habitus can a regular technique chart be followed without adjusting technique for anything but body part thickness?
4. Define *atrophy:*
5. What technique adjustment is required for a chest radiograph or *expiration?*

What proportion or percentage of adult patients fall within the "average" thickness range for technique purposes, for the following procedures:

6. Lumbar Spine AP:
7. Sinuses PA:

8. Foot AP;
9. Barium Enema AP:
10. Why do positive contrast agents work?
11. Your technique chart lists 200 mA at one-fourth second for a 24-cm L-spine. You are doing an L-spine on a very thin 16-cm patient. What *total mAs* should you use:
12. On the above patient, what new mAs would you use for a *lateral view,* assuming that the above mAs was correct for the AP view:
13. What is the optimum kVp for penetrating iodine:
14. What is the optimum kVp for penetrating barium:
15. Why do large patients reduce contrast

in the image?

16. What are the average measurements in cm for the torso in AP and lateral projections?

17. List the five general types of materials that are demonstrated on radiographs.

18. Muscular patients require (more, less, or equal) technique when compared to fatty patients of the same measured size:

19. Define *callus*:

20. For average patients, what percent of the body is composed of fluids:

21. What part of the body changes *least* in size from infant to adult:

22. What type of skull presents the greatest difference in technique between the PA and the lateral projections?

23. All measurements of body parts should be taken along the path of the _____.

24. The skin of a fluid-distended abdomen feels _____.

25. Bone stops how many x-rays for every x-ray stopped by soft tissue:

Chapter 11

PATHOLOGY AND CASTS

THE CONDITION OF THE PATIENT is the greatest variable the radiographer faces in producing quality radiographs. In addition to being aware of the normal variations in body habitus, tissue composition, age, bony structure, stage of respiration, presence of contrast agents, and thickness of body parts, discussed in the last chapter, one must also be conscious of abnormal changes due to pathology or medical intervention.

The radiographer must determine the image details that are to be accentuated and, if necessary, make suitable adjustment in the exposure factors. No matter what departures from the normal there may be in the radiographic density of these details, they must be clearly demonstrated if a correct radiologic identification is to be made of existing disease or trauma. When an abnormal *increase* in tissue absorption takes place, the radiographic density *decreases* from the normal value. When a *decrease* in tissue absorption occurs, a corresponding *increase* over the normal in radiographic density takes place.

The radiographer should ascertain the reason that each procedure was ordered, because this knowledge often includes information that bears upon technique selection and can thus prevent repeated exposures. To obtain this information, the radiographer should review the x-ray requisition prior to every procedure, and also obtain a brief verbal history from the patient if possible. In situations that are unclear, additional information may be obtained from the patient's chart. Radiographers should have at least a rudimentary ability to interpret patient charts. Careful observation of patients frequently provides readily apparent signs of conditions that bear on technique selection. It should be emphasized that obtaining pertinent patient history and assessing conditions that affect radiographic technique are the responsibility of the *radiographer*, not the referring physician or radiologist.

Not all diseases are radiographically visible. Many do not appreciably affect the densities present in the image, and are therefore of no concern in determining techniques. For a pathological condition to require a technique adjustment, it must substantially alter the presence and amount of one of the five radiographically demonstrable materials: Air, fat, fluid, bone or metal.

ADDITIVE DISEASES

Abnormal conditions which lead to an increase in *fluid, bone,* or *metal* are, for radiographic purposes, generally considered as *additive conditions.* They require added exposure, or increased technique factors, in order to be properly demonstrated. In the

162

case of excessive bone tissue or metals, the increase in technique is necessitated mostly because of their high average atomic numbers (large atoms). For fluid accumulation in the lungs (Fig. 11-1), an increase in factors is required because the fluid is nearly a thousand times more dense that the air which is normally present (there are one thousand molecules of fluid for every molecule of air). Fluid distention of the abdomen, on the other hand, does not substantially change atomic numbers nor tissue density, but results in an increase in part thickness constituting a bolus of nearly pure liquid, and requires *more* technique than the *four-centimeter rule* would normally dictate. In each of these cases, more x-ray photons are absorbed by the body tissues, and if an increase in technical factors is not

effected, an underexposed, light radiograph will result.

For additive diseases, technique may need to be increased from 35 percent (one-third) to over 100 percent (doubling) if the disease is in an advanced stage. *As a rule of thumb, increase overall technique by 50 percent for additive diseases in an advanced stage—this is in addition* too adjustments for part thickness. Since many of these diseases change the content of minerals in tissue, a change in penetration is indicated. In such cases, the kVp should be altered using the 15 percent rule, rather than increasing mAs. An 8 percent increase in kVp will be equivalent to a 50 percent increase in mAs.

Table 11-1 lists those diseases which are commonly encountered in radiography and which may require substantial increas-

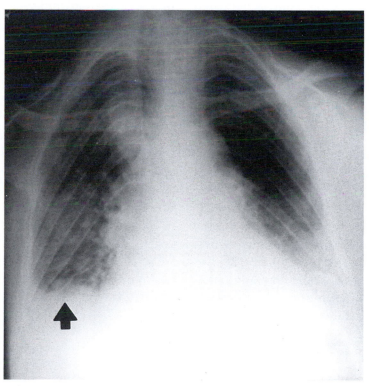

Figure 11-1. Radiograph using increased technique for a patient presenting with cardiomegaly (enlarged heart) as well as a pleural effusion (note fluid level at base of right lung).

Table 11-1
ADDITIVE DISEASES REQUIRING INCREASED TECHNIQUE

Acromegaly: 8-10% kVp	Osteochondroma: 8% kVp
Actinomycosis: 50% mAs	Osteopetrosis: 8-12% kVp
Ascites: 50-75% mAs	Paget's Disease: 8% kVp
Carcinomas, fibrous: 50% mAs	Pleural Effusion: 35% mAs
Cardiomegaly: 50% mAs	Pneumoconiosis: 50% mAs
Cirrhosis: 50% mAs	Pneumonia: 50% mAs
Edema, pulmonary: 50% mAs	Syphilis: 50% mAs
Hydrocephalus: 50-75% mAs	Tuberculosis, pulmonary: 50% mAs
Hydropneumothorax: 50% mAs	
Osteoarthritis (Degenerative Joint Disease): 8% kVp	

es in technique. The recommended adjustment is given for each, *assuming that the disease is well-advanced.* Naturally, the radiographer must modify this recommended change upward or downward upon assessing each individual patient.

Acromegaly, osteoarthritis, osteochondroma, osteopetrosis, osteomyelitis, Paget's disease, and advanced syphilis involve either excessive bone growth or the replacement of cartilagenous tissues with bone. In the case of osteoarthritis, even though there is degeneration within the bones themselves, bony spurs grow into the joints and bone tissue replaces normal cartilage and fluid in the joints, necessitating a net increase in technique. In the case of actinomycosis, fibrous carcinomas, cardiomegally (Fig. 11-1), cirrhosis, pneumoconiosis, and pulmonary tuberculosis, the growth or overexpansion of dense fibrous tissues replaces normal tissue. For ascites, pulmonary edema, hydrocephalus, hydropneumothorax, pleural effusion, and pneumonia, the accumulation of abnormal amounts of body fluids or the displacement

of aerated tissues in the lungs with fluid requires greater radiographic techniques.

It is well to reiterate the difference between fluid distention of the abdomen and obesity. When the abdomen is truly distended due to ascites or severe infection, the skin is tight and rather hard to the touch. The technique required may be slightly more than the *four centimeter rule* dictates. The radiographer should begin by measuring the abdomen and increasing technique from average according to the rule. If the distention is pronounced, an additional 30 percent increase in the resulting mAs is called for. For hypersthenic patients with very loose, flaccid skin that is soft to the touch, technique increases due to measured thickness will be somewhat less than the *four centimeter rule* dictates. This rule is an average and applies to variations in thickness which are attributable to mixtures of additional musculature, fluid, and fat. The skin of these average patients may be somewhat loose, but will not feel unusually soft on palpation.

DESTRUCTIVE DISEASES

Abnormal conditions which lead to an increase in *air* or *fat*, or to a *decrease* in nor-

mal body fluid or bone, are radiographically considered as *destructive conditions.* These

Table 11-2

DESTRUCTIVE DISEASES REQUIRING DECREASED TECHNIQUE

Aseptic Necrosis: 8% kVp	Hyperparathyroidism: 8% kVp
Blastomycosis: 8% kVp	
Bowel Obstruction: 8% kVp	Osteitis Fibrosa Cystica: 8% kVp
Cancers, osteolytic: 8% kVp	Osteomalacia: 8% kVp
	Osteomyelitis: 8% kVp
Emphysema; 8% kVp	Osteoporosis: 8% kVp
Ewing's Tumor: 8% kVp	Pneumothorax: 8% kVp
Exostosis: 8% kVp	Rheumatoid Arthritis: 8% kVp
Gout: 8% kVp	
Hodgkin's Disease: 8% kVp	

require a reduction from typical exposure techniques in order to be properly demonstrated. Both air and fat are significantly less dense than fluid, and absorb fewer x-ray photons.

For destructive diseases, overall technique may need to be reduced by 30 to 50 percent. *As a rule of thumb, destructive diseases require a 30 percent decrease in mAs, or a 5 percent reduction in kVp.* Table 11-2 lists destructive diseases commonly found in radiography, and the recommended technique reduction for each.

Aseptic necrosis, various bone carcinomas, Ewing's tumor, exostosis, gout, Hodgkin's disease, hyperparathyroidism, osteitis fibrosa cysitca, osteoporosis, oseo-

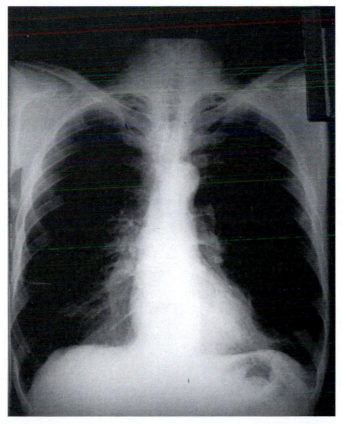

Figure 11-2. Radiograph using decreased technique for a patient with emphysema (note overdistention of lungs with air).

malacia, osteomyelitis and rheumatoid arthritis result in either a demineralization of bone or an invasive destruction of the bone tissue. Less penetration is required to secure optimum image contrast, so generally the kVp should be reduced for these diseases. In blastomycosis, yeast-like fungi produce gas pockets within tissues, while bowel obstructions, emphysema (Fig. 11-2) and pneumothorax are processes which essentially "trap" air or gas within body cavities. Due to their extremely low physical densities, gases are radiolucent and allow radiation to pass through to the film. Dark radiographs result unless technique is reduced.

TRAUMA

The challenges in determining optimum radiographic techniques for most trauma victims relate to the above discussion of disease conditions, particularly as regards the presence of excess fluids or gasses within the tissues. For example, pneumothoraces are common to trauma patients and, due to excessive aeration, require a reduced technique. Internal bleeding in the abdomen or hematomas in the brain may require a 30 percent increase in mAs, while blood pooling in the lungs can necessitate increases from 30 to 100 percent more than normal.

POSTMORTEM RADIOGRAPHY

Experienced radiographers learn to expect considerable pooling of blood and fluids in dead bodies, particularly in the head, thorax, and abdomen. An increase in technique, typically 35 to 50 percent, may be anticipated and should be applied on the very first exposure. Even shortly after death, blood and fluids begin to pool in the lungs as they follow simple gravity. Since postmortem radiographs are normally taken with the body recumbent, these fluids will pool across the entire lung field. In addition, bear in mind that postmortem chest radiography is by definition an *expiration* chest technique. Without the normal air insufflation of the lungs, an increase in technique is indicated. So, there are *two* distinct reasons to expect a needed increase in technique. *Postmortem chest techniques must be increased by at least 35 percent (one-third)*, and may require a 50 percent increase, depending on the amount of time since death. If this 35 to 50 percent rule is not applied on the very first exposure taken, a repeated exposure will very likely be needed.

SOFT-TISSUE TECHNIQUE

Normally, bullets and metallic foreign bodies do not need to be penetrated by the x-ray beam for radiographic localization. Any increase in technique would merely reduce the radiographic visualization of the tissues around the foreign object. However, many small foreign bodies such as slivers of wood, glass or metal, or swallowed bones are better visualized by using a reduced *soft-tissue technique.*

Metal and most types of glass are actually highly radiopaque and present little problem to demonstrate, yet very small slivers of the same can be difficult to detect. Chicken bones or similar objects which may become lodged in the laryngopharynx are often not very dense in cortical bone and have only slight radiographic contrast. Wood splinters are especially troublesome: because of the air pockets they contain, they may show up early on as a slightly *darker* air density, radiolucent against the soft tissue background. But in a brief period of time, wood splinters will absorb fluid from the surrounding tissues and become very difficult indeed to distinguish from tissue itself. The technique employed must be tailored to demonstrate soft tissue, rather than the usual bone tissue.

To maximize the visualization of these small foreign objects, image contrast must be enhanced *and* overall density must be lightened up. A reduction in kVp accomplishes both of these objectives at the same time (Fig. 11-3). There should be no attempt to "compensate" for the drop in kVp by adjusting mAs. *As a rule of thumb, for soft tissue techniques, subtract 15 to 20 percent of the kVp from the average technique, **without** changing the usual mAs.* In addition to demonstrating small foreign bodies, such technique show any damage to soft tissues. Soft tissue visualization is most frequently called for in radiography of the hands and the neck. For example, a common traumatic condition from automobile accidents is called *padded dash syndrome.* PDS may be

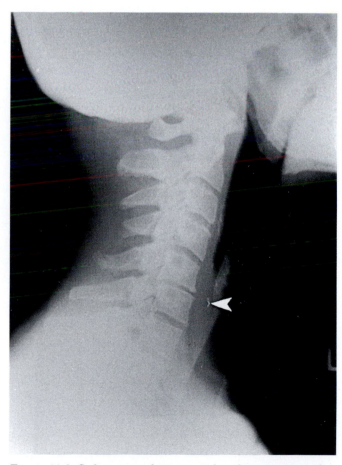

Figure 11-3. Soft tissue technique used to demonstrate a sliver of glass (arrow) in the neck. From a cervical spine technique, the kVP was decreased from the usual 76 kVp to 64 kVp, all other factors unchanged (15 mAs, 3-phase machine, 200-speed screens).

described as soft tissue damage in the anterior neck caused during a frontal impact when the victim lurches forward striking their neck against the padded dashboard. For padded dash syndrome, soft tissue views of the neck, especially the lateral, should be obtained along with a follow-up CT scan.

CASTS AND SPLINTS

Radiographic techniques must certainly be adjusted upward for most casts and splints. But to determine the extent of this increase, one must take into consideration the composition of the materials used, their thickness and configuration, and whether they are wet or dry. Radiographs taken after a limb of the body has been set and casted are called *postreduction radiographs.*

Full plaster casts require a minimum doubling of overall exposure factors from the usual technique for the body part. This can be accomplished either by doubling the mAs or by increasing the kVp by 15 percent. For example, suppose that 5 mAs at 60 kVp secured a proper exposure for the AP view of the normal foot. The same foot in a dry plaster cast would require 10 mAs at 60 kVp or, alternatively, 5 mAs at 69 kVp (using the 15 percent rule).

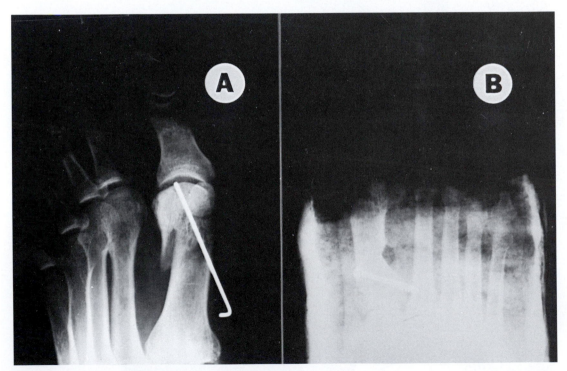

Figure 11-4. Bilateral radiographs of the feet taken during surgery on the same patient, demonstrating wet plaster cast technique adjustment. (A) was taken of the uncasted left foot using 10 mAs at 62 kVp. The right foot (B) had just been casted in thick, wet plaster. Technique used for (B) was 16 mAs at 70 kVp, an overall increase in *total technique* of approximately three times that of the uncasted foot. (The nearly 15% increase in kVp equivalent to a doubling, plus a mAs increase about half-way to another doubling.)

Full plaster casts which are still wet, having just been applied, require *three* times the overall technique (Fig. 11-4). To achieve this, the mAs may be tripled, the kVp may be increased by about 22 percent, or a combination of the two may be employed such as doubling the mAs with an additional 8 percent increase in kVp.

Unusually thick plaster may be applied around the femur or the torso. A full cast of this type which is dry will require a *tripling* of the usual technique. A plaster cast of this thickness that is still wet can require as much as *four times* the original technique.

Often, "half-casts" are secured to a limb by wrapping a partial cast with an Ace™ bandage. For this situation, use a *50 percent increase* in technique. That is, half again as

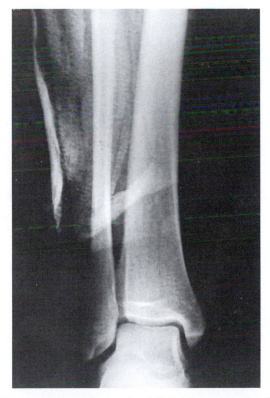

Figure 11-5. Radiograph of distal leg in a mixed fiberglass/plaster cast, using 50% more mAs than usual for an uncasted leg. Factors: 66 kVp, chart technique (uncasted): 6.8 mAs, actual mAs used: 10 mAs.

much mAs, or approximately 8 percent more kVp. Remember to employ the increase only when the projection of the part of interest passes through the cast material—on a lateral view of the forearm in a half-cast, the bones may not actually be covered by the cast material, and a normal technique may be used.

Fiberglass mesh has become popular as a casting medium. Ironically, fiberglass is so radiolucent that it allows almost all of the x-ray beam to pass through it unaffected. Normal techniques may be used in most cases. If the fiberglass is very thick, such as might be used on a thigh cast, a slight increase, not to exceed 30 percent in mAs or 5 percent in kVp, may be in order.

In modern trauma care, it has become common to mix fiberglass and plaster in roughly equal proportions to make casts. For casts of this type, a general rule of thumb is to increase mAs by *50 percent* or kVp by 8 percent (Fig. 11-5). Plastic materials may require increases from 30 to 50 percent.

Projections must sometimes be made through splints of wood or aluminum. Such splints may require from 35 to 50 percent increases in overall technique. Whether the splint is applied to one side or to both sides of the limb, the radiographer must assess

Table 11-3

TECHNIQUE INCREASES FOR
CASTS AND SPLINTS

4 x mAs or 30% kVp	Plaster, thick and wet
3 x mAs or 22 kVp	Plaster, medium and wet Plaster, thick and dry
2 x mAs or 15% kVp	Plaster, medium and dry
50% mAs or 8% kVp	Plaster half-cast, dry Fiberglass/plaster full cast Plastic splint Wood splint
No increase needed	Fiberglass, pure Inflatable air splint

the *total thickness* of wood or other material to be traversed by the x-ray beam. The mAs should be increased by 35 percent (one-third) for one-half inch of wood, or by 50 percent (one-half) for one inch. As a rule of thumb, *increase mAs by 50 percent for wood or aluminum splints.* Solid plastics are similar to wood. Inflatable air splints, however, require no change in technique.

The radiographer should be thoroughly familiar with these technique rules for splints and casts, and commit them to memory. For assistance, they are summarized in Table 11-3.

SUMMARY

1. Radiographers are responsible for using x-ray requisitions, patient charts, verbal histories and careful observation to acquire *preliminary information* which may bear upon technique selection.
2. *Additive diseases* require an increase in technique, typically 50 percent, while destructive diseases require a decrease, usually 30 percent.
3. *Fluid* distention, or pooling of fluids such as in postmortem cases, requires increasing technique from 30 to 50 percent greater than usual, in addition to 4-centimeter rule adjustments.
4. For *soft tissue techniques,* decrease kVp 15 to 20 percent from the normal, without any other compensation.
5. Plaster *casts* require double the usual technique and can require much more. Half-casts, fiberglass/plaster combinations, and wood splints usually require a 50 percent increase in technique.

REVIEW QUESTIONS

1. How much would you increase your total technique from the chart technique for a humerus in a dry plaster cast?
2. What technique change would be required for a lateral projection of a femur splinted with two one-half-inch pieces of wood?
3. What technique change is required for an extremity in a pure fiberglass cast?

For each of the following pathologies, state whether the kVp should be increased for more penetration, or decreased for less penetration:

4. Osteoarthritis (degenerative joint disease):
5. Hyperparathyroidism:
6. Osteochondroma:
7. Hydrocephalus:
8. Emphysema:
9. Hydropneumothorax:
10. Pneumoconiosis:
11. Ascites:
12. A fluid-distended abdomen requires _____ (more, less, or equal) technique than a fatty abdomen of the same thickness.
13. Postmortem chest radiographs require _____ (more, less, or equal) technique than normal.
14. If the usual technique for a lateral cervical spine is 15 mAs at 76 kVp, what mAs and what kVp would be used for a *soft tissue technique* lateral neck?
15. For destructive diseases, generally technique should be _____ by _____.
16. Fresh wood slivers appear as a _____ density against the soft tissue background.

Chapter 12

SCATTERED RADIATION AND IMAGE FOG

THE EFFECTS OF scattered radiation are among the most misunderstood concepts in radiography. This chapter will consolidate all of the aspects of this topic covered in previous chapters. The relationship of x-ray beam interactions within the patient to the resulting image qualities on the radiograph are rather complicated, and a careful review of Chapters 3 and 4 (Qualities of the Image, and Interactions of X-Rays Within the Patient) may be helpful.

DESIRABLE GRAY SCALE VERSUS FOG

An important concept learned in Chapter 3 is that extended gray scale is a desirable, *indeed an essential*, component of the radiographic image. Any portion of the image which is blank white presents no information at all (except at its edges), and is diagnostically useless. (Figure 6-14 in Chapter 6 illustrates such a radiograph, with unpenetrated barium in the stomach.) The same may be said for portions of the image that are pitch black–they are diagnostically useless. The ideal radiograph possesses a range of gray shades from a very dark gray to a very light gray, with no blank areas within the anatomy. This means that every type of tissue depicted must be at least *partially* penetrated by the x-ray beam.

Optimum kVp results in at least some penetration of the beam through *all* tissues, resulting in a fairly long gray scale. An image with long gray scale has many different shades of gray and depicts many different types of tissue. *Quantitatively, an image with long gray scale has more information in it than a short-scale image.* Of course, gray scale can be *too* long, but unless all tissues are penetrated to some degree, the gray scale is too short.

Reasonably long gray scale is, therefore, desirable. Such images contain much information but are not immediately appealing to the eye. They have an overall gray appearance. It is important to understand that the apparent "grayness" of such images is *not due to fog*. Figure 12-1 compares an unfogged image with long gray scale to a fogged image. Not every "gray" radiograph is a fogged radiograph. Optimally long gray scale is desirable, fog is not.

Gray scale is, by definition, the opposite of contrast. *Image contrast is reduced at a higher kVp. This would be true whether scattered radiation were present or not.* Fog can, however, *contribute* to lower image contrast in a very destructive way. There are several ways in which an image can be fogged, but the most important of these to the radiographer is scatter radiation.

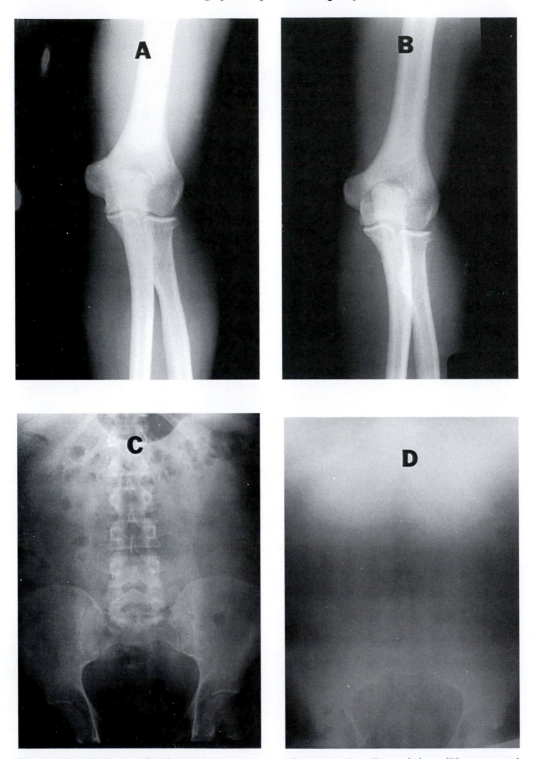

Figure 12-1. Radiographs demonstrating gray scale versus fog. From (A) to (B), increased "grayness" is due to a desirable increase in penetration and gray scale, with no fog present. From (C) to (D), increased "grayness" is due to fog.

SECONDARY VERSUS SCATTER RADIATION

Secondary radiation is radiation produced when the primary x-ray beam interacts with atoms in the body, tabletop, or other objects, and emitted *by the object*, not by the x-ray tube. In physics, *secondary* radiation and *scattered* radiation are often synonymous. But, for medical imaging, a distinction must be made.

Even when grids are used, much of the radiation reaching the film is *secondary* radiation which is emitted from within the body. Grids only eliminate that secondary radiation which has been *scattered* significantly, which has *changed direction* enough to be visibly destructive to the image.

Not all secondary radiation is significantly scattered. Some is emitted in a forward direction, close enough to the original direction of the primary beam that it does not *visibly* change the image. Such radiation will pass through a grid, and may be considered as constructive to the visible image. For imaging purposes, *scatter* radiation should be considered as only those rays which have *significantly changed direction* from the primary beam and are visibly destructive to the image.

CAUSES OF SCATTER FOG

Almost all scatter radiation is caused by the Compton interaction, as described in Chapter 4. Let us briefly consider each of the three factors that increase the amount of scatter radiation reaching the film. They are:

1. High kVp levels (Chapter 6)
2. Large field sizes (Chapter 9)
3. Large body part thicknesses (Chapters 10 and 11)

High kVp Levels

At high kilovoltages, slightly *less* scattering interactions actually occur within the patient (Chapter 4, Fig. 4-6). However, that scatter radiation which *is* produced has higher energy and is emitted in a more forward direction. With an increased *proportion* of scattered x-rays penetrating through to the film, and with an increased *proportion* of them directed toward the film, *the net result is an increase in scatter radiation **reaching the film**, thus increasing image fog.*

But, high kVp settings are required to obtain adequate *penetration* for the radiographic studies using contrast agents and for those body parts with high proportions of bone tissue. Furthermore, high kVp is frequently desirable in order to produce sufficiently long *gray scale* in the image. In most cases, these two benefits far outweigh the gradual increase in fog at higher kilovoltages. Therefore, the selection of kVp should be based primarily upon the penetration and gray scale desired, with scatter radiation only as a secondary consideration.

Large Field Sizes

Chapter 9 describes how larger field sizes allow greater amounts of exposed tissue to generate more scatter radiation (Fig. 9-4), while the concentration of the primary beam is unaffected (Fig. 9-5). Excessive proportions of scatter radiation are also produced from the x-ray table any time the light field is allowed to extend well beyond the anatomy. As long as the field size is adequate to include all anatomy of interest, there is *no benefit* to further increasing the field size, and no reason for accepting an image fogged in this manner.

Large Part Thicknesses

Larger patients or larger body parts present more exposed tissue to generate scatter radiation, even while the primary beam is further attenuated (Chapter 10). The loss of useful rays combined with the increased scatter result in a dramatic increase in visible image fog.

For some procedures (particularly fluoroscopic procedures), the radiographer or radiologist may be able to reduce tissue thickness by using a *compression paddle* or similar compression device. But for the most part, tissue thickness is outside the control of the radiographer.

Of these three causes of scatter radiation, the high kVp levels have advantages which outweigh the fog produced, and tissue thicknesses are not under the radiographer's control, leaving *field size limitation (collimation) as the primary method of preventing scatter radiation.*

Two methods are available to help eliminate scatter radiation *after it has been produced* but before it reaches the film and fogs it. These are the use of grids, discussed in the next chapter, and the use of the "air gap technique," discussed in Chapter 19.

EFFECTS ON DENSITY AND CONTRAST

Scattering is a *random* event, and therefore, when it occurs in sufficient quantity, it results in a relatively *even density deposit across an area of the film.* (Of course, by inverse square law, this deposit will gradually decrease at greater distances from the scattering source; nonetheless, a silver deposit will result both directly under the scattering object and under adjacent structures (Fig. 12-2).

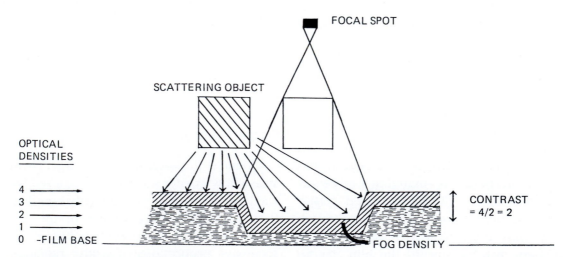

Figure 12-2. Effect of scatter radiation upon image contrast. Prior to fogging, background density is 3.0, density under object of interest is 1.0, and contrast is 3/1 = 3. After scatter radiation lays down additional "blanket" density of 1.0, background density is now 4.0 and image density is 2.0. Contrast for this fogged image is 4/2 = 2, reduced from the original contrast of 3.

Figure 12-2 is a density trace diagram (see Chapter 24) showing the "blanket" effect of scatter fogging. The diagram is a cross-section of the thickness of silver deposit on the x-ray film. A thicker silver deposit would be seen as a darker density on viewing the radiograph. The white box represents a high-contrast object, such as a bone, being projected onto the film and showing a lighter density. Contrast is measured as the *ratio* of the background density to the density under the object of interest. At the left of the diagram optical density levels are listed; the optical density of the background would normally measure 3, and the density of the bone image 1. The normal contrast of the image should be 3/1 = 3.

However, if a scattering object is placed within the x-ray beam near to the object of interest, the scatter radiation produced lays down a roughly even blanket of density across the image, covering *both* the area directly under itself and adjacent areas under other structures such as the hypothetical bone. In the diagram, this added fog density has an optical density value of 1, which is added to all other densities. Thus, the background density is increased from 3 to 4, and the bone image density is increased from 1 to 2. The image contrast *after fogging* is now 4/2 = 2.

Fogging has diminished the measured contrast from 3 to 2. Contrast in the image has clearly been reduced by scatter fog.

Ironically, even though image gray scale is considered as the opposite of contrast, fogging reduces *both* gray scale and contrast. The reduction of gray scale from the laying down of this *blanket fog density* is demonstrated using a step wedge image in Figure 12-3. Note that when the layer of fog is superimposed over the step wedge image, you can count fewer density steps of density. Gray scale has been reduced. Yet, at the difference between each pair of steps has also been reduced, showing that contrast has also been reduced. This may seem like a contradiction, but it really is not if one remembers that gray scale is composed of "good" grays in the image which were produced by penetration of the desirable x-ray beam signal, whereas fog is composed of "bad" grays which are produced by random, destructive scatter radiation. As the number of gray shades in the image is diminished by fog, useful information is also diminished.

Further, since fog increases density anywhere it occurs on the film, the addition of fog density to those areas normally depicted as dark grays may be sufficient to turn them pitch black, resulting in a loss of image information. Fog increases density, but in a *destructive way*, reducing image quality. Fog is *completely destructive* to the image in terms of density, contrast, and gray scale.

It is possible for a radiograph to be both *light* and *fogged* (Fig. 12-4). This frequently occurs with very large patients. The large volume of tissue results in excessive scattered radiation, which would normally fog and darken the film, but, at the same time, such thicknesses of tissue reduce the amount of primary radiation reaching the film. The total exposure to the film is reduced, yet a greater *percentage* of that exposure is attributable to fog densities. The result is "washed out" appearance, underexposed and gray at the same time. Such radiographs are of little diagnostic value.

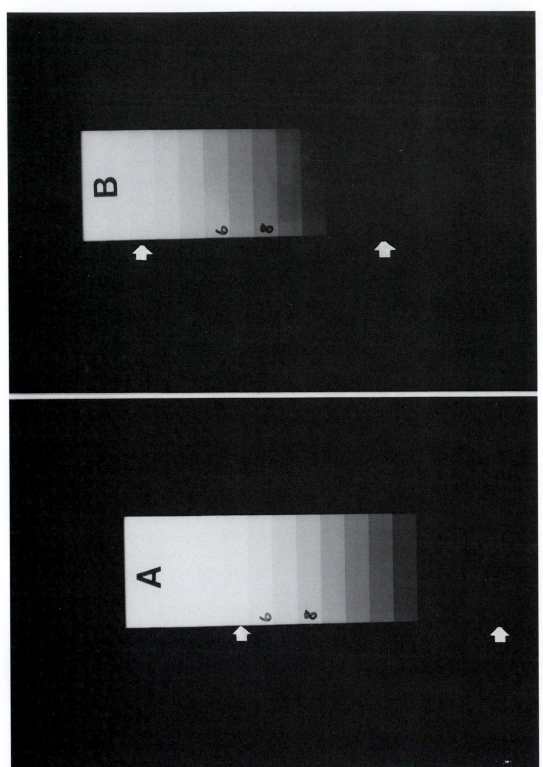

Figure 12-3. Even slight scatter fogging in image B has reduced gray scale: In good lighting, one can count 12 steps from pitch black to white in A, but only 11 steps from pitch black to white in B. This is because the darkest grays in B are lost as they turn to pitch black from the fog.

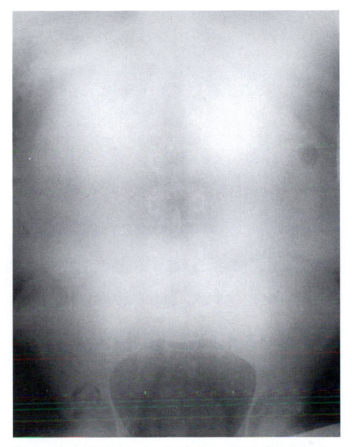

Figure 12-4. Radiograph of a large patient demonstrating both fog and underexposure. An image can be light and yet fogged.

FOG VERSUS BLUR

There is also a common misconception that scattered radiation "undercuts the edge" of an image, causing it to become "blurred." It has even been asserted that grids reduce blur by eliminating scatter radiation. These are false and misleading statements. As described in Chapters 3 and 24, the *resolution* of details (the ability to distinguish them as separate from each other) is reduced by a loss of contrast, but this is due to less *visibility*, not to a lack of geometrical integrity. The sharpness of recorded detail at the edges of an image depends upon the width of the *penumbra*.

Anything which does not change the spread of the penumbral shadow cannot be said to affect sharpness.

Scatter is a completely random phenomenon. It does not "select" the edges of the image to affect, but simply lays down a blanket of density over the *entire* image. Blurring, on the other hand, is geometrically predictable through penumbra and absorption diagrams and relates specifically to the edges of the image as projected from the x-ray tube. Scatter, emanating from the patient, cannot and does not affect the alignment of the primary rays project-

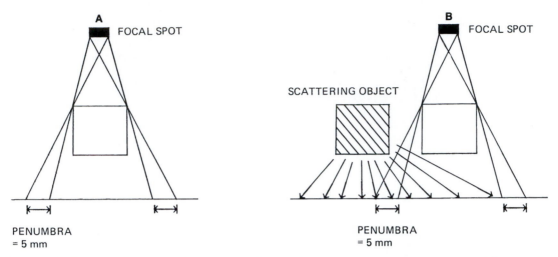

Figure 12-5. Diagram illustrating that scatter radiation does not affect sharpness of recorded detail. The spread of the penumbral shadow is 5 mm prior to fogging (A), and is still 5 mm after fogging (B). Although *visibility* is reduced by the scatter, blur is unchanged and sharpness is equal.

ed from the x-ray tube.

To develop this concept, let us separate a fogging event and the projection of the original image in time. A film may certainly be fogged before or after the x-ray exposure is made. For example, it may be fogged in the dark room during storage. Would such a fogging event affect the way that the edges of the image were projected onto the film during the actual exposure? Clearly, the answer is no. The visibility of the image would be compromised because of the fogging, but the projection of the penumbra and umbra of the image during regular exposure is affected only by *primary beam geometry*.

Figure 12-5 illustrates that scatter radiation is a phenomenon separate from the geometry of penumbra formation, and does not change image sharpness or blur. Figure 3-15 in Chapter 3 demonstrates that images can be fogged without blur, or blurred without fog. Because scatter is random in nature, it cannot affect *any* of the geometrical factors in the image—sharpness of recorded detail, magnification, or distortion.

Scatter does affect all three of the visibility functions in an image: It increases density, it increases image noise (fog), and it reduces image contrast. Thus, the overall resolution of the image is destroyed. This is all due to a loss of *visibility*, not to any loss in sharpness.

Image fog is properly classified as a form of noise, because it is an extraneous density that impedes the visibility of the desired image, just as any artifact would "get in the way." In the hierarchy of image qualities (Fig. 3-18) fog should be listed as a visibility factor under "noise."

SCATTER AND RADIATION EXPOSURE

While it is not within the scope of this text to fully discuss all of the implications of scatter radiation exposure and protec-tion methods, it is important to point out that scattered radiation is the main source of *occupational* exposure to the radiographer, as well as a substantial portion of the dose received by the patient. Therefore, the reduction and control of scatter production is essential not only for image quality, but also for radiation protection purposes.

Equipment operators must use the three cardinal principles of protection from scattered radiation: minimize exposure time, maximize distance, and use appropriate shielding. Also, remember that the least amount of scatter radiation produced is emitted at right angles to the central ray. *The safest location to stand in an exposed area is to the side of the x-ray beam*, not behind it.

SUMMARY

1. Optimally long *gray scale* is desirable in an image and should not be confused with fogging.
2. Not all *secondary radiation* should be considered as "scatter," only that portion which has been substantially changed in direction.
3. The three *causes of scatter radiation* are high kVp levels, large field sizes, and large tissue thicknesses. Of these, *field size* should be considered as the major *controlling* factor.
4. Scatter radiation creates a relatively even density deposit across the entire film area called *fog*. This fog density reduces image contrast and *also* destroys image gray scale.
5. *Fog* generally increases the overall *density* of the image. Nonetheless, by gross underexposure, it is possible for an image to be both light and fogged.
6. Fog has no relationship to blur or *sharpness of recorded detail.* However, it does reduce the *visibility* of image edges because of the destruction of contrast, and the overall *resolution* of the image is degraded.
7. Scatter fog is a form of image *noise,* impeding the visibility of the desired image.
8. Scatter radiation is the main source of *occupational exposure* to the radiographer, and an important component of patient dose as well. The safest place to stand during mobile radiography is at 90 degrees or right angles to the central ray, where scatter radiation is least intense.

REVIEW QUESTIONS

1. An image can appear gray overall and still be of high quality if the "grayness" is due to _____.
2. List the *three* causes of scatter radiation:
3. Considering these three causes of image fog, what is the most important way for the radiographer to prevent excessive scatter radiation?
4. List the two methods by which scatter radiation can be reduced or eliminated *after* it has been produced.
5. High kVp levels actually result in *less* scattering interactions in the patient. Give *two* reasons why image fog increases anyway with high kVp:
6. What method can sometimes be used to reduce scatter production due to tissue thickness:
7. Fog always has what effect upon image contrast:

8. Is there a direct relationship between scatter fog and image sharpness?

9. Fog _____ (increases, decreases, or has no effect on) image resolution.

10. In the hierarchy of image qualities, fog would be classified as a type of image _____.

11. Where is the safest location to stand in relation to the central ray of the x-ray beam during a mobile procedure?

12. Unless *all* tissues are penetrated to some degree by the x-ray beam, gray scale is too _____.

13. Scatter radiation affects all three of the _____ functions in a radiographic image.

14. The main source of *occupational* exposure to the radiographer is scatter radiation from the _____.

15. Fog always has what effect upon image gray scale:

Chapter 13

GRIDS

UNTIL GUSTAV BUCKY invented the grid diaphragm in 1913, the only control for scatter radiation was by means of various shaped single- and double-aperture diaphragms and cones inserted at the portal of the x-ray tube. Although these devices proved of value, large amounts of scatter radiation could not adequately be controlled in radiography of thick body tissues.

The function of the Bucky grid is to absorb scatter radiation that has already been produced in the patient's body tissues before it reaches the film. This required that the grid be placed *between* the patient and the film. The grid is a flat rectangular plate containing alternating strips of lead foil separated by a radiotransparent interspacer material. Figure 13-1 shows a cross-section cut-away view of a grid plate; it can be seen that when the grid plate is lying flat or horizontal, the lead strips point vertically toward the x-ray tube. The lead foil strips are approximately 0.005 inch thick. These strips are vertically aligned to the fanning primary beam of x-rays so that, in use, most of the focused remnant beam of x-rays will pass *between* these strips to reach the film, while most of the unfocused, randomly scattered radiation will strike the lead strips broadside and be absorbed (Fig. 13-1).

The grid as Dr. Bucky invented it was not too practical at first because it was used in a stationary position and the grid pattern on the radiograph was quite course. If you carefully examine Figure 13-7 in the latter portion of this chapter, you can see the white lines that occur as artifacts on the final image when these grid strips are visible. It was for Dr. Hollis Potter, of Chicago, to solve the problem and place the Bucky grid on a practical basis. This was accomplished by *moving* the grid during the exposure and making the grid strips thinner. By moving the grid during the exposure, all grid lines were blurred out of the image. The first commercial moving grid was announced in 1920 and became known as the Potter-Bucky diaphragm. R. B. Wisely, of the Kodak Research Laboratories, presented scientific data in 1920 firmly establishing the effectiveness of the Potter-Bucky diaphragm in eliminating scatter radiation, reducing fog, and enhancing contrast dramatically in the radiographic image. This was one of the few historical milestones in the search for better radiographic results.

Types of Grids

There are two general types of grids: stationary and moving. When a modern *stationary* grid is used, an image of the grid strips appears on the radiograph as a series of evenly spaced fine white lines (Fig. 13-7). In grids containing 60-80 lines per inch, these grid lines are barely perceptible at normal viewing distances. However, improvements in design have made possible grids containing 110 lines per inch which are virtually invisible at similar view-

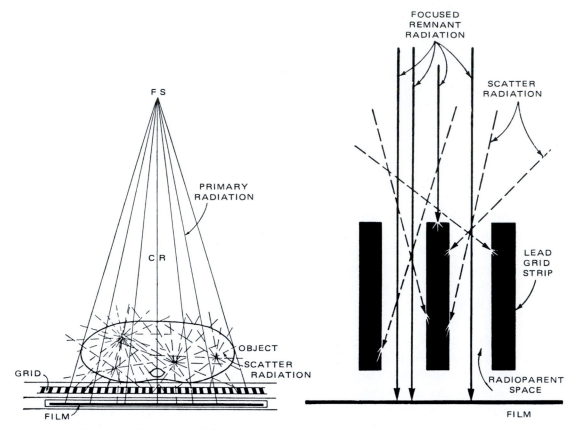

Figure 13-1. Diagrams illustrating (*left*) function of Potter-Bucky diaphragm in absorbing scatter radiation before it reaches the film; (*right*) details of grid construction.

ing distances. The moving grid is used extensively for routine radiography. The stationary grid is frequently employed in mobile radiography or other circumstances where it is difficult or impossible to apply a moving grid.

Among modern moving grids in the Potter-Bucky mechanism, there are two types of movements used. The *reciprocating* grid uses a motor which drives the grid plate back and forth during the exposure in a direction perpendicular to the grid lines, effectively blurring them from the final image. The *oscillating* grid mechanism moves the grid in a circular motion. Either way, the grid lines are effectively blurred out of the image, reducing noise. Having eliminated the grid lines as a form of image

noise, the moving grid is extremely effective in stopping scatter radiation, removing fog from the image, and thus enhancing image contrast.

GRID RATIO

Grid ratio is the major factor in the efficiency of a grid in cleaning up scatter radiation. The *grid ratio* is defined as the relation between the *height* of the radiotransparent interspaces between these lead foil strips (or the strips themselves) and the *width* of the interspaces. The formula for grid ratio is:

$$\text{Grid Ratio} = \frac{H}{D}$$

where H is the height of the lead strips and D is the distance between the strips. For example, an 8:1 grid ratio means that the spaces between the lead strips are tall and narrow, 8 times taller than they are wide.

Example: What is the grid ratio for a grid that is 3 millimeters thick and has interspaces between the lead strips which are 0.5 millimeters in width? The "thickness" of the grid plate, stated as 3 mm, corresponds to the *height* of the lead strips. Applying the formula, then:

$$\frac{H}{D} = \frac{3 \text{ mm}}{0.5 \text{ mm}} = 6$$

Answer: The grid ratio is 6:1

Obviously, the grid ratio may be increased by increasing *H* or by decreasing *D*: The height of the strips could be increased; however, this would result in a thicker grid plate which might not then fit into the Potter-Bucky mechanism or other devices. The more practical way of achieving a high grid ratio is to reduce the spaces between the lead strips. This means there will be more lead strips per inch and more lead in the grid overall.

The 8:1 ratio grid has great efficiency because only secondary radiation that is traveling approximately parallel to the primary radiation can reach the film. The most commonly used grids generally have ratios of 8:1, 10:1, and 12:1. A grid ratio of 16:1 is still more efficient, but it requires great accuracy in positioning, with an accurate SID and near perfect alignment of the x-ray tube, the patient and the film. With lower grid ratios, less fog is eliminated but greater latitude in positioning and SID is permissible.

EFFECT ON CONTRAST

The sole purpose for which the grid was invented is to *restore contrast* in the final image. Image contrast is reduced by scatter radiation fog and is increased in proportion to the amount of scatter radiation eliminated. Employment of a grid shortens the gray scale so that images are produced exhibiting higher contrast; the greater the grid ratio, the higher is the contrast obtained. For example, a radiograph made with a 4:1 ratio grid has lower contrast than one made with an 8:1 ratio grid because the 4:1 grid has lower efficiency in fog cleanup.

Demonstration No. 1

The manner in which contrast is affect when using a stationary grid is illustrated in Figure 13-2. Radiograph *A* exhibits some evidence of fog even though a field of correct size and 80 kVp were employed with 5 mAs. Effective reduction of the fog, radiograph *B*, was obtained by using a stationary grid, 100 kVp and 5 mAs for this radiograph.

Demonstration No. 2

Screen radiographs of the frontal sinuses were made in Figure 13-3. Radiograph A was made with a large cone—the high density is due to excessive scatter radiation fog. Radiograph B was made with a small cone of correct size—definite improvement in image quality is apparent. For radiograph C, a cone of correct size *and* a stationary grid were employed—the cone reduced the amount of tissue irradiated, thereby reducing the scatter radiation produced, and the grid absorbed most of the scatter radiation

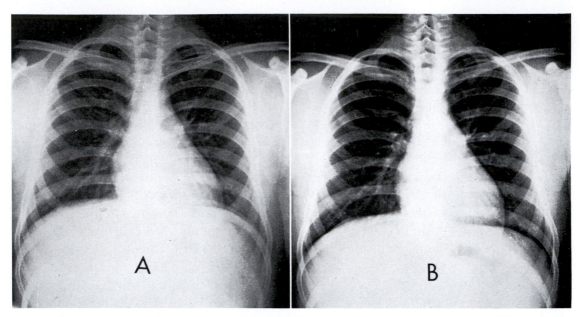

Figure 13-2. Two screen radiographs of a 22-cm PA chest demonstrating the elimination of fog and contrast improvement attained with a stationary grid (B).

that might have reached the film. This teamwork resulted in a good radiographic quality.

INDICATIONS FOR GRID USE

Since scattered radiation is generated both by high kVp and by large tissue thick-nesses, both of these considerations determine *when* a grid should be used. Body parts with thicknesses greater than about 12 cm typically produce enough scattered photons to visibly fog the image. This is the size of a large knee, and although some radiologists prefer tabletop non-grid techniques for knees and others prefer grid

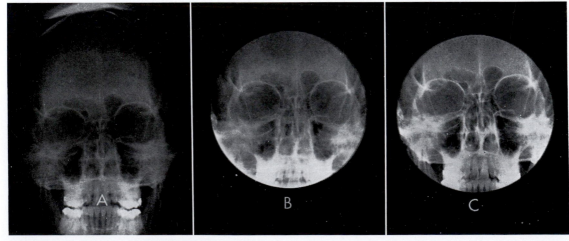

Figure 13-3. Screen radiographs of the frontal sinuses demonstrating contrast enhancement. Factors: 70 kVp; Radiographs A and B: 15 mAs; radiograph C: 62.5 mAs, stationary grid.

techniques, anything *larger than the knee* should generally be exposed using a grid. This includes all femurs and shoulders. Extremities smaller than the shoulder or the knee do not produce enough scatter radiation to pose a real threat to the image, and should be done non-grid. *Anatomy larger than 12 cm thick should be radiographed using a grid.*

Consulting Table 6-1 in Chapter 6, it is found that kVp levels in the 70 to 76 range are needed to adequately penetrate the larger extremities such as the shoulder and femur. A related rule of thumb for grid use is that *grids should generally be used on any procedure utilizing more than 70 kVp.*

The particular grid ratio selected depends primarily upon the typical kVp levels used on a radiographic unit, or in other words, upon the types of procedures most commonly done in that radiographic room. For procedures typically done in the 70 to 80 kVp range, a 6:1 grid is recommended. At the other extreme, a 16:1 ratio grid should be used on dedicated chest units using 110-120 kVp, where the tube is center-locked to the bucky and thus guaranteed to be well-centered and aligned. For most general procedures done with the cassette in the Bucky tray of a standard radiographic table, typical kVp levels range from about 76 to 90 kVp. Therefore, most radiology departments install 8:1 or 10:1 grids in the Potter-Bucky mechanisms of their tables and chest boards. The detailed recommendations for grid ratios, according to kVp, are listed in Table 13-3.

GRID EFFICIENCY

Grid Frequency and Lead Content

Closely related to the grid ratio is *grid frequency* and *lead content.* Grid frequency is the number of lead strips counted per inch when scanning transversely across the grid. The most commonly used grids have frequencies of about 80 lines per inch, but grid frequencies can range from 60 lines per inch up to as much as 110 lines per inch. It is generally taught that the more lead strips there are, that is, the more *concentrated* they are, the more efficient the grid. This is true, *assuming* that nothing else is changed in the grid, such as its overall plate thickness (the height of the strips).

However, it is possible to achieve higher grid frequencies in *two* distinct ways: The lead strips themselves can be made thinner, or the interspaces between them can be made narrower. If the spaces between the strips are made narrower, an increased grid ratio will result unless the height of the lead strips were also reduced. If the height in the lead strips were reduced proportionately (by making the grid plate thinner), it will cancel out the effect of narrowing the interspaces and the grid ratio will remain the same (Fig. 13-4). No difference in efficiency will occur. In other words, if the grid plate is thinner, it is possible to increase grid frequency *without* changing grid ratio. In such a case, there is no gain in effectiveness. Thus, *grid ratio is much more important than grid frequency in determining effectiveness.*

On the other hand, *if* the thickness of the grid plate is maintained, preserving the height of the interspaces, then an increase in grid frequency will result in a higher grid ratio, and the grid will be more effective (Fig. 13-5). Clearly, effectiveness cannot be improved by increasing grid frequency *unless* the grid ratio is improved thereby.

The *lead content,* which can be measured

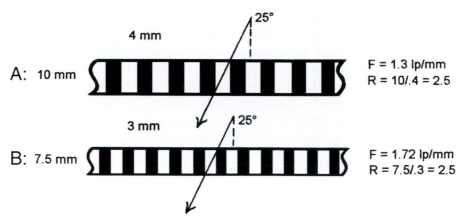

Figure 13-4. Due to narrower interspace, Grid B has a higher grid frequency than grid A; nonetheless, since the height in the lead strips was also reduced proportionately by making the grid plate thinner, there has been no change in grid ratio. Note that the selectivity, indicated by the maximum angle at which scatter radiation can pass through, is unchanged. No difference in grid efficiency has occurred.

in grams per square inch, or as total grams for the entire grid, is sometimes cited as an indication of a grid's efficiency. Clearly, at a higher grid frequency with more lead strips per inch, there will be more *total* lead content in a grid. However, more total lead content could *also* result from simply using thicker lead strips. It is possible to have thicker lead strips, and maintain the grid ratio if the grid plate is thicker, as shown in Figure 13-4 by simply comparing *A* to *B*

rather than *B* to *A*. In this case, again, there is no real gain in efficiency. Finally, note that with thicker lead strips, more of the *primary* x-rays will be absorbed as they strike the lead strips end-on. This is not desirable. Thus, *grid ratio is much more important than lead content in determining effectiveness.*

Although it can be true that more lead content or a higher grid frequency improves the performance of a grid, these

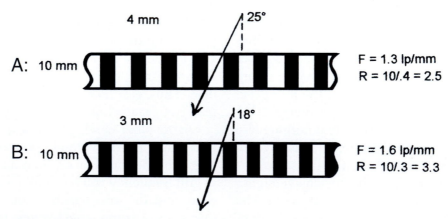

Figure 13-5. Due to narrower interspace, Grid B has a higher grid frequency than grid A. In this case, the thickness of the grid plate is maintained, so that the result is an increase in grid ratio. The selectivity, indicated by the maximum angle at which scatter radiation can pass through, is increased, and grid efficiency is improved. The key to grid efficiency is the *grid ratio.*

assumptions are not *always* true. The key factor is in how any of these changes ultimately affect the *grid ratio*. The grid ratio is at the heart of the efficiency question.

Bucky Factor

The *Bucky factor* is defined as the ratio of the exposure (mAs) required with a grid to the exposure required without the grid in order to maintain an equal density. Historically, some authors have suggested that it can be used as a measure of grid effectiveness. Yet, as explained above, a grid can have more lead content in it without necessarily being more efficient. The simple fact that a particular grid requires more technique is *not* a reliable indication of its effectiveness at all, and can even indicate poor construction. The Bucky factor is *useful* in technique conversions, as will be demonstrated later in this chapter.

There are two reliable and valid methods of measuring grid efficiency. They are grid *selectivity* and the *contrast improvement factor.*

SELECTIVITY

The *selectivity* of a grid is mathematically defined as the ratio of the primary beam transmission to the scatter radiation transmission through the grid:

$$\text{Selectivity} = \frac{\text{Primary transmission}}{\text{Scatter transmission}}$$

Selectivity can be extrapolated from direct measurements of radiation taken with ion chambers. Since it takes into account that the objective of a grid is to attenuate scatter radiation *without* attenuating primary radiation, the selectivity ratio is an excellent measure of actual grid effectiveness.

CONTRAST IMPROVEMENT FACTOR

For the radiographer, the *contrast improvement factor* is the most important, practical measure of grid effectiveness. The purpose of the grid is to improve image contrast. The *CIF* directly measures this. Image contrast can be readily measured by a radiographer using a densitometer, by simply dividing one measured density step (from an aluminum step wedge) into another in the presence of a scatter-generating object. The contrast improvement factor may be formulated as:

$$\text{CIF} = \frac{\text{Measured contrast with the grid}}{\text{Measured contrast without the grid}}$$

Table 13-1 is a condensed excerpt from

Table 13-1
CONTRAST IMPROVEMENT FACTORS (NON-GRID = 1)
FOR VARIOUS RATIO GRIDS AT DIFFERENT RANGES OF kVp

Grid ratio	None	2:1	4:1	6:1	8:1	10:1	12:1	14:1	16:1
kV					Relative contrast*				
70	1	2.0	3.0	4.0	4.8	5.0	5.3	5.5	5.8
95	1	1.5	2.0	3.0	3.3	3.5	3.8	3.9	4.0
120	1	1.3	1.5	2.3	2.5	2.8	3.0	3.2	3.3

*Contrast relative to that with no grid using a 20 cm thick water phantom and a test pattern.
(Reprinted with permission of the National Council on Radiation Protection and Measurements, NCRP Report No. 102.)

Report No. 102 of the National Council on Radiation Protection and Measurements, showing the typical contrast improvement factors for various grid ratios at selected kVp levels. It can be seen that contrast is improved from 2.5 times (for high kVp and low grid ratio) up to as much as 6 times (for low kVp and high grid ratio). These are very impressive measurements indeed, and they confirm that the grid is one of the most effective means of enhancing image contrast by the elimination of scatter radiation.

GRID RATIOS AND TECHNIQUE COMPENSATION

Grids with narrower spacing between the lead strips in relation to their height are more *selective* in absorbing scatter radiation, and only those secondary photons which are very close to the original direction of the primary beam will be able to pass through the interspaces without striking a lead strip. To minimize the the number of *primary* photons being attenuated, the high-ratio grid must be more perfectly centered and aligned with the central ray. Even when this is done, the high-ratio grid will absorb so much more radiation that technique increases are necessitated to maintain image density. The radiographer must know what magnitude of adjustment is required at each grid ratio.

Bucky Factor

Technique conversions for using grids are derived by comparing the mAs required when using the grid to the mAs required without the grid in order to maintain a given image density. This is, by definition, the *Bucky factor* alluded to earlier. The formula for the Bucky Factor is:

$$\text{Bucky Factor} = \frac{\text{mAs with grid}}{\text{mAs without grid}}$$

When changing from a non-grid approach to a grid technique, the mAs should be multiplied by this factor to prevent the final image turning out too light.

This can be a controversial subject, and there seem to be as many different tables for grid conversion techniques as there are authors. It must be taken into account that grids have evolved somewhat over the years, primarily in regard to refining the materials used in the interspaces between the lead strips and making the strips themselves thinner. Progress has been made in reducing the absorption of the primary x-ray beam, and workable technique conversions for modern grids are of less magnitude than some older publications suggest. Table 13-2 presents the Bucky factors, or technique conversion factors, taken from Report No. 102 of the National Council on Radiation Protection and Measurements. *Cahoon's Formulating X-Ray Techniques* recommends Bucky factor numbers considerably lower than these, based upon actual radiographic images of scatter-producing anatomy rather than ion chambers or step-wedge images. The author's experience, and one students may find, in performing laboratory experiments on grid Bucky factors, is that Cahoon's figures seem more accurate, and the figures in Table 13-2 may be overstated for practical radiography.

As with other technique factors discussed throughout this text, in practice the radiographer needs a simple set of a few conversion factors that can be readily memorized for daily use. One cannot very well memorize the entire Table 13-2, and we are compelled to search this table for *average conversion factors for common grids at typical kVp levels*, and to further round these figures out for easy memorization. Many

Table 13-2
TECHNIQUE CONVERSION FACTORS (BUCKY FACTORS) FOR VARIOUS RATIO GRIDS AT DIFFERENT RANGES OF kVp

Grid ratio	None	2:1	4:1	6:1	8:1	10:1	12:1	14:1	16:1
kV					Bucky factor				
70	1	1.1	2.7	3.3	3.5	3.8	4.0	4.3	4.5
95	1	1.1	2.7	3.4	3.8	4.0	4.3	4.6	5.0
120	1	1.1	2.7	3.5	4.0	4.5	5.0	5.5	6.0

(Reprinted with permission of the National Council on Radiation Protection and Measurements, NCRP Report No. 102.)

textbooks, especially older ones, have recommended figures that are in line with the *120 kVp* conversions listed in Table 13-2. They have thus concluded that mAs should be multiplied by as much as 5 times for a 12:1 grid and 6 times for a 16:1 grid and suggested these figures as *averages*. They are clearly not averages, for only a few types of radiographic procedures are done at 120 kVp. These figures would apply accurately to the grid chest procedure performed with a dedicated chest unit and little else in modern radiography.

By far, most grid procedures are performed in the range of 70 to 95 kVp. This would include all types of procedures from the knee, femur, and shoulder to spines, skulls, and even air-contrast barium procedures. Hence, in terms of deriving a few practical rules of thumb, the figures in Table 13-3 for *70 to 95 kVp* should logically be consulted. Grid ratios of 2:1, 4:1 are extremely rare in actual use. Therefore, we shall focus on those factors from the 6:1 grids up through the 16:1 ratio. Rounding these figures, the simple Table 13-3 may be recommended for commitment to memory. Generally, a 6:1 grid requires approximately 3 times the mAs. Bucky grids in radiographic tables and chest boards usually range from 8:1 to 12:1 in ratio. The 8:1 grid requires roughly $3\frac{1}{2}$ times the non-grid mAs, while the 12:1 requires 4 times

the mAs. The 16:1 grid generally requires 5 times the mAs.

Figure 13-6 demonstrates lucidly the application of these recommended factors. Since contrast also changes in these images, it is important to focus on a single medium-level density in comparing the accuracy of the Bucky factors from Table 13-3: This is found in the mid-orbit as indicated on the radiographs. In Radiograph B, the mAs was only doubled for a 6:1 grid (less than indicated in Table 13-2), yet the image turned out darker than expected. This is consistent with *Cahoon's Formulating X-Ray Techniques*, which recommended a factor of only 2 for the 6:1 grid based on actual radiographic images. The remaining radiographs all bear out the recommended numbers well: In

Table 13-3
TECHNIQUE CONVERSION FACTORS (BUCKY FACTORS) AND RECOMMENDED kVp RANGES BY GRID RATIO

Grid Ratio	mAs Conversion Factor	Recommended kVp Range
Non-Grid	1	Less than 70
6:1	3	70-80
8:1	3.5	80-90
12:1	4	90-110
16:1	5	110-120
Tabletop to Bucky: 3-4X		70-110

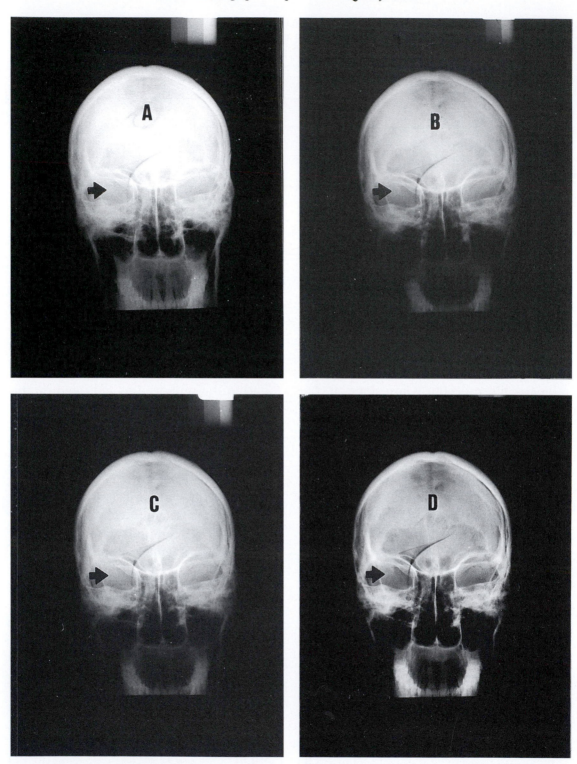

Radiograph C, tripling the mAs restored the orbital density very closely for an 8:1 grid - the recommended value is 3.5.

Radiograph D utilized the recommended factor from Table 13-2 of 4 times for a 10:1 grid and turned out somewhat dark. Note in

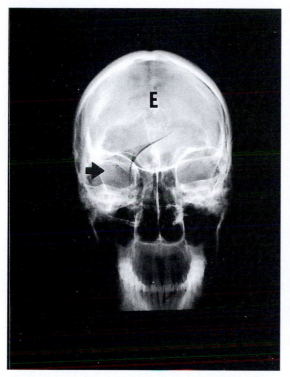
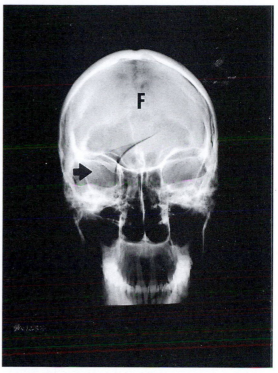

Figure 13-6. Radiographs of a PA skull demonstrating the accuracy of the "grid conversion factors" in Table 13-3 in maintaining image density at various grid ratios. The increasing contrast at higher grid ratios must not be confused with average density: To properly evaluate these images, compare a medium density area such as the intra-orbital density marked by the black arrow. (A) was exposed nongrid with 4 mAs at 76 kVp. Factors used include: (B) 6:1 grid: *Double* to 8 mAs, 76 kVp, (C) 8:1 grid: *Triple* to 12 mAs, 76 kVp, (E) 12:1 grid: *Four times* original technique: 14 mAs, 80 kVp, and (F) 15:1 grid: *Five times* original technique: 20 mAs, 76 kVp. *Note*: Older textbooks recommend 4X technique for a 10:1 grid, 5X for a 12:1, and 6X for a 15:1. These factors are too high for modern grids–Note that in (D) the technique was increased by 4 times for a 10:1 grid, showing excessive density within the orbit (arrow), as compared to the other five exposures.

particular radiographs E and F, where the rules of thumb from Table 13-3 worked almost perfectly: Four times the mAs for the 12:1 grid, and five times the mAs for the 16:1 grid, using mid-range kVp levels.

The 6:1 grid is generally encountered only for mobile bedside radiography or other stationary grid applications where the Potter-Bucky mechanism cannot be accessed. It is common for gridded cassettes and for "wafer" grids that may be attached to the front of a film cassette. The 16:1 grid, at the other extreme, is only recommended for use with *dedicated* chest units where the central ray is permanently center-locked and aligned to the grid. The Bucky factor of 6 would be applied only in this scenario where a dedicated chest unit is employed. It may be stated that *for grids commonly used in the Bucky tray, the conversion factors range from 3 to 4.* This is an easily remembered range, 3 to 4 times the mAs, and useful on a daily basis. *Changing from the tabletop to the Bucky, increase mAs by 3 to 4 times; When changing from the Bucky tray to the tabletop, reduce mAs to 1/3 or 1/4.*

Note that moving grids, such as in the Potter-Bucky mechanism, absorb slightly more radiation than stationary grids of the same ratio. This difference is too slight, however, to warrant a separate list of conversion factors.

Grid conversion factors are extremely controversial in the literature–the author has found no fewer than *six different* tables of recommended Bucky factors. In an attempt to concisely summarize, the following statements regarding grid conversions may be made with confidence:

1. *Grid conversion factors can range from 3 to 6 times the mAs.*
2. *For the most common practical applications using the most common grid ratios, grid conversion factors range only from 3 to 4 times the mAs.*
3. *For tabletop-to-Bucky conversions, use 3 to 4 times the mAs.*

A more complicated conversion problem is encountered when changing from one grid ratio to another. Once the rounded Bucky factors are memorized, all that is needed is to make a *ratio* out of the two factors in question, keeping the grid you are changing *to* on top as the numerator and the grid you are changing *from* as the denominator.

Example: When changing from 6:1 grid to a 12:1 grid, mAs should be increased by what proportion?

Solution: $\dfrac{\text{To}}{\text{From}} = \dfrac{12{:}1 \text{ Factor}}{6{:}1 \text{ Factor}} = \dfrac{4}{3} = 4/3$

mAs should be increased to 4/3 the original amount
Increase mAs by 1.33 X or about 33 percent

Example: When changing from an 8:1 grid to a 16:1 grid, mAs should be reduced by what proportion?

Solution: $\dfrac{\text{To}}{\text{From}} = \dfrac{8{:}1 \text{ Factor}}{16{:}1 \text{ Factor}} = \dfrac{3.5}{5} = 0.7$

mAs should be reduced to 0.7 times the original amount
Reduce mAs by 30 percent to 70 percent of the original amount

Milliampere-seconds should generally be used to compensate for density loss during the application of grids. Changes in kilovoltage will slightly alter the contrast of the radiograph, which is precisely what the grid was employed to control.

For a question of image *density*, simply invert the formula used for technique conversions, placing the grid you are changing *from* on top as the numerator and the grid you are changing *to* as the denominator.

Example 1: Changing from a tabletop non-grid approach into the Bucky tray with an 12:1 grid, if the technique is *not* compensated, how dark will the radiograph turn out compared to the original?

Solution: $\dfrac{\text{From}}{\text{To}} = \dfrac{\text{NG}}{12{:}1} = \dfrac{1}{4}$

The radiograph will turn out 1/4 as dark as the original
The density will be 25% of the original

Example 2: Changing from a 12:1 grid to a 6:1 grid, if the technique is *not* compensated, how dark will the radiograph turn out compared to the original?

Solution: $\dfrac{\text{From}}{\text{To}} = \dfrac{12{:}1}{6{:}1} = \dfrac{4}{3} = 1.3$

The radiograph will turn out 1.3 times darker than the original
The density will be increased by 33%

Try the following exercises for practice, and check your answers from the Appendix.

EXERCISE #12

What would the new *density* be if technique is unchanged and the grid ratio is changed from:

1. Non-grid to 6:1 =
2. 16:1 to non-grid =
3. 8:1 to 16:1 =
4. Bucky to Tabletop =

By what factor must *technique* be changed from the original to maintain density when changing the grid ratio from:

5. Non-grid to 6:1 =
6. 16:1 to 6:1

7. 12:1 to 16:1 =
8. 12:1 to 8:1 =

EFFECTS ON OTHER QUALITIES

Sharpness of recorded detail and the other recognizability functions are based upon beam projection geometry—distances, areas, angles, etc. But, as discussed in the previous chapter, scatter radiation is generated at random distances from the film and in random directions and, therefore, can have no predictable geometrical effect on the image. Scatter reduces the *visibility* of edges of details in the image by destroying their contrast, but does not affect the *sharpness* of those edges. Similarly, a perfectly sharp image may exist on a billboard, yet due to the lack of light, you may not be able to see it—it is technically sharp, but not visible.

Because scattered radiation can play no geometrical role in image formation, the use of grids, designed only to absorb scatter, cannot have any geometrical effect on the image either. The direction of *primary* radiation is not altered as it passes through a grid. Beam projection geometry is unchanged.

Neither are magnification or distortion affected by the use of a grid. Grids should be considered to affect only the visibility functions of the image. However, an indirect problem arises when the Potter-Bucky diaphragm is used: Since the Bucky tray holds the film normally 2 or 3 inches below the tabletop (and as much as 4 to 6 inches on some machines, especially tomographic units), an increased object-image receptor distance results. Sharpness is thereby reduced and magnification slightly increased, but it is the increased OID that is directly responsible for these effects rather than the use of the grid. The use of wafer grids, which are attached to the front of a cassette, poses no such problem with changing OID.

GRID CUT-OFF

The lead strips of a grid absorb some of the primary x-rays along with many of the scattered rays. With a stationary grid, this absorption will leave white lines in the image, called *grid lines*, where a loss of information occurs. Although these grid lines can be minimized by the use of proper alignment and distance, they can never be completely eliminated when stationary grids are used. The employment of the Potter-Bucky diaphragm blurs out the grid lines, but there is still some loss of density called *grid cut-off*, caused by the absorption of the remnant radiation. Special care must be taken when using stationary *wafer* grids

and *grid cassettes* to keep the interference of grid lines to a minimum. When improper distances are used or when the beam is not properly aligned to a stationary grid, the grid lines recorded become much wider than necessary, obscuring larger amounts of information from the image (Fig. 13-7).

GRID RADIUS

Due to the fact that x-ray beams diverge or spread out as they approach the film, most grids in modern use are *focused*, that is, the lead strips are tilted more as they move away from the center of the grid, such that

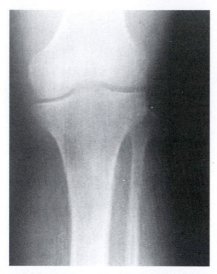

Figure 13-7. Radiograph of a knee with the central ray off-centered laterally 2 inches using a 12:1 stationary grid. Thin, vertical white lines are grid lines, most visible in the middle of the film.

they are always pointing toward the source of the x-rays–the x-ray tube focal spot (Fig. 13-1, left). This tilt of the lead strips is called *canting*.

With a focused grid, the *grid radius* is defined as that distance from the grid at which lines drawn from the canted lead strips, with their various degrees of tilt, would converge to a focal point or *convergent point*. Since there is some margin for error, actual grid radii are given as ranges rather than as one specific number. The two most common such ranges are 36-42

inches and 66-74 inches, obviously designed for the commonly used source-image receptor distances of 40 inches and 72 inches. The x-ray tube must be placed at a distance from the grid within the grid radius designated. If it is not, excessive grid cut-off will occur, with the lead strips absorbing much more *primary* radiation than desired and creating grid cutoff on the radiograph. This occurs because peripheral x-rays strike the grid strips broadside. Figure 13-7 shows how placing the x-ray tube either too close to the grid or too far away from it will result in the same grid cutoff and loss of information.

Parallel grids have no canting of the lead strips. Each strip points straight up, Figure 13-8, left. Therefore, parallel grids have a radius of infinity–the further the x-ray tube is away from the grid, the more parallel the primary rays will be to the lead strips in the grid. For this reason, grid cutoff problems

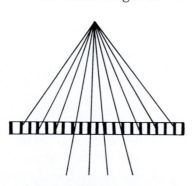

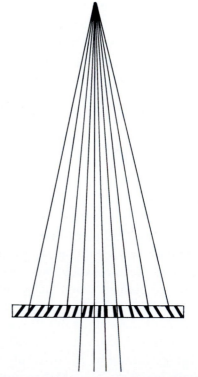

Figure 13-8. Diagram illustrating grid cut-off from placing the x-ray tube too close to a parallel grid (*left*), or outside the grid radius on a focused grid (*right*).

never occur by having the tube too far away from a *parallel* grid. Placing the x-ray tube too close, however, causes the beam divergence to be great, an inordinate amount of primary radiation is absorbed toward the periphery, and severe grid cutoff with a loss of information occurs (Fig. 13-8, left).

Any time the SID used is not within the grid radius, the density pattern resulting on the radiograph will be a darker strip of density down the middle of the lengthwise axis of the film, with a loss of density toward both lateral sides equally, as long as other factors and centering are correct (Fig. 13-9).

Demonstration No. 1

The radiograph in Figure 13-9 was produced without using a phantom or patient in the beam, and with a somewhat exaggerated distance change, in order to demonstrate better the effects of using improper source-image receptor distances that are not within the grid radius. The ratio of the grid used was 15:1, focused grid, 85 lines per inch, with a radius of 36-42 inches. The SID used was 20 inches, too close to the grid. Note that density is lost equally toward both lateral sides of the film. Upon close examination, it is seen that the density loss is due entirely to severe grid lines where no information is recorded under the lead strips. It can also be surmised that the grid cutoff created is more severe for the higher-ratio grids than for the lower-ratio grids even though the distances used were the same. More *selective* grids, with higher grid ratios, have shorter ranges for their grid radii, within which the SID must fall. There is less margin for error, and the distance actually used must be more exact. The same types of mistakes will cause more sever grid cutoff and information loss with a high-ratio grid.

The proper placement of the stationary grid is also critical in minimizing grid cut-

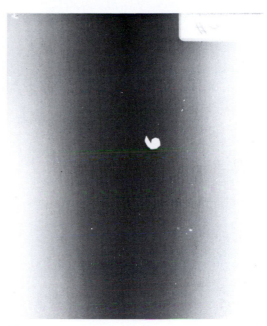

Figure 13-9. Radiograph demonstrating grid cut-off from placing the x-ray tube at 20 inches SID with a 12:1 40-inch radius focused grid.

off and information loss. With wafer grids, a common error is to place the grid upside down over the film cassette. With a focused grid, the effect is to *obliterate* the densities toward both lateral sides of the film equally. This effect is similar to placing the x-ray tube outside of the grid radius, but much more severe in its appearance (Fig. 13-10).

ALIGNMENT OF THE BEAM AND GRID

When performing mobile radiography with stationary grids, two other problems commonly occur: First, the grid and film may be tilted so that they are not perpendicular to the central ray (equivalent to angling the central ray transversely across the lead strips). Second, the grid and film may be off-centered transversely in relation to the central ray. Off-centering or angling *across the lead strips* has the same effect: while there may be some loss of density toward both sides of the film, the loss will be obviously greater toward one side than the other, as

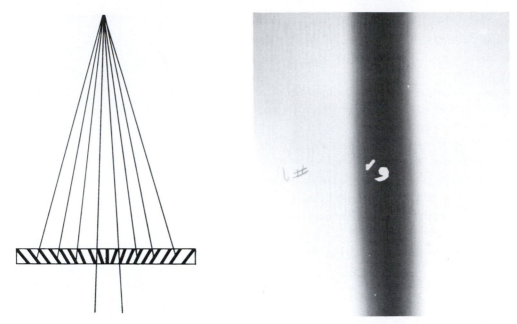

Figure 13-10. Diagram and radiograph showing the grid cut-off caused by placing a focused stationary grid upside down.

illustrated in Figure 13-11 and demonstrated in Figure 13-12. Again, these problems become more severe when working with high-ratio grids than with low-ratio grids.

Only when off-centering or angling the central ray *across* the strips, perpendicular to them, do visible grid cutoff problems occur. Tube angles and intentional off-centering *can* be used when done along the long axis of the grid strips. This is precisely what allows cephalic and caudal tube angles than run longitudinal to the x-ray table, since the grid strips in the Bucky also run longitudinal. The x-ray tube must never be angled transversely across the table while the film is in the Bucky tray. A typical application of intentional off-centering may be found in mobile radiography for skull injuries, as shown in Figure 13-13. Often, the patient is on his or her back and a lateral radiograph of the skull must be taken *cross-table* or using a *horizontal beam projection.* If a 10 x 12 inch cassette with a grid is placed in the normal fashion relative to the skull, the lead strips will be running vertically. With the grid in this position, note that in a superior-to-inferior relation to the patient's head, the central ray must be centered perfectly to the grid even though it may be off-centered to the head—otherwise grid cutoff will occur. Yet in a *vertical dimension* it is permissible to center properly to the head, even though the central ray is not centered strictly to the grid, because *this* off-centering runs along the direction of the grid strips. If the head is built up on a sponge to ensure that the occipital bone is included on the radiograph, the central ray may be recentered vertically at will.

SPECIAL GRIDS

In mobile radiography, a device of considerable help is the grid cassette, a cassette with a grid built into it. These cassettes are very expensive and care must be taken not

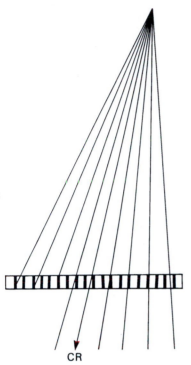

CR

Figure 13-11. Diagram illustrating grid cut-off from angling or off-centering the x-ray beam across the grid strips, or by tilting the grid crosswise.

Figure 13-12. Radiograph demonstrating the grid cut-off caused by off-centering the central ray by two inches across the strips of a 15:1 stationary grid. The effect of angling the beam or tilting the grid would be similar.

to drop them, which can damage the grid or screens inside. When using grid cassettes, the centering and angling considerations just discussed must be carefully followed. Due to the higher probability of off-centering or off-angling in mobile radiography, grid cassettes and wafer grids with a lower grid ratio of 6:1 are most common. This allows some additional margin for error in positioning before grid cutoff becomes noticeable.

The *crosshatch grid* and the similar *rhombic grid* shown in Figure 13-14 are occasionally used in biplane angiography or similar procedures, where there is a high level of cross-scattering radiation from film changers and the table. Centering and alignment must be perfect in *all* directions for these types of grids. If such a grid is constructed with all the lead strips in the same plane, the *Moire grid artifact* occurs: there is a loss of density at each *junction* of the lead strips, causing a pattern of white stellar artifacts on the image. To avoid this artifact, these grids must be constructed as two linear grids, one place above the other, so there are no actual intersections of lead strips.

REVERSE-CASSETTE TECHNIQUE

A "trick-of-the-trade" that has emerged in recent years is the use of a cassette *placed in reverse position* so that the remnant radiation must pass through the *back* of the cassette, in lieu of a grid. The back of modern cassettes usually includes a thin sheet of lead foil intended to reduce backscatter radiation from reaching the film. This foil

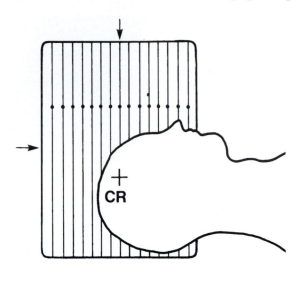

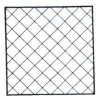

Figure 13-14. Diagram of crosshatch and rhombic grid patterns.

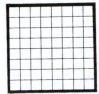

Figure 13-13. Diagram of centering problems encountered in portable cross-table grid-cassette radiography of the skull. The CR must be centered to the grid crosswise even thought this may place it off-centered to the skull in a superoinferior direction. The CR may be centered to the anatomy, however, in a posteroanterior direction even though doing so places it off-centered to the grid lengthwise.

acts as a *filter* in the remnant beam, and since scatter radiation has lower energies than the primary beam, it tends to filter out more scatter radiation than primary radiation, thus improving the overall primary-to-scatter ratio.

This *post-filtration* technique does work in improving image contrast, and can be utilized where-ever a 6:1 ratio grid might be recommended, particularly in mobile (portable) radiography. It requires an increase in overall technique just as a low-ratio grid would. This approach, however, cannot compete with the effectiveness of medium-to-high ratio (8:1 to 12:1) grids such as are normally used in the radiology department and should not be used for general radiography.

SUMMARY

1. Grids should be used on anatomy thicker than 12 cm or when more than 70 kVp is used. They dramatically reduce the *scatter* radiation in the remnant beam, minimizing image *noise*.

2. Since scatter radiation fogs the film, its removal by grids contributes to increased image *contrast*. The higher the *grid ratio*, the greater the contrast improvement. This is the purpose of the grid.

3. Grids also cause a loss in *density* which must be compensated for by increasing mAs from 3 to 5 times. The higher the grid ratio, the greater the loss of density and the more technique adjustment is required to maintain density.

4. *Technique* adjustments for changing grid ratios may be calculated by making simple ratios using the memorized Bucky factors.

5. Grids have no effect upon the *recognizability* functions in the image—sharpness of detail, magnification or distortion. Neither scatter radiation nor grids have any direct relationship to the sharpness of the image.

6. Grids must be placed facing up, perfectly centered to the beam crosswise across the strips, and kept perpendicu-

lar to the beam. Also, the x-ray tube must be placed at the recommended distance within the *grid radius*. Failure to do any of these four things results in severe *grid cutoff* and a loss of density. The higher the grid ratio, the more critical these alignment factors become.

7. Grid *effectiveness* is best measured using the *contrast improvement factor* from actual radiographs. Selectivity is also a valid measure. While grid effectiveness can be affected by changes in grid fre-

quency and overall lead content, the most important determining factor is the *grid ratio*.

8. The technique conversion factor (Bucky factor) for most *Bucky grids* falls between 3 and 4 times the mAs. When changing from the Bucky tray to a tabletop exposure, reduce mAs to 1/3 to 1/4 the original.

9. The *reverse-cassette* technique can be used to advantage in mobile bedside radiography in place of a low-ratio grid.

REVIEW QUESTIONS

1. What is the purpose of a grid, in regard to image quality?
2. A grid has a frequency of 40 lines per cm. It is 1 mm (1/10 cm) thick. What is the grid ratio?
3. What is the purpose of the Potter-Bucky diaphragm?
4. From an original mAs of 60, changing from a 12:1 grid ratio to a 6:1 grid, what should the new technique be to maintain density?
5. Explain the difference between grid ratio and grid radius:
6. Using a stationary grid, the radiograph shows grid cut-off and thicker grid lines toward one side of the film. Name *two* possible causes:
7. When changing from the tabletop to the Bucky tray, assuming a Bucky grid ratio of 8:1, what would the new density be compared to the original density if technique is not adjusted.
8. If a mobile cross-table lateral skull was performed on a grid cassette with the lines running vertically, the x-ray beam was centered horizontally but not vertically since the patient's head was raised on a sponge, the grid had a radius of 40 inches and a ratio of 8:1, and the SID used was 55 inches in order to get

around emergency equipment, describe what single problem would appear on the finished radiograph:
9. What material is most commonly used for grid interspaces?
10. At what minimum kVp level should grids be used?
11. Define grid *selectivity*:
12. What is a "linear grid"?
13. What factor is best used to actually measure the efficiency of a grid?
14. When changing from an 8:1 grid to a 15:1 grid, and adjusting the mAs to maintain equal image density, what will happen to *patient skin dose*?
15. If grids remove poorly-directed scatter radiation, why don't they improve image *sharpness*?
16. Grid efficiency can be enhanced generally by increasing what three factors?
17. Define "convergent point" as it relates to a grid:
18. In what year did Bucky invent the grid?
19. What grid ratio is recommended for kVp levels from 90 to 110?
20. What is defined as the ratio of transmitted primary radiation to transmitted scatter radiation?
21. Define the Contrast Improvement Factor:

Chapter 14

INTENSIFYING SCREENS

X-RAY INTENSIFYING screens are radiographically indispensable. Although they introduce some measure of detail unsharpness in the image, their value in radically reducing patient exposure and reducing motion unsharpness is of prime importance. Less than 1 percent of the x-rays striking an x-ray film is absorbed by the emulsion to expose it; the balance fails to perform any useful radiographic work. The absorption of the x-rays by the emulsion primarily governs the formation of the latent image. It is obvious, therefore, that a means for fully utilizing this small percentage of energy is desirable. This may be accomplished by the use of x-ray intensifying screens that serve to increase the effect of the x-radiation on the sensitized emulsion by means of fluorescence, thereby reducing the exposure. Certain chemicals have the ability to absorb x-rays and instantaneously emit light. This property is called *fluorescence*.

HISTORICAL

Fluorescence was first systematically studied by Sir George Gabriel Stokes of Cambridge, England, in 1852. He showed that a large number of solid bodies and solutions possess the power of absorbing radiation of various wave lengths and then transforming and emitting it in such a manner that an increase in the wave length occurs. (Remember that an increase in wave length indicates a lower energy. Therefore, these materials simply "break" the absorbed radiation into "pieces" of lower energy and then emit these low energy waves.) For example, a solution of quinine sulfate was found to absorb ultraviolet rays and then emit them as visible blue rays. As might naturally be expected—and which later proved to be true in Röntgen's discovery—the extremely short wave length of the rays above the visible violet of the spectrum caused them to be absorbed by most fluorescent bodies and to be emitted as visible light rays of longer wave length. Stokes applied this principle in other experiments by employing a sheet of paper coated with a paint made from pulverized crystals of barium platinocyanide—another fluorescent chemical. There were a number of other investigations conducted with fluorescent materials from this time up to discovery of the x-rays, but little knowledge was added to the discoveries made by Stokes.

At the time of his discovery, Röntgen was searching for light rays beyond the visible spectrum, and the nature of the experiment which he was making at the time with low-pressure discharge tubes in a darkened room led him to cover the tube completely with black paper. When the

200

tube was excited, he noticed that a barium platinocyanide fluorescent screen lying on a table a few feet away glowed brightly. The covered discharge tube precluded any possibility of the effect being due to ordinary or ultraviolet light, and he reasoned that there must be some strange radiation emanating from the tube. Objects that were interposed between the energized tube and the screen caused images to appear. Since this strange light caused the screen to fluoresce, it became possible to photograph and record the images. Röntgen then made those first radiographs, which have become very familiar to us.

Development of Fluorescent Chemicals

Röntgen's discovery of x-rays by means of the fluorescent screen served as a new means to further intensive research in the study of fluorescent compounds. In fact, subsequent experimental work with x-rays and various fluorescent crystals finally led Becquerel to the discovery that uranium or its compounds constantly emitted radiations which were very similar to x-rays in that they penetrated opaque objects, ionized gases, and also caused fluorescence.

To understand more fully the development of the fluoroscopic and intensifying screen, some knowledge relative to the modern conception of fluorescent compounds is necessary.

Edison's Work

In the period, January to March, 1896, Thomas Alva Edison ambitiously tested some 8,500 different materials in his efforts to build a new incandescent lamp. Finally, from among 1,800 which fluoresced, he discovered that the fluorescence of calcium tungstate crystals has approximately six

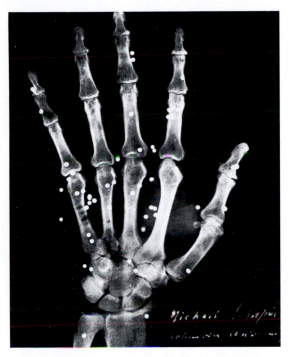

Figure 14-1. First radiograph of the hand using a fluorescent screen to enhance the x-ray exposure, made in 1896 by Professor Michael Pupin.

times more intensity than barium platinocyanide. He then recommended the use of this salt for x-ray fluoroscopic screens in March of 1896. Edison prepared his calcium tungstate screens by mixing the crystals with collodion and spreading a thick layer upon paper; later, cardboard was employed, and on occasion, thin sheets of aluminum.

FIRST USE OF INTENSIFYING SCREENS

At the time of the discovery of x-rays, Professor Michael Pupin of Columbia University had been keenly interested in the work conducted in Germany on discharge-tube phenomena; consequently he was one of the few persons in 1896 who had any equipment adequate to produce x-rays. Pupin immediately began to study these rays and accomplished a tremendous amount of experimental work. In addition, a large number of patients were sent to him for examination by the local physicians. The exposures necessary for him to employ were very long and he made every effort to increase the efficiency of his apparatus so that he could shorten the exposure. This he accomplished in February of 1896 by sandwiching together a photographic plate and a fluorescent screen that Thomas Edison had sent to him. He then made an exposure of a hand in a few seconds that formerly had required an hour's exposure. A large number of buckshot were revealed in the image (Fig. 14-1). Subsequent improvement in fluorescing power of the fluoroscopic screen by Edison, and its application to radiography by Pupin, meant much to radiology, for it made possible shorter exposures and consequently increased the life of those fragile, unstable x-ray tubes then in use.

SCREEN AND CASSETTE CONSTRUCTION

THE INTENSIFYING SCREEN

In modern intensifying screens, the fluorescent crystals used are suspended throughout a layer of plastic similar to the way that film emulsion suspends crystals of silver bromide. This "emulsion" of phosphor crystals is finely coated onto sheets of flexible polyester. The screens may be mounted in pairs in the top and bottom of light-proof cassettes, so that radiographic film can be sandwiched between them. Each screen consists of the plastic *base*, a *reflective layer*, the *phosphor layer*, and a *protective coat* of thin, clear plastic to prevent scratches (Fig. 14-2). The total thickness of modern intensifying screens is about 0.4 mm.

Base

The polyester plastic base of the intensifying screen ranges in thickness, depending on the brand, from 180 to 250 micrometers, roughly one-quarter of a millimeter. The base must be durable, yet flexible enough to allow good contact across the entire surface of the film. It must be homogeneously radiolucent to the x-ray beam so that no artifacts are created in the image. It must also be chemically inert so that there is no chance of it discoloring the emulsion in contact with it. Such discoloration of the emulsion would interfere with the light emission of the screen.

Reflective Layer

Light produced by the phosphor crystals in the emulsion is emitted isotropically, in all directions. Although much of the light is emitted toward the film, light emitted "sideways" and "backwards" away from the film is lost and lowers efficiency. For general-use screens, a very thin layer of titanium dioxide or a similar white, reflective substance is spread over the screen base. This layer acts as a mirror, reflecting the light that is emitted in a direction away from the film back toward the film, maximizing the benefit of fluorescence.

Unfortunately, light reflected from this layer has a longer distance to travel before reaching the film, so it spreads out slightly more than the light emitted directly toward the film and contributes to penumbra or *blur*. (See Figure 14-13 demonstrating variations of the crossover effect.) For this reason, some brands of "fine" screens or "extremity cassettes" designed for high res-

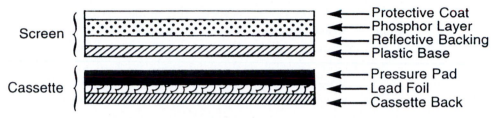

Figure 14-2. Diagram of the components of an intensifying screen and cassette.

olution of detail do not employ the reflective layer.

Phosphor Layer

The *phosphor layer* consists of fluorescent crystals suspended uniformly within a plastic *binder* solution which is coated onto the base and allowed to dry. This is the "active layer," the primary functional part, of the intensifying screen. The phosphor crystals used must be efficient at absorbing x-rays and re-emitting that energy as visible light. Several specific phosphors are used, and these will be discussed in detail later. The phosphor layer must be durable and flexible. Its thickness varies considerably with the "speed" or intended used of the screen, and may range from 80 to as much as 250 micrometers.

Protective Coat

A thin protective super-coating of tough plastic, sometimes called the *T-coat* or *tough-coat*, about 20 to 25 micrometers thick, serves two functions: It gives some protection to the delicate phosphor layer from damage during the loading of films, handling and cleaning, and it helps to prevent artifacts caused by static electricity discharges from friction during film loading. The T-coat must be clear and transparent to the light emitted by the phosphor crystals, and must be very thin. Therefore, great care must be taken in handling

screens, since abrasive cleaners, fingernails, and film edges can all still easily penetrate this layer and damage the phosphor layer.

THE CASSETTE

The *Cassette* is designed to be a light-proof case for the radiographic film and to hold the film and intensifying screens in proper placement to each other. It must be thin and light-weight for easy handling, yet it must have a sturdy, durable frame and rigid, inflexible covers so that the contact of the flat surfaces of film and screens inside it is protected. Care must be taken not to drop cassettes, as the resulting damage can lead to warped backing and consequent poor film/screen contact, which destroys the sharpness of the image and can render the cassette useless.

The front of the cassette must made of material that is as uniformly radiolucent as possible, yet sturdy. New graphite carbon-fiber and plastic materials have proven ideal for these needs, especially in low-kilo-voltage mammography. Older cassettes may have bakelite or aluminum fronts. The back of the cassette is the "lid" one opens to load and unload film, and includes latches for secure closure of the cassette. The cassette back is frequently made of a stronger material than the cassette front, since radiolucency is not essential "behind" the film. In most cassettes, the back cover includes a thin sheet of lead or copper foil

(Fig. 14-2). The purpose of this foil is to absorb *backscatter* radiation which is produced in the Bucky tray, film holder, table or wall immediately behind the cassette. Backscatter radiation from these sources behind the cassette can fog the radiograph, especially during exposures of large body parts.

Many modern cassettes are made with a slight curvature to the lid which can be seen when it is opened, a concave bending away from the open cassette. As the cassette is closed on a film, the effect of the curve is to squeegee out any air pockets to better ensure uniform film/screen contact. Intensifying screens may be mounted inside the front and the back of the cassette. Fine-detail or slow-speed cassettes may have a screen mounted on only one side, usually the back or lid. For regular dual-screen cassettes, some manufacturers designate which screen is to be mounted in front and which in back by labeling them along the edge. This indicates that the back screen is thicker than the front. Since some of the radiation is absorbed by the front screen, the actual exposure to the back screen is always less. To compensate for this and ensure identical radiographic densities on both sides of the film, the back screen is slightly faster than the front one by making it thicker. Some manufacturers make the two screens in the pair identical. But, for those who make them different thicknesses, it is essential to mount them correctly as labeled.

Pressure Pad

Wherever an intensifying screen is mounted, there will be a felt or foam rubber pressure pad between the screen and the cover. The *pressure pad* or *supportive backing* is of critical importance: Its function is to guarantee sufficient, uniform pressure when the cassette is closed to assure complete contact of the screens with the film across their entire surfaces. Figure 14-2 shows a cross-sectional diagram of the various layers within a typical screen cassette, including both the screen and the cassette itself.

EFFICIENCY OF THE PHOSPHOR LAYER

To produce density on the radiographic film, an intensifying screen must perform the following three operations in order: (1) absorb x-rays; (2) convert the energy from these x-rays into visible light rays that will expose the film, rather than dispersing it as some other form of energy; and (3) successfully emit the produced light out of the phosphor layer and to the film. In measuring the efficiency of intensifying screens, radiographic physics textbooks categorize these processes using various terms: For example, "Intrinsic efficiency" has been used to describe the ability to both absorb and convert the x-ray energy, while "screen efficiency" has been used to describe the ratio of light produced which escapes the screen (emission). "Quantum detection efficiency" and "attenuation coefficient" are both terms used to describe absorption. To simplify the following discussion for the student, we shall use only three terms, strictly defined by each of the three essential processes:

Absorption Efficiency: The ability of the phosphor layer to absorb x-rays

Conversion Efficiency: The inherent ability of the phosphor chemical to convert x-ray energy into visible light rays, rather than dispersing it as some other form of energy that does not significantly affect the film

Emission Efficiency: The ability of the produced light to escape the phosphor layer and reach the film to expose it

Let us now examine the various characteristics of the intensifying screen phosphor layer, how they affect each of these three processes, and the results in overall screen efficiency:

THICKNESS OF THE PHOSPHOR LAYER

A common method used by manufacturers to produce screens of different *speeds* (efficiencies) is to make the phosphor layer thicker or thinner. For a particular phosphor type or screen brand, thicker phosphor layers are the main method for achieving higher speeds. Which of the three processes defined in the previous section are affected by phosphor layer thickness? Just as thicker patients absorb more radiation, so thicker phosphor layers will absorb more x-rays, and more light will then be produced by the screen. This is simply due to the fact that more atoms have been placed "in the way" of the x-ray beam, and so the likelihood that a particular x-ray will be absorbed increases. Absorption efficiency increases.

Note that with a thicker phosphor layer, some of the produced light will have to travel farther to escape the screen itself—this light may "run into" other phosphor crystals on its way out. Since it is more difficult for produced light to penetrate out of the phosphor layer and reach the film, the *emission efficiency* is slightly lowered. This effect is very minor, however, when compared with the great increase in *absorption efficiency*. The net result is that thicker phosphor layers emit much more light, because of increased x-ray absorption.

PHOSPHOR DENSITY

The configuration (shape) of some types of phosphor molecules allows them to be packed more tightly together within a crystal. Thus, there will be a higher *concentration* of molecules in each crystal. This is described as a higher molecular density or physical density (mass per volume of space). There are simply more atoms *per cubic millimeter* for the x-rays to "run into," and absorption goes up proportionately. The physical density of the phosphor molecules is an important reason why "rare earth" screens were such an improvement over the old technology.

Interestingly, manufacturers have recently developed new gross shapes of the entire *crystals themselves*, such as *flat-shaped* crystals. In this way, it is sometimes possible to pack the crystals closer together within the binder substance, and still maintain a good uniform distribution. This may be thought of as the "crystal density" of the phosphor layer, and it has the effect of proportionately increasing the absorption of x-rays. Whether packing the crystals closer together, or packing the molecules within each crystal closer together, an increase in phosphor density enhances the *absorption efficiency* of the screen.

ATOMIC NUMBER OF PHOSPHOR ELEMENTS

"Large" atoms, those with a high atomic number (Z#), have many more electrons in their "shells." However, their actual *diameter* as measured across the outermost shell only increases very slightly when compared to atoms of low atomic number. This is because, as protons are added to the nucleus and electrons added to shells, the shells collapse in closer and closer to the nucleus. In other words, atoms with a high atomic number are not so much "larger" as they are more "concentrated." This increased concentration of electrons within the space around the nucleus is referred to as the atom's *electron density*. Atoms of high atomic number have a more *dense cloud of electrons* around them. This means that an x-ray passing through the space of such an atom will be much more likely to strike an electron and be absorbed by it. Thus, high atomic number elements absorb x-rays much more efficiently than low atomic number elements. It is for this reason that high atomic number elements are sought after as phosphors for intensifying screens.

Table 14-1 lists the highest atomic number element used in each of the most common types of intensifying screens for comparison—note that these are all elements "high up" on the periodic chart, with 56 or more electrons. The use of high atomic number elements increases the *absorption efficiency* of the screen.

K-EDGE EFFECT: Directly related to the atomic number is the binding energy of the K-shell in these atoms. The K-edge effect may be thought of as an *exception* to rule that higher atomic numbers increase absorption. Ironically, if the atomic number is *too high*, as is the case with calcium tungstate, so that the K-edge binding energy is well above the average x-ray beam energies, then absorption due to the photoelectric effect may be *lost*. This is fully explained in a following section, but is mentioned here because it is directly related to the atomic number of the elements used in the phosphor layer.

CRYSTAL SIZE

Historically, larger crystals were sometimes used to increase the *absorption* efficiency of a screen. However, this method increased mottle effects and caused a loss of resolution of fine details, and it is no longer employed because of these limitations.

CHEMICAL COMPOUND USED FOR PHOSPHOR MOLECULE

Thomas Edison tested hundreds of chemical compounds to determine which was most efficient at *converting* x-ray energy

Table 14-1

HIGHEST ATOMIC NUMBER ELEMENTS USED IN SCREEN PHOSPHORS

Phosphor Molecule	*Highest Z# Element:*	*Atomic Number*
Barium Fluorochloride	Barium	56
Lanthanum Oxybromide	Lanthanum	57
Gadolinium Oxysulfide	Gadolinium	64
Calcium Tungstate	Tungsten	74
(Various Activators:	Niobium-Terbium	41-65)

into visible light. He concluded that calcium tungstate, with its intense emission of blue light, was best suited for use in radiographic intensifying screens to expose film. This compound was the standard for many decades, well into the 1970s. With enhanced chemical technology and knowledge, it was found that several "rare earth" elements when treated with trace amounts of terbium, thulium, europium, or niobium as chemical activators (catalysts), were *2 to 4 times* more efficient than calcium tungstate in converting x-ray energy into fluorescent light. Thus, if two phosphor layers of equal thickness are compared, the activated rare earth chemical will produce more light than the calcium tungstate. This is a higher *conversion efficiency*, and is due entirely to the chemical properties of the molecules. Several types of phosphor compounds are now used in different brands of intensifying screens, each having a different intrinsic conversion efficiency.

ADDITION OF DYES TO PHOSPHOR LAYER

A color dye may be added to the phosphor binder in order to reduce the amount of light reaching the film from distant points within the phosphor layer and improve sharpness of detail. The diffuse light which produces penumbra (blur) around a detail is emitted at a greater angle and must travel a greater distance to reach the film than light which is emitted directly toward the film. When just the right amount of dye is added, direct light will just escape the screen while much of the diffuse light will be absorbed by the dye before escaping and reaching the film (Fig. 14-3). Thus, penumbra is reduced and sharpness enhanced.

However, a price is paid for the improved resolution: The speed of the

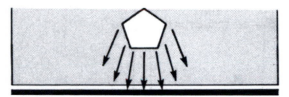

Figure 14-3. Diagram of the effect of adding dye to the binder of high-detail intensifying screens. On average, light only penetrates through the dye a limited distance, indicated by the length of the arrows. Only the light traveling most directly downward toward the film escapes, thus reducing penumbra and increasing sharpness of detail. Since overall light output is reduced, screen speed is lowered, and increased techniques are required.

intensifying screen is substantially reduced, since less total light is reaching the film. In turn, this necessitates increased techniques which result in higher exposures to the patient. This increased exposure is acceptable when used on distal extremities. Cassettes with these types of screens used to be called "detail" cassettes because of the enhanced sharpness of details they produced. They are now generally referred to as "extremity cassettes."

Under normal room lighting, one can open a detail or extremity cassette and easily recognize the yellow or gray appearance of a screen with such a dye added. Which of the three types of efficiency do added dyes affect? The answer is the *emission efficiency* of the screen, since they reduce the amount of produced light that escapes from the screen.

THE REFLECTIVE LAYER

When a reflective layer is added behind the phosphor layer in an intensifying screen, or when the reflectivity of this layer is somehow improved, more of the produced light will reach the film. Improved reflectivity, then, also increases the *emission efficiency* of a screen.

kVp DEPENDENCE AND
K-EDGE EFFECT

At some time in your life you have likely seen how some types of rocks glow in the dark or *phosphoresce*. Each different phosphorescent mineral emits its own characteristic color of light—one emits green light, another yellow, and so on. A particular mineral always emits the same color of light. The same holds true for the *fluorescence* of the phosphor crystals used in intensifying screens—each chemical emits a characteristic *color* or *wavelength of light*. The nature of these phosphor chemicals is to always emit the *same wavelength* of light. The wavelength of a ray of light (its color) is a direct manifestation of its energy, so we might re-phrase this to say that a particular phosphor always emits light photons of the same *energy*.

This is the very key to how intensifying screens work: The energy of a single incoming x-ray photon will be *split* by the phosphor into hundreds of light photons, each one having exactly the same energy. For example, a calcium tungstate screen always emits blue-violet light rays having about 3 volts of energy each. How much light will be produced from a single x-ray photon of 30 kilovolts? The 30 kilovolts of energy, or 30,000 volts, will be *split* into units of 3 volts each. The law of conservation of energy requires that the *total* amount of energy after this event be equal to the original amount (10,000 photons at 3 volts each equals 30,000 volts total). Theoretically, then, some 10,000 blue light rays will be emitted from this single x-ray!

In reality, the above calculation is oversimplified, because it assumes a 100 percent conversion efficiency for the phosphor chemical. The real conversion efficiency for various phosphors is much less, from 5 percent to 20 percent. The remaining energy is dispersed as heat. Assuming a 5 percent conversion efficiency for calcium tungstate, the actual amount of light emitted would be 10,000 x 5 percent = 500 light rays. Further, remember that this light is emitted isotropically in all directions from the phosphor crystal, and only a portion of it is directed toward the film, even with the use of a reflective backing in the screen. Also, some of the light is absorbed before it escapes the screen, and some penetrates through the film without being absorbed. Perhaps 100 light photons will ultimately expose the film due to each single x-ray photon striking the intensifying screen. Still, this is a very impressive increase in overall efficiency. The invention of intensifying screens in 1896 reduced patient exposures a *hundred fold*, and was truly an historic event in medical imaging.

This same phenomenon, that a screen always emits the same energy of light regardless of the energy of the incoming x-ray photon, causes the output of the screen to be *kVp-dependent*. Figure 14-4 illustrates this effect. When a higher keV x-ray photon strikes a phosphor crystal, the crystal will split that energy into *more* light photons, all with the same energy, rather than emitting higher-energy light rays, which would change their color. Whereas a 30-keV x-ray would be split into 10,000 light rays of 3 volts each, a *60-keV* x-ray would be split into *20,000* light rays, still at 3 volts each. Therefore, as kVp rises, the intensifying screen increases its actual output of light and glows brighter. This can be demonstrated easily by opening any screen cassette in the laboratory, exposing it to various kVp levels at equal mAs, and observing the brightness and color of the light emitted. The color of the light does not change, but the higher the kVp, the brighter the screen glows. While converting x-rays into light, the screen has con-

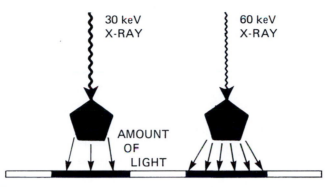

Figure 14-4. Diagram of the kVp-dependence effect of intensifying screens. The energy of a single x-ray is "split" by the phosphor crystal into tens of thousands of light photons, always of the same color and same energy. Note that if the keV of the single incoming x-ray is doubled, the *amount* of light photons emitted will double, resulting in a greater exposure to the film.

verted *energy differences* into *intensity differences* (as if the mA had been increased rather than the kVp). The film is exposed to more light photons, rather than higher energy photons. The kVp-dependence effect is classified as a change in the *conversion efficiency* of the screen.

The kVp-dependence effect is *slightly* offset by the fact that at higher kVp levels, the x-ray beam is more penetrating and less x-rays are absorbed by the screen. There is a drop in *absorption efficiency* at higher kilovoltages, but the increase in conversion efficiency due to kVp-dependence is much greater. Because the increased *conversion efficiency* at higher kVp levels is so much greater than the loss of absorption and K-edge effects, the *net change in screen speed is a dramatic increase at higher kilovoltages, resulting in darker radiographic densities.*

Radiologic physics textbooks use absorption graphs to depict an irregularity in the absorption of x-rays by intensifying screens known as the *K-edge* effect. As kVp is increased, there can be a sudden surge in the screen's absorption of x-rays just when the kVp surpasses the binding energy of the K-shell electrons in the screen. (Binding

energy is how "tightly" the electrons are held in orbit.) Intensifying screens absorb x-rays primarily by the photoelectric effect (Chapter 4). This surge in absorption is due to the fact that the photoelectric effect is prevalent when the x-ray beam energy is just slightly above the K-shell binding energy. Generally, as kVp is increased, there is more penetration and *less* absorption. The K-edge effect is an *exception* to this rule. Figure 14-5 graphs this relationship: Note that the absorption curve steadily drops as keV increases, *except when the keV crosses the K-edge for tungsten.*

In the older calcium tungstate screens, this "surge" of increased absorption occurred at about 69 keV, the K-shell binding energy for the element tungsten. This might have caused havoc with technique selection, except for the fact that the *average* energies within the x-ray beam are well below this K-edge energy. Recall from Chapter 1 that the *average* energy of the Bremsstrahlung x-rays in the beam is about one-third of the set kVp. The Bremsstrahlung spectrum is added (dotted line) in Figure 14-5 to show that *most* of the x-rays even in a 100-kVp beam have energies

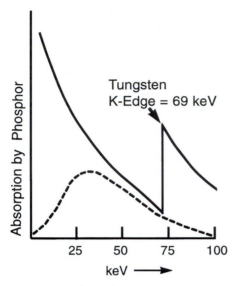

Figure 14-5. Graph of the K-edge effect for tungsten in calcium tungstate screens (solid curve) with the, x-ray spectrum for a 100 kVp beam added (dashed curve.) Note that at this kVp, most x-rays are produced in a range of 20 to 50 keV, where the absorption of the screen is quite poor (and less than the K-edge absorption.) At the K-edge of tungsten, where absorption suddenly spikes to a high level, there are only a few x-rays being produced. Thus, the absorption of the screen is poorly matched to the actually energies of the x-rays.

averaging around 35 keV and ranging from 20 to 50 keV, well below the K-edge. Only a small portion of the beam, those few x-rays above 69 keV, are subjected to this "sudden surge of absorption." Thus, the K-edge effect for calcium tungstate screens was only noticeable at very high kVp's and generally of little consequence in setting techniques. It did, however, mean that the overall absorption of radiation by calcium tungstate screens was not very efficient.

SUMMARY

Besides all of the factors just discussed, *anything* which increases the *exposure rate* to the intensifying screen will, of course,

result in more light output from that screen. The key word here is the *rate* of exposure, since the apparent brightness of a glowing screen is in reality the *rate* of light emission from it. The milliampere station selected by the radiographer controls the rate of exposure, and higher mA values will cause the screens to glow brighter. Increased exposure time has no effect on the output rate of the screen—it glows with the same steady brightness. But, naturally, since the screen would glow for a longer period of time, the exposure time must be factored into the end *total* of light exposure to the film. The effects of kVp-dependence have just been discussed; in addition to these effects, recall that within the x-ray tube itself, higher kVp's result in the production of greater amounts of Bremsstrahlung radiation. This means that at higher kVp's, the rate of x-ray exposure to the screens has also increased and this results in even more light output from those screens.

Having covered the variables that bear upon the actual light *output* of a screen, we should observe that only those characteristics which are inherent to the screen structure itself ought to be considered as affecting the *screen speed*. The speed of a screen is published by the manufacturer as a numerical value, 100, 200, and so on. If screen B has twice the speed of screen A, then screen B will be expected to emit twice as much light *under identical exposure conditions.* When factors that alter the exposure *to* the screen are considered, such as increased mA, bear in mind that even though the light *output* of the screen may increase or decrease accordingly, this does not constitute a change in the inherent *speed* of the screen. Table 14-2 summarizes all of the variables affecting the output of intensifying screens, and is helpful in clarifying these relationships.

Table 14-2
VARIABLES AFFECTING INTENSIFYING SCREEN OUTPUT

I. Inherent Screen Speed
    A. Absorption Efficiency
        1. Thickness of Phosphor Layer
        2. Physical Density of Phosphor Layer
        3. Average Atomic Number (Z) of Phosphor
        4. K-Edge of Phosphor
    B. Conversion Efficiency
        1. Chemical Compound Used as Phosphor
    C. Emission Efficiency
        1. Reflective Backing (use of, effectiveness of)
        2. Added Dye (use of, effectiveness of)
        3. Thickness of Phosphor Layer (binder material)
II. Exposure Factors (affecting remnant beam)
    A. kVp
    B. mA
    C. All Beam Attenuators (filters, patient, grid)

EFFICIENCY OF RARE EARTH SCREENS

The *rare earth screen* made its debut in the 1970s and has since become the standard of practice, much more commonly used now than calcium tungstate screens. Rare earth screens are so named because in most cases the phosphors utilized are based upon elements with atomic numbers between 57 and 71 on the periodic chart of the elements, known as the *rare earth elements.* Various compounds of yttrium, lanthanum, gadolinium, and barium have been used. When special "activators" such as the elements niobium, thulium, or terbium are added to these compounds, a maximum fluorescent response is achieved upon exposure to x-rays. The two most widely used compounds in screens are thulium-activated lanthanum oxybromide and terbium-activated gadolinium oxysulfide.

Table 14-1 lists the highest atomic numbers of the elements in several of these compounds. Note that the first three of these compounds, marketed as rare earth screens, all have atomic numbers *lower* than that of the old calcium tungstate screens. If screen speed were solely dependent upon the atomic number of the material, we would expect the rare earth screens to be *less* efficient than the older calcium tungstate screens. Clearly, in rare earth screens, there must be other factors which compensate for these lower atomic numbers, and then beyond compensating, go on to result in a faster overall speed. Indeed, there are at least *three* such factors. They are the K-edge effect, phosphor density, and inherent conversion efficiency.

K-Edge Effect

Ironically, the lower atomic number of the rare earth elements places their K-edge at a lower energy as well. As shown in Figure 14-6, this actually *improves* overall absorption: To demonstrate, consider the fate of those photons having 40 kV of energy. The beam spectrum curve in both Figures 14-5 and 14-6 shows that there are many more photons at this energy than, say, at 80 kV. (Remember that *most* x-rays

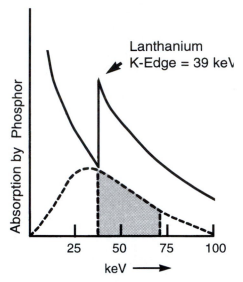

Figure 14-6. Graph of the K-edge effect for lanthanum in a rare earth screen (solid curve) with the x-ray spectrum for a 100 kVp beam added (dashed curve.) Note that the K-edge for lanthanum is much more closely matched to the peak of the x-ray beam than the K-edge of tungsten shown in Figure 119. Those x-rays produced between 39 and 69 keV (shaded representing the two different K-edges) are much better absorbed than they were in tungsten. Gadolinium, yttrium and terbium also have lower K-edges similar to this one.

in the beam average only about one-third the energy of the kVp.) If more of these 40-kV photons can be captured by the screen, efficiency will improve dramatically. Compare the position of the K-edge for calcium tungstate in Figure 14-5 to that for Lanthanum Oxybromide in Figure 14-6. In the calcium tungstate, there is *no* photoelectric absorption of 40-kV x-rays by the *K-shell.* In Figure 14-5, the absorption curve at 40 kV represents photoelectric interactions occurring primarily in the *L-Shell.* (The K-shell is absorbing x-rays above 69 keV, but there are only a few x-rays at these energies.)

For lanthanum oxybromide, Figure 14-6 shows that 40-kV x-rays are slightly above the K-edge. This is the ideal situation for

photoelectric interactions to occur in the K-shell. These x-rays have just enough energy to knock K-shell electrons out of their shell without any left-over scatter radiation, and so they will be completely absorbed by the K-shell electrons. With the addition of K-shell absorption, the overall absorption curve spikes sharply upward. At *40-kV,* more photons are absorbed by lanthanum than by tungsten, even though lanthanum has a lower atomic number. The same is generally true for all photon energies in the shaded area of the beam spectrum in Figure 14-6. Compared to calcium tungstate, there will be increased absorption of those x-rays ranging in energy from 39 kV to 69 kV.

Phosphor Density

The configuration (or "shape") of rare earth molecules allows for the phosphor molecules to be more "tightly packed" together. They are more concentrated within a volume of space than the calcium tungstate molecules can be. Clearly, this will result in additional absorption of x-rays, as there are simply more molecules per cubic millimeter for the x-rays to "run into."

Conversion Efficiency

Calcium tungstate has an inherent conversion efficiency of only 5 percent. Only 5 percent of x-ray energy is converted into emitted visible light, the rest is dispersed as heat. Gadolinium and lanthanum compounds have a conversion efficiency of almost 20 percent, nearly four times that of calcium tungstate. This improvement is simply characteristic of the chemical molecules used.

Table 14-3 compares the absorption efficiency and conversion efficiency of two dif-

Table 14-3
WHY RARE EARTH SCREENS ARE FASTER

Screen Type	Absorption Efficiency	Conversion Efficiency
CaWO4 Par	20%	5%
CaWO4 High	40%	5%
Rare Earth Phosphors	60%	20%

ferent thicknesses of calcium tungstate screens and a typical rare earth screen. In comparing the two calcium tungstate screens, note that the *absorption efficiency* is doubled for the "high-speed" screen; the only difference between these two screens is that the high-speed screen is *thicker*, which affects its absorption. Since the same chemical is used, conversion efficiency is equal. The rare earth screen, however, shows a dramatic increase in *both* absorption efficiency (60%) and conversion efficiency (20%). The improved absorption is due to both the K-edge effect and increased phosphor density. These two improvements are so effective that they compensate for the lower atomic number of the rare earth elements, and go well beyond that to bring about a net increase in absorption. The very high conversion efficiency multiplies these factors still further, resulting in a family of intensifying screens that are *two* to *eight* times faster than calcium tungstate.

This improvement has dramatically reduced patient exposures in modern radiography.

SPECTRAL MATCHING

Radiographic films are designed to be most sensitive to specific colors of light. The old calcium tungstate screens emitted blue-violet light, and film was designed to be most sensitive to this color. Most rare earth screens emit light wave lengths that are centered in the *green* portion of the spectrum. Special film was designed for use with these screens, which is most sensitive to green light. Any mis-matching of screen emission with film sensitivity, placing blue-sensitive film in a green-emitting screen, or green-sensitive film in a blue-emitting screen, will result in some loss of efficiency and the resulting radiograph will turn out *underexposed.*

Some barium and lanthanum compounds emit blue light rather than green. Barium is not a true rare earth element, but barium compounds are frequently marketed as "rare earth" screens. Therefore, one must be careful to determine the color of light emission and film requirements when considering the purchase of any "rare earth" imaging system.

SCREEN SPEEDS AND DENSITY

The function of the intensifying screen is to intensify the effect of x-ray exposure upon image density. *Speed* refers to a screen's ability to produce density with a given exposure to x-rays. The higher the speed of the screen, the more density will be produced at a given exposure. Higher speeds reduce the patient dose, since lower exposure settings will produce adequate radiographic density.

The speed of an intensifying screen is derived from the *intensification factor*, the factor by which exposure can be reduced to obtain a similar density when using the screen. The intensification factor is mathematically expressed as:

$$IF = \frac{\text{Exposure required without screen}}{\text{Exposure required with screen}}$$

For example, if a direct, non-screen exposure required 300 mAs to produce a density of 2.0, and an exposure with *Screen A* required 10 mAs to produce the same density, the intensification factor for *Screen A* would be 300/10 = 30. The *speed* of *Screen A*, then, is 30 times faster than direct exposure.

Although the intensification factors for different types and speeds of screens can be used to compare their effectiveness one to another, it has become conventional to compare all of the other screens to the *par speed calcium tungstate* screen rather than to direct exposure technique. In doing so, manufacturers fixed a speed figure for *par* screen at *100*. Thus, a screen that is one-half as fast as a par-speed screen would be assigned a relative speed of *50*, one that is twice as fast would be considered a *200-speed* screen, and so on. Table 15-1, in the next chapter, is an example of various speeds obtained with different combinations of Kodak™ screens and film when compared to the 100-speed par speed film and par-speed screen combination.

A *relative density* factor for different speeds of screens can be obtained by simply deleting the two zeros in the relative speed; For example, a 200-speed screen will produce a radiographic density 2 times darker than the 100-speed par screen using the same technique. All other factors equal, a 300-speed screen will produce a density 3 times darker, 400-speed will be 4 times darker, and so on. A 50-speed screen will produce one-half the density, a 25-speed screen one-fourth.

Depending on the particular brand name of the rare earth screen used, other speeds will be encountered. The exact speeds for these screens must be obtained from the manufacturers. Although some rare earth screens boast a speed as high as 1200 (12 times the par speed), these are rarely used for two very important reasons: First, their speed is usually increased from that of the regular rate earth screen by using a thicker phosphor layer, which results in a real loss of sharpness in the image. Second, their speed is so excessively high that quantum mottle will become visible on the image, due to the grossly reduced mAs values used. Because such a speed cannot generally be recommended for medical use, it is not listed in Table 14-5. The 800-speed screen can present these same two problems for the same reasons, and is only recommended for pediatric or other procedures wherein it is essential to minimize exposure time and *in which sharpness of detail is not of primary concern.*

Table 14-4

TRADITIONAL IMAGE RECEPTORS
TECHNIQUE CONVERSION FACTORS BY SCREEN SPEED

Screen Speed (Density Fx)	Descriptive Name	mAs Conversion Factor
2	Direct Exposure Holder	50
50	Slow or Detail Speed	2
100	Par or Medium Speed	1
200	High Speed	1/2 (.5)
300	High-Plus or Ultra-High Speed	1/3 (.33)

Table 14-5
RARE EARTH RECEPTORS
TECHNIQUE CONVERSION FACTORS BY SCREEN SPEED
COMPARED TO CONVENTIONAL PAR SPEED SCREENS

Screen Speed (Density Fx)	Descriptive Name	mAs Conversion Factor
80	Extremity Cassette	1.25
300	Medium Speed	1/3 (.33)
400	Regular Speed	1/4 (.25)
800	High Speed	1/8 (.125)

TECHNIQUE CONVERSION FACTORS

Table 15-1 only presents a sample, one of three pages listing the many different speeds of screen-film combinations available from this one manufacturer. Of course, there are several other manufacturers of intensifying screens with their own various speeds available. In daily clinical practice, it is of great utility to have memorized typical technique conversions for those screens which are most common. As was done with grids in the last chapter, by focusing only on the most common types of screens and rounding values, a simplified system can be developed which lends itself to easy memorization. In this way, Tables 14-4 and 14-5 are derived, presenting useful rules of thumb for technique.

Unfortunately, different descriptive names for screen speeds are often used by the manufacturers in labeling their screen cassettes rather than the numerical speed. This can be somewhat confusing; for example, the Kodak *Medium* rare earth screen has an actual speed of 300, while the Kodak *Regular* rare earth screen has a speed of 400. Because these numerical speed values are often *not* labeled on cassettes, some of the most commonly used descriptive names have been included in Tables 14-4 and 14-5. To reinforce this information, some of the descriptive names are also used in the practice exercises in this chapter, mixed in with numerical speeds.

Although the par-speed calcium tungstate screen is almost out of use in modern radiology departments, it continues to be the standard against which all other screen speeds (including rare earth screens) are measured. This is well, for the resulting figures are much easier to work with mathematically than if all screens were compared to, say, the rare earth regular speed as a standard.

Tables 14-4 and 14-5 list rounded out conversion factors to facilitate memorization. Depending on the brand, rare-earth (fine-detail) cassettes have a speed approximately **one-fifth** that of regular rare earth cassettes. This conversion is encountered frequently and should be memorized: *When changing from regular rare earth to an "extremity" cassette, the mAs should be increased five times. When changing from an extremity cassette to a regular cassette, reduce mAs to 1/5.* In Table 14-5, extremity cassettes cassettes are listed as having a mAs conversion of 1.25 times the technique required for the old par speed screens, while regular screens are listed at 0.25. Dividing 1.25 by 0.25, we obtain a ratio of 5 to 1. In other words, the regular screens are 5 times faster than the extremity cassette. In a similar way, technique conversions for all changes in screen speed can be found by simply making a ratio out of these *mAs* factors from Tables 14-4 and 14-5, dividing one into the other.

To adjust technique when changing from one screen speed to another, make a ratio out of the two corresponding mAs conversion factors from Table 14-4 or Table 14-5, placing the screen factor you are changing *to* as the numerator over the factor you are changing *from*. This formula will yield the factor by which the original technique must be adjusted (multiplied).

Example No. 1: Change from a regular rare earth screen to a rare earth high-speed cassette. What change in technique is needed to maintain density?

$$Solution: \quad \frac{To}{From} = \frac{R.E.\ High}{R.E.\ Regular} = \frac{.125}{.25} = 0.5$$

One-half (0.5) the mAs is required with the high-speed rare earth cassette

Example No. 2: Change from a direct exposure holder to a rare earth regular screen cassette. What change in technique is needed to maintain density?

$$Solution: \quad \frac{To}{From} = \frac{R.E.\ Regular}{Direct\ Exposure} = \frac{.25}{50} = 0.005$$

One two-hundredth (0.005 X) the mAs is required with the regular rare earth cassette

To solve *density* problems, the above formula may be inverted, with *from* on top and *to* on bottom, or, simply invert the answers resulting from the above technique conversions. In the above problems, *Example No. 1* would result in twice the density *if* the technique were not compensated, *Example No. 2* would result in 200 times the density *if* the technique were not compensated. However, probably the simplest way to solve for density is to *use the screen speeds themselves*, placing the screen speed factor you are changing *to* on top as the numerator and the factor you are changing *from* as the denominator. For

example, changing from a 50-speed screen to a 250-speed screen, the latter will produce a density 250/50 = 5 times darker, using the same technique. In order to maintain density, technique would need to be cut to 1/5.

Example No. 3: Change from a high-speed calcium tungstate screen to a direct-exposure film holder. If technique is *not* compensated, what will the density change be?

$$Solution: \quad \frac{To}{From} = \frac{Direct\ Exposure}{High} = \frac{2}{200} = 0.01$$

The density will turn out 1/100th as dark as the original

Example No. 4: Change from a slow-speed calcium tungstate screen to a rare earth regular screen. All other factors equal, what will the density change be?

$$Solution: \quad \frac{To}{From} = \frac{Regular}{Slow} = \frac{400}{50} = 8$$

The density will turn out 8 times darker than the original

The effect of increasing screen speed upon radiographic density and the use of density factors in adjusting technique to maintain density at various screen speeds is demonstrated in Figure 14-7.

Try the following exercise for practice, and then check your answers from the Appendix.

EXERCISE #13

Conventional calcium tungstate screens are abbreviated below as *CaWO4* screens.

What would the new *density* be if technique is unchanged and screen speed is changed from:

1. 300-speed to 75-speed:
2. Direct Exposure to Slow CaWO4:
3. High-speed CaWO4 to Rare Earth Regular:
4. Par CaWO4 to Slow CaWO4:
5. Rare Earth Extremity Cassette to Rare

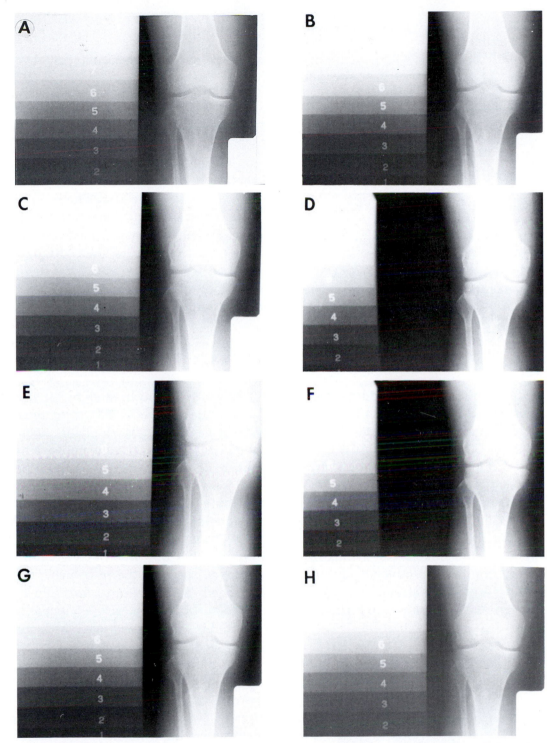

Figure 14-7. Radiographs of a knee and step wedge demonstrating the accuracy of the technique factors given in Tables 14-4 and 14-5 in maintaining overall density with various speeds and types of screens. Note in particular step #5 on the step wedge, a medium density value. All were taken at 70 kVp. Factors: (A) direct exposure using 500 mAs (50 times par), (B) slow screen using 20 mAs (double par), (C) par screen using 10 mAs, (D) high-speed screen using 5 mAs ($^1/_2$ par), (E) high-plus screen using 3.3 mAs ($^1/_3$ par), (F) "regular" rare earth screen using 2.5 mAs ($^1/_4$ par), (G) "medium" rare earth screen using 3.55 mAs (1.4 times "regular"). (H) is a rare earth "extremity" screen using 18 mAs (6 times "regular"): Note that this is slightly darker than (F), (observe step #3). *Five* times the mAs used on the "regular" rare earth screen is the exact conversion factor, as listed in Table 14-5.

Earth Regular:
6. Regular Rare Earth to Medium Rare Earth:

What change in the original *technique* would be required to maintain image density when changing screen speed from:

7. 50-speed to 250-speed:
8. High-plus $CaWO_4$ to Direct Exposure:
9. Rare Earth Regular to Rare Earth Extremity Cassette:
10. Slow $CaWO_4$ to Rare Earth Extremity Cassette:
11. High-speed $CaWO_4$ to Par $CaWO_4$:
12. Direct Exposure to Regular Rare Earth:

Influence of Temperature

The fluorescent property of screens excited by x-rays decreases as the temperature increases. At 95°F. screens emit less fluorescent light than at 70°F. One might assume that this fact is important radiographically. Actually, it is not, for the x-ray sensitivity of the x-ray film used with screens increases with the temperature. Since film and screens are used in combination at a given temperature, the screen effect balances the film effect and there is no need to observe the differences from a practical radiographic standpoint.

EFFECT ON CONTRAST

Screen radiography produces higher contrast in the image than can be attained by direct exposure when using the same kilovoltage. The higher contrast is a characteristic response of the emulsion to the fluorescent screen light. Also, the front screen tends to absorb some of the longer wave length secondary radiation emitted by the patient, thereby reducing the level of fog on the image. A comparison between contrasts produced on direct exposure (A) and on screen exposure (B) employing 50 kVp is shown in Figure 14-8.

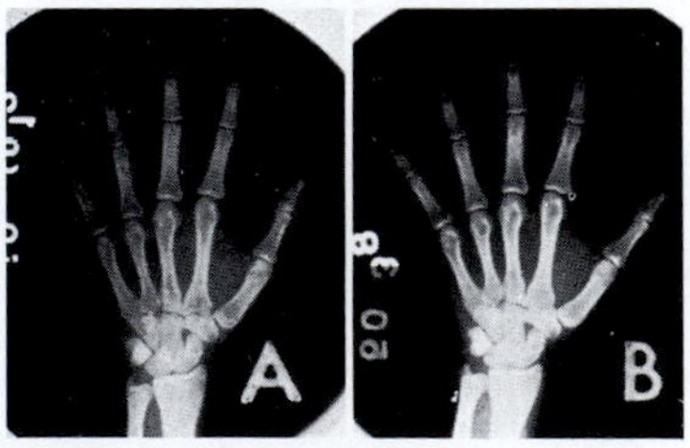

Figure 14-8. Radiographs of a hand showing the dramatic increase in image contrast when changing from a direct exposure technique (A) to a medium speed intensifying screen with screen-type film (B).

The change from a modern 80 speed extremity cassette to a 400-speed regular rare earth cassette is dramatic enough (about 5 times faster) that the improvement in image contrast is notable. Both of these screens are widely used, and thus are available to any student who wishes to duplicate the demonstration in Figure 14-9. An improvement in image contrast may not always be obvious when changing from one screen speed to the next higher adjacent speed, such as from a medium rare earth to a regular rare earth; consequently, some authors have shied away from making a categorical statement about the relationship between screen speed and image contrast. Yet, it should be clear from both Figures 14-8 and 14-9 that any substantial increase in screen speed makes the contrast enhancement quite visible. Thus, it can be confidently stated that *generally, increasing screen speed increases image contrast.*

The effect of increasing image *contrast* is not very notable from one speed of screen to the next. It is quite visible when comparing screen exposures to direct non-

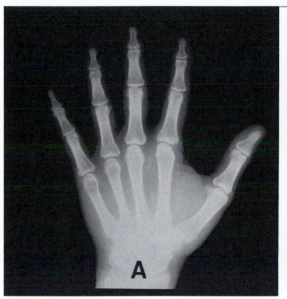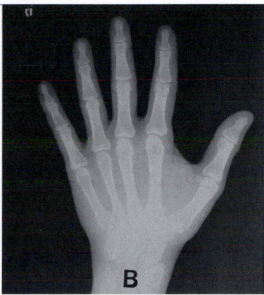

Figure 14-9. Radiographs of the hand showing a higher contrast image A, using a regular rare earth screen versus the visibly reduced contrast of image B taken with an "extremity cassette."

screen exposures. This is due to the fact that x-ray film has a higher inherent contrast when exposed to light rather than when it is exposed to x-rays and also to the fact that screen output is kVp dependent:

Higher kV x-ray photons result in *more* light being emitted by the screen than low kV photons. Since scatter radiation averages much lower energy than the primary beam, it will not be as effective in producing light when it strikes the intensifying screen. Proportionately less light will be produced by scatter than by primary radiation. Therefore, the effect of scatter radiation on the overall image will be somewhat less notable. With scatter contributing less to the overall image, contrast is increased when screens are used.

EFFECT ON SHARPNESS OF RECORDED DETAIL

Loss in image sharpness always ensues when screens are employed, because the fluorescent light diffuses across image boundaries within the body of the screen itself. No matter how fine a crystal is used in screens, its fineness does not compare with that of the film emulsion crystals. Any radiograph made with screens cannot compare favorably as to detail sharpness with a radiograph made without screens. However, when screens are not used, patient movement may occur during the longer exposure times required whether the part is immobilized or not. Screens should always be employed whenever there is a possibility of movement, and the exposure time should be as small as possible.

SCREEN-FILM CONTACT

Close contact between the active surfaces of the screens and the emulsion surfaces of the film is essential so that sharp-

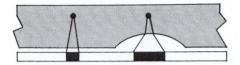

Figure 14-10. Diagram illustrating the effect of poor film-screen contact from a warped screen. Light refracts as it passes through from the screen into the air bubble, spreading the penumbra. In addition, the increased distance to the film allows further penumbral spread. Sharpness of detail is lost.

screen and film surfaces inside. Any time visible light passes through an *interface* or boundary between two very different media, the light will bend or *refract* (Fig. 14-10). This diffusion of the light is made worse by the increased distance to the film created by the air pocket. The result is a spreading of penumbral edges or blur, and a severe loss of image sharpness.

THICKNESS OF PROTECTIVE COAT

The protective coating of varnish or plastic is necessary to protect the screen emulsion somewhat from scratches. However, the coating adds to the distance through which light from the screen must travel to reach the film, so it must be as thin as practically possible. If the protective coat is thick, the light from the screen will spread out more before it reaches the film,

ness of detail will not be impaired. Poor or uneven contact allows the fluorescent light to spread and produce blurring of the image. For that reason each pair of screens is placed in a rigid holder (cassette) so that they will be in direct contact with the film. Any damage to the cassette from dropping it or otherwise abusing it can bend or dent this structure, causing air-gaps between the

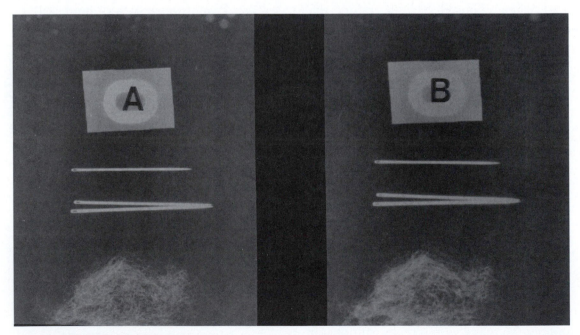

Figure 14-11. Radiographs of steel wool and needles to demonstrate the enhanced sharpness of a rare earth extremity cassette, A, to a rare earth regular-speed screen, B. Note that even though B shows increased contrast within the steel wool, individual fibers of the steel wool and the eyes of the needles are better resolved in A with the extremity screen system. (Reprinted with permission of Eastman Kodak Company, Screen Imaging, Image Insight Workbook #3.)

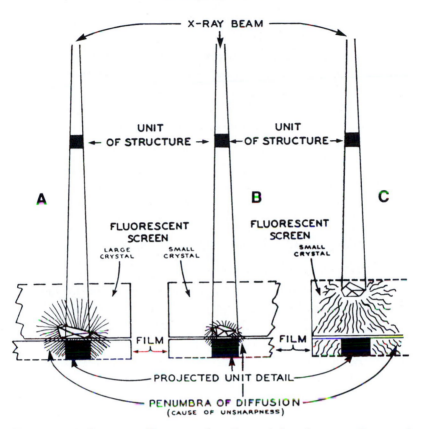

Figure 14-12. Diagrams illustrating the effects of phosphor crystal size and phosphor layer thickness upon image sharpness: (A) larger phosphor crystals increase penumbra, reducing sharpness, (B) smaller crystals increase sharpness, (C) thicker phosphor layers result in some crystals being located further from the film, allowing more penumbral spread and reducing sharpness.

contributing to penumbra and reducing sharpness.

SCREEN SPEED

Sharpness of detail generally decreases with higher screen speeds. While changing from one screen speed to the next may not cause a notable change, the difference between direct-exposure (non-screen) technique and screen technique, or that between a detail or extremity cassette and a high-plus or rare-earth screen, is marked (Fig. 14-11). Most screen speed increases are accomplished by using thicker emulsions. This places some of the crystals far-

ther away from the film (deeper in the emulsion) so that penumbral light from each crystal diverges more before reaching the film. Increasing the size of the phosphor crystals is another method used to increase screen speed. Larger crystals also result in greater penumbral spread of light from the screen to the film. Whether from thicker emulsions or from larger crystals, the result is less distinct edges of the recorded image and sharpness of detail is lost (Fig. 14-12). However, these distances and penumbral changes are microscopic, and in comparison with factors such as OID or focal spot size they are relatively minor. Changing from calcium tungstate to

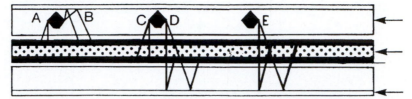

Figure 14-13. Diagram of geometry of screen light emission and cross-over effects: (A) direct emission of light from phosphor crystal to nearest film emulsion minimizes penumbral spread; (B) light reflected off reflective layer of screen spreads more before reaching film, reducing sharpness; (C) *simple crossover* with light passing through film to opposite emulsion increases penumbra; (D) *reflective crossover* with light passing to opposite screen's reflective backing, then back to film with severe penumbral spread; (E) *compound crossover* with light reflecting back and passing through film base a *second* time to opposite emulsion, with severe penumbra.

rare-earth screens does not present a problem with detail loss, because the efficiency is achieved by using chemicals such as lanthanum oxybromide, gadolinium oxysulfide or barium fluorochloride, which have higher absorption and conversion efficiency for x-rays, rather than by increasing emulsion thickness.

Binder Dyes

An effective method used to increase the sharpness of intensifying screens (at the expense of speed) is to add a color dye to the binder. Many detail screens have a yellow dye. Just as colored glass stops some light from passing through, this dye prevents those light photons which are diverging more (and thus have a longer distance to travel before escaping the binder) from being emitted. Since the beams escaping are those travelling a straighter course, sharpness is improved (Fig. 14-3).

CROSSOVER EFFECT

When duplitized film is used, a *crossover* effect occurs whereby light from one screen may pass through the film base to the opposite emulsion, or even on through to the other screen's reflective backing and then reflect back to the film emulsion. This increases penumbral divergence of the light and thus reduces detail (Fig. 14-13). For this reason, some extremity cassettes or other high resolution cassettes have only one screen so as to improve sharpness of recorded detail by eliminating crossover.

As much as 30-40 percent of film exposure can be due to light crossing over to the opposite emulsion. With the increased penumbral divergence that this causes, image sharpness is *significantly* reduced by the crossover effect, so manufacturers have used several different approaches to improve on this problem: The addition of an *anti-crossover dye* between the film base and the emulsion has rendered some improvement by absorbing light escaping the first emulsion. The recent development of *tabular grains* (flat-shaped silver bromide crystals) in the film emulsion has also assisted—these flat crystals lie broadside to the light rays (and x-rays) and capture more of the incoming light in the first emulsion. Finally, manufacturers offer extremity cassettes or other high-resolution cassettes which have only *one intensifying screen* in them. This prevents light from reflecting back and forth between the reflective layers of two opposing screens until the film emulsion captures it. Hence, whenever image sharpness is paramount, *single-screen* cassettes with *single-emulsion* film are strongly recommended, and *tabular grain* film should be used.

Since both the x-ray film and the binder layer in the intensifying screen are relatively translucent to the light emitted by the screen phosphors, there are in fact several variations or types of crossover, which might be described as *simple crossover, reflective crossover,* and *compound crossover.* These are illustrated as *C, D,* and *E* in Figure 14-13 along with diagrams of normal and reflected light divergence from the intensifying screen. In Figure 14-13, *A* illustrates the normal amount of light divergence from a phosphor crystal in the intensifying screen to the nearest film emulsion layer. This divergence may be considered as a *penumbra* diagram, and is directly proportional to the amount of *blur* in the image. In *B,* light is emitted backward from the phosphor crystal, but its direction is reversed by the reflective layer in the screen, steering it back to the film. Because of the increased distance of travel as the light traverses through the screen, it diverges much more before reaching the nearest film emulsion, thus spreading penumbra and increasing blue. This effect, however, would not be considered as a true crossover event.

In Figure 14-13C, *simple crossover* is illustrated: The light emitted from the phosphor crystal heads directly to the film, but passes *through* the first emulsion (without striking a silver-bromide crystal) and on through the film base to the *opposite* emulsion. Strictly speaking, this is *simple crossover,* and has resulted in more divergence and blur by the time the light traverses through the film. *Simple crossover is best reduced by the use of tabular grain films with an anti-crossover dye added to them.*

In Figure 14-13D, the light manages to penetrate all the way through the film *and* the phosphor layer of the opposite screen to its reflective layer; the light is then reflected back to the nearest emulsion of the film. The extended distance traveled results in *substantial* divergence of the light, and *significant* blur in the image. This effect might be termed *reflective crossover.* In *E* and *F, compound crossover* is diagrammed, where the light, having traversed all the way to the opposite screen's backing, is reflected back to the film but passes through the nearest emulsion *again* to the opposite film emulsion, or may even transmit all the way to the original screen's backing and be reflected a second time. Naturally, these last two scenarios represent only the smallest fraction of crossover occurring; yet when they do occur, they are extremely detrimental to the image sharpness.

Reflective and compound crossover are best reduced by the use of single-screen cassettes with single-emulsion film properly loaded. The lack of an opposing emulsion in the film eliminates the capture of light that has undergone increased divergence from simple crossover, as well as *parallax* unsharpness from the superimposing of two images in two emulsions, discussed in the next chapter. It has become somewhat common practice to utilize single-screen cassettes but to load them with duplicated film—this defeats the purpose of using this special cassette, because simple crossover is still present across the two film emulsions. *Whenever a single-screen is employed, single-emulsion film should also be used, and properly loaded.* Proper loading of single-emulsion film requires that the emulsion-side of the film be in direct contact with the screen. If the film is loaded backward, light divergence through the film base will still result in simple crossover blurring. The emulsion side of a single-emulsion film can be recognized under darkroom lighting because it is *dull* in appearance, whereas the non-emulsion side has a glossy, reflective sheen to it.

The key to the extent of blue created by crossover events is the total linear *distance* traveled by the light. Some manufacturers have added a layer of *anti-crossover dye* to the base of the film which reduces some of the crossover effect.

EFFECTS ON OTHER QUALITIES

Shape distortion and magnification of the *gross* image are not affected by screen speed, because there are no significant distances involved on the microscopic level of individual crystals in the screen and film, which are in direct contact. (It may be said that sharpness of edges is lost because the edges spread out, but this is not the same process as magnifying the gross image, so that you could actually measure a larger image with a ruler.)

Very high screen speeds, particularly the rare-earth speeds, may indirectly lead to quantum mottle in the image by dramatically reducing the mAs needed. As thicknesses and concentrations of crystals are increased in order to produce extremely high speed screens, there is a greater probability that phosphor crystals may clump together, causing an uneven distribution of the crystals throughout the screen. This will also lead to a grainy "mottled" appearance in the final radiographic image, called *material or receptor mottle*. Thus, very high-speed screens may lead to two types of image mottle: quantum mottle and material mottle.

SCREEN LAG

As previously mentioned, the property of fluorescence in a substance is its ability to emit radiation of one quality when stimulated by radiation of another quality. A common example is the luminous paint employed on instrument dials to render them visible in darkness. Such paints are excited by tiny quantities of radioactive material included in a paint mixture consisting usually of zinc sulfide or a sulfide of some other metal. *Phosphorescence*, however, is another phenomenon comparable to fluorescence.

In a fluorescent material, the glow of light only takes place as long as the substance is excited by radiation. In a phosphorescent chemical, the glow continues for an appreciable period *after* the exciting radiation is cut off. A typical example is the action of x-rays on an intensifying screen showing screen lag or afterglow. In such an example, the glow of light continues after the x-rays are turned off. When screen lag is present, the radiographer cannot reload his cassette immediately for an image made by the previous exposure would be recorded on a fresh unexposed film. The second radiograph might contain two images if the afterglow from the first exposure was sufficiently strong in intensity. It is possible for an afterglow to remain for months after exposure if the screen is of poor quality. Fortunately, the rigid production controls employed in the manufacture of modern screens precludes the use of fluorescent chemicals that exhibit phosphorescence. In good-quality screens, the intensity of fluorescence must rapidly reach its peak as the x-rays strike the crystals and should cease immediately upon termination of the exposure.

Intensifying screens tend to develop screen lag as they age, and very old cassettes should be discarded for this reason.

A test of persistent screen phosphorescence (test for screen lag) may be made by exposing the lower lumbar vertebral area laterally with 85 kVp and an appropriate mAs value at an SID of 40 inches. The exposed film is removed from the cassette and replaced by another film. The second film is left in the cassette for 10 to 15 minutes, and then processed. If no image is produced, the problem of phosphorescence does not exist with respect to the screens tested.

SPECIAL SCREENS

Special *gradient* screens have been developed which gradually increase speed from one end to the other. This gradation of speed is accomplished by gradually increasing the thickness of the emulsion in most cases. Similar to the use of compensating filtration, such screens are designed for radiography of anatomy which changes in thickness substantially across its length.

The most common application of the gradient screen is in the 36-inch-long cassette for use on thoraco-lumbar spine radiography in evaluation of scoliosis patients. These long cassettes should be marked *high speed* on one end and *par speed* on the other end. They should always be placed in the wall mount, with the par speed or slower-speed end at the top and the high-speed end at the bottom. In this fashion the density at the lumbar spine will be enhanced to an adequate level, while the less sensitive screen emulsion at the upper thoracic spine region will produce less density appropriate to the smaller thoracic vertebrae and thinner shoulder area. Placing this type of cassette upside down will certainly result in a repeated exposure, as the lumbar end of the spine will be grossly underexposed and the thoracic end excessively overexposed. This type of screen is also occasionally used when a single radiograph of the entire leg is needed, placing the high-speed end at the thigh/pelvis region.

CARE OF SCREENS

As screens influence the quality of the radiograph, their proper care is important. The fluorescent light emitted by intensifying screens obeys the laws of light, and any foreign matter on a screen will absorb light during the exposure and cause objectionable marks in the radiograph. Consequently, bits of paper, lint, and dust should be carefully removed and dirt and stains should never be allowed to remain on the surfaces of the screens. To avoid scratches and finger marks, the active surfaces should not be touched or handled except in washing. Cassettes may be stored in the processing room, but they should be kept at a safe distance from chemicals and all other possible sources of contamination or damage. Developer stains cannot be removed from screens. Therefore, as a safeguard, handle cassettes away from chemicals in the processing room. They should be kept closed when not in use.

SUMMARY

1. By converting x-rays into visible light, intensifying screens multiply the exposure effect of the x-ray beam and reduce the required *patient dose* to obtain diagnostic images.

2. As screen speed increases, image *density* is increased for a given exposure. Non-screen direct-exposure techniques require excessive amounts of radiation and, therefore, should only be used on the distal extremities.

3. As screen speed increases, image *contrast* is enhanced. This effect is not very visible from one screen speed to the next, but it is remarkable when changing from direct-exposure film holders to intensifying screens.

4. Increasing screen speed *usually* causes a loss of *sharpness* in image detail, because most speed increases are accomplished with more or thicker emulsion crystals or screens. Changing from calcium tungstate to rare-earth screens is an exception to this rule, because more effective chemicals are used. But changing from one rare-earth speed to a faster rare-earth speed is accomplished by thicker or more emulsion again and, therefore, reduces sharpness. Thicker protective coatings also reduce sharpness.

5. Intensifying screens have no effect upon the *magnification* or *shape distortion* of the gross image, because they are in direct contact with the film.

6. Screen *lag* or phosphorescence occurs in old screens and renders technique uncontrollable.

7. Screen *speed* is measured by the *intensification factor*. It increases with *kVp* and decreases with temperature.

8. The light output from a screen is affected by its thickness, phosphor density, the average atomic number of the phosphor, the inherent conversion efficiency of the phosphor chemical used, the addition of dyes, the K-edge of the phosphor, and the kVp used.

9. Rare earth screens are much faster than calcium tungstate screens because (1) they take advantage of the K-edge effect, (2) they have a higher phosphor density, and (3) they have a much higher conversion efficiency.

10. Very high-speed screens can lead to both the appearance of quantum mottle and material mottle in the image.

11. *Crossover* effects cause a substantial loss of sharpness when using intensifying screens. These include simple, reflective, and compound crossover. These effects are minimized by the use of single-screen cassettes in conjunction with properly-loaded single-emulsion film.

REVIEW QUESTIONS

1. List the components of an intensifying screen:

2. When an intensifying screen phosphoresces after the x-ray exposure terminates, what is this called?

3. When changing from a cardboard holder direct exposure to a rare earth extremity cassette, to what factor will patient exposure be decreased after the technique has been adjusted?

4. If par speed is assigned a speed number of 100, what is the relative speed for:
   a) "High" speed
   b) "Slow" speed

c) Rare Earth "Regular" speed

5. Why is a high-speed calcium tungstate screen faster than a par-speed calcium tungstate screen?

6. Why is a "extremity" or detail-speed calcium tungstate screen sharper than a par speed calcium tungstate screen if both have the same thickness of emulsion?

7. What is conversion efficiency?

8. Which type of screen efficiency is increased by using a thicker emulsion?

9. What is the crossover effect?

10. What is the purpose of the pressure pad in a cassette?

11. When changing from a 400 speed rare earth screen to a 1200-speed rare earth screen of the same phosphor, what image quality is *reduced*?

12. Leaving the same technique, how much darker will a high-speed screen exposure be than:
    a) a slow-speed screen?
    b) a direct exposure holder?

13. Why must green-sensitive film be used with rare earth screens?

14. How do very high-speed screens contribute to image mottle?

15. What is a gradient screen?

16. What is the difference between fluorescence and phosphorescence?

17. What effect does increasing kVp have on screen speed?

18. List the three general types of efficiency for intensifying screens.

19. How can rare earth screens be faster than calcium tungstate screens, when rare earth elements have lower atomic numbers than tungsten?

20. Who first sandwiched x-ray film between two intensifying screens?

21. Phosphor crystals in an intensifying screen are suspended in a plastic _____ layer.

22. Cassette lids (backs) are usually slightly curved in order to assure good _____.

23. A thicker protective coating on a screen would have what effect on image penumbra?

24. What percentage of film emulsion exposure is due to crossover light?

25. Light which has transmitted all the way to the opposing screen and returned to the film would be best classified as which type of crossover?

Chapter 15

IMAGE RECEPTOR SYSTEMS

FILM-SCREEN COMBINATIONS

WHILE AN IMAGE may be formed on film by light, gamma rays, or other forms of radiation including x-rays, the properties of the latter in producing a radiographic image are of a distinct character. For this reason, x-ray film must be distinctly different from that used in photography. It has not been possible to manufacture a film that is solely sensitive to the action of x-rays and not to light. In fact, modern radiography depends greatly upon the use of the visible fluorescent light emitted by x-ray intensifying screens to augment the x-ray action on the film. Two general types of x-ray film are employed in medical radiography, *screen-type* film and *direct-exposure* film.

Screen-Type

Film that is particularly sensitive to the *fluorescent* light of x-ray intensifying screens is known as screen-type x-ray film. The visible fluorescent light from screens amplifies the direct action of the x-rays. When used with intensifying screens, screen-type film is much faster than the direct-exposure type. When screen-type film is used without intensifying screens, however, it is about half as fast as the direct-exposure type. Nonetheless, it is frequently exposed without screens: In radiography of the smaller thicknesses of the body such as the hand, ankle, etc., screen-type film provides

a wider range of densities than when it is employed with screens. Because of its lower sensitivity to direct action of the x-rays, the background density of the processed radiograph is usually less than that of the direct-exposure type.

Direct-Exposure Type

Direct-exposure film (no-screen film) is especially sensitive to the *direct* action of the x-rays. It is used only for the thinner body parts. Its silver content is greater and the film has a higher inherent contrast than the screen-type film when directly exposed.

Direct exposure film has such thick emulsion that it cannot be run through the rollers of automatic processors. Since automatic processors are nearly universal in medical radiography, direct exposure film has become generally obsolescent, but may still be found for specialized uses.

Orthochromatic Film

The development of intensifying screens utilizing the rare-earth elements as phosphors necessitated the manufacture of a new type of x-ray film. Film emulsion is designed to be chemically sensitive to a specific frequency or wave length of light. Since calcium tungstate screens emit a blue-violet light wave length, regular

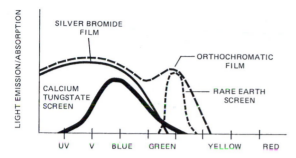

Figure 15-1. Graph of intensifying screen light emission spectra superimposed upon film sensitivity spectra. Any mismatching results in a loss of density. Note, for example, that rare earth screens are centered over the green portion of the light spectrum, while silver bromide film is centered over the blue-violet portion.

screen x-ray film emulsion was chemically compounded to be sensitive to this color. True rare-earth elements, however, emit a wave length of light centered mostly in the green portion of the spectrum (Fig. 15-1). *Orthochromatic* x-ray film was developed for use with rare-earth screens in order to efficiently convert this green light into image density.

Since many radiology departments now have both green-sensitive film and blue-sensitive film stored in their darkrooms, it is important for radiographers to take care not to mix screen and film types. If orthochromatic film is used in calcium tungstate screens, or if regular film is used in rare earth screens, the result will be insufficient density. Uninformed attempts to correct such a situation by increasing techniques will only lead to unnecessary patient exposures until the real error is found.

FILM COMPOSITION

X-ray film consists of an *emulsion* of finely precipitated silver bromide crystals suspended in gelatin that is coated on *both* sides of a transparent blue-tinted polyester support called the *base*.

Film Base

The base furnishes support for the emulsion and provides the correct degree of stiffness for handling.

At various times attempts were made to improve the overall quality of film by tinting the film. The purpose was to emphasize contrast and thus make it easier to visualize the densities present in the image. The colors used or locally applied were various shades of green, pink, orange, or blue.

The first commercialized (patented) method to be applied to x-ray film in America was described in 1933 by George A. Scanlan and Charles Holzwarth of Parlin, New Jersey who introduced a blue tint in x-ray film. The idea became popular with radiologists because they found that the presence of the blue tint slightly emphasized contrast differences. Modern x-ray film is blue tinted. An additional dye may be added to the film base to reduce the crossover effect of intensifying screen light discussed in the last chapter.

Subcoating. After the base is made, it is covered on both sides with a thin adhesive-type material so that the sensitive emulsion will adhere to the base. This is called the subcoating and prepares the base for emulsion coating.

Emulsion

The *emulsion* itself starts with gelatin. Next, virgin silver is dissolved in nitric acid to form silver nitrate; then the silver nitrate solution is mixed with potassium bromide and gelatin to produce an emulsion of silver bromide crystals. It is then coated on both sides of the film base. After drying, the surfaces of the emulsion coatings are specifically treated to prevent surface abrasion.

The purpose of the silver emulsion is to

absorb radiation during an x-ray exposure and produce a latent image. The degree of exposure depends upon the intensity of the radiation *emerging* from the object that is interposed between the focal spot of the x-ray tube and the film, to reach the film.

A most important discovery in the manufacture of photographic sensitive materials occurred many years ago as previously mentioned when gelatin was found to be an ideal medium for suspension of silver salts. Its ability to withstand action of the developer and fixer solutions at the processing temperatures normally employed without affecting the distribution of the silver crystals within it was most important. The fact that it assisted in the sensitization of the emulsion came as an after development.

Gelatin for photographic purposes is extracted from calf or cattle skins. In the early days of photography some gelatin was found to be good and some not. A study of this fact revealed that cattle grazing on pasturage containing mustard plants retained microscopic traces of sulfur in their hides, which in turn was carried in the gelatin obtained from them. Moreover, the silver bromide crystals suspended in this kind of gelatin were much more sensitive to the action of x-rays or light than crystals obtained in gelatin having no trace of sulfur. Film manufacturers obviously cannot depend upon the vagaries of bovine grazing habits when making film, but the problem was solved by adding the proper amount of natural synthetic mustard oil and now, other chemicals, to the emulsion formula.

An important physical property of gelatin is that in both liquid and solid forms it is clear and transparent so that no optical impairment of the image occurs when it is used in film manufacture. Another favorable characteristic is the fact that when incorporated in the emulsion, it can swell considerably in a cool solution without dissolving thereby permitting action of the processing chemicals on the silver crystals without altering their places in the emulsion; afterwards the gelatin can be shrunk and hardened in the fixing bath so that the radiograph can be washed and dried. The influence of gelatin on sensitivity varies with different gelatins; therefore the gelatin must be carefully selected. Increased sensitivity can be given to the emulsion by adding certain substances to the gelatin during manufacture.

Emulsion Coating

In the coating operation, the film base is passed at high speed through a trough containing the sensitive emulsion where it acquires a coating of uniform thickness. The coated film next passes into a chamber of cold air where the emulsion is chilled to a jelly. It then traverses other chambers where it is dried and a nonabrasive coating is applied. It is then tested and spooled into a huge roll. The finished film is finally cut to the various sizes required by the radiologist. Each emulsion layer is about one-thousandth of an inch in thickness. Since x-rays pass readily through x-ray film–and also through x-ray intensifying screens when used–an emulsion layer is coated on *both* sides of the film base, providing thereby a greater effect upon exposure to x-rays than would be possible with an emulsion coated only on one side.

T–COATING. The emulsion is protected by the very thin, non-abrasive coating of varnish. This "tough-coat" or T-coat guards against emulsion damage from scratches. It must be thin enough, however, to easily wash away upon development. The four main component layers of duplitized x-ray film are illustrated in Figure 2-1, Chapter 2.

LATENT IMAGE FORMATION

The silver bromide crystals in the emulsion are composed of alternating atoms of silver and bromine with a few "free" silver ions (atoms) mixed in (Fig. 15-2A.). Exposure to x-rays ionizes the atoms, liberating electrons (negative ions) and breaking the bonds between the atoms (Fig. 15-2B).

In manufacture the emulsion is treated with silver sulfide or other chemicals which constitute "impurities" within the silver bromide crystals. These altered molecules reside on the surface of the crystal at sites called *sensitivity specks* (Fig. 15-3A). Sensitivity specks have the ability to "trap" electrons, and provide the future sites for the beginning of the development process

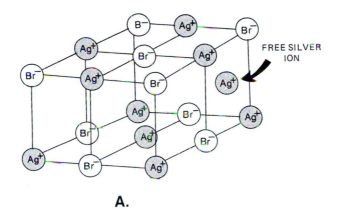

A.

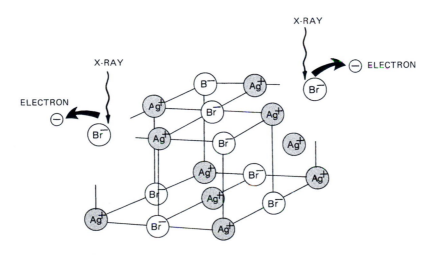

B.

Figure 15-2. Cubical structure of silver bromide crystal showing (A) alternating atoms of silver and bromine, and a free silver ion. X-rays ionize atoms, breaking the chemical bonds between them and liberating electrons (B). In Figure 15-3, these liberated electrons are shown as negative charges, and free silver ions as positive charges.

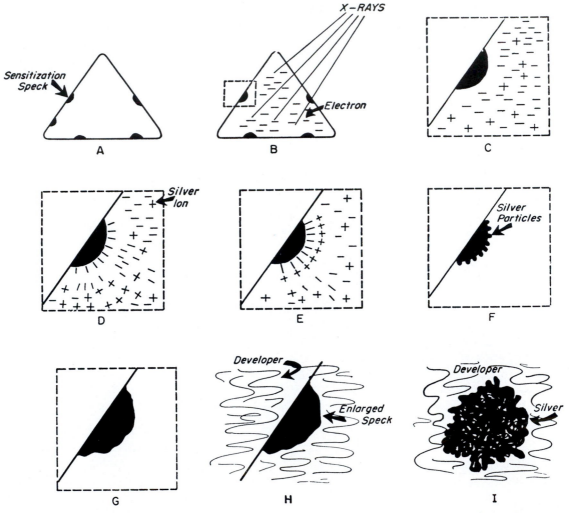

Figure 15-3. Changes occurring within the silver bromide crystal upon exposure and development. Electrons liberated by exposure (B) accumulate around the positive sensitivity speck (D). Free silver ions then attach to the sensitivity speck (E), forming a clump of silver (F). During processing (H and I), additional silver atoms "broken" from the crystal by developer solution continue to attach to the clump, making it grow in size.

leading to a visible image. Development only can be continued by the *growth* in size of these specks and *not* by the formation of new specks. Crystals that do not possess sensitivity specks cannot develop.

The general aspects of latent image formation and visible image development are diagrammatically shown in Figure 15-3. A complete silver bromide crystal, composed of thousands of atoms, is shown in (A), with sensitivity specks (impurities) on the sur-

face. Exposure to x-rays (B) ionizes atoms, releasing free electrons as also shown in Figure 15-2B. Enlarging our view of a sensitivity speck (C), it is seen that it soon traps many of the free electrons (D), acquiring a strong negative charge. Free or "migrant" silver atoms (see Fig. 15-2A) have a positive charge, and are attracted to the negatively charged sensitivity speck. They move slower than the free electrons, and arrive at the sensitivity speck later, attaching themselves to it (Fig. 15-3E), and forming a clump of silver particles (F). The amount of silver deposit depends on the amount of exposure. If sufficient silver accumulates around the speck, it will act as a development center making the entire crystal potentially developable. This constitutes the *latent image* (G).

Upon chemical development (H), the rest of the crystal is attacked by reducing chemicals that separate the remaining silver and bromine atoms from each other, pulling the bromine out into the developer solution. The remaining silver accumulates around the various sensitivity specks, forming a large clump of black metallic silver (I) which remains on the film, composing an image. If the quantity of x-rays that strikes the crystal happens to be insufficient, the sensitization speck will not grow to the point where it can break down the entire crystal upon development. The fully exposed crystal will usually develop and be reduced to black metallic silver within the normal time of development at a given temperature.

FILM SPEED

The shorter the exposure required in making a high quality radiograph, the faster the film is said to be. As with intensifying screens, films come in various speeds and contrast/gray scale characteristics. Generally, a "high"-speed film is about twice as fast as a "medium"-speed film. *Relative speeds*, using a value of 100 for "medium," are usually determined using 80 kVp exposures, and accurately compare one film's speed to another. These must be obtained from each film manufacturer.

Film can be made more sensitive or "faster" by increasing crystal size, crystal concentration, or overall emulsion thickness. New tabular-shaped crystals have resulted in improved crystal concentration. However, such advances in the shape and size of the crystals themselves are rare indeed.

Generally, since the concentration and size of crystals in the film are optimized for sharpness of detail in most cases, speed differences are usually attained by changing emulsion thickness. Chemical changes may be used to alter speed, contrast and gray scale characteristics. In selecting a film type, its compatibility with the intensifying screens it will be used with must also be taken into account.

Reciprocity Law

The reciprocity law was discussed in Chapter 5 on mAs. It implies that exposure rate (mA) may be exchanged with exposure time and still get the same film exposure, as long as the total *mAs* is equal. In radiography, reciprocity holds strictly true for direct exposure of the film to x-rays; however, when intensifying screens are used, it is found that extremely short exposure times (less than 0.05 second) or extremely long exposure times the response of the film can be somewhat *less* than the total mAs is expected to produce, and the image may turn out slightly light. This is because in order to chemically convert a silver bromide crystal into a developable grain, only one x-ray photon is required, but for light photons from an intensifying screen, more than on photon is required. Reciprocity law failure is more pronounced when using *high-speed films*. Technically, the reciprocity law "fails" for x-ray film exposed to light from intensifying screens when extreme exposure times are used. It may be noticeable when using very high-speed film.

Fortunately, reciprocity law failure has been largely compensated for by the characteristics of modern x-ray film emulsion and is seldom encountered in modern radiography. In general radiography, the approximate density produced on the film may be assumed to be directly proportional to the total exposure received by the film.

Shelf-Life of Film

Faster-speed films are more sensitive, not only to regular exposure, but also to scatter radiation, background radiation, and other environmental fogging variables such as high temperatures and humidity during storage. Most manufacturers list the expected good *shelf-life* or a recommended expiration date on each box of film. Film stock for a radiology department must be purchased in relatively small quantities over short periods of time for this reason. The longer the film is stored, the greater the background fog present prior to use. High-speed films have a much shorter shelf-life due to their high sensitivity, and must be rotated even more frequently.

IMAGE RECEPTOR SPEED

Films and screens must always be considered *together* in selecting a receptor system that will produce the desired image characteristics. Some applications are focused on high speed to minimize patient dose, such as in angiography, others emphasize long gray scale such as chest screening radiography, others demand high contrast, and still others focus on maximum sharpness of detail. Each manufacturer provides a selection of different film/screen combinations to fit these various needs (Table 15-1).

When considering receptor system speed, especially in view of patient exposure, the *total system speed must be considered by multiplying the film speed by the screen speed and dividing by 100*. For example, if a 100-speed screen were used with a 50-speed film, the overall receptor system

Table 15-1
COMBINED SPEEDS FOR KODAK™
ORTHOCHROMATIC FILMS AND RARE EARTH SCREENS

Kodak™ Films	Lanex Fine Extremity	Lanex Fine General	Lanex Medium	Lanex Regular	Lanex Fast
T-Mat G	80	100	300	400	600
T-Mat L	80	100	300	400	600
T-Mat H	–	–	600	800	1200
Ortho G	80	100	250	400	600

(Reproduced by permission from Kodak flyer.)

speed would be 100 x 50/100 = 50. If a 200-speed screen were used with a 200-speed film, the overall receptor speed would be 200 x 200/100 = 400. What is the overall speed for a 30-speed screen and a 50-speed film? The answer is 15.

Within a particular radiology department, a standardized single speed of film is normally utilized, and only screen speeds are varied. So in making technique adjustments, usually one needs only to consider the screen speed changes. In situations where different speeds of film are used, radiographers should be aware of the technique adjustments required by considering overall receptor speed.

When manufacturers attempt to increase film speeds by using larger crystals or higher concentrations of crystals, the crystals can clump together and cause a *grainy* appearance in the image, called *film mottle.* Such films will always present noise in the image and should be avoided.

FILM CONTRAST AND LATITUDE

X-ray film is manufactured with inherent contrast characteristics that are most suitable for the type of radiograph it is designed to produce. It is axiomatic that different kinds of x-ray films made by one manufacturer or those made by another manufacturer yield different contrasts even though the same developer and processing procedures are employed. Two general types of medical x-ray film are normally employed that can yield any one of several kinds of radiographic contrast depending upon the manner in which the films are exposed. The use of either type is based primarily on the speed and image definition requirements for the various projections.

Screen-type film possesses an emulsion that is particularly sensitive to the fluorescent light emitted by x-ray intensifying screens. It is less sensitive to the direct action of x-rays. The characteristics of this film are such that a relatively *higher* contrast is obtained when it is exposed with intensifying screens than when the same film is directly exposed to x-rays at the same kilovoltage.

When two posteroanterior radiographs at 50 kVp and 36" SID are made of a body part such as the hand (Fig. 15-4), one with 1.5 mAs and intensifying screens (*Left*) and the other without them (*Right*) at 40 mAs, the images differ materially in contrast and sharpness of detail. In the case of the screen exposure, bone details exhibit greater contrast, but there is some loss in image sharpness. The soft tissues show higher density and in some areas details cannot be easily visualized because of some opaque densities. The radiograph made *without* screens, however, will show a lower contrast and greater detail sharpness, while the densities representative of *all* tissues are translucent. However, screens should always be employed in radiography of the heavier body parts and where shortness of exposure is necessary to stop movement.

It should be noted that *high-latitude* films

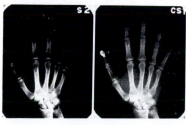

Figure 15-4. Two radiographs of the hand showing increased contrast resulting from use of intensifying screens (*left*), less contrast and higher latitude without screens (*right*).

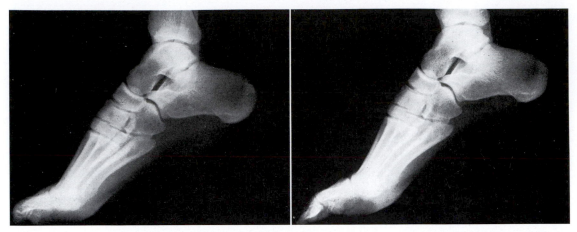

Figure 15-5. Radiographs of the foot employing the same kVp, (*left*) with high latitude film, (*right*) with short latitude film. Note the lower contrast with the high latitude film.

are often recommended to produce long gray scale images, such as in screening chest radiography. These films produce low contrast and long gray scale (Fig. 15-5) to maximize the amount of information recorded. They therefore allow a greater margin for error in setting exposure tech-niques, that is, they have *high exposure lati-tude*, which reduces repeat rates.

Solarization

Extreme overexposure of radiographic film can lead to a bizarre *reversal* of the

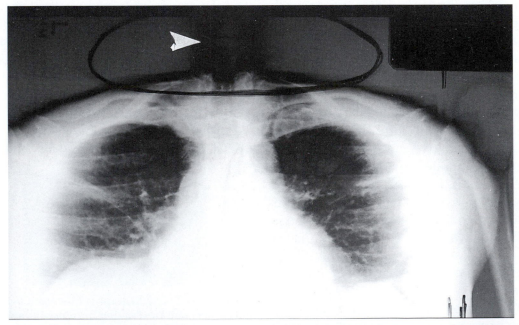

Figure 15-6. Radiograph exhibiting solarization in the neck area and edges of the shoulders, due to extreme overexposure in a duplicator unit. Note that the bones in these areas are dark.

image densities (Fig. 15-6) in which structures such as bone which normally appear "white" will be dark, and the background density lightens. This effect is called *solarization.*

GEOMETRIC FACTORS

Film with emulsion coated on both sides is called *duplitized* film. When observing the duplitized radiograph, one is actually looking at *two* superimposed images, one in each emulsion, with a microscopic distance between them imposed by the film base. When recorded by an angled beam, one of the two images will be shifted in relation to the other. This shift is known as *parallax.* The double image will result in reduced sharpness of detail.

Thicker film emulsions and larger crystals also result in less sharpness of detail and can contribute to mottling. A thicker film base separates the two emulsions at a greater distance, and thus contributes to *parallax* unsharpness. These effects are *microscopic* in magnitude. They are so minor in comparison with the effects of intensifying screens, focal spot size, distances and motion that the choice of radiographic film is not a serious consideration in controlling sharpness of detail. Film should be selected entirely upon the basis of its speed and contrast characteristics.

The image resides in the film emulsion, and there can be no distances or angles involved therein. Hence, the type of film used has no relation to magnification and shape distortion.

Halation

Any time light passes from one medium into another, such as from air into water, a certain percentage of the light will be reflected from the surface separating these two media. When exposing an x-ray film in a screen cassette, not all of the light from the screens passes completely through the film. After entering into the film, a small amount is reflected at the back surface rather than passing back into the air. This reflected light comes back to the opposing

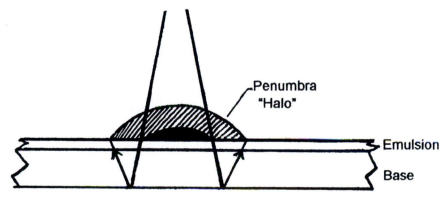

Figure 15-7. Diagram of *halation* unsharpness: Light from an intensifying screen passing through to the non-emulsion side of the film is reflected back to the emulsion side, spreading the penumbra as it travels.

emulsion, causing a slight "halo" effect around image details. The result is a destructive loss of recorded detail. This slight "halo" effect is termed *Halation* (Fig. 15-7).

Halation is particularly pronounced with single-emulsion film. A special coating is applied to the nonemulsion side of the film to reduce this effect. When using single-screen cassettes with single-emulsion film, the film emulsion must be placed in direct contact with the screen, and the special coating must be placed opposite the screen. The correct sides of the film can be easily identified even in dark room lighting, because the *emulsion side is dull, while the coated side is glossy.* The dull side of the film should always face the intensifying screen.

Material Mottle

Image mottle is defined as a "grainy" appearance to the image, a form of image noise. In Chapter 5 we learned that *quantum mottle* appears when low mAs values are used, due to the randomness of the distribution of x-rays within the beam. A very similar effect occurs when either a film or an intensifying screen is poorly manufactured, allowing the silver bromide crystals in the film or the phosphor crystals in the screen to clump together. The emulsion of the film is designed to provide a colloid suspension which holds these crystals evenly distributed throughout the emulsion thickness, and the emulsion must be perfectly coated onto the film. This is much like trying to make Jello™ with cherries suspended in it–they have to be added at exactly the right time and temperature. The binder in the phosphor layer of an intensifying screen must do the same, suspending the phosphor crystals in an even pattern throughout. If the crystals settle to the bottom or stick together in clumps or, when exposed, these large dark clumps become visible in the image as mottle.

Mottle caused by the characteristics of the receptor system is properly called *receptor mottle* or *material mottle*–it is caused by the materials used rather than by the x-ray beam. Material mottle may be further subdivided into *screen mottle* and *film mottle*. It is not unusual for cheaper brands of film, in particular, to present problems with material mottle.

FILM HOLDERS

All types of film holders serve the primary function of protecting the film from light, and cassettes also provide a support system for intensifying screens that should assure direct film/screen contact across the entire area of the film.

There are many types of special purpose cassettes, including curved cassettes for knee, hip, and shoulder radiography; grid cassettes with the grid built into the cassette; and 36-inch cassettes for scoliosis studies or long bone measurement.

The front of the cassette must be rigid and durable, but radiolucent to the x-ray beam. Cassettes with radiolucent (nonmetal) backs that include a sheet of lead foil can be placed in reverse position if necessary to reduce scatter radiation much like a grid would. This is actually a *filtration* technique, but since scatter radiation has less energy than the primary beam overall, more scatter than primary radiation will be filtered out by the lead foil and contrast is enhanced. This method is workable for medium-sized anatomy such as skulls, cervical spines and proximal extremities, but should never be used on torso anatomy where only the effectiveness of a high-ratio grid will suffice to clean up the scatter radiation generated.

SUMMARY

1. The use of higher-speed film types results in increased image *density* for a given exposure.
2. Higher film speeds also produce slightly increased *contrast.*
3. Higher film speeds lead to a reduction in *sharpness* of image detail, because more or thicker emulsions or larger crystals are used.
4. Film speed has no effect upon *magnification* or *distortion* of the gross image, because the image resides within the emulsion.
5. In all of the image qualities, the above effects must never be considered alone but always in connection with the use of intensifying screens. It is the complete screen/film combination, as a *receptor system,* which determines the final image results.
6. Film sensitivity *type* must be properly matched with the screen emission type being used—that is, ortho film with rare-earth screens, regular film with calcium tungstate screens, and direct-exposure film with direct-exposure holders—in order to prevent a loss of density.
7. *Latent image* formation occurs when x-rays ionize silver bromide crystals, releasing free electrons to accumulate at the *sensitivity speck* and attract migrant silver ions.
8. *Halation* is a halo effect caused by reflected light from the back surface of the film, and is most pronounced on single-emulsion films.
9. In loading single emulsion films into cassettes, the *dull* side (the emulsion side) should face the cassette screen.
10. Cassettes must be carefully handled to prevent damage that can lead to poor screen/film contact or light leaks.
11. Placing cassettes backward to reduce scatter should only be done on medium-sized anatomy, not torso anatomy.
12. *Solarization* is a reversing of the image densities due to extreme overexposure.
13. *Material mottle* is a grainy appearance to the image caused by the clumping together of crystals when film or screens are poorly manufactured.
14. Failure of the *reciprocity law* occurs when using intensifying screens at extreme exposure times but is not a significant problem in modern radiography.

REVIEW QUESTIONS

1. Clumping together of large crystals in high-speed films can lead to what type of image noise?
2. What is the total receptor system speed for a 200-speed film in a 300-speed screen?
3. Switching from 50-speed film to 200-speed film, how much darker will the image be using the same technique?
4. What effect do faster speed films usually have on image sharpness?
5. How do high-latitude films help reduce repeat rates?
6. What special type of unsharpness is

caused by duplitizing film?

7. Define "halation":

8. Why do plastic and fiber cassettes have a sheet of lead foil in the back?

9. Reversing cassettes should never be substituted for a grid when radiographing _____ anatomy.

10. What imperfection must a silver bromide crystal have in it to develop into a silver image?

11. Image density will _____ (increase, decrease, or not be affected) when film is mismatched with screens.

12. What is used as a flexible but firm colloidal suspension for silver bromide crystals in film emulsion?

13. The shelf-life of high-speed films is _____ than that of regular speed films.

14. What is solarization, and what causes it.

15. What is the term for film that is sensitive to the green light emitted by rare earth screens?

16. What is the cause of material mottle?

Part III

GEOMETRICAL FACTORS

Chapter 16

FOCAL SPOT SIZE

THE TERM *focal spot* is normally used to refer to the area on the x-ray tube anode from which x-rays are emitted, as seen from the viewpoint of the film. This area is determined by the width of the beam of electrons striking the anode and by the *bevel* or angle of the surface of the anode where the electrons impact.

The relation of the anode bevel angle to image qualities is discussed in the next chapter. The stream of high-speed electrons from the x-ray tube filament is *focused* onto a small area on the anode surface, hence the name *focal spot*. The projected focal spot is smaller than a pinhead, and all useful x-rays are emitted from this small area. Because the anode surface is beveled (angled), the apparent size of the focal spot depends upon the direction from which it is observed. For the purposes of this chapter, only the *effective* or *projected* focal spot size will be discussed. This is the size of the focal spot as seen from the viewpoint of the x-ray film or image receptor. Image quality is determined only by the *projected* focal spot size.

EFFECT ON SHARPNESS OF RECORDED DETAIL

The focal spot of the x-ray tube is comparable to the light source employed in shadow formation. The influence of the focal spot on detail is confined to image sharpness. With all other factors constant, *the smaller the focal spot, the sharper the recorded detail. The size of the focal spot is inversely proportional to image sharpness.* A large focal spot, although capable of withstanding high electrical energies, does not produce the sharpness of detail that is characteristic of tubes with a small focal spot. It is advantageous to use, whenever possible, a smaller focal spot with smaller tube capacities or a rotating anode tube.

The effect of focal spot size upon the sharpness of recorded details is illustrated in Figure 16-1 using a line-pair test pattern.

Note that smaller line pairs can be recognized when using the smaller focal spot. Increasing focal spot size reduces image sharpness because the penumbra at the edges of the details is increased (Fig. 16-2). With more penumbra, a blurry image results. Note in Figure 16-2 that as penumbra grows from larger focal spots, it spreads *inward* as well as outward, invading the umbral shadow so that the umbra shrinks in size.

When excessively large focal spots are used in conjunction with long object-film distances, it is possible for the umbral shadow to shrink to the point of disappearing entirely, so that a blurry patch of penumbra is the only image left on the film and information is lost.

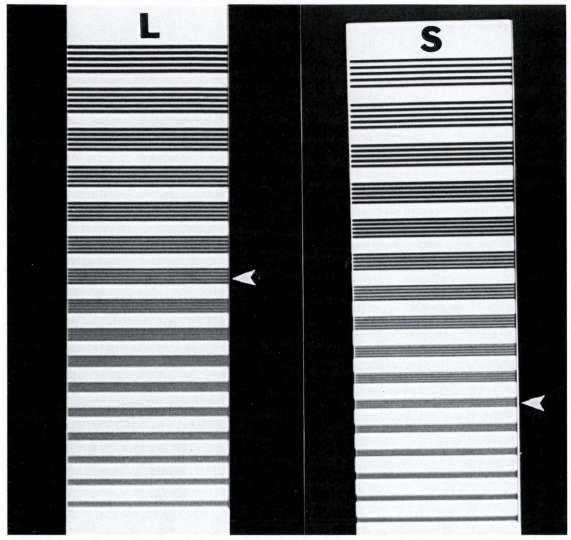

Figure 16-1. Radiographs of resolution template exhibiting the.increase in sharpness and greater number of line pairs resolved using a small focal spot (S) as compared to a large focal spot (L).

PENUMBRA

X-rays can be emitted at various angles and from different points within the area of the focal spot, and yet record the same edge of an object on the film. This means that the same edge of the object will actually be recorded several times in various different locations on the film (Fig. 16-3). This "spreading" of the edge constitutes blur or *penumbra*. Figure 16-3 demonstrates why penumbra occurs in radiography. Note that all x-rays emitted at the same angle as beam "A" but from other regions of the focal spot (dashed lines) are subject to absorption by this object. All x-rays emitted at the same angle as beam "B" but from different regions of the focal spot (dotted lines) will reach the film unattenuated.

Inbetween beams "A" and "B", different amounts of x-rays are absorbed by the object depending on their angle and point of origin within the focal spot. In other words, between "A" and "B" absorption of

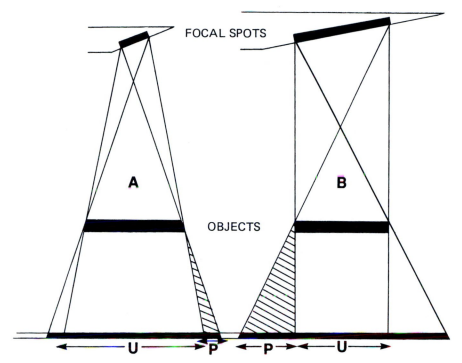

Figure 16-2. Diagram illustrating that larger focal spot sizes increase penumbral blur (p) but actually shrink the umbra (u). Note that the penumbra is directly proportional to the focal spot size—tripling the focal spot triples the penumbral spread or blur.

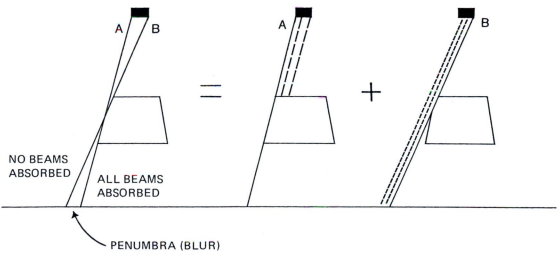

Figure 16-3. Diagram illustrating creation of penumbra. All x-rays parallel to *A* but emitted from the focal spot to the right of it (dashed line) are subject to absorption by the object. None of the beams parallel to *B* but emitted to the left of it (dotted lines) are subject to absorption by the object. Between *A* and *B* some beams are subject to absorption by the object and others are not. This *partial* absorption causes a partial shadow celled *penumbra.*

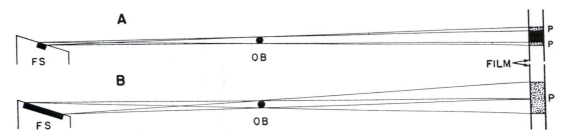

Figure 16-4. Diagram illustrating disappearance of umbral image when the object of interest is significantly smaller than the focal spot size used.

the x-ray beam is *partial*, increasing toward the object. This causes the edge gradient known as geometrical penumbra. Hence, "penumbra" may be thought of as a *partial absorption* process (bearing in mind that "partial" refers to a portion of the total amount of x-rays which the object in question is capable of absorbing, not to a portion of the total x-ray beam).

Focal spot is directly proportional to penumbra: Doubling the FS doubles the penumbra (Fig. 16-2).

WHEN THE FOCAL SPOT IS GREATER THAN THE OBJECT

Occasionally, an opaque object in the tissues may have a diameter less than that of the tube focal spot. If there is sufficient unsharpness caused by a long OID and a short SID, the entire object may be visualized as a diffuse gray area. This condition is

diagrammatically represented, Figure 16-4, in which a small object (OB) at an extended object-film distance is shown projected by a larger focal spot (B). If details composed the object, all image details would be blurred and indistinguishable, having only the gross shape of the object. If scatter radiation undercut the object, the blurred details would be superimposed by fog, and any suggestion of image might then be entirely eliminated.

This effect is of great significance in angiography, because vascular embolisms and other pathology of interest may be smaller than the projected focal spot used and, therefore, would not be visibly recorded on the image, leading to misdiagnosis.

In A, the object is shown projected by a focal spot *smaller* than the diameter of the object. The image would then contain some details but with small blurred margins.

EFFECT ON MAGNIFICATION

The relationship of focal spot size to magnification of the image is a source of confusion for many radiographers. A review of Figure 16-2 will illustrate that the penumbral portion of the image spreads outward with larger focal spots, which may be misinterpreted as causing the image to grow in size. This fact has led many to

believe that larger focal spots magnify the image. But such a notion ignores the additional fact that the umbra, the clear portion of the image, actually shrinks in size with larger focal spots, also shown in Figure 16-2.

A practical experiment with changing focal spot sizes will demonstrate that the measured size of the *gross* image of a bone or other anatomical structure does *not* change with focal spots. Magnification of the image should be defined as an expansion of the size of *both* the *umbra* and the *penumbra*. There can be no magnification when the umbra (the most important part of the image) is actually shrinking in size. If both the umbra and the penumbra expand,

magnification is present.

A clear understanding of the nature of the penumbra helps explain the apparent contradiction between the diagram in Figure 16-2 and the actual results seen on radiographs. Remembering that penumbra is a spreading of the *edge* of an image both outward and inward, it may be surmised that the human eye will tend to locate the

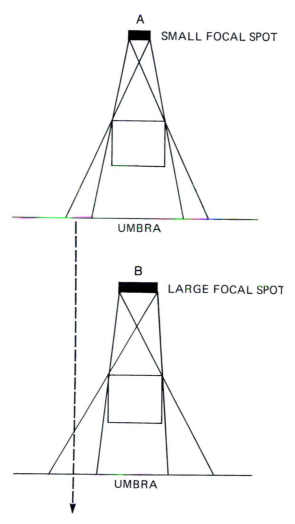

Figure 16-5. Diagram illustrating how the human eye locates the edge of an image at the mid-point of the penumbra regardless of the amount of penumbral spread. Hence, the apparent *size* of the image does not change with differences in focal spot.

edge of the image in the *middle* of the penumbral shadow (Fig. 16-5). Since the penumbra grows inward by an equal amount as it grows outward, its midpoint does not change location. A radiographer measuring the image will line up a ruler at this midpoint in the penumbral edge because the density change in the outer portions of the penumbra is too diffuse to see well. He will thus obtain the same measurement regardless of focal spot size.

To reiterate, an increase in focal spot size will lead to a growth in the blur or penumbra at the edges of an image only. The umbra does not increase in size but actually shrinks. Sharpness of detail is affected, but the magnification of the gross image size is *not*. There is no relation between focal spot size and magnification.

EFFECTS ON OTHER QUALITIES

Focal spot size has no relation to distortion of the shape of the image, because it is not related to alignment or angles.

The focal spot has no controlling effect over the visibility functions of the image—density and contrast. A common misconception is that larger focal spots allow greater tube output, because the larger focal spot sizes are only available with the greater milliamperage settings on the mA knob. Small focal spots may only be used with low milliamperage because the excessive heat created by focusing a large number of electrons into a small area of the anode can damage the anode surface. But at a selected milliamperage, if a larger focal spot were used, *the same number of electrons would still be used to strike the anode.* So the output—the intensity of the x-rays emitted from the tube—remains the same and density is unaffected. The focal spot is a geometrical rather than an electrical factor and has no influence on the energy levels in the x-ray beam. Therefore, it can have no effect upon contrast.

Noting that focal spot size affects *only* the sharpness of detail in a radiographic image and does not affect any other image qualities, focal spot size becomes the *prime controlling factor* over sharpness of detail. While the various distances involved in aligning the x-ray tube, patient and film have an affect upon image sharpness, they also affect other qualities such as magnification, density, contrast, and noise. *The focal spot is the only technical factor which exclusively affects sharpness of detail.*

SUMMARY

1. Increasing the focal spot size results in more penumbra at the edges of an image and, therefore, reduces *sharpness* of recorded detail. Focal spot size is a primary control over sharpness, because it affects sharpness exclusively. FS size is directly proportional to blur or penumbra.

2. Focal spot size does *not* affect *magnification* of the gross image. Although penumbra spreads with larger focal spots, the umbra actually shrinks. For magnification to be apparent, the umbra must be enlarged.

3. Focal spot size has no relationship with gross image *distortion*, because it does

not relate to alignment nor angles.

4. Focal spot size has no effect upon image *density*, *contrast*, or *noise* because these image qualities are not related to geometry. Focal spot changes are strictly geometrical in nature and cannot bear upon total output or energy of x-rays.

REVIEW QUESTIONS

1. What is the *only* quality that the focal spot size really controls?
2. What is the focal spot?
3. Explain *why* larger focal spots do *not* produce more x-ray intensity in the beam, resulting in a darker film image.
4. *Why* do larger focal spots *not* increase magnification of the gross image size?
5. The smaller the focal spot, the _____ the spread of penumbra.
6. Images of small details can be made to effectively disappear when the focal spot is _____ than the object.
7. Cutting the focal spot size to one-half the original, the amount of image sharpness is exactly _____.

Chapter 17

THE ANODE BEVEL

THE ANODE *bevel* refers to the angle of the target surface of the anode in relationship to a vertical line drawn perpendicular to the axis of the x-ray tube. The angle of this surface affects both the relative size of the focal spot produced (the *line-focus principle*) and the relative distribution of the intensity of the x-rays within the beam (the *anode heel effect*).

LINE-FOCUS PRINCIPLE

The size of the projected effective focal spot is controlled by the width of the beam of electrons striking the anode and the angle of the anode bevel. To control the width of the electron beam, modern x-ray tubes have two different cathodes: large and small. The actual stream of electrons is considerably wider than the resulting projected focal spot.

If the anode bevel angle were exactly 45 degrees, the resulting effective focal spot would be the same width as the beam of electrons impinging on the anode surface (Fig. 17-1). It is desirable, however, to reduce the size of the effective focal spot to achieve finer sharpness of details in the image, as explained in the preceding chapter. This is accomplished by the *line-focus principle*, which states that beveling the anode at angles steeper, or more nearly

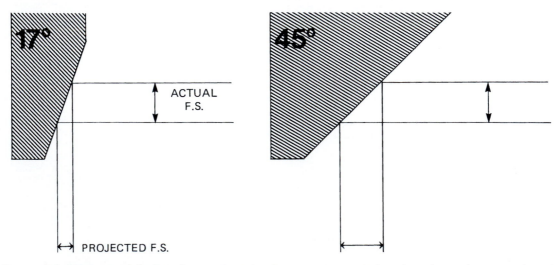

Figure 17-1. Diagram of the line-focus principle. By using an anode bevel angle much steeper than 45 degrees, projected focal spots much smaller than the actual focal spot can be obtained.

vertical, than 45 degrees will cause the effective focal spot to be smaller than the actual focal spot (Fig. 17-1). This procedure allows for greater levels of image sharpness to be achieved, while maintaining adequate dispersal of heat generated over the area of the target so that anode damage does not occur. Most target angles are around 15-17 degrees. Angles steeper than this, such as those used in some special procedures tubes, can lead to severe anode heel effect and limitations on film size.

Typical *large* focal spots vary from 1 to 2 millimeters in size, while typical *small* focal spots range from 0.5 to 1 millimeter. *Fractional* focal spots used in special tubes can be as small as 0.2 mm.

From the diagram, Figure 17-2, it may be seen that the size of the projected focal spot varies with the angle at which it is projected from the target. When the projected focal spot is nearly perpendicular to the face of the target, it is large (4). As the angle decreases toward the central ray, the projected focal spot becomes smaller. The focal spot as projected at the central ray (2) is characteristic of the rated or effective focus of the tube. As the projected focal

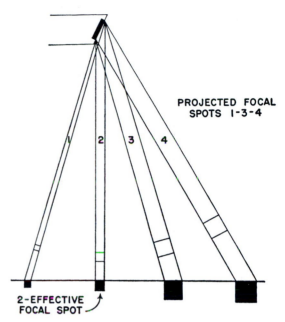

Figure 17-2. Diagram illustrating how the size of the focal spot varies with the angle at which it is projected from the target.

spot moves anode-wise from the central ray, it becomes smaller (1) until it reaches the limits of the anode side of the beam. Actually, at routine SID's, the differences in sharpness from one end of the film to the other are difficult to determine visually.

ANODE HEEL EFFECT

Many radiographers have occasionally been puzzled by radiographic density differences which could not always be attributed to the incorrect use of exposure factors. For example, an anteroposterior radiograph of a thoracic spine would show overexposure in the upper thoracic area and underexposure in the lower thoracic area (Fig. 17-6). This regional lack of density balance is often caused by improper alignment of the long axis of the x-ray tube to the body part so that the "heel" effect of the anode was manifested in its worst form.

This inherent characteristic of all x-ray tubes—the "heel" effect—may be employed to advantage in a limited manner to balance radiographic densities in the image.

WHAT "HEEL" EFFECT IS

The "heel" effect is a variation in x-ray intensity output along the longitudinal tube axis (depending upon the angle of x-ray emission from the focal spot). The intensity diminishes fairly rapidly from the central ray toward the *anode* side of the x-ray beam; on the *cathode* side of the beam, the intensity increases over that of the central ray and then slightly diminishes.

X-rays produced at a given point inside the anode have less distance to travel if they exit in a direction perpendicular to the anode bevel surface (toward the cathode) than if they exit straight down or toward the anode end of the tube (Fig. 17-3). The anode acts as its own filter. Output is greater towards the cathode end of the tube. Figure 18-6, in the next chapter, demonstrates this actual diminution of intensity toward the anode in the beam of x-rays.

Using short SID's (30 inches) and large film areas, its effect is most advantageous, particularly where decided differences in tissue densities require the balancing of radiographic densities to avoid over- and underexposures within the same image. The "heel" effect is more apparent when using steeper, more acute anode bevel angles than more obtuse ones. For example, in order to achieve smaller focal spots and greater sharpness in special procedures suites, special x-ray tubes with anode bevel angles of 7-10 degrees from vertical are often employed. Average tube anode angles in the diagnostic department are around 17 degrees from vertical. With the steeper angle used in the special procedures tube, the anode heel effect becomes so severe with large field areas that the maximum film size used must be limited. This is the primary reason that the largest films used in angiography and similar special procedures is the 14 x 14-inch film, rather than the 14 x 17-inch film.

The anode heel effect is also more pronounced with large focal spots than with small ones, because the difference in thickness of anode material through which the x-rays must escape is greater from one end of the focal spot to the other.

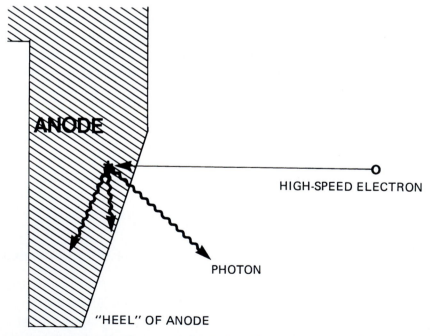

Figure 17-3. Diagram of the anode heel effect. X-ray photons traveling towards the cathode have less metal to penetrate out of, so beam intensity is greater in this direction.

DISTRIBUTION OF X-RAY INTENSITY OVER FILM AREA

The approximate percentage of x-ray intensity emitted by a tube at various angles of emission may be determined directly from photographic measurements of the radiographic blackening of an x-ray film. For radiographic purposes, this procedure is adequate and gives an indication of the approximate percentage of intensity variation to be expected when the x-ray beam falls on specific areas of different sizes of x-ray films at various SID's.

The mean values of radiographic density measurements obtained from many intensities emitted by various x-ray tubes are graphically shown in Figure 17-4. This diagram shows radii emanating from the target face, drawn at 4° intervals from 0° to 40° and intercepting horizontal lines representing various SID's. At the termination of the radii at the bottom of the chart, the mean intensity values in percentages are indicated. For convenience, the intensity at the central ray (CR) is assumed to be 100 percent. To the left, or anode side of the central ray, the intensities diminish in value, while those to the right or cathode side, increase moderately and then decrease slightly.

A radiographic illustration of the differences in intensity is shown in Figure 17-5. A wire mesh was placed on a 14 x 17-inch film. The long axis of the tube was aligned on the center film axis, and the anode portion of the beam was directed toward the top edge of the film. An exposure at a film distance of 20 inches caused the upper portion of the image of the mesh to have less density than the bottom portion where the cathode portion of the beam exposed the film.

INTENSITY-FILM AREA RELATION

Consulting Figure 17-4, the vertical dotted lines beginning just below the diagram of the cathode and terminating at the 72-inch SID distance line, indicate various film lengths. Source-image receptor distances are shown as solid horizontal lines. The respective intensity values created by the radiation emitted at various angles of x-ray emission at various SID's is shown at the bottom. For example, on the 48-inch SID line the outermost pair of vertical lines representing the 36-inch length of film passes outside the limits of the x-ray beam. In order to make use of the entire range of intensities on this length of film, it would be necessary to employ a source-image receptor distance of 49 inches. All intensity radii would intercept at this distance; consequently, if an exposure were made, the entire range of intensities would be expected to become evident, let us say, on a radiograph of an entire spine. Since the minimal intensity in the anode portion of the beam, approximately 31 percent, is emitted in advance to the angle indicated as 0°, it is obvious that the portion of the spine having the least tissue density (the neck) should be exposed by this portion of the beam, and the heavier portion (the lumbar vertebrae) should be exposed by the cathode portion of the beam.

When radiographs on large film are made at relatively short SID's, the percentage distribution of x-ray intensity delivered to a particular size of film at a known source-image receptor distance should be known. This knowledge will aid in correct alignment of the tube and part to the film at

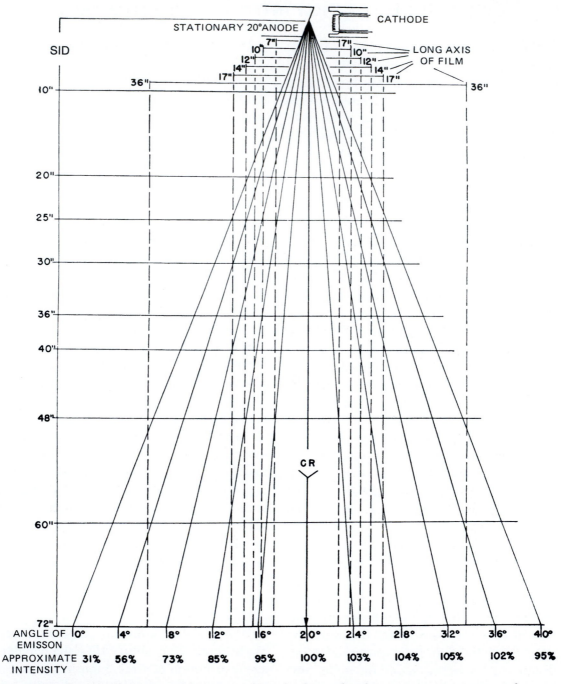

Figure 17-4. Graphic illustration of the mean values of radiographic density measurements over the x-ray beam at different source-image receptor distances obtained from many intensities emitted by various x-ray tubes.

the most favorable SID. Radiographic densities cannot be balanced if only the intensity of the central ray is considered.

Example 1. An example of the "heel" effect is demonstrated by a radiograph, Figure 17-6, *Left*, of the thoracic vertebrae

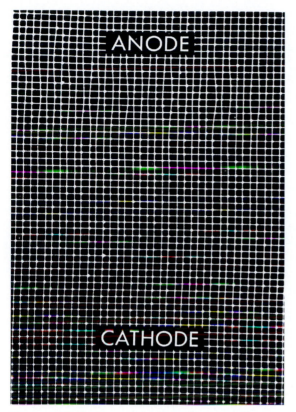

Figure 17-5. Radiographic illustration of the anode heel effect using a wire mesh image. Note that the cathode end of the film is somewhat darker than the anode end.

in which the cathode portion of the beam was directed cephalically. Note the high density in the upper thoracic region and the insufficient density in the lower thoracic vertebrae. By correctly applying the "heel" effect, a radiograph, Figure 17-6, *Right*, was obtained in which all the densities were properly balanced in the image because the anode portion of the beam was directed cephalically. Note that the densities are less in the upper thoracic region and greater in the lower thoracic area.

Example 2. To demonstrate the influence of the source-image receptor on the "heel" effect, a series of anteroposterior radiographs of the humerus, Figure 17-7A-D, were made. Radiograph A was made with a SID of 20 inches and the anode portion of the x-ray beam was directed cephalically. Note the underexposure of the upper portion of the humerus and the overexposure of the distal end. The intensity of the radiation passing to the heavier end of the humerus was insufficient and that portion of the beam passing to the thinner distal end overexposed the area. Radiograph B was made with the same exposure factors after the tube axis was rotated 180°. It may be seen that all densities have been approximately equalized. Radiograph C was made with a 40-inch SID and the anode portion of the beam was directed cephalically.

Note that, because the center portion of the beam only was employed, there was little variation in intensity and all areas have a fairly uniform density. Yet, radiograph D, also made with a 40-inch SID after the tube axis was rotated 180°, shows no improvement over the densities depicted in radiograph C. This example demonstrates that as the SID increases, the "heel" effect diminishes.

RULE. When body parts of unequal thickness or tissue density are to be recorded the following rule should be observed.

Align the long axis of the x-ray tube with the long center axis of the part and film, and direct the cathode portion of the x-ray beam toward the anatomic area of greatest tissue density or thickness.

It should be observed that the "heel" effect diminishes with an increase in the SID and with the use of small size films, since the more uniform intensities of radiation exist in the neighborhood of the central ray. Its greatest effect is observed when the source-image receptor distance is relatively short, when a large film is employed and the body part is unequal in thickness or tissue density.

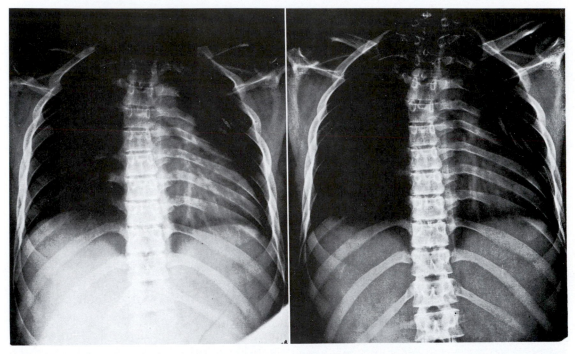

Figure 17-6. Screen-grid radiographs of the AP thoracic spine demonstrating the density variation caused by the anode heel effect. (*Left*) cathode portion of beam directed toward the head. (*Right*) cathode portion of beam directed toward the thicker abdomen, resulting in more balanced densities throughout the T-spine.

SUMMARY

1. The line-focus principle demonstrates that the steeper the anode bevel angle, the smaller will be the projected focal spot size, and therefore greater *sharpness* of recorded detail will be obtained and smaller anatomical images may be recorded. A resulting disadvantage is that smaller field sizes may have to be used.

2. The *anode heel effect* demonstrates that the anode acts as its own filter and, due to the anode surface bevel, results in less image density toward the anode end of the radiograph. For this reason, when radiographing anatomy of variable thickness, the thinner end of the anatomy must always be placed toward the anode end of the tube.

3. The anode heel effect is more visible with steeper anode bevel angles, larger focal spots, shorter distances, and longer field sizes.

REVIEW QUESTIONS

1. Using an anode bevel angle of less than 45 degrees causes the projected focal spot to be smaller than the actual focal spot. This relationship is called the _____.

2. At the "anode-end" of the film the pro-

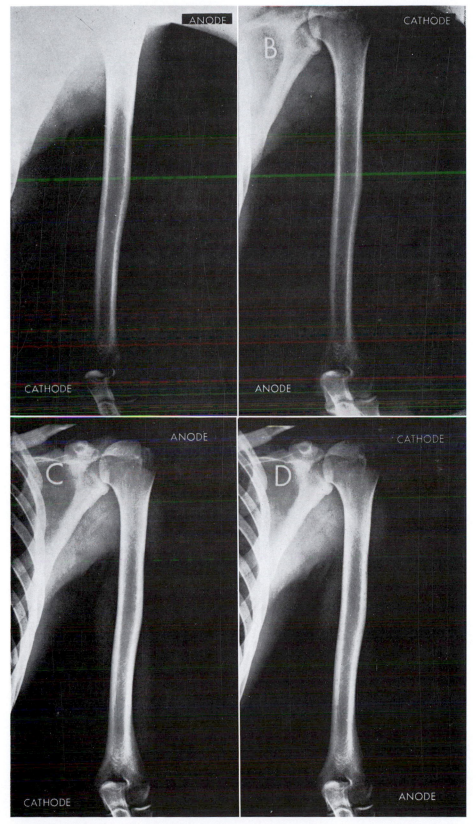

Figure 17-7. Radiographs of humerus illustrating the heel effect at (A and B) 20 inches SID and (C and D) 40 inches SID. Note that the effect is worse at the short 20 inch distance used in (A) and (B). The most balanced view is (D), taken at 40 inches and with the cathode at the thicker end of the humerus.

jected focal spot is _____ than the cathode end.

3. In the anode heel effect, explain *why* less x-rays exit the anode toward its own side of the tube than toward the cathode.

4. For an AP thoracic spine radiograph, place the patient with the head toward the _____ end of the x-ray tube.

5. A "fractional" focal spot in a special procedures x-ray tube is usually in what size range?

6. At a shorter SID, the collimator must be opened up to cover the same field size and the anode heel effect is _____ (increased, decreased, or not affected).

Chapter 18

SOURCE-IMAGE RECEPTOR DISTANCE

THE DISTANCE FROM the x-ray tube to the film or other image receptor is very important because it has substantial influence upon three image qualities: (1) radiographic image density, (2) magnification of the size of the projected image, and (3) the sharpness of recorded detail. Since this distance is also easily manipulated by the radiographer, it has come to be considered by many as a *fourth* prime factor of radiography, along with mA, exposure time, and kVp.

Source-image receptor distance, abbreviated *SID*, is known by many names. It is sometimes called the *target-film distance* (*TFD*) or the *focus-film distance* (*FFD*). It is measured from the *focal spot* or *target* on the x-ray tube anode to the film holder.

ESTIMATING SID

The source of x-radiation is the surface of the anode within the x-ray tube, located roughly in the middle of the cylindrical tube housing. In mobile radiography or when a measuring tape is not immediately available, the SID may be estimated by extending one arm so that the fingertips are at the middle of the tube housing (not the collimator). *For an average male in the United States, 40 inches will correspond to the distance from the fingertips to the opposite side shoulder of the body.* With the fingertips at the tube, the film or image receptor should be about at the opposite shoulder. *Extending both arms, 72 inches will be slightly more than the distance from fingertip to fingertip.*

For the average U.S. female radiographer, the same guidelines may be used, only measuring to the collimator rather than to the tube. Obviously, one must adjust these rules of thumb if one is much shorter or taller than average, but these guidelines are particularly useful for mobile radiography.

EFFECT ON SHARPNESS OF RECORDED DETAIL

When the x-ray tube is moved farther away from the film and object, the amount of blur or penumbra produced at the edges of the image diminishes. As illustrated in Figure 18-1, this occurs because those beams recording the edges of the image are more vertical—nearer and more parallel to the central ray. Thus, the SID has a direct effect upon image sharpness: The longer the SID, the sharper the image, and vice versa. As a rule then, the maximum feasible SID should always be used in order to optimize image sharpness.

In practice, several considerations limit the SID we can use: When radiographing patients recumbent on the table with a vertical beam, the technologist cannot reach the tube if it is too high. (When using the upright chest board, in *most* cases, one has the option to use 72 inches SID on expo-

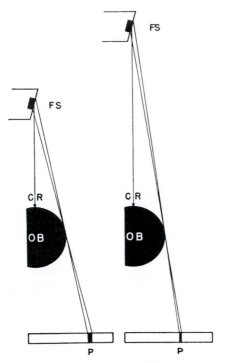

Figure 18-1. Diagram illustrating that longer source-image distances minimize penumbral shadows and thus improve sharpness of detail.

sures that would normally be done at 40 inches SID, since the tube can be easily moved horizontally, and the increased

sharpness only benefits the image.) The main limitation is that the greater the SID, the more technique is required to maintain image density. For large anatomy, extreme distances would result in high techniques that might damage the x-ray tube. If exposure time is used to increase technique, the probability of unsharpness caused by patient motion increases. Given these constraints, the maximum *feasible* SID should be used.

It is important to understand that, in reality, it is the *source-object distance*, the *SOD*, that is directly responsible for these effects upon image sharpness. Any calculations to predict image sharpness or unsharpness must employ the SOD rather than the SID. The specific geometry controlling image sharpness is discussed in Chapter 20. It may be stated that *image sharpness is directly proportional to the SOD*. Any increase in the SID will always result in an increase in the SOD, as long as the distance between an object and the film is maintained. The increased SOD will, in turn, enhance image sharpness as demonstrated in Figure 18-2.

EFFECT ON MAGNIFICATION

At a set object-image distance, *increasing the SID results in less magnification* of the image size. The diagram in Figure 18-3 clearly shows that when a longer SID is employed, not only is there less penumbra produced, but the clear umbral portion of the image is reduced in size as well. For all objects which lie at any significant distance from the film, the magnification produced is quite noticeable (Fig. 18-4). For most applications, magnification is undesirable, and generally the maximum practical SID should be used to minimize magnification.

As long as the object is placed directly on the film cassette, as in tabletop radiography, the effects of SID changes become insignificant. But, any anatomy which cannot be placed directly upon the film, such as organs in the middle of the body, will be significantly magnified and blurred by a shorter SID.

The control of magnification by using long source-image distances is of special importance for routine chest radiography. More than one-half of all chest radiographs are ordered primarily to determine heart size and condition. Magnification is always present to some degree in radiographic

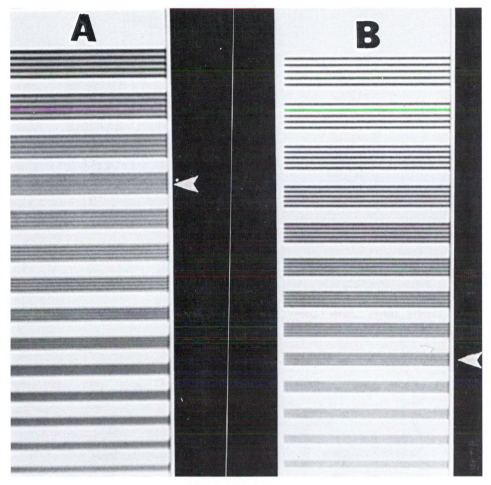

Figure 18-2. Radiographs of resolution test template taken with a fixed OID of 8 inches. Arrows demarcate blur points. For Exposure A, 24 inches SID was used to obtain an SOD of 16 inches, resolving 1.23 line pairs per millimeter. For Exposure B, the SID was increased to 40 inches in order to obtain an SOD of 32 inches, resolving 2.46 line pairs per millimeter, and showing a directly proportional relationship between the SOD and image sharpness.

projections. For heart size measurements to be accurate, the magnification of the projected heart "shadow" must be negligible. The heart is relatively anterior in the body, closer to the sternum than to the patient's back. Routine chests are done in posterior-anterior projection in order to place the heart as close as possible to the film, but because a significant distance is still present between the heart and the film, the SID must be increased well beyond the usual 40 inches.

The use of extended distances in order to eliminate visible magnification is recommended for chest series whenever possible—the recommended SID is 96 inches (8 feet), and dedicated chest units are usually installed with the x-ray tube permanently set at 96 inches. When chest series are performed with general radiographic units, 72 inches is conventionally used. Slight visible magnification of the heart is present at 72 inches, but it is at an acceptably low level for most diagnostic purposes.

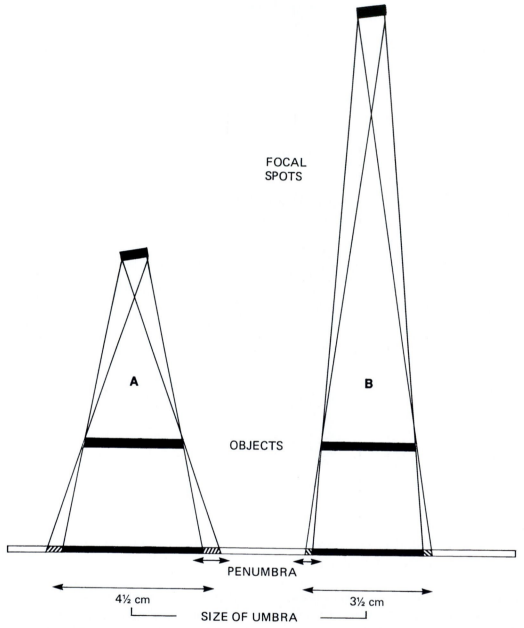

Figure 18-3. Diagram showing how longer SID's reduce the size of *both* the umbra and the penumbra, reducing magnification of the image; (A) 40 inches SID, (B) 72 inches SID.

There are occasions when the magnification and blurring effects of a short SID may be used to advantage. A visibility problem is created any time the anatomy of interest is superimposed by contrasty anatomy which is not of interest. This prob-lem can often be resolved by using positioning and beam angles to project the image *around* the obstructing anatomy. In the case of the sternoclavicular or temporomandibular joints, the contrasty bones of the upper side of the head present a

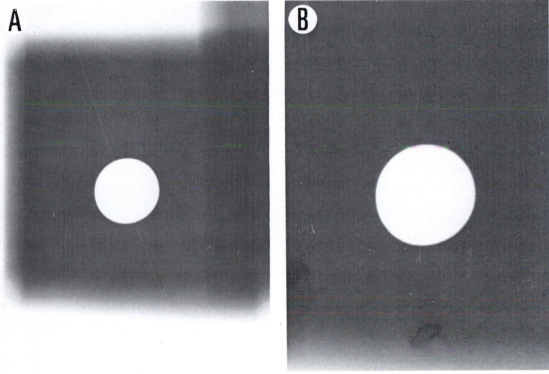

Figure 18-4. Radiographs demonstrating magnification of an object from short SID, with a fixed OID of 4 inches; (A) 40 inches SID, (B) 20 inches SID.

problem which is not adequately solved by angles. A short SID in the range of 26-30 inches should be used on all such procedures and techniques adjusted appropriately. The short SID will both magnify and blur the upside bones to the extent that the anatomy of interest on the down side, against the film, will be more visible through it. The anatomy of interest which is against the film is affected only in a negligible amount. The combination of positioning, angling the beam and using a short SID will result in the highest-quality radiograph. This technique may also be used in other similar cases such as with the sternoclavicular joints and sternum, which are superimposed by the contrasty spine and ribs.

EFFECT ON SHAPE DISTORTION

Shape distortion is a complex function of the alignment and angling of the x-ray beam and the shape of the object being radiographed. It is thoroughly discussed in Chapter 21. Only effects directly attributable to distance will be discussed at this point.

Figure 18-4 demonstrates that although changes in SID will affect the magnification of an image, the shape of the image does *not* change as long as the object is centered in the x-ray beam and the beam is not angled. A circular object will still be circular (not oval) and a square will still be a square (not a rectangle).

Reviewing the definitions of magnification and distortion, it will be recalled that shape distortion only occurs when the measurement of an object in one dimension changes more than that in the opposite dimension—length changes more than width or vice versa. As long as both dimensions, length and width, increase by the same ratio, it may be said that the image is magnified but not distorted. Changes in SID do not distort the shape of an image.

Some confusion has resulted in this area, because an image which is *already* distorted is more obvious when it is also magnified. Consider a spherical object which is being projected onto the film by an angled beam as an oval-shaped image. Distortion of the shape has already been caused by this tube angle. Reducing the source-image distance will magnify the total image. Both the length and the width of the oval will increase by proportionate amounts. However, the ratio of length/width is still equal, and *shape* has not changed. The distance change is not responsible for any distortion which may be present but only for the magnification of the total image size. Images may be *both* distorted in shape and magnified in size, but each of these problems results from a different cause. Distortion of shape is never *caused* by changes in SID. It may, however, be made more apparent because of the magnification effect of SID changes.

EFFECT ON DENSITY

Intensity directly influences radiographic density; any change in distance will cause a change in density when other factors are constant. *Only a 20 percent change in distance will cause a visible change in image density and will require an adjustment in technique*, a fact the radiographer must be aware of.

Since x-rays conform to the laws of light, they diverge as they are emitted from the focal spot, and, proceeding in straight paths, cover an increasingly larger area with *lessened* intensity as they travel from their source. This principle is illustrated in the diagram (Fig. 18-5). It is assumed that the intensity of the x-rays emitted at the focal spot (FS) remains the same, and that the x-rays cover an area of 4 square inches on reaching the horizontal plane (C) which is 12 inches from FS. When the source-image distance is increased to 24 inches to plane D or twice the distance between FS and C, the x-rays will cover 16 square inches—an area 4 times as great as that at C. It follows, therefore, that the intensity of the radiation per square inch on the plane at D is only one quarter that at the level C.

The diminution of intensity of the x-ray beam as it travels further and further away from the focal spot in accordance with the inverse square law may be observed in the radiograph (Fig. 18-6). This image was produced by placing one edge of a 14 x 17-inch film contained in an exposure holder at the portal of the x-ray tube. An exposure was made and the film processed. The top of the image was at the tube portal. Note the high density in this area. As the radiation coursed downward along the film, the x-ray intensity gradually diminished, hence the loss in radiographic density as the SID increased. The difference in density along a horizontal plane through the beam from the anode to the cathode side is due to the "heel effect" (see Chapter 17).

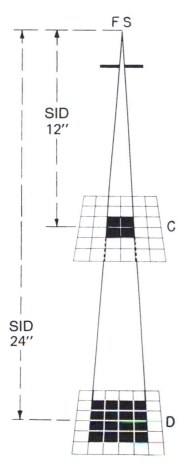

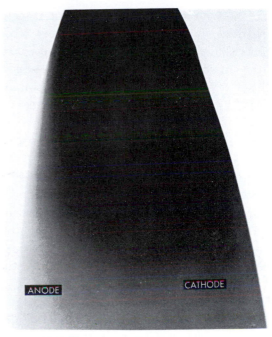

Figure 18-6. Flash x-ray exposure with film placed vertically in beam to demonstrate decrease in intensity of radiation as distance increases from the source. The anode heel effect is also noted in this radiograph toward the anode end of the exposure field.

Figure 18-5. Diagram illustrating the inverse square law. Doubling the distance allows the beam to spread out over a four-fold area, reducing exposure to one-quarter.

THE INVERSE SQUARE LAW

This relationship between distance and radiographic density follows the *inverse square law*, which may be stated as:

$$\frac{\text{Original density}}{\text{New density}} = \frac{(\text{New SID})^2}{(\text{Original SID})^2}$$

Let us apply this formula to the distance change illustrated in Figure 18-5 as an example. In this case, the original distance was 12 inches, and the new distance is 24 inches. Let us assign the original density a value of 1.0, and find how the new density would compare—The formula should be set up as follows:

$$\frac{1}{\text{New Density}} = \frac{(24)^2}{(12)^2}$$

and solving:

$$\frac{1}{X} = \frac{576}{144}$$

$$576X = 144$$

$$X = 144/576$$

$$X = 0.25$$

The new density will be 25 percent, or one quarter, of the original. This agrees with the diagram in Figure 18-5, for there are four times as many squares across which the x-ray beam has spread. Each square must have one-fourth the original exposure.

Simple inverse square law problems can be solved mentally by simply applying the *name of the law* to the *proportional change in distance. Invert* the change, then square it. For example, if the distance is reduced to one-half the original, what would the resulting density be? Mentally invert one-half–this is two. Now square two. The radiograph will be four times darker if it is exposed at one-half the distance and no compensation is made. One third the distance results in nine times the exposure, tripling the distance results in one-ninth the exposure, and so on.

Try the following brief exercise, and check your answers from the Appendix.

EXERCISE #14
Use the inverse square law to solve these problems:

From	To
1 40" SID	72" SID
Density = 1	Density = _____
2. 60" SID	72" SID
Density = 1	Density = _____
3. 50" SID	36" SID
Density = 1	Density = _____
4. 72" SID	96" SID
Density = 1	Density = _____

The inverse square law works because the x-ray beam *fans out* across greater areas as it travels, and to find an area, one must square the length of its sides. The following experiment and Figure 18-5 demonstrate the effect of increasing distance upon image density when all other factors are kept constant.

EXPERIMENT NO. 1–SID DENSITY RELATION

Purpose. To demonstrate the relation between source-image receptor distance and radiographic density.

Theory. Any change in SID influences the intensity of radiation. The intensity varies inversely as the square of the SID. Since changes in SID produce changes in intensity, radiographic density changes.

Procedure

1. The SID-density relation was demonstrated by making a series of three radiographs of the hand using a screen exposure with 50 vKp at a fixed 50 mAs. Only the SID was altered as follows:

Exposure No.	SID
1	25 inches
2	36 inches
3	48 inches

Comment. It may be observed that *as the SID increased, the radiographic density diminished* because the intensity of the x-radiation reaching the film diminished (Fig. 18-7).

THE SQUARE LAW

Distance changes should usually be compensated for by using mAs, rather than kVp. Changes in distance alter the intensity of the x-ray beam–energy levels or penetrating ability are not affected. Adjusting the mAs restores the original intensity of the beam, without changing its quality. If kVp is used to compensate, the altered penetration of the beam will lead to different contrast levels in the image, an undesirable side-effect.

Whereas the inverse square law is used to predict image density, the *Square Law* is used to compensate technique so that den-

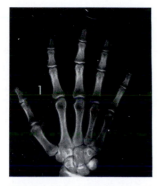 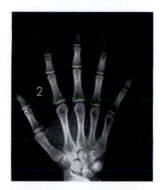 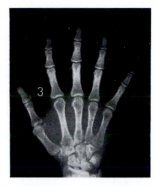

Figure 18-7. Demonstration of effect of increasing SID on radiographic density on hand radiographs. Note the loss of density at increased distances: (A) 25 inches SID, (B) 36 inches SID, and (C) 48 inches SID, all other factors equal.

sity is maintained when distance changes. The formula for the square law is

$$\frac{\text{Original mAs}}{\text{New mAs}} = \frac{(\text{Original SID})^2}{(\text{New SID})^2}$$

Simply stated, the change in technique should be equal to the square of the change in distance. If the distance were doubled, as illustrated in Figure 18-5 the technique change required to maintain density would be *2 squared* or 4 times the original. Suppose 20 mAs had been used for the exposure taken at 12 inches in Figure 18-5. What new mAs would be required for an exposure taken at 24

inches? Using the formula:

$$\frac{20 \text{ mAs}}{X} = \frac{(12)^2}{(24)^2}$$

$$\frac{20 \text{ mAs}}{X} = \frac{144}{576}$$

$$144X = 20(256)$$
$$144X = 11,520$$
$$X = 11,520/144$$
$$x = 80$$

At 24 inches, 80 mAs would be required to maintain the original density level. Note that this is four times the original mAs. Table 18-1 was derived using this formula.

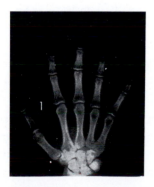 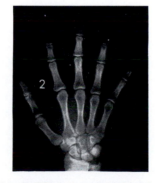 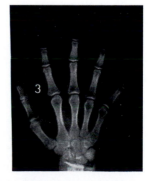

Figure 18-8. Demonstration of time-SID relation on hand radiographs, maintaining density by using the adjustment factors in Table 18-1. Factors: (A) 25 inches SID with 25 mAs, (B) 36 inches SID with 50 mAs, and (C) 48 inches with 90 mAs, all other factors equal.

Table 18-1

mAs MULTIPLYING FACTORS FOR USE WHEN SID IS CHANGED

Original SID	New SID								mAs Multiplying Factors
	20"	25"	30"	36"	40"	48"	60"	72"	
20"	1.00	1.56	2.25	3.22	4.00	5.76	9.00	12.96	
25"	.64	1.00	1.44	2.07	2.56	3.68	5.76	8.29	
30"	.44	.69	1.00	1.44	1.77	2.56	4.00	5.76	
36"	.31	.48	.69	1.00	1.23	1.77	2.77	4.00	
40"	.25	.39	.56	.81	1.00	1.44	2.25	3.24	
48"	.17	.27	.39	.59	.69	1.00	1.56	2.25	
60"	.11	.17	.25	.36	.44	.64	1.00	1.44	
72"	.08	.12	.17	.25	.31	.44	.69	1.00	
	mAs Multiplying Factors								

If the original mAs is unknown, a "1" may be placed in the formula, and the resulting number will be a *factor* by which mAs must be multiplied.

Experiment No. 2 and Figure 18-8 prove that the square law works in maintaining density. Note that, from exposure #1 to exposure #3, the distance is nearly doubled (from 25 inches to 48 inches), while the mAs was nearly quadrupled (from 25 mAs to 90 mAs). Inspection of the resulting radiographs in Figure 18-8 reveals a constant density level.

Following this experiment are three examples of applying the square law, one for an adjustment in exposure time, one for total mAs, and one for a mAs adjustment factor.

EXPERIMENT NO. 2–TIME-SID DENSITY RELATION

Purpose. To demonstrate the interrelation of time of exposure and source-image distance to radiographic density when all other factors are constant.

Theory. The time required for a given radiographic density is directly proportional to the *square* of the SID when all other factors are constant.

Procedure

1. The time-SID relation may be demonstrated by making a series of three screen radiographs of the hand employing the following materials and exposure factors:

Factors	kVp:		50		
	mA:		50		
Variable Factors	Exposure No.	SID		Time	mAs
	1	25 inches		¹/₂ sec.	25
	2	36 inches		1 sec.	50
	3	48 inches		1⁸/₁₀ sec.	90

Comment. In comparing these radiographs, (Fig. 18-8) it may be seen that the densities are approximately the same because suitable exposure time compensation has been made for each SID change in accordance with the square law. Since the SID has a material effect on radiographic density, it is recommended that once an SID is established for a given projection that it should be considered a constant. When some unusual need arises for varying the SID, the square formula should be used to equalize density.

EXAMPLE NO. 1–TIME AND SID

RULE. The exposure time required for a given radiographic density is directly proportional to the *square* of the SID when the remaining factors are constant. This rule may be expressed by the following formula for the purpose of solving the exposure problems:

$$\frac{\text{Original Time}}{\text{New Time}} = \frac{\text{Original SID}^2}{\text{New SID}^2}$$

Example. Assume that an exposure time of 10 seconds (T_1) and an SID of 30 inches (D_1) have been used, and it is desired to decrease the SID to 24 inches (D_2). What exposure time (T_2) would be required?

Solution. T_1, D_1, and D_2 are known; T_2 is unknown. The following working equation adapted from the above basic formula should be employed to solve the problem:

$$T2 = \frac{(T_1)(D_2)^2}{(D_1)^2}$$

$$T2 = \frac{10 \times 24^2}{30^2} = \frac{10 \times 4^2}{5^2} = 6.4 \text{ sec. Answer.}$$

EXAMPLE NO. 2–MAS AND SID

RULE. The mAs required to produce a given radiographic density is proportional to the *square* of the SID when the remaining factors are constant. This rule may be expressed by the following formula for the purpose of solving exposure problems:

$$\frac{\text{Original mAs}}{\text{New mAs}} = \frac{\text{Original SID}^2}{\text{New SID}^2}$$

Example. Assume that an exposure of 10 mAs (M_1) at an SID of 25 inches (D_1) is

employed. The SID is increased to 60 inches (D_2). What mAs (M_2) must be employed to maintain the same radiographic density?

Solution. M_1, D_1, and D_2 are known; M_2 is unknown. The following working equation adapted from the above formula should be used to solve the problem:

$$M2 = \frac{M_1(D_2)^2}{(D_1)^2}$$

$$M2 = \frac{10 \times 60^2}{25^2} = \frac{36000}{625} = 57.6 \text{ mAs. Answer.}$$

To facilitate the mathematics involved, Table 18-1 may be employed to determine mAs values when common SID values are changed. For example, under the column headed "Original SID" find 25 inches. Find the vertical column headed by the new SID of 60 inches. Where these two columns intersect will be found the mAs multiplying factor 5.76. Multiply the original mAs of 10 by 5.76. The answer is 57.6 mAs.

EXAMPLE NO. 3–TECHNIQUE CHANGE FACTOR AND SID

RULE. The factor by which technique must be changed to maintain a given density is proportional to the *square* of the SID when all other factors are constant. This rule may be expressed by the formula:

$$\frac{1}{X} = \frac{\text{Original SID}^2}{\text{New SID}^2}$$

Example: Suppose the SID is increased from 40 inches to 60 inches. The technique chart lists a technique for 40 inches. What change would need to be made in the mAs from the chart to maintain adequate density at 60 inches SID?

$$\frac{1}{X} = \frac{40^2}{60^2}$$

Since the actual mAs is not given, place a 1 for "mAs$_1$" D$_1$ is 40 inches and D$_2$ is 60.

$$\frac{1}{X} = \frac{1600}{3600}$$

Square the distances

$$1600(X) = 3600$$

Cross-multiply.

$$X = \frac{3600}{1600}$$

Isolate X by dividing both sides of the equation by 1600.

$$X = 2.25$$

This is the *factor* by which mAs should be changed

The 40-inch technique should be increased 2.25 times to maintain density at 60 inches SID.

The solutions to square law problems are always the inverse of those for solving inverse square law problems. For example, if a distance change would result in twice as dark a film by the inverse square law, then the technique that would be required in order to maintain the original density at the new distance would be one-half the mAs. If the density change can be predicted, simply invert this change to find the technique adjustment.

Try the following exercise and check your answers from the Appendix. You will need to find square roots to solve for the distance in numbers 7 and 8. Calculators are allowed!

EXERCISE #15

Use the square law to solve these problems:

1. $\frac{5 \text{ mAs}}{50" \text{ SID}}$ = $\frac{\text{_____ mAs}}{60" \text{ SID}}$

2. $\frac{2.5 \text{ mAs}}{40" \text{ SID}}$ = $\frac{\text{_____ mAs}}{72" \text{ SID}}$

3. $\frac{2.5 \text{ mAs}}{60" \text{ SID}}$ = $\frac{\text{_____ mAs}}{20" \text{ SID}}$

4. $\frac{12 \text{ mAs}}{96" \text{ SID}}$ = $\frac{\text{_____ mAs}}{30" \text{ SID}}$

5. $\frac{25 \text{ mAs}}{96" \text{ SID}}$ = $\frac{\text{_____ mAs}}{40" \text{ SID}}$

6. $\frac{40 \text{ mAs}}{80" \text{ SID}}$ = $\frac{\text{_____ mAs}}{36" \text{ SID}}$

7. $\frac{180 \text{ mAs}}{96" \text{ SID}}$ = $\frac{20 \text{ mAs}}{\text{_____ SID}}$

8. $\frac{45 \text{ mAs}}{90" \text{ SID}}$ = $\frac{5 \text{ mAs}}{\text{_____ SID}}$

RULES OF THUMB FOR DISTANCE CHANGES

Although the inverse square law is important to understand, in practice, radiographers rarely use a calculator or pencil to apply it accurately–rather, when doing a mobile procedure at 60 inches SID, for example, they will likely make a mental estimate of the increase in technique required when compared to the usual 40-inch SID. This section provides some simple rules of thumb which, if committed to memory, will greatly improve your accuracy in making this kind of technique adjustment.

A handful of distances (30 inches, 40, 60, 72 and 96 inches), applies to more than 95 percent of radiographic procedures. By taking the most commonly used 40 inches as a standard and comparing the others to it, rules of thumb are easily derived and learned.

It helps to think of distance changes in factors of two, that is, doublings and halvings. For example, the square law formula shows that if SID is increased from 40 inches to 80 inches (a doubling), the technique must be increased by 4 times in order to maintain density. However, by thinking of this quadrupling of the technique as *two doublings*, rules of thumb can be formulated for other distance changes:

Think of increasing the SID from 40 inches to 60 inches as going *half-way to doubling* the SID. That is, 60 inches is halfway from 40 to 80. Since 80 inches would require two doublings of technique, 60 inches will require one-half of that increase, or *one doubling*. For a 60-inch projection, double the mAs used at 40 inches.

In a similar manner, 30 inches can be considered as half-way to cutting 40 inches in half. A 20-inch distance would require one-fourth of the overall technique, or two halvings. Thus, 30 inches requires only one halving of the 40-inch technique.

Table 18-2 summarizes these rules of thumb for the most used distances. A column listing the actual solution based on the square law formula is provided as well so that you can see how close these rules of thumb are for accuracy. Keeping in mind that density must be changed by at least 30 percent to see a visible difference, the rules of thumb are clearly accurate enough for practical use.

Radiographers performing mobile procedures must be especially wary of the fact that only a 20 percent change in SID will result in an unacceptable density level unless technique is adjusted. A classic example occurs when a radiographer who places the mobile unit at the foot of the patient's bed for an AP chest exposure asks another radiographer for a technique. If the advice-giver is used to placing the mobile unit alongside the bed, he may be using as little as 55-60 inches SID. Using his technique at 72 inches (x-ray tube near the foot of the bed) will result in such a light exposure that a repeat will be needed. *A ten-inch difference in SID is always significant enough to require a technique adjustment.*

By far, the most useful of these rules of thumb will be those for 60 inches and 72 inches because these distances are frequently used both in mobile procedures and in the radiology department. For mobile procedures, the rules of thumb can be taken one step further to derive a technique for 50 inches SID:

Considering 50 as the half-way to 60, the technique would be increased half-way to doubling, or increased 50 percent. By the square law formula, the needed increase is 1.57 times the original. The rule of thumb rounds it to 1.5 times. Radiographers assigned to mobile units should remember that *compared to the usual 40-inch technique, a 50-inch SID requires a 50 percent increase in overall technique* (preferably using mAs), *a 60-inch distance requires a doubling, and a 72-inch distance requires a tripling.*

Since chest radiography is commonly performed with the 72-inch SID, it is well to emphasize that the 72-inch distance requires 3 times the 40-inch technique, and that a 40-inch distance requires one-third of the 72-inch technique. This relationship is frequently encountered in performing upright or decubitus abdomen radiographs along with chest radiographs. Remember that the *relationship between a 40-inch SID and a 72-inch SID is a factor of 3.*

These rules of thumb can also be used to solve for density problems, if you remember to invert them (make fractions out of them). For example, if the distance is increased from 40 inches to 72 inches, and the technique is NOT compensated for this

Table 18-2
RULES OF THUMB FOR DISTANCE
CHANGES STARTING AT 40 INCHES

New Distance	Technique Change Computed by the Square Law	Rule of Thumb Technique Change
30 inches	0.56	1/2
40 inches	1.0 (standard)	1
60 inches	2.25	2 x
72 inches	3.24	3 x
80 inches	4.0	4 x
96 inches	5.76	6 x

change, how dark will the radiograph be? Simply invert the factor for 72 inches from Table 18-2. The answer is that the new radiograph will have one-third the density of the original. A radiograph taken at 60 inches without compensating technique would be one-half as dense as a 40-inch radiograph, and so on.

Complete the following exercise *mentally, using the rules of thumb*. Note that those starting at 60 inches or 30 inches can also be solved in your head, if you analyze the distance changes as doubling, halving, half-way to doubling, or half-way to halving. Check and review your answers using the Appendix.

From	To Maintain Density
1. 25 mAs	_____ mAs
40" SID	72" SID
2. 15 mAs	_____ mAs
40" SID	60" SID
3. 7.5 mAs	_____ mAs
40" SID	80" SID
4. 6 mAs	_____ mAs
40" SID	96" SID
5. 60 mAs	_____ mAs
40" SID	20" SID
6. 30 mAs	_____ mAs
40" SID	30" SID
7. 2.5 mAs	_____ mAs
30" SID	60" SID
8. 12.5 mAs	_____ mAs
30" SID	45" SID

EXERCISE #16

Use the technique rules of thumb to solve these problems:

EFFECT ON CONTRAST

Although the intensity of both the secondary and the primary radiation in a beam changes as the inverse square of the distance changes made, they both change by the same proportion. Therefore, at any distance in the beam, the *ratio* of scattered x-rays to primary x-rays will remain the same. Since there is no change in the relative proportion of scatter in the beam, image contrast will not be affected (see Fig. 18-8). Two adjacent densities may both be lighter or darker, but the ratio of difference between them will be unchanged.

Source-image receptor distance, as a controlling factor over density, is similar in its effects to mAs. Both simply control the intensity of the beam. Like mAs, very extreme changes in SID leading to a blank underexposed film or to an overexposed film will clearly destroy the contrast of the image. But within the diagnostic ranges of distances used in real practice, SID is not a consideration in controlling contrast.

SUMMARY

1. A longer SID reduces penumbra and therefore increases *sharpness* of recorded detail. Increasing the SID extends the SOD. Sharpness is *directly proportional to the SOD.*

2. A longer SID reduces the amount of image *magnification*. Magnification is *inversely proportional* to the SID.

3. Source-image distance is not directly related to alignment of the beam and

part and does not affect shape *distortion*. Once shape distortion is present in the image, the magnification effect of distance may make it more or less noticeable. But distance changes do not cause distortion.

4. Increasing source-image distance reduces image *density* by the inverse square law, because the area over which the x-rays are distributed spreads out with distance.

5. Regarding *technique*, the square law may be used to accurately compensate mAs values for changes in SID.

6. SID has no effect upon image *contrast* within typical diagnostic ranges, because the numbers of x-rays penetrating through the patient, interacting by Compton effect, and interacting by photoelectric effect, are all changed by the same proportion, so that the ratio between them is unaffected.

7. An SID of 96 inches is recommended for routine chest radiography, to reduce magnification of the heart.

REVIEW QUESTIONS

1. Decreasing SID _____ penumbra. (Increases, decreases, or has no effect on)

2. Why would you intentionally use a short SID on such procedures as sternoclavicular joints or temporomandibular joints?

3. List the *three* image qualities which are affected by changes in SID.

4. Image density is related to changes in the SID by the _____ law.

5. If the density of one radiograph is 4 times greater than that of another, all other factors equal, the SID must have been changed to a factor of _____ the original.

6. A technique chart lists $1/20$ second for a procedure using 40 inches SID. At an SID of 80 inches, what new time would be required to maintain density?

7. As a rule, the _____ feasible SID should always be used.

8. Increasing SID _____ magnification. (Increases, decreases, or has no effect on)

9. Any change in distance of _____ percent or greater will require an adjustment in technique.

10. What is the recommended SID for a dedicated chest unit?

11. Changing from 72 inches SID to 40 inches SID, technique must be adjusted to _____ the original.

12. Image sharpness is directly proportional to which distance?

13. Image magnification is inversely proportional to which distance?

Chapter 19

OBJECT-IMAGE RECEPTOR DISTANCE

OBJECT-IMAGE RECEPTOR DISTANCE is a crucial factor in controlling radiographic image quality. Although it is primarily a geometric, *recognizability* factor, it affects most of the aspects of the radiograph, directly or indirectly, in dramatic fashion. When the object is placed directly upon the radiographic film, all of the image qualities are optimized. Relatively small changes, such as placing the film four inches away from the anatomy, result in large effects on density, contrast, sharpness, and magnification. Therefore, every effort should be made to minimize the OID on all radiographic procedures.

EFFECT ON SHARPNESS OF RECORDED DETAIL

When the object is at some distance from the film as shown in diagram, Figure 19-1, the sharpness is not as great as it is when the object is next to the film. *The larger the object-image distance, the greater the penumbra grows, and therefore the less the sharpness of recorded detail.* Image sharpness and OID are inversely proportional. The use of Bucky grids requires a slight increase in object-image distance, causing a small amount of image unsharpness to be introduced.

Example. The series of four radiographs of a hand, Figure 19-2, was made in which all factors were constant except the object-image distance. Radiograph A was made with the hand on the film; B, the OID was 2 inches; C, 6 inches; and D, 8 inches. Note that as the OID increased, the edges of the carpal and metacarpal bones can be seen to have become more blurred, thin joint spaces between the carpals are less distinct, and there is less detail visible within the bone marrow. Sharpness has been reduced, resulting in a loss of information.

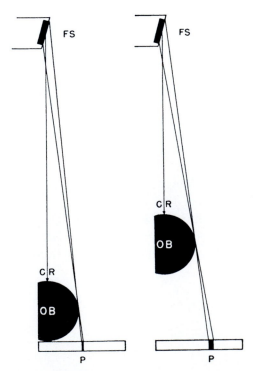

Figure 19-1. Diagram of effect of increasing OID. (*Right*) penumbra spreads at large OID, reducing sharpness.

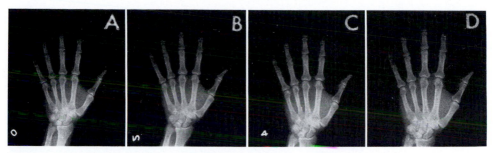

Figure 19-2. Radiographs of hand demonstrating that OID increases (B through D), magnification and unsharpness at the edges of the bones become apparent. Factors: (A) no OID, (B) 2 inches OID, (C) 6 inches OID, (D) 8 inches OID.

EFFECT ON MAGNIFICATION

Magnification in the radiographic image is a normal occurrence. The degree of enlargement is a function of the source-image and object-image distance.

When the object is close to the film, enlargement is minimal. When the center of the part is traversed by the central ray, normal magnification occurs. Whether the SID is great

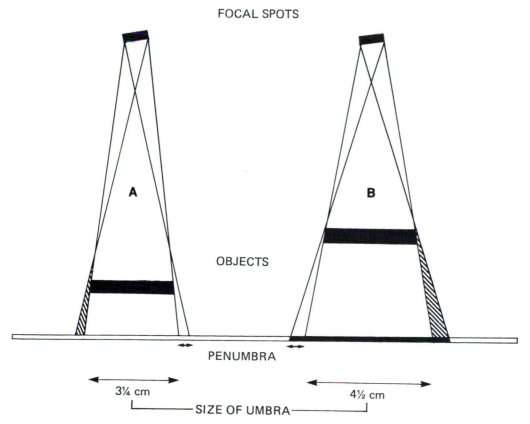

Figure 19-3. Diagram illustrating effect of increasing OID upon image magnification of the overall image. (B) both umbra and penumbra expand at greater OID.

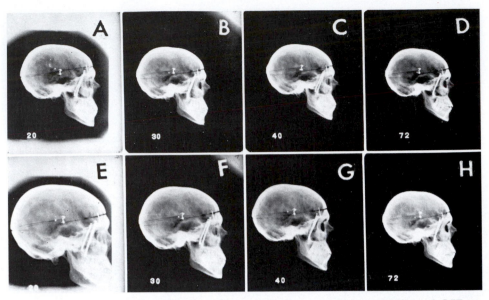

Figure 19-4. Radiographs of dry skull illustrating the interrelation of SID and OID in controlling magnification of the image. .SID's are marked on each radiograph. The top series was taken with no OID, the bottom series with 4 inches OID. The least magnification is at (D) with 72 inches SID and no OID, the greatest magnification is at (E) with 20 inches SID and 4 inches OID.

or small, the image will always be magnified when a large OID exists (Fig. 19-3).

The use of a long SID in these situations serves only slightly to increase the sharpness of definition and decrease the image size. Therefore, the film should always be placed as near the object as possible.

The following example will illustrate the effects of simple magnification when the OID and SID are varied.

Example. Two series of lateral radiographs of a dry skull, Figure 19-4, were made in which the OID and SID were varied as indicated on the radiographs. The dry skull was placed directly on the exposure holder in radiographs A-D, Top. Note that as the SID was increased, the images became smaller. Radiographs E-H, Bottom: the various source-image distances were the same as in Figure 19-4, Top, but the OID was increased to 4 inches in each case. This entire series was magnified as compared to A-D.

EFFECT ON SHAPE DISTORTION

As with SID, changes in OID do not affect shape distortion. Changes in OID only cause changes in magnification, as previously described.

Distortion will occur from improper beam-part-film alignment. Once distortion is created by these types of problems, a longer OID will make that distortion more apparent by magnifying it. But the shape, measured as the ratio of length to width, will not change. Changes in object-image distance do not *create* distortion.

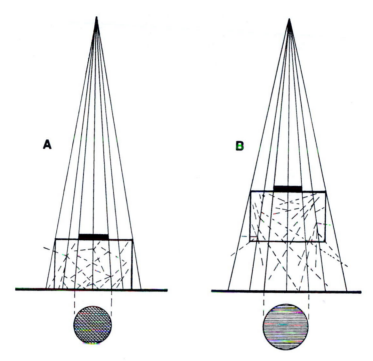

Figure 19-5. Diagrams demonstrating the effect of scatter radiation from a block of paraffin on the image of a coin: (A) When the coin is on top of the emitter, scatter edition from the paraffin fogs the coin image. (B) When the block and coin are moved away from the film, the fog density is reduced, because the scatter radiation is allowed to spread out (by the inverse square law).

EFFECT ON CONTRAST

The emission of scatter radiation and its influence on the image may be simulated radiographically by the use of paraffin—a material that generates large quantities of scatter radiation. A block of paraffin $2\frac{1}{2}$ x 6 x 10 inches may be used for this purpose.

Two principal conditions under which scatter radiation fog may be produced on film are illustrated by the series of diagrams and radiographs shown in Figures 19-5 and 19-6.

WHEN OBJECT IS NEAR FILM

When the emitter is placed on the film and a coin is mounted on its top (Fig. 19-5A), the radiograph will show the image of the coin to be fogged by the scatter radiation that undercuts the object. This diagram and radiographic example (Fig. 19-6A) demonstrate that images of objects in or on an emitter, located at a distance from the film will be fogged when the emitter is adjacent to the film.

WHEN OBJECT IS DISTANT

When the emitter together with the disc on its top is moved away from the film (Fig. 19-5B), the degree of fog in the image will be *less* than that shown in Radiograph (A) (Fig. 19-6), since the scatter radiation reaching the film has been diminished by reason of its greater distance from its source.

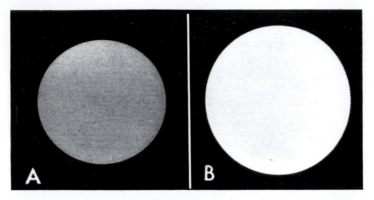

Figure 19-6. Radiographs of a disc on a paraffin block demonstrating the effects diagrammed in Figure 19-5. (A) fogged image of disc, (B) reduction of fog due to placing the disc and paraffin block 5 inches off of the film.

Therefore, *by increasing the distance between the emitter-disc combination and the film, the intensity of the scatter radiation reaching the film diminishes.*

Since the scattered photons spread out more as they move away from the object, they are less concentrated in any given area on the film (Fig. 19-7). In fact, at a large OID, some scatter misses the film entirely. Primary photons which have penetrated the object are travelling in a nearly vertical direction and maintain the same concentration over a given area on the film that they would have had with no OID. This means that the *ratio* of scatter to primary photons striking a given area on the film is reduced. *With less fogging, image contrast is enhanced.*

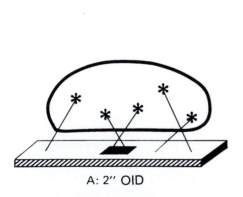

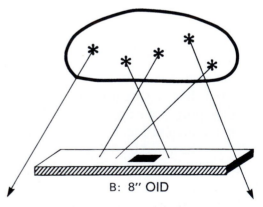

Figure 19-7. Diagram of effect of increasing OID (air gap technique) upon both density and contrast. As OID increases (B), scattered photons *miss* a given area (the black square) because of greater divergence. The scattered rays to the far sides completely miss the film. With the reduced concentration of scatter, contrast is improved, while density is reduced.

EFFECT ON DENSITY

The diagram in Figure 19-7 and the radiographs in Figure 19-6 demonstrate the effect of increasing the object-image distance on image density as well as contrast. *Since the scatter x-rays diverge more* before reaching the film, they are less concentrated in any given area of the film; consequently, *a loss in density occurs.* At significant object-image distances, an increase in mAs is required to maintain image density at a diagnostic level.

AIR GAP TECHNIQUE

Because of its contributory effect on image contrast, a large OID may be occasionally used to advantage in combatting image fog. A common application of this concept is found in chest radiography of very large patients. When an excessive amount of scatter fogging is present on the radiograph, a repeat exposure may be taken, with the patient placed six to eight inches away from the film. This procedure is called the *air gap technique* and is effective in restoring a portion of the desired image contrast.

But, the air gap technique creates problems with other image qualities which must be compensated for. First, since the anatomy will be magnified considerably, the largest practical SID should be used along with the high OID in order to compensate for some of the magnification. A minimum of 72 inches, and ideally 96 inches, SID are suggested. Sharpness of detail lost from the OID will also be partially restored in this manner. Second, the loss of image density from both the high OID and from the inverse square effect of an increased SID must be compensated for by an appropriate increase in mAs.

SUMMARY

1. Increasing the object-image receptor distance results in the growth of penumbra at the image edges and thus reduces *sharpness* of recorded detail. Sharpness is *inversely proportional* to the OID.
2. Increasing object-image distance also *magnifies* the image.
3. Increasing object-image distance has no direct effect upon shape *distortion* in the image. If distortion is already present from poor alignment of the beam and part, the magnifying effect of a larger OID may make it more noticeable. But a larger OID does not *cause* distortion.
4. Increasing the object-image distance reduces image *density*, because scattered radiation produced within the patient diverges more and loses intensity before reaching the film.
5. Increasing the object-image distance enhances image *contrast*, because scattered radiation reaching the film is reduced while the primary rays penetrating the patient remain at the same intensity.
6. The *air gap* technique is recommended for very large patients, in order to restore some of the image contrast. However, magnification and unsharpness also result.

REVIEW QUESTIONS

1. Always use the _____ feasible OID.
2. The greater the OID, the _____ the image contrast.
3. The greater the OID, the _____ the image sharpness.
4. Explain *how* increased OID enhances image contrast.
5. List the three essential steps to the "air gap technique":
6. Which image quality is inversely proportional to the OID?

Chapter 20

DISTANCE RATIOS

THE PREVIOUS TWO CHAPTERS have discussed SID and OID separately, explaining the results in image qualities when one of these is changed and *all* other factors are kept equal. This approach works well when considering image *visibility* qualities such as density and contrast. But when examining the *geometric* qualities of sharpness and magnification, the SID, SOD, and OID should be considered *in relation to each other*. For example, a proportionate change in the SID may completely offset the magnifying effects of a change in the OID.

Both sharpness and magnification are actually determined and controlled by *similar triangle geometry* and can be calculated by forming *ratios* between the appropriate distances. Similar triangles are defined as triangles whose respective corners are of the same number of degrees. When a ratio is made between the same part of two similar triangles, it will always be equal to the ratio formed between any other part of the two triangles. For example, the ratio between the heights of the two triangles will always equal the ratio between their bases. The geometry of the x-ray beam forms similar triangles between the tube, object and film, with the height of each triangle representing a distance–SID, SOD or OID. Certain ratios between these distances can be used to predict changes in both sharpness and magnification of the image.

MAGNIFICATION: THE SID/SOD RATIO

Figure 20-1 depicts the similar triangle geometry of *magnification*. Two similar triangles are formed, one by the SID and the film, the other by the SOD and the object, both sharing the apex "X" at the focal spot of the x-ray tube. *Magnification is simply defined as the ratio between the size of the image and the size of the object.* In Figure 20-1, the size of the image is represented by M_1, the base of triangle *XCD*, and the object is represented by M_2, the base of triangle *XAB*. The ratio between M_1 and M_2 should equal the ratio between the distances D_1 and D_2 (the heights of the triangles):

$$\frac{M_1}{M_2} = \frac{D_1}{D_2}$$

By definition, the ratio M_1/M_2 is the factor of magnification and may be abbreviated M. Since D_1 is the *SID* and D_2 is the *SOD*, these may be substituted and a formula for radiographic magnification derived as:

$$M = \frac{SID}{SOD}$$

Magnification is determined and controlled by the ratio SID/SOD. If the SID/SOD ratio is 2.0, this means that the projected image is

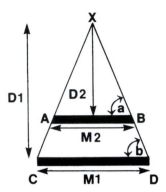

Figure 20-1. Diagram of similar triangle geometry for magnification: Triangles XAB and XCD are similar (angle a = angle b). AB represents an object or the aperture of a collimating device. CD represents the image or the field size at the film. The ratio D_1/D_2, or SID/SOD, will determine the factor of magnification (M_1/M_2).

magnified twice as large as the real object. If the ratio is 1.5, the image is half-again as large, or 50 percent larger, and so on. *Magnification is directly proportional to the SID/SOD ratio.* Note that the *OID* is not used in calculating magnification. In Figure 20-1, the OID does not represent a triangle, but rather a trapezoid formed by the points *A, B, D and C.* It cannot be used for calculations. When the OID is given in a problem and the SOD is not, you must first subtract the OID from the SID to obtain the SOD, then work the formula.

Example No. 1

With an SID of 30 inches and the object placed 20 inches away from the film, how much will the image be magnified?

First, find the SOD as:
SID - 0ID = 30 - 20 = 10

$$\frac{SID}{SOD} = \frac{30}{10} = \frac{3}{1} = \text{Magnification Factor of 3.0}$$

Solution: The image will be three times as big as the real object.

Example No. 2

An image measures 8 inches across. A 30-inch SID was used along with an SOD of 20 inches. What is the size of the original object?

$$\frac{SID}{SOD} = \frac{30}{20} = \frac{3}{2} = \text{Magnification Factor of 1.5}$$

Solution: The image size, given as 8 inches, is 1.5 times larger than the real object. Designating the real object as X then 8 = 1.5 times X:

$$1.5(X) = 8 \text{ and}$$

$$X = \frac{8}{1.5} = 5.3 \text{ inches}$$

The real object is 5.3 inches in width.

Note that any change in SID, SOD, or OID will be exactly offset by a *proportionate* change in one of the other distances. For example, suppose that the OID and the SID are *both* doubled: As shown in Figure 20-2, this results in the SOD also being doubled, and the SID/SOD ratios are maintained equal, $(40/38 = 80/76)$. Magnification will be identical as long as the distances are changed proportionately so that they offset each other.

Try the following exercise for practice, then check your answers in the Appendix.

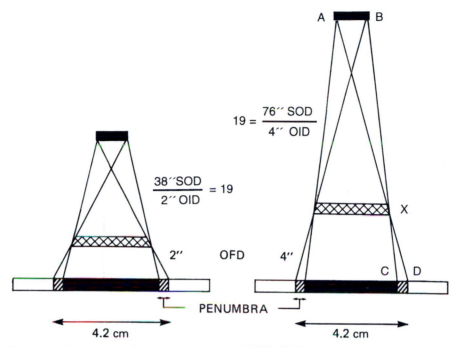

Figure 20-2. Diagram showing a doubling of SID, SOD and OID. As long as the ratios between these distances are maintained, there is no change in sharpness nor in magnification: Relative Sharpness (SOD/OID) = 38/2 = 76/4 = 19. Magnification (SID/SOD) = 40/38 = 80/76 = 1.05.

SHARPNESS: THE SOD/OID RATIO

The sharpness of recorded detail in the image is also determined by similar triangle geometry, but in this case a pair of triangles are formed by the penumbra diagram at each edge of the image as shown in Figure 20-2. Note that in Figure 20-2, triangle *XAB* and triangle *XCD* are inverted to each other with their common apex, *X*, being the edge of the projected object. The height of triangle *XAB* represents the *SOD*. Triangle *XCD* represents the *OID*. If the object were moved twice as far away from the film, triangle *XCD* would stretch twice as high, and the penumbra *CD* would spread exactly twice as much. Penumbra or blur is directly proportional to the OID.

THE "GEOMETRIC UNSHARPNESS" FORMULA

As demonstrated in the last chapter, image blur or unsharpness is directly proportional to the OID. In Chapter 16, we learned that blur is also directly proportional to the size of the focal spot. In Chapter 18 we learned that blur is *inversely proportional* to the SOD. All three of these relationships can be mathematically expressed by the *geometric unsharpness formula* used in many textbooks:

$$\text{Unsharpness} = \frac{\text{FS x OID}}{\text{SOD}}$$

EXERCISE #17

Magnification ratios are calculated identically for both the light field/x-ray field size and also for the magnification of an object being radiographed. For each of the following, three factors are given—solve for the fourth, using the ratio SID/SOD. Don't forget to subtract the OID when needed to get the SOD:

	Width of Distal End of Cone or Collimator	Width of X-Ray Field at Film	SID	SOD
1.	8 inches	_____	60 inches	30 inches
2.	6 inches	_____	60 inches	45 inches
3.	_____	10 inches	60 inches	20 inches
4.	1 inch	9 inches	72 inches	_____
5.	5 inches	15 inches	_____	60 inches

	Width of Light Field on Patient's Surface	Width of X-Ray Field at Film	SID	**O.I.D.**
6.	8 inches	_____	60 inches	40 inches
7.	10 inches	_____	24 inches	8 inches
8.	4 inches	5 inches	_____	6 inches
9.	_____	12 inches	96 inches	84 inches
10.	4 inches	6 inches	96 inches	_____

	Width of Actual Object	Width of Object's Image on Film	SID	SOD
11.	10 cm	_____	80 inches	20 inches
12.	6 cm	_____	100 inches	80 inches
13.	_____	24 cm	96 inches	72 inches
14.	8 cm	12 cm	60 inches	_____
15.	12 cm	18 cm	_____	60 inches

Theoretically, one can calculate the actual size of penumbral spread due to geometrical penumbra in millimeters, given the focal spot size in mm and the two distances. For example, if the OID is 10 cm and the SOD is 40 cm, how much geometrical penumbra would be produced by an 0.5mm focal spot? The calculation would be 0.5 x 10/40 = 5/40 = 0.125 mm of penumbral spread. Unfortunately, the actual *total penumbra* produced in an image includes *absorption penumbra* which must be added to the *geometrical penumbra*. This is explained fully in Chapter 24. Therefore, the geometrical penumbra formula is of limited practical application. It is useful in comparing only the *geometrical* unsharpness between different techniques using varied distance and focal spot combinations.

SHARPNESS OF RECORDED DETAIL

"Geometrical sharpness" may be mathematically expressed by simply inverting the above unsharpness formula. It would then state:

$$\text{Sharpness} = \frac{\text{SOD}}{\text{FS x OID}}$$

Theoretical calculations can also be made for *relative* sharpness values. For example, two techniques are compared, *A* using an 0.5 mm focal spot, 40 cm SOD and 10 cm OID, and *B* using an 0.4 mm focal spot, 50 cm SOD and 25 cm OID. Which produces a sharper image?

$$A = 40/0.5 \times 10 = 40/5 =$$
8 (relative sharpness value)
$$B = 50/0.4 \times 25 = 50/10 =$$
5 (relative sharpness value)

Solution: A is sharper than B
(8/5 = 1.6 times or 60 percent sharper)

More importantly, though, this formula may serve to remind us that sharpness is directly proportional to SOD, and inversely proportional to FS and OID. In Figure 20-2, the OID was doubled, which would normally double the blur and cut sharpness to one-half. However, the SID was also doubled in Figure 20-2, and this resulted in twice the SOD. On the left, the SOD/OID ratio is $38"/2" = 19$. On the right, the SOD/OID ratio is $76"/4" = 19$. The distances, having been changed proportionately, offset each other exactly, and result in the same ratio. The sharpness is therefore mainlined equal, and so is the magnification, as you can see in Figure 20-2. As long as the SOD/OID ratio is maintained, no geometrical changes will be noted in the image.

VISIBILITY FUNCTIONS

Distance ratios are not directly related to the visibility functions in the image.

Since increases in SID and increases in OID both decrease image density, the loss of density is exaggerated when both are increased. Since SID has no effect upon image contrast, and increasing OID enhances contrast, increasing both will result in a net increase in contrast.

MACRORADIOGRAPHY (MAGNIFICATION TECHNIQUE)

As discussed in Chapter 19, in most radiographic practice the object-image distance (OID) should be kept as small as possible in order to minimize magnification and preserve sharpness in the image. There are some applications, most notably for angiography and mammography, in which a magnified image is desired as a way of enhancing its visibility. For example, cerebral angiography is commonly performed with an intentional OID of 8 to 10 inches. With the usual 40-inch SID, the SID/SOD ratio will be 1.25 to 1.33 achieving 25 to 35 percent magnification of the vessels of the brain. For the 8-inch OID, the formula would be:

$$\frac{SID}{OID} = \frac{40}{32} = 1.25 \text{ magnification factor}$$

$(1.25 - 1) \times 100 = 25$ percent magnification

In this case, the loss of image *sharpness* caused by the high OID must be compensated for with some factor other than distance. Focal spot size is ideal, since it affects only sharpness. *Microfocus* x-ray tubes, with focal spots from 0.1 to 0.3 millimeters in size are therefore used. With the smaller focal spot, sharpness of recorded detail is restored to the normal level even though the image is magnified. The smallest available focal spot should always be used when performing magnification technique. This method is called *macroradiography*, meaning "big radiography."

SUMMARY

1. The SID/SOD ratio is the primary controlling factor over *magnification.* Magnification is *directly proportional* to the SID/SOD ratio.
2. The SOD/OID ratio is the primary controlling factor over *sharpness of recorded detail.* Image sharpness is *directly proportional* to the SOD/OID ratio.
3. A *relative geometric sharpness value* may be calculated with the formula S = SOD/FS x OID.

4. *Geometric unsharpness* may be calculated with the formula U = FS x OID/SOD.
5. Distance ratios are not related to shape distortion, density or contrast in the image. When determining density or contrast changes, SID and OID should each be considered separately.
6. In *Macroradiography,* fractionally small focal spots are employed to restore most of the sharpness which is lost by using an air gap OID.

REVIEW QUESTIONS

1. Aside from the effects of focal spot, the sharpness of an image is *directly* proportional to the ratio of the _____ _____ distance divided by the _____ _____ distance.
2. If the SID is 40 inches and the SOD is 20 inches, the projected image of the object will be magnified by a factor of _____.
3. An original technique is used with an SID of 40 inches and an OID of 2 inches. If the *OID* were increased from 2 inches to 3 inches, what new SID would be required in order to *completely* eliminate the blurring effects of the OID change.
4. An original magnification ratio is 50 percent. If the *SID* and *OID* were *both* tripled the new magnification ratio will be _____.
5. What are the two essential steps to performing macroradiography (magnification technique)?

Chapter 21

BEAM-PART-FILM ALIGNMENT

THE ORIENTATION of the central ray of the x-ray beam, the anatomy being radiographed, and the film, in relation to each other, their shapes, angles, and centering are all alignment factors which relate to positioning in controlling the geometrical integrity of the recorded image. Blanket statements such as "Angling the x-ray beam *always* causes shape distortion" are misleading. The effects of beam-part-film alignment on the image are complex and must be discussed on a case-by-case basis for the sake of accuracy.

OFF-CENTERING VERSUS ANGLING

Off-centering of either the central ray or the part in relation to each other places the part in the diverging peripheral rays of the beam. These peripheral rays angle away from the central ray. The further they are from the central ray, the more angled they are from it. Therefore, off-centering has identical effects to angling the beam or part (Fig. 21-1). Although the following demonstrations are all produced by angulation, equivalent effects are caused by off-centering.

EFFECT ON SHAPE DISTORTION

The traditional rule of keeping the part parallel to the film and the central ray perpendicular to both the part and the film effectively minimizes shape distortion in the image. But, this ideal situation is possible in not more than 70 percent of the radiographs commonly taken. The remainder of cases consist of anatomy which cannot

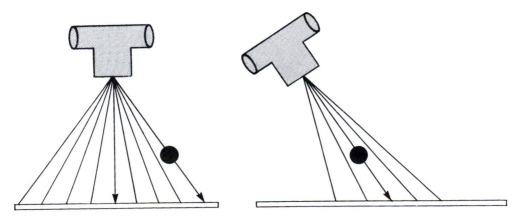

Figure 21-1. Diagram showing how off-centering the x-ray beam has an equivalent effect of angling the beam, since off-centering places the object in diverging rays.

be placed parallel to the film or the necessity of angles to desuperimpose overlying structures. In these cases, shape distortion must be minimized and keeping the beam perpendicular to the film or part is not always applicable in doing so. There are four major factors which affect shape distortion in the image: (1) the shape and thickness of the object being radiographed, (2) the centering of the central ray with respect to the object, (3) the angle formed between the central ray and the long axis of the object, and (4) the angle formed between the long axis of the object and the film. All of these must be understood in controlling distortion.

SHAPE OF THE ANATOMICAL PART

The shape of the anatomical part or object being radiographed affects the degree to which its image is distorted by changes in beam-part-film alignment.

Objects that are spherical or cubical in shape distort under more circumstances than do flat, wedge-shaped or tubular objects. Further, when the x-ray beam is angled, spherical or cubical objects which have no distinct long axis will be more distorted than flatter objects whose long axis parallels the film. Examples of anatomical parts which are spherical or cubical include the cranium, the femoral condyles, the heads of the femur and humerus, the vertebrae, and the tarsal bones.

Objects which are flat, such as the sternum and scapulae, wedge-shaped, such as the sacrum and anterior teeth, or tubular, such as the shafts of the long bones and the ureters, may not distort significantly with tube angles as long as their long axis is maintained parallel to the plane of the film. Thus, the shape of an object has a direct bearing upon the occurrence of visible shape distortion when the beam is angled or off-centered.

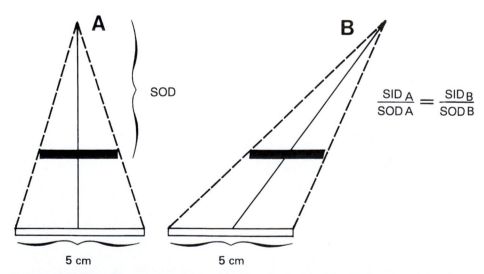

Figure 21-2. Diagram demonstrating that angling or off-centering the x-ray beam against a thin, flat object may not cause visible shape distortion if the object is kept parallel to the film, since the ratios of SID/SOD are maintained. Only relatively thick objects exhibit noticeable shape distortion.

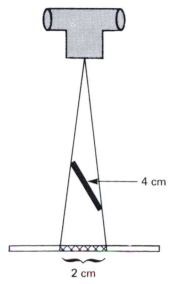

Figure 21-3. Diagram of foreshortening distortion caused by tilting the object while the beam and film are kept perpendicular.

OBJECTS WITH
A DISTINCT LONG AXIS

When a relatively flat, wedge-shaped, or tubular object is kept parallel to the film, angulation of the central ray may not lead to appreciable shape distortion (Fig. 21-2). This is because at *any* given ray in the beam, the angle will have caused SOD to increase by the same proportion as the SID. The SID/SOD ratio is therefore unchanged across the beam of x-rays and there is no distortion.

When a flat, wedge-shaped or tubular object is tilted in relation to the film, *foreshortening* distortion will occur (Fig. 21-3). The image recorded is shorter in the axis of the tilt than the real object is. This can cause misleading information on the radiograph. (Since a spherical or cubical object has no identifiable long axis, its orientation in relation to the film is of no consequence.)

If a flat, wedge-shaped or tubular object is tilted in relation to the film, and the central ray is angled to place it perpendicular to the long axis of the object (Fig. 21-4), *elongation* distortion occurs in the axis of the tilt. Again, misinformation is recorded on the radiograph.

Ceiszynski's Law of Isometry

Since tilted objects present distortion regardless of whether the central ray is placed perpendicular to the film or perpendicular to the object (foreshortening on the

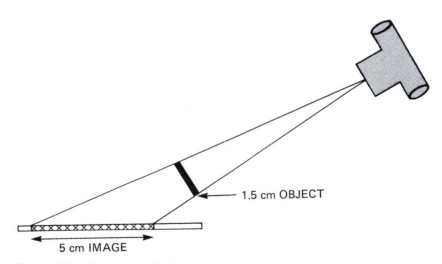

Figure 21-4. Diagram of elongation distortion caused when the beam is directed perpendicular to an object that is tilted in relation to the film.

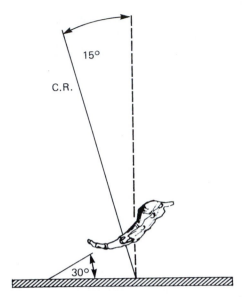

Figure 21-5. Ceiszynski's law of isometry applied to the AP sacrum projection: To minimize shape distortion of an object that cannot be placed parallel to the film, angle the beam one-half of the part/film angle. The sacrum lies at a 30-degree angle, the CR should be angled 15 degrees.

one hand and elongation on the other), the minimal distortion must be achieved at some angle between these two extremes. *Ceiszynski's Law of Isometry* states that an *isometric* angle, equal to one-half of the angle formed between the object and the film, will eliminate or minimize distortion. A classical example of the use of isometric angles is found in radiography of the AP sacrum. The sacrum is a fairly flat wedge-shaped object. Note that although the normal sacrum lies at an angle of 30-35 degrees from the film when a patient is lying supine, positioning atlases recommend the use of a 15-degree cephalic angle of the central ray, one-half of the anatomical angle, for the AP projection (Fig. 21-5). This angle minimizes shape distortion of the sacrum.

Figure 21-7 demonstrates these various effects radiographically, using a coin for a flat object.

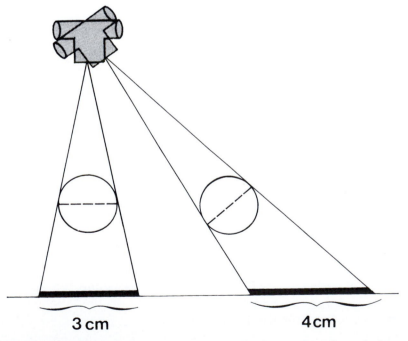

Figure 21-6. Diagram showing elongation distortion of a spherical object when the x-ray beam is angled or off-centered.

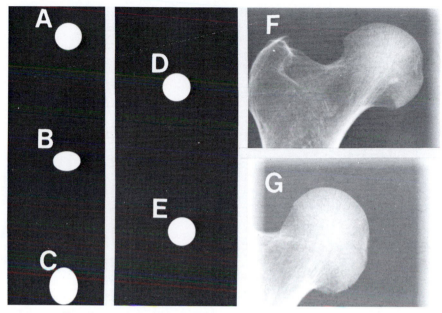

Figure 21-7. Radiographs demonstrating various cases of shape distortion: (A) flat coin parallel to film with beam perpendicular to both showing no distortion; (B) coin tilted and beam perpendicular to film showing foreshortening; (C) coin tilted and beam perpendicular to *coin* showing elongation; (D) coin angled 45 degrees to film, beam angled isometrically at 22.5 degrees showing no distortion; (E) coin parallel to film and beam angled 30 degrees to both showing no noticeable distortion because coin is flat and thin; (F) spherical head of femur in normal projection; and (G) angulation of beam 30 degrees showing elongation distortion of femoral head.

OBJECTS WITHOUT A DISTINCT LONG AXIS

Angling (or off-centering) the central ray distorts spherical or cubical objects. This occurs because, since they have no true long axis, the x-ray beam sees an artificial axis which is always perpendicular to itself. Thus, when the beam is angled, the same effects occur as if if a linear object were tilted to the film and distortion occurs (Fig. 21-6). These effects on actual radiographs are shown in Figure 21-7.

OFF-CENTERING AND BEAM DIVERGENCE

As mentioned at the beginning of this chapter, placing objects off-centered away from the central ray of the x-ray beam positions them within diverging, angled beams. Thus, the effects of off-centering are similar to those for off-angling, that is, shape distortion does occur. However, the most one can off-center an object in a 17-inch wide field is 8 inches from the C.R. The actual beam divergence at this point is only about 20 degrees, while the angle used to produce the distortion evident in Figure 21-7G was 45 degrees. If the field size could be opened wide enough to accommodate exposing an object so far off-center that it was in a 45-degree diverging beam, the

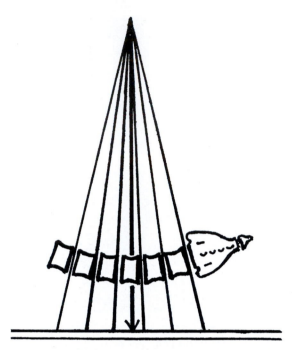

Figure 21-8. Diagram demonstrating that a *moderate* amount of "sagging" on the lateral projection of the lumbar spine actually aligns the joint spaces with the diverging x-ray beam. Building up the spine so that it is horizontal results in partially closing off these joint spaces. In positioning geometry, it is essential to remember the fan-shaped divergence of the x-ray beam.

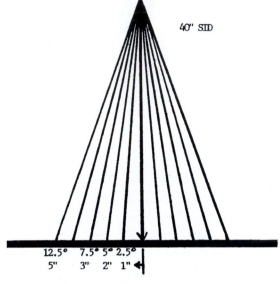

Figure 21-9. Beam divergence at 40 inches SID is *2.5 degrees per inch* (1 degree per cm) in any direction away from the central ray. This can be used to great advantage in positioning.

resulting distortion would be identical. The distorting effects of off-centering may seem less than those of off-angling, but this is only because off-centering is so limited in range.

Beam divergence can be used to advantage if it is well understood, yet most textbooks have thus far failed to even address the topic, much less quantify it, as will be done here. Lumbar spine radiography provides several examples. For the lateral projection of the L-spine, many positioning texts strongly recommend building up the waist portion of the patient's body on sponges or sheets until the spine itself is parallel to the film. This is supposed to better open the joint spaces as the x-ray beams pass through them. Figure 21-8 illustrates

why this is faulty reasoning: The central ray of the x-ray beam is the *only* ray that is perpendicular to the film. The best way to allow the remaining rays, which are *fanning out* or diverging, to pass cleanly through these joint spaces is in fact to *allow some "sagging" of the spine*, rather than completely "correct" it. Certainly, *excessive* sagging of the spine must be compensated, but a normal, moderate amount is in fact desirable in lining these joints up with a divergent x-ray beam. There are many other examples of positioning modifications which similarly take advantage of beam divergence, such as using the PA rather than the AP projection for an L-spine series, or exposing the hands in AP rather than PA position when the patient's fingers cannot be fully

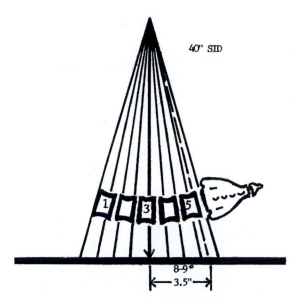

Figure 21-10. Example of applying the beam divergence rule-of-thumb. If the L5-S1 joint space is open on the *routine lateral* projection, then the indicated angle for the *spot lateral L5-S1 joint* is approximately *9 degrees caudal.* (The common 5-degree caudal angle would be underestimated.)

straightened out.

A *beam divergence rule of thumb* can be established—Experimentation has demonstrated that *for a 40-inch SID, the divergence of the x-rays is 2.5 degrees for every inch off-centered in any direction from the central ray* (Fig. 21-9). (Nicely, this comes to 1 degree of divergence per centimeter off-centered.) For a 72-inch SID, beam divergence is about 1.5 degrees per inch off-centered.

A beautiful example of the practical value of this rule is found again in lumbar spine radiography. There is a positioning rule of thumb which states that is the L5-S1 joint is nicely opened on the *routine lateral L-spine view,* a caudal angle should be employed when centering directly on this joint for the L5-S1 "spot" view. This rule is based on beam divergence, and works well; yet those who use it frequently *underestimate the amount* of angle indicated. By using the *beam divergence rule of thumb,* this

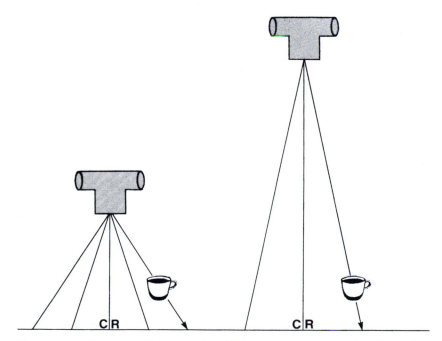

Figure 21-11. Diagram illustrating how SID becomes a controlling factor (but not a causing factor) when shape distortion is already occurring due to off-centering: By increasing the SID (*right*), the object is projected by more vertical beams, thus reducing shape distortion.

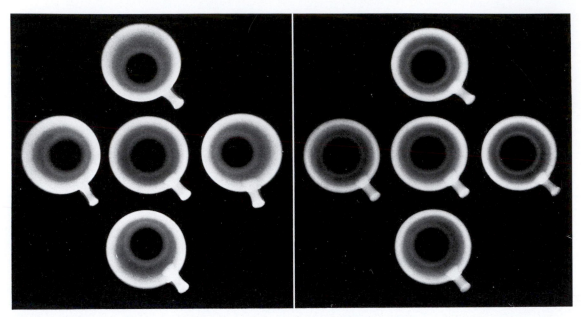

Figure 21-12. Radiographs of several mugs demonstrating the contributing effects of SID when distortion is already present. Note the centering of the darker area within each cup: (*left*) Using 30 inches SID, peripheral cups are distorted, while (*right*) using 72 inches SID this effect is diminished. Also, note that the cup centered in the CR is not distorted at either distance, because it is not in a diverging beam.

amount can be quantified with confidence as shown in Figure 21-10. Centering for the routine lateral L-spine is to the mid-body of L-3, about 1 inch above the iliac crest. On average, the L5-S1 joint lies about 3½ inches below this point. The actual amount of beam divergence at this point on the routine lateral view can be found by simply multiplying this distance by 2.5 degrees of divergence per inch. This comes to 2.5 x 3.5 = 9 degrees of divergence. That is to say, on the *routine lateral view*, the angulation of the beam which is passing through the L5-S1 joint is about 9 degrees. If that joint is nicely opened, the indicated caudal angle for the "spot" lateral is not the standard 5 degrees, but almost 10 degrees.

By both quantifying and more fully appreciating the effect of beam divergence, positioning skills can be greatly improved. Accurate centering as well as angulation, and compensation between the two using

the rule of thumb, are essential to keeping shape distortion to a minimum.

In the case of off-centering objects in the beam, using shorter source-image distances may indirectly lead to exaggerated distortion problems as follows: When a shorter SID is used, the radiographer must often open the collimator or otherwise increase the field size to avoid cutting off anatomy of interest. In doing so, objects that are placed at a given distance away from the central ray will be recorded on the film by more peripheral beams that are more angled from the central ray (Fig. 21-11). In effect, these objects have been angled against more, and if they are relatively thick objects they will be distorted in shape more (Fig. 21-12). Therefore, off-centering of objects in the x-ray beam causes more severe distortion problems at short distances than at long distances.

EFFECT ON DENSITY

Angling the central ray, part, or film does not directly affect image density. However, angling the C.R. *without* compensating the tube-to-tabletop distance results in an increased SID. The longer SID then leads to a loss of density, as described in Chapter 18. The distance change, not the angle itself, causes the density loss. To compensate for this reduction in density, use the rule of thumb: *One inch less tube-to-tabletop distance for every 5 degrees of CR angle.* It is not necessary to apply this rule at tube angles of 15 degrees or less, since the density loss at these angles is negligible. This rule serves to maintain an actual SID of 40 inches.

Tilting or angling the part may result in an effective increase or decrease in part thickness as measured through the central ray location. This will change image density accordingly. The change in density is due to the effectively changed part thickness and not to the angle itself.

EFFECTS ON OTHER QUALITIES

All of the preceding diagrams on distortion demonstrate the effects of alignment changes caused in *one* axis only—the axis of the angle or off-centering shift. In the opposite axis, across or perpendicular to the angle or off-centering shift, no change occurs. This may be documented by comparing the crosswise *width* of the sphere in Figure 21-7G, which does not change even though elongation distortion is occurring. Since magnification is defined as an increase in the *total* image size across *both* axes, it may be said that beam-part-film alignment does not affect magnification.

Misalignment can also be seen in these same radiographs to not affect sharpness of detail at image edges. Neither magnification nor sharpness are affected by alignment changes, because the ratio of the SID/SOD remains equal in all of the rays across an angled or off-centered beam. Any SID increase resulting from CR angles is accompanied by an equivalent SOD increase, so that the ratio between them is unchanged (Fig. 21-2). As described in Chapter 20, as long as this ratio remains equal and the focal spot is not changed, no change in sharpness or magnification will occur.

Alignment of the beam, part and film is strictly geometrical in nature and has no effect upon the ratio of scatter radiation produced within the patient or upon the penetration characteristics of the beam. It cannot, therefore, have any relationship to image contrast.

SUMMARY

1. *Distortion* of the shape of an image is absent when the x-ray beam, part and film are centered, the part is parallel to the film and the beam is perpendicular to the film.

2. *Off-centering* of either the central ray or the part results in the same effects as angling the beam.

3. Angling or off-centering the beam against spherical or cubical objects

causes *elongation* distortion.

4. When a relatively flat, tubular, or wedgelike object is tilted in relation to the beam and film, *foreshortening* distortion occurs.

5. If the beam *and* object with a long axis are equally angled to the film, *elongation* distortion occurs.

6. When a flat or linear object cannot be made to parallel the film plane, an *isometric angle* of the central ray of the beam, one-half of the object-to-film angle, should be used to minimize distortion.

7. If a relatively flat, wedge-shaped, or tubular object is kept *parallel* to the film, angling the beam may not result in visible distortion of its shape.

8. Angulation of the beam or part does not directly affect radiographic *density*. However, effective patient thickness, and distances if uncompensated for, may be changed in the course of angling the beam or part. These changes may then affect image density.

9. To compensate for distance changes from beam angulation so that density may be maintained, use the rule of thumb *one inch for every five degrees* in adjusting tube-to-tabletop distance.

10. Angulation of the beam or part has no effect upon image *contrast, magnification,* or *sharpness of detail.*

11. Beam divergence for a 40-inch SID is 2.5 degrees per inch in any direction from the central ray.

REVIEW QUESTIONS

1. As long as the body part is placed parallel to the film, the central ray should always be _____ to the film to minimize shape distortion.

2. Why is off-centering of the central ray similar in its effects to angling the x-ray beam?

3. Why do positioning atlases suggest a 15-degree cephalic angle for the AP sacrum projection, when the average sacrum lies at 30-35 degrees from the plane of the film?

4. Which of the following would distort *most* in shape with a 35-degree angle of the central ray: the head of the femur, the shaft of the femur, or the sternum?

5. If a flat object is angled in relation to the film, and the x-ray beam is angled to place the central ray perpendicular to the object, what type of image distortion occurs?

6. The distorting effects of off-centering an object within the x-ray beam are indirectly worsened if a _____ (long or short) SID is used.

7. If you angle the x-ray beam 20 degrees, the tube-to-tabletop distance must be changed from 40 inches to _____ inches in order to maintain a 40-inch SID and avoid loss of image density.

8. If the x-ray beam is angled 35 degrees, and the tabletop-tube distance is left at 40 inches, an increase in mAs will be required to maintain image density, NOT because of the angle itself, but because of:

9. List the four aspects of beam-part-film alignment which affect image shape distortion:

10. Why will the cranium distort more with an angled x-ray beam than the head of a femur, even though both are spherical in shape?

11. State Ceiszynski's Law of Isometry:

12. What is the angle of beam divergence at a point 3 inches cephalic to the cen-

tral ray?

13. Why is it *not* desirable to have the lateral lumbar spine built up on sponges to the point that all joint spaces are perpendicular to the film?

Chapter 22

GEOMETRIC FUNCTIONS OF POSITIONING

POSITIONING, at its most fundamental level, is a geometrical factor affecting the recognizability of the image details. Every specific position has as its purpose one of the following objectives:

1. To increase sharpness of recorded detail by placing the anatomy of interest closer to the film.

2. To reduce magnification by placing the anatomy of interest closer to the film.

3. To minimize distortion of the shape of the anatomy of interest by optimizing the alignment of the anatomy with the x-ray beam and the film.

4. To increase the visibility of the anatomy of interest by desuperimposing other overlying, contrasty anatomical structures which are not of interest and, therefore, represent *noise* in the image.

PROJECTION ROUTINES

The diagnostic radiograph is dependent upon proper positioning of the patient before exposure. This is facilitated by the use of standard projections. Such projections produce images that reveal the maximum amount of diagnostic information with a minimum of distortion. An accurate idea of the anatomic arrangement of the internal structures with relation to some external landmark aids materially in positioning the patient. A convenient method is to visualize the part as though it were transparent, so that the usual structures which appear on the radiograph may be identi-

fied in relation to an external landmark. The relation of the central ray to the part to be examined, and to the film, must be carefully considered in each projection. Imperfect centering of the part on the film and alignment of the tube to the part are the causes of image distortion. The requirements of radiography are such that slight differences in position do not necessarily rule out the diagnostic value of the radiograph. A certain degree of latitude in routine may be permissible, because the radi-

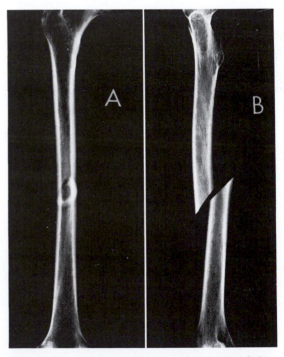

Figure 22-1. Radiographs of a dry femur, (A) in AP and (B) in lateral projections emphasizing the importance of a second projection at right angles to determine misalignment of a fracture.

298

ologist ordinarily can make satisfactory adjustment by reason of his experience and knowledge. However, in order to secure reliable diagnostic results, it is best to conform to a procedure which is precise and accurate.

To derive the maximum information concerning the size and shape of body parts and foreign objects in relation to their position in the body, projections should be made from different directions. The need for multiple views is clearly demonstrated in Figures 22-1 and 22-2.

In routine radiography, two views, each at right angles to the other, are made as shown in Figure 22-1, wherein posteroanterior and lateral views of the femur are illustrated.

These radiographs demonstrate the value of two opposing projections. In radiograph A, a portion of the image appears abnormal. When viewed at right angles, it may be seen in radiograph B that the ends of the bone are not united but are quite distant to each other, yet their ends were projected so that their images were superimposed.

To determine the nature of a foreign

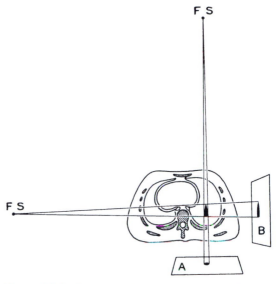

Figure 22-2. Diagram illustrating the need for two projections to determine the true nature of a foreign body, in this case a bullet which appears only as a circular density on the AP projection.

body, two views are also necessary (Fig. 22-2). In this diagram an anteroposterior radiograph would show a foreign body as a circular object (image A). Another, when viewed at right angles to the original projection (image B) would show by its shape that the foreign body was a bullet.

SUMMARY

1. Radiographic *positioning* is essentially a geometrical factor designed to increase sharpness of recorded detail, minimize magnification, minimize shape distortion, or desuperimpose overlying structures.

2. *Standardized* projections, including at least two views at right angles to each other, are necessary for complete diagnosis.

REVIEW QUESTIONS

1. When the contrasty spine is obscuring the gall bladder because of the particular position used, and if interest is only in the gall bladder, the spine then is considered as what type of undesirable image quality?

2. Explain why two views must be taken at right angles to each other as standard radiographic procedure, and give an example:

3. State the four objectives of positioning:

Chapter 23

MOTION

MOTION OF A BODY part being examined directly influences sharpness of recorded image detail. Motion may be voluntary on the part of the patient, or may be involuntary. The only means for controlling the effects of motion are (1) patient cooperation, (2) immobilization of the part being examined, and (3) short exposures.

Voluntary motion may take several forms. The noncooperative child who needs restraint is common. The patient who does not understand the manner in which he is to cooperate is usually the fearful one. A satisfactory explanation of the procedure usually suffices to create confidence. When in doubt, immobilize the part and use short exposures.

Involuntary motion is normally associated with the physiologic activity of the body tissue. Respiration produces movement of the thorax and its contents so that short exposures are mandatory (Fig. 23-1). The normal adult respiratory rate is 16 to 18 respirations per minute; in some pulmonary or cardiac lesions, the rate may be greater; in the newborn, it may be 30 to 40 per minute. Respiration also influences in some degree the viscera adjacent to the diaphragms.

Movement of the heart and great vessels is an important factor in radiography of the chest. The pulsation of the arterial system

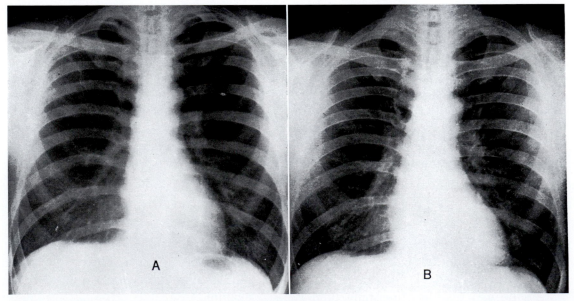

Figure 23-1. Radiographs of the PA chest demonstrating blurring of pulmonary and mediastinal anatomy due to movement (A) compared to a properly exposed film (B).

in all parts of the body at the rate of about 5 to 8 meters per second creates various degrees of movement in the tissues they supply.

Esophageal peristalsis begins about 1 second after the initial swallowing act. The rate of travel is not the same at all levels. In the first 7 to 8 centimeters of its course, the rate is rapid (1 second); in the next 7 centimeters, the rate is 1 to 2 seconds; and in the lower segment, the rate is about 3 seconds. Solid or semisolid food takes between 6 and 7 seconds to pass from the mouth to the stomach. When liquids are ingested, the rate is relatively more rapid. Movement of the gastrointestinal tract requires proper use of exposure time to avoid unsharpness in the image. Motion of the stomach exhibits great individual variations. In some stomachs, the peristaltic wave travels rapidly and lasts 10 to 15 seconds. In others, the wave may occupy as much as 30 seconds to move from its origin to the pylorus. The slower waves, however, are more common. Peristalsis in the small intestine is about 10 centimeters per second; the colonic rate is very slow.

The gallbladder exhibits rhythmic contractions that may last 5 to 30 minutes. Contractions also occur in the common bile duct.

In the urinary tract, peristaltic waves begin at the kidney and extend to the urinary bladder at the rate of 20 to 30 millimeters per second or 3 to 6 contractions per minute.

To summarize, there are four general categories of motion: (1) peristalsis, (2) heart motion, (3) breathing motion, and (4) voluntary or involuntary movement of the body itself or its limbs. The effects of the first three are localized to specific areas on the final image. Body movement certainly has the greatest effect on the overall image.

EFFECT ON SHARPNESS OF RECORDED DETAIL

The influence of motion in producing image unsharpness is diagrammatically shown in Figure 23-2. In this illustration, the object moved during the exposure resulting in unsharpness in the margins of the image. A typical radiographic example of patient movement is shown in a radiograph of the hand (Fig. 23-3). Note the blurring of all image details and the double edges.

Immobilization

Immobilization is imperative in radiography, for differential diagnoses depend upon the visualization of sharp, undistorted images. Movement should be practically eliminated during the exposure in order to avoid blurring of details in the image.

Composing the Patient

The responsibility of keeping the part immobile is the job of the radiographer, not the patient, for movement may occur consciously or unconsciously. Respiration and body tremor are physical conditions that are important enough to warrant close attention. To some patients, the mere fact it is necessary to lie on a table for an x-ray examination is perturbing. Some may show signs of trembling. A few words of assurance will help to restore peace of mind. Too much cannot be left to the patient in the matter of keeping still during the exposure because most patients are not familiar with the requirements for making a radiograph. Frequently, they are nervous and afraid; so it is the job of the radiographer to

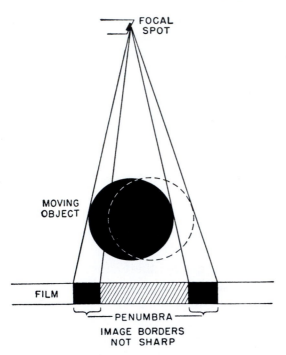

Figure 23-2. Diagram illustrating the influence of motion in producing image unsharpness.

put the patient at ease—so that he will be comfortable, mentally and physically. When the patient is passive and relaxed as a result of his comfort, he will be most cooperative. The radiographer's task does not end there, however, for much of his success is dependent upon the closeness and the firmness with which the part is juxtaposed to the filmholder and the method of immobilization used. Even with the short exposures now possible, immobilization is necessary. There is no usable exposure so short as to fail to record uncontrollable or involuntary tremor of the area under examination. Proper immobilization assures comparison of symmetrical parts, for it also serves to prevent involuntary rotation of the part. The tube carriage always should be locked in position, because its vibration is a common cause for blurred radiographs.

Immobilization Methods

There are a number of good methods for immobilizing the body part: sandbags, compression bands, cones, and special clamps, etc. Many of these devices for immobilization are found in the modern laboratory. An important aspect of immobilization is compression of tissues, particularly in the abdomen. By displacing some of the tissues, less scatter radiation is produced and better contrast attained.

Exposure Time

In pediatric procedures and other situations where some motion is expected, it is essential to minimize the exposure time. As a rule of thumb, *to freeze motion, exposure time should not exceed 1/30 (0.033) second.*

EFFECT ON CONTRAST

Motion of the x-ray tube, patient, or film during the exposure causes extraneous densities from other structures to be superimposed over the anatomy of interest. If this overlapping of adjacent densities is severe, the differences between them becomes less distinct and image contrast is reduced. If the motion is slight, the loss of contrast only occurs in the peripheral portions of each density area (tissue type) but is nonetheless sufficiently destructive to image quality to render it unacceptable. Note in Figure 23-1 that in radiograph A where motion blurring occurred, the contrast in the peripheral portions of the heart shadow against the density level of the surrounding lung tissues is not as great as it is in radiograph B, where no motion

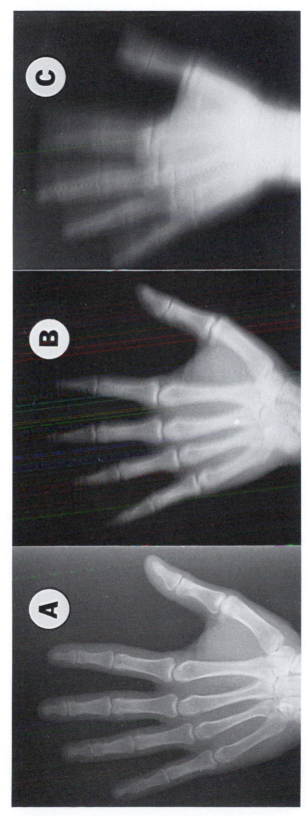

Figure 23-3. Radiographs of the hand showing (A) a sharp and high contrast image; (B) a blurred image due to motion, but still possessing high contrast in some areas; and (C) a severely blurred image showing the destruction of contrast as well as sharpness.

occurred.

Motion is the only variable which may affect image contrast *without* doing so through the mechanism of scattered radiation proportions in the remnant beam. Motion is not related in any way with the production of scatter radiation. But since sufficient levels of blurring will lead to excessive overlapping and superimposition of image densities, these densities tend to cancel each other out and contrast may be lost.

The hand radiographs in Figure 23-3 demonstrate how the effect of motion on contrast is dependent on the severity of the motion. Radiograph B shows the effect of moderate motion when compared to the sharp radiograph A. While B is obviously blurred, any change in overall image contrast is arguable. In radiograph C there is severe motion and a gross loss of contrast is apparent when compared to A: The finger bones are a "washed out" darker gray, while the tissues of the palm are a "washed out" very light gray.

The mechanism by which this superimposition process can result in reduced contrast is fully described in the next chapter. Breathing, heart motion and peristaltic motion are usually *not* sufficient to affect overall image contrast, but whole body motion can certainly destroy it. Although it should not be considered as a *controlling* factor over image contrast, *motion generally reduces contrast* in the image.

EFFECT ON DENSITY

Since motion causes adjacent densities on the radiograph to overlap each other, there is clearly an effected change in the density of some small, *confined* areas of the radiograph. However, in discussing radiographic density, we normally refer to the *overall* density of the radiograph, or, in other words, the average density. Further, the overlapping of densities may not alter the overall average density of the image. For example, the mixing of a white area over a black area will result in a medium-gray density. It is not then said that the black area became *more white* and that the white area became *more black*, but simply that a new density has been created in place of the two originals, namely, the gray. The new gray density has exactly the same *average* density measurement as the average density between the original black and white.

The effects of motion on density are at best completely unpredictable and at worst nonexistent. Therefore, *motion should not be considered to be a controlling factor over image density*. To confirm this fact, observe Figure 23-1 once again and note the similar densities present in both radiographs despite the presence of motion in one.

EFFECT ON OTHER QUALITIES

There is a very common misconception that motion causes shape distortion in an image. True elongation or foreshortening of an image are caused only by alignment changes as discussed in Chapter 21. When motion occurs, new images are actually created in the radiograph by the interaction between the anatomy present and the motion itself. The most common of these new images are the familiar *streaks* seen in the image when doing linear tomography or when the tube, patient or film is moved in one direction during the exposure. The streaks and other similar artifacts are *false images*, not distorted images.

These *false images, created by the geometrical interaction between the anatomy present and the movement of the tube, part or film, may be categorized as image noise.* Noise is any unwanted and deleterious information in the image which impedes the visibility of the desirable information. Any false image is a form of noise.

When motion is very slight, the shape of the image will be still recognizable although the edges are blurred. Again, this is a blurred image, not a distorted one. True distortion only occurs from changes in beam-part-film alignment.

For the same reasons, it may be said that *motion has no direct relationship to image magnification.* If motion results in an average distance from the film which is greater than normal, magnification may be present. But, in this case the change in distance, not the motion itself, causes the magnification.

SUMMARY

1. Motion destroys *sharpness* of image detail by expanding penumbra at image edges. It is the most destructive factor affecting image sharpness.
2. Severe motion can destroy image *contrast* by superimposing the various densities.
3. Motion has no direct relation to *overall* image *density.*
4. Motion does not cause *magnification* nor shape *distortion* of the gross image.
5. Motion does create *noise* in the form of *false images* on the radiograph.
6. To freeze motion, exposure time should not exceed 1/30 (0.033) second.

REVIEW QUESTIONS

1. Motion has the *most* detrimental effect upon which image quality:
2. List two internal body functions which may result in involuntary blurring of the radiograph, even though the breath was properly held:
3. Explain why excessive motion can reduce image contrast:
4. Sometimes the relationship between the movement of the x-ray tube during tomography and the shape of the anatomy *produces* streaks or other images on the radiograph which do not represent any real anatomical structure. Such images are classified as:
5. Name the three methods of reducing the probability of motion leading to visible blur on the radiograph:
6. As a rule of thumb, to freeze motion, exposure time must not exceed:

Part IV

COMPREHENSIVE TECHNIQUE

Chapter 24

ANALYZING THE RADIOGRAPHIC IMAGE

WE HAVE NOW COVERED some twenty types of variables which affect the quality of the radiographic image prior to processing it. We have described how each variable affects the six primary radiographic qualities: Density, contrast, noise, sharpness of recorded detail, magnification, and distortion. This material is frequently taught in reverse order, taking each image quality and then listing all of the variables that affect it. By using this approach in this chapter, it will serve as a comprehensive review.

We have been further limited by treating each quality and each variable one at a time. In reality, several of the image qualities and the variables affecting them are intimately related to each other in rather complex ways. The overall ability of an imaging system to bring out the maximum number of details in an image, or the most visible information, is called its *resolution*. Resolution determines the overall quality of the image. The ways in which image qualities interrelate to produce a highly resolved image will be discussed later in this chapter.

The ability to critique the technical quality of finished radiographs is essential for radiographers to keep patient dose due to repeated exposures at a minimum. This ability will also be discussed.

VISIBILITY FUNCTIONS

The visibility of a radiographic image depends upon three things only—its density, its contrast and the presence of any noise. These qualities were defined and illustrated in Chapter 3. We shall briefly review the variables affecting each.

DENSITY

Milliamperage

Milliamperage is directly proportional to image density. For example, doubling the mA from 100 to 200 will double the apparent darkness of the radiograph, if all other factors are kept constant and no compensations are made. During the exposure, x-rays are emitted from the tube at twice the *rate*, and the x-ray beam is therefore twice as *intense*.

Exposure Time

Exposure time is also directly proportional to density. If no compensation is made, increasing the time from $1/20$ second to $1/10$ second, or from 0.35 to 0.7 second, will double the density.

Milliampere-Seconds (mAs)

The total mAs is the product of mA and

exposure time. It controls the total density resulting on the film in a directly proportional fashion. Doubling the mAs doubles the density. To see a visible difference in image density, mAs must be altered by at least $1/3$ or 30 percent.

In producing a total mAs value, mA and exposure time are inversely proportional to each other. A doubling of the mA may be compensated for by halving the exposure time to achieve the original density. *The total mAs is the prime factor for controlling image density*, because it does not directly affect other image qualities.

Kilovoltage-Peak

Kilovoltage-peak directly affects image density. However, this relationship is *exponential* rather than *proportional*. That is, a small increase in kVp results in a large increase in image density. The relationship follows the *15 percent rule*: A 15 percent increase in kVp causes twice as dark a radiograph (100 percent darker). A 15 percent decrease in kVp results in an image one-half as dark.

Two useful correlaries follow: An 8 percent increase in kVp increases density by one-half or 50 percent, and a 5 percent change in kVp is the minimum required to see a visible difference in image density.

The 15 percent rule should be used when compensating for mAs changes. To maintain the original density when the mAs is doubled, reduce kVp by 15 percent. Kilovoltage can be used for density compensations, but is not recommended as a control for density. *Optimum kVp*, however, is essential to allow the production of adequate density: kVp affects density because it controls the *proportion* of the original x-rays which are able to penetrate through the body and reach the film. Adequate density cannot be produced without suffi-

cient penetration.

Machine Phase and Rectification

The type of electrical generators and rectifiers used in x-ray equipment affects the output intensity of the x-ray beam, as well as its average energy, and directly bears upon the resulting density of the image. Operated at the same mAs, three-phase equipment produces twice the density when compared to single-phase machines.

Constant potential generators such as battery-powered mobile units, and high-frequency generators can be equal to or somewhat higher than three-phase units in their efficiency. They often require less kVp to obtain the same density levels. Half-rectified units require four times the mAs used on a three-phase unit in order to achieve adequate density.

Protective Filtration

Excessive filtration in the x-ray beam can lead to a visible reduction in image density, due to its absorption of x-rays. However, the removal of filtration (or a small increase in it) will not visibly affect the density of radiographs in daily practice, because the body of the patient will absorb nearly all of what the filtration "missed."

Compensating Filtration

Compensating filters, such as wedges and troughs, are specifically designed to even out the density on radiographs of anatomy with irregular thickness or absorption characteristics. These filters are as much as five times thicker than protective filtration, and thus result in visible density effects. If they were inappropriately used on regular anatomy, the thicker end of the filter would result in less image density. They can be used to advantage on irregular anatomy, however, to produce more consistent densities across the radiograph.

Field Size Limitation

Collimation of the field size to smaller, confined areas results in a loss of image density. Density may drop by one-third to one-half, depending on how drastic the change is, and should be compensated for by a corresponding increase in mAs. The loss in density is brought about because less tissue is exposed, producing less scatter radiation. Even though the intensity of primary radiation is maintained, the reduction in scatter radiation results in a lower total exposure to the film, and a visible drop in density.

Patient Status and Contrast Agents

Larger body part thicknesses result in a loss of image density, simply because more radiation is absorbed within the patient and less reaches the film. The *four-centimeter rule* should be used to compensate for deviations in patient thickness from the average of 22 cm measured anterior-to-posterior and 30 cm laterally. For every increase of 4 cm, mAs should be doubled. For patients who are thinner than average, cut mAs in half for every 4 cm.

The radiographer must be observant of body habitus, anthropological factors and condition in deriving appropriate techniques to maintain density. Large muscular patients require a much greater increase in technique than hypersthenic patients. Fluid distention requires more technique than obesity. Brachiocephalic skulls often require more technique than average. Expiration chest radiographs require more exposure than the normal inspiratory views.

The main technique consideration when contrast agents are introduced into body cavities is to obtain the optimum kVp to achieve penetration of some of the x-rays through the contrast bolus. Iodine compounds require at least 80 kVp, while solid-column barium studies require over 100 kVp with a corresponding reduction in mAs, and air-contrast barium studies about 90 kVp. These compensations are necessary to "see through" the contrast bolus to obtain maximum information, and the bolus should thus appear as a very light gray rather than blank white. Blank areas on the radiograph contain *no* information and are diagnostically useless.

Pathology and Casts

Additive diseases which increase the bone or fluid component of tissue require increases in technique, typically from one-third to one-half again as much. Destructive diseases which reduce bone or fluid content, or which increase gas or fat content, necessitate a technique reduction. Recommendations for specific diseases are presented in Chapter 11. Failure to make these compensations will result in densities that are either too light or too dark.

Casts and splints will result in inadequate image density unless technique is increased to compensate for them. Plaster casts require from 2 to 4 times the average technique, while half-casts, wood splints and similar devices require a 50 percent increase. Specific recommendations are given in Chapter 11. Using the 15 percent rule, kVp may be used to make these types of technique adjustments.

Extraneous Fog

Scattered radiation, from whatever source, always increases overall image density, and can thus contribute to overexposure. Since fog density is always destructive to the image, field size limitation, optimum kVp, grids, leaded masking sheets, and other methods must be used to control it.

Fogging of the radiograph can also occur from accidental exposure to light, heat or chemical fumes. All fog results in undesirable, darker density.

Grids

The use of grids always lightens the radiographic density unless compensated for. The higher the grid ratio, the more severe the loss of image density. The recommended compensation is an increase in mAs from 3 to 5 times that of a nongrid, table-top technique, depending on grid ratio. Chapter 13 lists specific recommendations.

Misuse of grids can lead to grid cut-off, an unacceptable loss of density over particular regions of the radiograph. Causes of grid cut-off include off-angling, off-centering, SID outside of the grid radius and grids placed upside-down.

Intensifying Screens

The use of intensifying screens always enhances radiographic density and allows the reduction of patient exposure by compensated techniques. If technique is not compensated, then the higher the speed of the screen, the darker the resulting image density. Special gradient screens can be used to even out the density for radiographs of body parts with irregular thicknesses.

State-of-the-art radiology departments currently use 400-speed "regular" rare earth screens. "Medium" rare earth screens are normally 300-speed, and "High-speed" calcium tungstate screens are typically 200 speed and require about double the mAs

from the 400-speed screen. "Extremity" screen cassettes usually require 5 times the technique for a "regular" screen, or 4 times the technique for a "medium" screen, to maintain density. There are many variations in screen speeds, types and brands. Specific compensating factors and special circumstances are described in Chapter 14.

Films

The higher the speed of radiographic film, the darker the image density will be for a given exposure level. Faster films allow lower mAs values in obtaining the same density. Films are designed according to the types of screens or exposure holders used with them, and the type of film must be appropriately matched according to manufacturer specifications, or a light density will result.

Anode Heel Effect

The anode heel effect results in a slight loss of density toward the end of the film nearest the x-ray tube anode. This is used to advantage for wedge-shaped anatomy by placing the thinnest anatomy toward the anode, but is detrimental to radiographs of regular anatomy.

Source-Image Receptor Distance (SID)

Image density is inversely related to distances in an exponential fashion. Small changes in distance cause substantial changes in density. The greater the SID (the distance from the x-ray source to the image receptor), the less the density. This relationship follows the *inverse square law* described in Chapter 18. Density will be inversely proportional to the square of the change in distance. For example, doubling the distance results in one-fourth the image density.

To prevent such dramatic changes in density, the *square law for technique* must be applied: Adjust the mAs according to the square of the distance change. For example, if the distance is doubled, the mAs should be quadrupled to maintain density.

Distance changes should be compensated with mAs rather than with kVp. Distance and mAs both affect the x-ray beam intensity without changing its quality (energy). An adjustment in kVp would unnecessarily change other image qualities besides density.

Object-Image Receptor Distance (OID)

Dramatic changes in object-image receptor distance can cause visible differences in image density. The larger the OID, the less the resulting density. When the air-gap technique is used, or whenever the OID cannot be minimized, an increase in mAs from one-third to one-half is required to maintain adequate density.

Processing

If an exposed radiographic film is developed for too long, at too high a temperature, or in chemicals that are too concentrated, it will turn out dark. Details of these relationships are explained in Chapter 37.

CONTRAST AND GRAY SCALE

Kilovoltage-Peak

Kilovoltage-Peak (kVp) should be considered as the prime factor for controlling radiographic image contrast and gray scale. It does so both through its effect upon x-ray beam *penetration* and upon the *proportion of scatter radiation reaching the film*. At higher kVp levels, more different types of tissue are penetrated by the x-ray beam and recorded as shades of gray. With more shades of gray present in the image, there is a smaller degree of difference from one shade to the next, therefore, contrast decreases. When long gray scale is desired, high kVp should be used. When high contrast is desired, low kVp should be used. Optimum kVp is the minimum kVp which still penetrates *all* tissues of interest. At this level, both contrast and gray scale will be balanced.

In addition to its penetration effects, high kVp also results in a loss of most photoelectric interactions in the tissues. The remaining image is then controlled mostly by penetrating rays and scattered rays. Also, more scatter radiation reaches the film because it is produced with higher energy and in a more forward direction. Image fog becomes more visible, and contributes to the reduction of apparent contrast.

Machine Phase

Three-phase and high-frequency generators produce a higher average x-ray beam energy. Penetration is enhanced, slightly lengthening the gray scale and slightly reducing the contrast in the resulting image.

Field Size Limitation

When the field size is collimated to a smaller area, image contrast is enhanced. Less exposed tissue is available to produce scatter radiation, but the primary beam concentration is unaffected. With a reduction in the proportion of fog in the image, contrast will increase.

Patient Status and Contrast Agents

With thicker patients, more exposed tissue is available to produce scatter radiation. Even as the primary beam is attenuated by the tissue mass, scatter increases, fogging the film and reducing contrast. Technique must be increased to maintain density, so the only ways to counter this fog are to use grids, collimate the field size, and if possible for chest radiographs use the air-gap technique.

Contrast agents are designed to enhance subject contrast by exaggerating differences in penetration through different tissues. Positive contrast agents absorb radiation, but should not stop *all* of the beam. Therefore, optimum kVp must be used for these agents to obtain partial penetration through them and maximize radiographic information. Negative agents are highly radiolucent and generally require a decrease in kVp to optimize both density and contrast levels in the image.

Pathology and Casts

Muscular or fluid-distended tissues produce much more fog than fatty tissues, and air produces almost no fog. Plaster casts produce additional scatter, especially when wet. The Radiographer should be aware of these effects in evaluating each patient.

Extraneous Fog

Anything that reduces the occurrence of photoelectric interactions in the patient, or that increases the occurrence of Compton scattering interactions, will result in more visible fog in the image, as explained in Chapters 4 and 12. Fog may also be caused from light, heat, chemical fumes or over-processing. Fogging destroys image contrast.

An important and interesting point is that *fog also destroys gray scale.* When all of the shades of gray are darkened by a blanket density, there will be a net loss in the number of shades present, because extremely light shades will no longer be present and shades that should have been dark gray will be black.

Grids

Grids were developed for the express purpose of restoring image contrast when larger body parts are radiographed. The large amounts of exposed tissue result in more scatter radiation produced. Grids eliminate much of this scattered radiation before it reaches the film, as described in Chapter 13. The higher the grid ratio, the more effective it is in "cleaning up" scatter, and the higher the resulting image contrast.

Intensifying Screens

Because of their magnifying effect on film exposure, the use of intensifying screens results in much higher image contrast than direct exposure techniques, as described in Chapter 14. Generally, high-speed screens produce somewhat higher contrast in the image than slow-speed screens; however, this is not *always* the case. Screens were developed to enhance density, and any effect they have on image contrast is a side-effect. Therefore, they are not of primary concern when regarding image contrast.

Radiographic Film

Generally, higher-speed films also produce higher image contrast. Film can be chemically treated to produce either longer gray scale or higher contrast, according to the needs of the diagnostician. The recommendations of manufacturers should be strictly followed when matching films and screens to obtain a desired image quality.

Object-Image Receptor Distance (OID)

When the OID is increased, leaving a gap between the body and the film, scattered radiation produced within the tissues and emitted at random angles is allowed to diverge more before reaching the film, in accordance with the inverse square law. The divergence of the primary beam, however, is unaffected by a change in OID. Hence, the concentration of scattered rays is reduced while the primary beam remains at the same intensity. A smaller proportion of the resulting image will be composed of fog, and contrast will increase. The intentional use of a large OID for the purpose of enhancing contrast is called the *air gap technique.*

Motion

Motion should not be considered as a *controlling* factor for image contrast. If it is severe enough, however, it can reduce contrast because of the superimposition of different densities across the image. This process is explained later in this chapter.

Processing

There are optimum times, temperatures and chemical concentrations for processing radiographic film, as described in Chapter 37. Although slight increases in any of these may increase contrast, excessive development time, temperature or chemical action will fog the film and destroy contrast as a rule.

NOISE

Milliampere-Seconds (mAs)

Insufficient mAs leaves such a light exposure reaching the film that the uneven distribution of x-rays within the beam becomes visible on the finished image. The resulting blotchy or freckled appearance in the image is called *quantum mottle*, and is a form of image noise because it interferes with the visibility of details.

Kilovoltage-Peak

Because of the loss of photoelectric interactions at high kVp levels, the remaining image is composed only of penetrating rays and scattered rays. Further, a higher proportion of those scattered rays that are produced will reach the film, because they have more energy and are emitted in a more forward direction. Fog in the image becomes more apparent. A high proportion of fog interferes with the visibility of image details. Therefore, high kVp may be considered as a contributor to image noise.

Field Size

Larger field sizes increase the amount of exposed tissue producing scatter radiation. The scatter creates noise in the image in the form of fog. This noise is reduced by limiting field size to the anatomy of interest.

Patient Status and Pathology

Large patients also increase the amount of exposed tissue creating scatter radiation, causing more noise in the form of image fog.

Artifacts and Casts

Artifacts include any object or substance inadvertently left within the passage of the x-ray beam which impedes visibility of image details. A few examples are objects or clothing left on the patient, removable devices on the patient's person such as dentures, objects left on the x-ray table or film, particles of dirt or paper inside intensifying screens, and contrast agents soaked into positioning sponges from previous spills. Casts and splints also interfere with the image quality, and constitute noise, even though they may not be removable.

Extraneous Fog

Fog on the radiograph, whatever the source, constitutes noise since it reduces visibility of details.

Grid Lines

Grid cut-off may be considered an extreme case of artifacts occluding the image. But stationary grids such as those taped to cassettes during mobile procedures will result in grid lines even when they are used properly. On close inspection, one can see the clear white lines where grid strips absorbed radiation, reducing the amount of information reaching the film. Grid lines interfere with details and are a form of noise.

Intensifying Screens and Film

The use of extremely high speed intensifying screens can lead to very low mAs values. As previously explained, this will lead to quantum mottle, a form of noise. Clumping of crystals in the manufacture of emulsions for screens or for radiographic film can cause a mottled appearance in the finished radiograph that is unrelated to the x-ray beam itself. This type of image noise is referred to as screen mottle or as film mottle, respectively.

Motion

In addition to its blurring effects, motion of the patient, the x-ray tube or the film during exposure can cause the production of false images such as streaks, described in Chapter 23. False images can obscure the anatomy of interest, and are a form of image noise.

GEOMETRICAL INTEGRITY (RECOGNIZABILITY)

The geometrical functions of an image are those qualities which allow correct recognition of the object it represents. There are three such functions fully defined and explained in Chapter 3: sharpness of recorded detail, magnification and shape distortion. The variables determining the integrity of the image by affecting these three qualities will be reviewed.

SHARPNESS OF RECORDED DETAIL

Focal Spot Size

The size of the focal spot should be considered as the primary control for sharpness of recorded detail in the image, for two reasons: (1) It is the only variable that *exclusively* affects sharpness, without affecting any other image characteristic; (2) it is readily manipulated by the radiographer. The smaller the focal spot, the sharper the recorded detail. The relationship is inversely proportional: If the focal spot size is reduced to one-half the original, sharpness of detail doubles.

Radiographers should be conscientious enough to utilize the small focal spot whenever high detail resolution is of essence, (for example, whenever "extremity" cassettes are used). The large focal spot must be employed whenever high techniques might overheat the x-ray tube.

Anode Bevel

Through the line-focus principle described in Chapter 17, steeper anode bevels (at a smaller angle from vertical) result in smaller projected focal spot sizes, and therefore contribute to sharpness of recorded detail.

Source-Image Receptor Distance (SID)

SID is directly proportional to the sharpness of recorded detail produced in the image. If the distance is doubled, the sharpness is doubled, provided all other factors are equal. SID should not, however, be considered as a primary control for sharpness, because it affects other image qualities as well, and because it cannot always be easily modified.

Object-Image Receptor Distance (OID)

When the distance from the object to the image receptor is increased, sharpness of recorded detail is reduced. If all other factors are kept equal, the sharpness is inversely proportional to the OID. When OID is doubled, sharpness is cut to one-half due to a doubling of the penum-

bra. The OID should always be kept at a minimum.

SOD/OID Ratio

The ratio of SOD to OID is directly proportional to sharpness of recorded detail, as discussed in Chapter 20. If both the SID and the OID are doubled, the SOD will also be doubled. The SOD/OID ratio will therefore be unchanged, and image sharpness will remain equal.

Positioning

If the body is positioned so that the anatomy of interest is further from the film than necessary, sharpness of recorded detail is diminished. This effect is due to a change in the OID where the "object" is restricted to the specific anatomy of interest. Radiographers must utilize those positions which place the anatomy as close as possible to the image receptor.

Motion and Exposure Time

Motion blurs the image and is therefore the prime enemy of sharpness of recorded detail. Radiographers must use communication skills, immobilization and short exposure times to reduce the probability of motion occurring.

Long exposure times are not the *direct cause* of motion. But in chest radiography, for example, heart motion is unavoidable, and can only be eliminated radiographically by the use of very short exposure times. In addition, the longer the time, the greater the chance for peristaltic motion, breathing motion or movement of the patient to occur. Therefore, exposure time should be considered as a *contributing factor* of motion during radiographic procedures. Generally, the shorter the exposure time, the sharper the recorded detail.

Intensifying Screens

The use of an intensifying screen always results in less sharpness of detail than the use of direct exposure holders, because light from a screen diffuses prior to reaching the film. When changing from one screen speed to a higher speed, image sharpness *may* be compromised depending on the manufacturing method by which the higher speed was achieved. If a thicker emulsion or larger crystals were used, sharpness will be reduced. If chemical differences were used, sharpness may be unaffected, or even enhanced if the resulting emulsion layer is thinner. As a general rule, the higher the speed, the less the sharpness.

Image Receptor Systems

Usually, the higher the speed of a radiographic film, the lower the sharpness of recorded detail. As with screens, chemical changes will not affect sharpness. But most speed differences in films are due to crystal size or emulsion thickness. Any increase in these will reduce sharpness.

Duplitized film is less sharp than single-emulsion film, because of the parallax effect of viewing two images in two separate emulsions.

Single-screen cassettes result in better sharpness of detail than double-screen cassettes, due to the elimination of the crossover effect described in Chapter 14.

MAGNIFICATION

Source-Image Receptor Distance (SID)

The SID is inversely related to magnification, but not proportional to it. A longer SID projects the image of the object with more parallel beams and results in less magnification. The reduction in magnification, however, is relatively small compared to the change made in the SID. The longest feasible SID should always be used to minimize image magnification.

Object-Image Receptor Distance (OID)

The OID is directly related to magnification, but again, is not proportional to it. The greater the OID, the greater the magnification. If the OID is doubled, the image size will not double, but it will increase (by about 30 percent). The OID should always be minimized to control magnification.

SID/SOD Ratio

The SID/SOD ratio should be considered as the primary controlling factor for magnification of the image size. The SID/SOD ratio is directly proportional to the magnification factor.

For example, a 20-inch SID and a 15-inch SOD yields a magnification factor of $20/15 = 1.25$ or 25 percent magnification. Doubling the SID to 40 inches without changing the object-film distance results in an SOD of 35 inches, and the magnification factor becomes $40/35 = 1.14$ or 14 percent magnification.

To minimize magnification of the image, the SID/SOD ratio should always be kept as low as possible. This is accomplished by long SID's and short OID's.

Positioning

Since positioning of the patient may place the anatomy of interest nearer to or further from the film, effectively changing the OID it can result in unnecessary magnification of the anatomy of interest. To minimize magnification, radiographic positioning should always be done with an eye to placing the anatomy of interest as close to the film as possible.

SHAPE DISTORTION

Beam-Part-Film Alignment and Positioning

The *only* variable which affects shape distortion in radiography is beam-part-film alignment. Nonetheless, this variable has several aspects including positioning of the patient, the actual shape of the anatomy of interest, centering of the central ray, angulation of the x-ray beam, and proper placement of the film holder or image receptor. Beam-part-film alignment is the controlling factor for distortion.

If the anatomy of interest is thick and spherical or cubical in general shape, any distortion of it will be exacerbated. If it is thin and flat, linear, tubular, or wedge-shaped, with a distinct long axis, then distortion effects will not be as severe. When the long axis of an object is angled in relation to the film, while the beam is perpendicular to the film, foreshortening distortion will occur.

When the object and the film are parallel to each other, any angling of the x-ray beam so that it is not perpendicular to them will cause elongation distortion. However, when the object is angled in relation to the film, distortion is minimized by using Ceiszynski's law of isometry: Angle the central ray one-half of the angle formed between the object and the film.

Off-centering of the central ray from the anatomy of interest causes distortion effects similar to angulation. Positioning must be performed with an eye to maintaining a perpendicular beam-film relationship and a parallel part-film relationship whenever possible.

RESOLUTION

In evaluating the overall quality of any image, the concept of resolution is of essence. A dictionary may define optical resolution as the "ability to distinguish the individual parts of an object or closely adjacent images," as being separate from each other. On a radiograph, in order for two small, closely adjacent details to be recognized as distinct and separate from each other, density and contrast must be optimal; sharpness of recorded detail must be high; and magnification, distortion, and noise must be minimal. *All of the image qualities affect resolution.*

To fully understand resolution, these six qualities must be considered collectively, in relation to each other, rather than individually. A helpful aid in studying these interrelationships is the density trace diagram.

DENSITY TRACE DIAGRAMS

Density trace diagrams are simple diagrams of a physical "cross-section" of the radiographic film emulsion after development. They demonstrate the thickness of metallic silver deposit remaining on different areas of the film. Where the thickness of the silver is great, the film would appear dark, thinner regions would appear gray, and areas with little or no silver thickness would appear nearly clear or "white."

Contrast can be defined as the ratio between two adjacent densities. This difference is shown on a density trace as the *vertical* distance through which the image edge drops (Fig. 24-1). This contrast measurement must be taken at the center of the image, as compared to the density outside

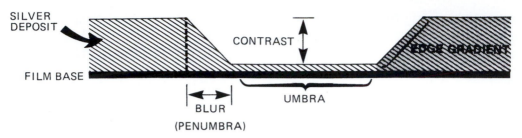

Figure 24-1. Density trace diagram. Image *contrast* is indicated by differences in the vertical depth of the silver deposit on the film, comparing the middle of the image to the background deposit. The *edge gradient* is the slope in the silver deposit at the edges of the image. Penumbra or blur is indicated by the *horizontal* spread of the edge gradient.

the image.

One can see that the density at the edge of a radiographic image does not drop straight down. Rather, it drops more or less gradually, forming a slope of decreasing silver deposit on the film. This slope is called the *edge gradient* (Fig. 24-1). The edge gradient can be measured by dividing the height of the slope by its width. For example, if the silver deposit drops 10 microns over a horizontal distance of 2 microns, the edge gradient is $10/2 = 5$ (A in Fig. 24-2). If it takes 4 microns of horizontal distance for the silver deposit to drop 10 microns, the edge gradient is $10/4 = 2.5$ (B in Fig. 24-2). A high edge gradient indicates a steep slope, a low edge gradient indicates a gradual slope.

The abruptness of the edge of a radiographic image is called its *acutance*, how *acutely* it drops off. Acutance is closely related to the sharpness of recorded detail. A steep edge gradient indicates high acutance, and results in a high level of image sharpness.

Sharpness is defined in terms of the *horizontal* distance through which the edge gradient passes. More precisely, the horizontal measurement of the edge gradient represents penumbra or blur from *un*sharpness (Fig. 24-1).

At this point, one can readily see that contrast and sharpness are closely related

to each other, because they both affect the slope of the edge gradient. In other words, contrast and sharpness are both essential to the *resolution* of image detail. Resolution of detail depends upon both sharpness and contrast.

Nonetheless, contrast and sharpness are different image qualities, and they must not be confused, even though they are related. Figure 24-2 illustrates the traces for various images with different contrast and blur levels. High contrast images can still have poor resolution if edges are blurred (Fig. 24B). Low contrast images can be sharp in spite of poor visibility (Fig. 24C).

Image resolution may be measured with the unit *line pairs per millimeter*, using a test template as shown in Figure 3-17, Chapter 3. Exposure of this device records alternating black and white lines on the film so that it can be visually determined which ones can be distinguished from each other, as shown in Figure 16-1, Chapter 16. The smaller the lines resolved, the more of them would fit into one millimeter. This measurement is called *spatial frequency*, the number of details that fit into a given *space* of one millimeter and still be visibly distinct. Spatial frequency depends on both contrast and sharpness. It is a direct measurement of overall image resolution that the radiograph can achieve.

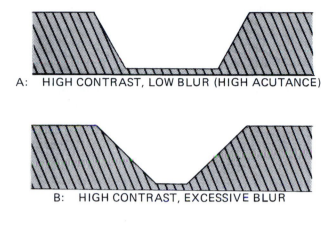

A: HIGH CONTRAST, LOW BLUR (HIGH ACUTANCE)

B: HIGH CONTRAST, EXCESSIVE BLUR

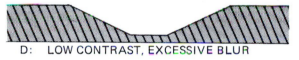

C: LOW CONTRAST, LOW BLUR

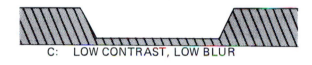

D: LOW CONTRAST, EXCESSIVE BLUR

Figure 24-2. Density trace diagrams for various contrast and sharpness levels. (A) is the best resolved image, with high contrast (vertical density drop) and high sharpness (steep edge gradients). (B) shows increased blur, but still has high contrast. (C) shows a loss of visibility low contrast, but has sharp edges. (D) is the poorest image, with both low contrast and excessive blur.

MODULATION TRANSFER FUNCTION

Physicists use a complex measurement of the total resolution capacity of an imaging system called *modulation transfer function* or *MTF*. A full discussion of MTF is not necessary for radiographers, but it is worth noting that MTF is very similar to density trace diagrams. If one were to expose a resolution test template (Fig. 3-17), the density trace diagram for the resulting silver deposits on the film would be essentially identical to an MTF graph. A high MTF indicates that the imaging system produces high resolution, and therefore provides images with maximum diagnostic information. A low MTF indicates poor overall image quality.

GEOMETRICAL PENUMBRA

X-rays can be emitted at various angles and from different points within the area of the focal spot, and yet record the same edge of an object on the film. This means that the same edge of the object will actually be recorded several times in various different locations on the film (Fig. 24-3). This

FOCAL SPOT

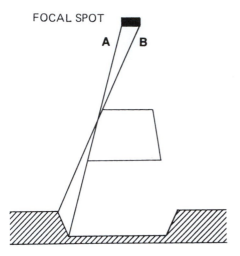

Figure 24-3. Density trace diagram illustrating geometrical penumbra. The extent of penumbra is represented by the horizontal spread of the edge gradient slopes.

"spreading" of the edge constitutes blur or *penumbra*, and is fully explained in Chapter 16 (see Fig. 16-3).

In Figure 24-3, between "A" and "B," absorption of the x-ray beam is *partial*, increasing toward the object. Hence, "penumbra" may be thought of as a *partial absorption* process (bearing in mind that "partial" refers to a portion of the total amount of x-rays which the object in question is capable of absorbing, not to a portion of the total x-ray beam).

Motion and Parallax Blur

Motion blur and parallax blur (from double-coated film) are actually both superimposition processes which result in *horizontal* spreading of the edge (Fig. 24-4). Motion should not be considered to affect image contrast unless it is so severe that this horizontal spreading crosses the middle of the image, effectively reducing the vertical component of the density trace at mid-image (Fig. 24-4B).

ABSORPTION PENUMBRA

"Absorption unsharpness" or "absorption penumbra" is a blurring of the edge of an image due to the relationship between the shape of the object being radiographed and the diverging x-ray beam. Suppose that several objects having different shapes, but made out of the same, homogeneous material, are to be radiographed:

The "ideal" shape for an object to be radiographed would be a trapezoid whose slanted sides coincide exactly with the angles of the diverging x-rays (Fig. 24-5A). All portions of the x-ray beam striking such an object will be attenuated by the same thickness of material. The density trace diagram in Figure 24-5 shows that there will be no blur due to absorption unsharpness at the edge of the image produced. Note that the black silver deposit on the film drops off straight down at the edge of this image. The image of the trapezoid is as "white" just inside the edge as it is in the middle. This "sudden" change in density at the edge of the image represents a sharp edge with no blur.

Imaging a *cube* of the same material (Fig. 24-5B) yields different results: Note that the lateral diverging x-rays pass through only a small thickness of material at the upper corners of the cube. Little absorption occurs, and the density trace shows a reduced but still dark deposit of silver. As inner beams pass through thicker portions, the density trace drops until the full thickness of the cube is reached at the lower corners (dashed line). On observing this image, the density would gradually change from dark to light as one scans across its edge. This effect is identical to geometrical blurring, even though it is caused by a different process.

Worse yet is the spherical object (Fig. 24-5C), whose full thickness is found only at

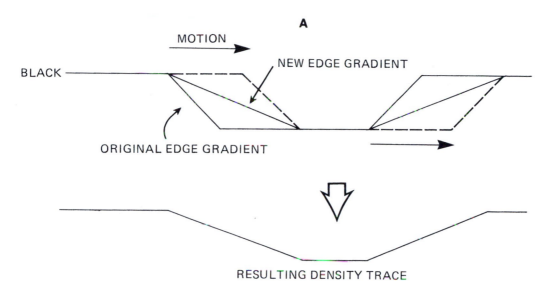

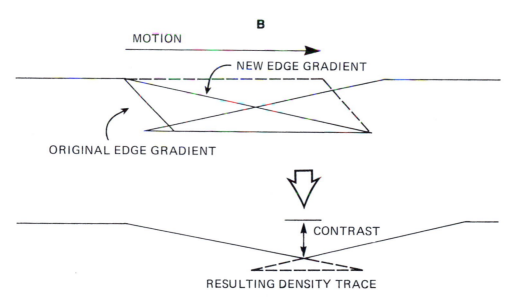

Figure 24-4. Density trace diagrams showing the effects of motion on image sharpness and contrast. Slight motion (A) increases the horizontal spread of the edge gradient, reducing sharpness, but contrast at the middle of the image is unchanged. With *severe* motion (B), the edge gradients may begin to overlap, causing a loss of contrast.

the center. The density trace shows that the drop in density is very gradual and the edges of the image very indistinct.

Referring to Figure 24-5, note that all three objects are of the same thickness in the center, and should have identical absorption and identical contrast at this point. Indeed, the density traces have dropped the same vertical distance in the center of each image.

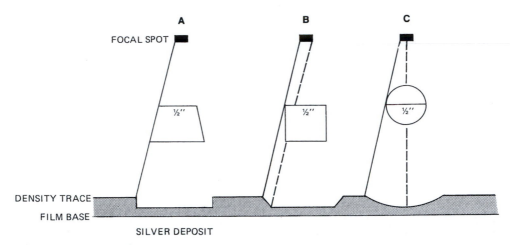

Figure 24-5. Density trace diagrams for absorption penumbra, using objects of equal thickness but different shapes. The trapezoid object (A) will produce *geometrical* penumbra as shown in Figure 24-3, but will have no *absorption* penumbra as shown here. The square object (B) absorbs most radiation at the thickest portion of its projected edge, causing a penumbral edge gradient. For a spherical object (C) the edge gradient (penumbra) extends to the middle of the image. This represents the most severe absorption penumbra.

TOTAL PENUMBRA

A representation of total blur or penumbra may be obtained by combining the diagram for geometrical blur with that for absorption blur (Fig. 24-6), using a cube or a spherical object. In this case, all beams are not absorbed at the inside penumbral line, but rather at the (dashed) absorption line. Within the penumbral (solid) lines, absorption varies primarily because the beams originate at different points within the focal spot. Within the dashed lines, absorption continues to vary, but strictly because of changing object thickness. *Total penumbra is comprised of geometrical penumbra plus absorption penumbra.*

MAGNIFICATION, DISTORTION AND NOISE

Magnification or distortion of an image does not cause any change in edge gradient. The slope of the edge will drop at the same rate. (Many of the same variables that create magnification also cause unsharpness, and it is easy to mistake the two as being directly related to each other, but they are not. If the magnification of an image is accompanied by increased blur, that is, if the expansion of the umbra is accompanied by an expansion of the penumbra, then adjacent details may overlap and image resolution will be lost. But, this loss of resolution is due to the *blurring*, which does affect the slope of the edge gradient, *not* to the magnification. Desirable magnification techniques, such as those used in angiography, can be employed without a loss of sharpness.)

Clearly, the enlargement of any image makes it more visible overall, but results in an inaccurate representation of its true size. The value of magnification depends on whether the diagnostic emphasis is on measurement or simple detection.

Noise, such as an artifact or fog, superimposes and obscures the visibility of the anatomy of interest. This does not change the slope of the edge gradient, but since details are obscured, overall image resolution is lost. The effects of scatter radiation are thoroughly discussed in Chapter 12.

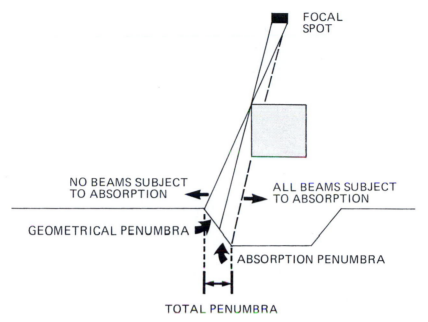

Figure 24-6. Density trace diagram combining the effects of geometrical penumbra and absorption penumbra in producing the total penumbra or total amount of blurring at the edge of the image.

CRITIQUING AND REPEATING RADIOGRAPHS

Radiographers must develop, primarily through experience, the ability to accurately assess the technical qualities of the finished radiograph—its density level, contrast, gray scale, noise level, sharpness of recorded detail, and any magnification or distortion present. This ability is *essential* to the control of unnecessary repeated exposures to the patient. A review of the radiographs used throughout this book, particularly in Chapter 3, should help.

The single greatest technical cause for repeated exposures is improper density levels. Exposed radiographs that are either too light or too dark account for *73 percent* of all repeats in radiology departments without quality control programs, and for *33 percent* of all repeats in departments with quality control (see Table 30-1, Chapter 30).

The following exercise is designed to help the student develop an ability to visu-

ally estimate the needed adjustment in overall technique when repeating an exposure that turned out too light or too dark. In each of two series of radiographs (Figs. 24-7 and 24-8), a radiograph with optimum density level is first shown for comparison. The following numbered radiographs were taken at precisely selected techniques at rounded out values, such as double the original mAs or one-third the original mAs. For each of the numbered radiographs, estimate the *overall technique change* required to restore density to the optimum level. All answers are in factors of 2, 3 or 4. Check your answers using the Appendix.

EXERCISE #18

Critiquing Radiographic Density

A: For the series of chest radiographs in Figure 24-7, compare each of the *numbered* radiographs to the *optimum* radiograph first

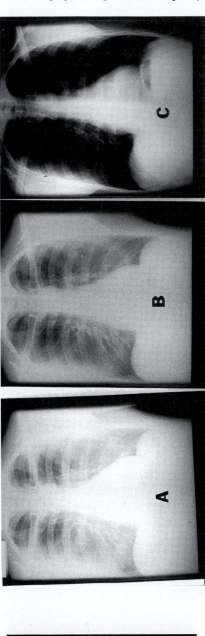

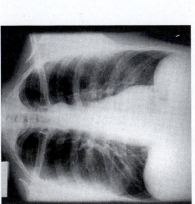

Figure 24-7. Chest radiographs: Estimate density change needed. Answers in Appendix II.

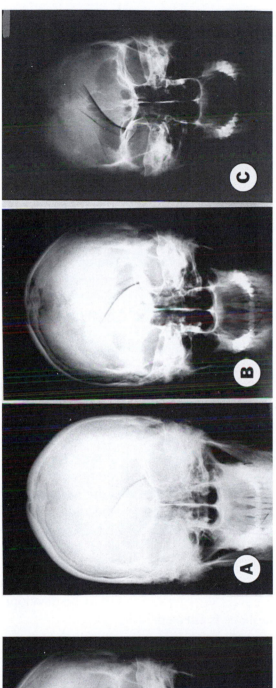

Figure 24-8. Skull radiogrpahs: Estimate density change needed. Answers in Appendix II.

shown. List the *factor* to which the density for each numbered radiograph should be changed to restore it to optimum density. The correct answer will be *4X, 3X, 2X, 1/2, 1/3* or *1/4.*

B: For the series of skull radiographs in Figure 24-8, compare each of the *numbered* radiographs to the *optimum* radiograph first shown. List the *factor* to which the density for each numbered radiograph should be changed to restore it to optimum density. The correct answer will be *4X, 3X, 2X, 1/2, 1/3* or *1/4.*

SUMMARY

1. Image *density* is affected by mAs, kVp, machine phase, filtration, field size, patient condition and casts, contrast agents, fog, grids, screen/film combinations, the anode heel effect, SID, OID, and processing.

2. Image *contrast* and gray scale are affected by kVp, machine phase, field size, patient condition and contrast agents, fog, grids, screens and film, motion, and processing.

3. Image *noise* can be caused by insufficient mAs, excessive kVp, excessive field size, large patients, fog, grids, screens and film, motion, and artifacts.

4. *Sharpness of recorded* image *detail* is affected by focal spot size and the anode bevel angle, SOD, OID, SOD/OID ratio, positioning, motion, and image receptor systems.

5. *Magnification* of the image is affected by SID, SOD, the SID/SOD ratio, and positioning.

6. *Distortion* of the image shape is affected by beam-part-film alignment, which includes angling and centering considerations, and positioning.

7. Image *resolution* depends upon *both* contrast and sharpness of recorded detail. A loss of either one of these qualities makes it more difficult to distinguish adjacent details. Resolution is determined by the *edge gradient* of the image, and can be measured by modulation transfer function (MTF) or by spatial frequency in line pairs per millimeter (LP/mm).

8. The *total penumbra* or total *blur* in an image is the sum of geometrical penumbra plus absorption penumbra.

9. One of the most fundamental skills for the radiographer is the ability to analyze proper image density to determine if a repeated exposure is indicated. Improper density can account for 1/3 to 3/4 of all necessitated repeats. This skill must be developed by practice.

REVIEW QUESTIONS

1. What variable is the primary *control* for image density?

2. What variable is the primary *control* for image contrast?

3. What variable is the primary *control* for sharpness of recorded detail?

4. What variable is the primary *control* for image magnification?

5. What variable is the primary *control* for distortion of image shape?

6. What effect do additive diseases or casts generally have upon image densi-

ty?

7. What effect does the anode heel effect have upon image density?

8. What variable is the primary *control* for image gray scale?

9. What form of noise destroys *both* image contrast and gray scale?

10. How can stationary grids contribute to image noise, even if they are properly aligned ?

11. Artifacts should be classified in the hierarchy of image qualities as _____.

12. Name *two* types of mottle that high-speed receptor systems might lead to:

13. Streaks caused by motion or by tomography should not be considered as distorted images but rather as _____ images, a form of image noise.

14. Positioning can be *indirectly* related to both sharpness and magnification because it can alter the _____ distance to the anatomy of interest.

15. As demonstrated with density trace diagrams, what *two* image qualities combine to determine image resolution (the ability to distinguish adjacent details as being separate)?

16. As demonstrated by density trace diagrams, what *two* types of penumbra combine to form the total penumbra of an image?

17. The quantitative measurement of the total resolution of an imaging system used by physicists is called:

18. Even for departments with quality control programs, one-third of all repeated exposures is caused by improper image _____.

19. What is the only shape of object that would produce *no* absorption penumbra when projected by an x-ray beam?

As a general review of the variables that affect each image quality, complete the following EXERCISE 19, and check your answers from the Appendix.

EXERCISE #19

Directions: For each technique change listed at the left, indicate the effect it will have upon each image quality by placing a plus sign in the box if it increases the image quality, a minus sign if it decreases it, or a zero if it is not a *direct* cause of changes in the image quality. Assume that all factors are maintained equal except the listed change. For example, when the x-ray beam is angled, assume that the SID is maintained equal through compensating tube-to-tabletop distance.

	Density	Contrast	Sharpness	Magnification	Distortion
Increase mA					
Increase Exp. Time					
Increase kVp					
Increase Filtration					
From 1-Phase to to 3-Phase or HFG					
Increase Field Size					
Increase Motion					
Increase Patient Size					
Increase Grid Ratio					
Increase Screen Speed					
Increase Size of Focal Spot					
Increase SID					
Increase OID					
Misalign or Misangle Beam					

Chapter 25

SIMPLIFYING AND STANDARDIZING TECHNIQUE

THE FUNDAMENTALS of exposure are easy to understand and there seems to be no reason why they should be made complicated. It must be realized that the radiologist is not so much interested in the occasional "beautiful" radiograph–or poor one–as he is with *uniform* radiographic quality. Such uniformity from day to day and year to year can only be achieved through complete control and standardization of exposure and processing procedures. The *appearance* of the radiographic images should always be fairly consistent. The busy radiologist should not be obliged to interpret radiographs made with a particular projection in which the image of a body part is seldom twice alike. The apparatus, x-ray tube, x-ray film, and processing chemicals have been scientifically designed so that radiographic standardization may be more readily employed to produce radiographs from which the radiologist can make competent interpretations.

The common lack of unanimity on the subject of radiographic exposure is aptly demonstrated by the numerous recipes advanced in the form of complicated exposure tables. The lack of systematic and workable exposure method becomes readily apparent when it is necessary to train a student in radiographic exposure.

Standardized projections of an anatomic part portray the structures always in the same manner. It has been demonstrated repeatedly that an essential point in the radiographic diagnosis often appears in an inconspicuous portion of the image. Therefore, a systematic analysis and evaluation of the *entire* image should always be made. This requires that the entire image should be diagnostically informative and that translucent silver deposits representative of the anatomic structures always be produced.

RADIOGRAPHIC QUALITY

Radiographic quality should be evaluated along realistic lines rather than upon the emotional response of the individual observer to the image. Quality results when sound judgment is employed in the selection of the exposure factors and in the manner in which the exposed x-ray film is processed. Also, there should exist a balance in compromise between the exposure factors employed, the clinical situation as it is presented to the radiographer, and the objective of the examination–the diagnosis.

When a radiologist views a good radiograph, he is not particularly interested in how it was produced. But, if the quality is not what he should reasonably expect, then the *practical* reasons for failure should be recognized and investigated.

CRITERIA

The following criteria for attaining satisfactory radiographic quality may serve as a guide to better radiography.

1. All image densities should be translucent when viewed before a conventional x-ray illuminator.

2. All portions of the image should have silver deposit. Areas devoid of silver deposit are diagnostically useless. Excessive silver deposits should be avoided for they obscure detail and also are diagnostically useless.

3. The part examined should be fully penetrated.

4. The *basic mAs* factor should be selected so as to provide the best overall radiographic density for the patient whose measurement is within the *average* thickness range.

5. Contrast and gray scale should be balanced such that differentiation between densities or details can be readily made.

6. Image details should not be obscured by scatter radiation or chemical fog.

7. Maximum sharpness and true shape and size of the image should be consistent with the clinical needs of the examination.

EVOLVING THE EXPOSURE SYSTEM

The foregoing chapters have described in detail the functions of x-ray exposure factors. From this material may be summarized essential features that can serve as a basis for formulating a standardized exposure system. The ideal should establish all factors as constants with the exception of one to be employed as a variable. Hence, kilovoltage should be regarded as the factor of penetration, exposure latitude and radiographic contrast; milliampere-seconds as the factor of radiographic density; and the focal spot size, SID, SOD, and OID as geometric factors influencing image sharpness, shape, and size. Thus, standardization of radiography resolves itself into three phases.

1. **Standardization of Exposure Factors.** The reduction of all exposure factors in a given projection to constants with the exception of one variable (mAs).

2. **Standardization of Projections.** A standard method for positioning the patient and projection of the central ray for a given procedure.

3. **Standardization of the Processing Procedure.** The reduction of time and temperature values to constants so that changes in radiographic density can more properly be attributed to exposure.

OPTIMUM (FIXED) KILOVOLTAGE TECHNIQUE

The bulk of modern radiography is expeditious effort. A standardized system for selecting and applying exposure factors therefore becomes a necessity. Such a system, however, must produce consistently good radiographic quality. The optimum kilovoltage technique satisfies these requirements. This technique was evolved to eliminate many complexities in the application of exposure factors and reduce them to simplicities. Specifically, it is based upon standardization of the processing procedure and the reduction of exposure factors to constants with the exception of one variable. The technic is based on the following general principles. By trial, a fixed or optimum kilovoltage is established for an average tissue thickness range and for a given projection. Once it has been found that the kilovoltage selected produces the most desirable amount of penetration and contrast for the given human part, irrespective of size, it is established as a constant. A basic mAs value is then decided upon that will produce the required amount of radiographic density within the average range. When a patient is classified as outside the average thickness range—smaller or larger—the basic mAs value is adjusted. All other factors, including processing, are constants.

TECHNIQUE

In working out an optimum kilovoltage technique, each projection must be considered individually. It must be understood that for a given thickness of a particular body part, the wave length of the x-rays employed to penetrate the tissues must be adequate or, in other words, *optimum*. The amount and kind of tissue—the relation of bone to soft tissue—and its penetrability by x-radiation must be evaluated. Measurement of the part must be made along the course traversed through the tissues by the central ray, and the average range of measurements verified by checking many individuals. On the basis of this information, a kilovoltage is selected that will thoroughly penetrate the part, irrespective of size, and produce a satisfactory contrast. Once established as optimum for the projection, it should not be changed unless the conditions under which the kVp was established are changed.

With the kVp fixed, a basic mAs or density value must be established for the average thickness range of the part. In deriving mAs values for thicknesses outside the average range or for variations in the physiologic or pathologic state of the tissues, a rule of thumb for density changes by mAs is employed. The source-image distance need seldom be changed and may, in most cases, be considered a constant.

When the wave length is optimum, a lower mAs value is usually more adequate for the exposure than that habitually employed for the same purpose with the lower kilovoltages. Less mAs, of course, permits a greater number of radiographs to be made in a given projection before the limit of radiation safety is reached. The overall radiographic density produced by this method is uniform from case to case—a point of considerable diagnostic value because any differences from the normal density may then be attributed to abnormal changes within the tissues. Duplication of results is easy to attain in followup cases. The technique may be employed with any type of rectified or self-rectified apparatus. Whatever the type of generator, the only variable factor to adjust is the mAs; all other factors are constant.

Role of Thickness Ranges

Average thickness ranges are actually guides for establishing basic mAs values for various projections since approximately 85 percent of all patients fall within these ranges. However, thickness ranges have been established for a number of projections shown in Table 10-1, Chapter 10. The approximate frequency in percentage with which these thicknesses appear is also listed.

Illustrated in Figures 25-1 and 25-2 are groups of unretouched radiographs in which, for the respective projections the exposure factors were identical since the thicknesses of the parts in each case were

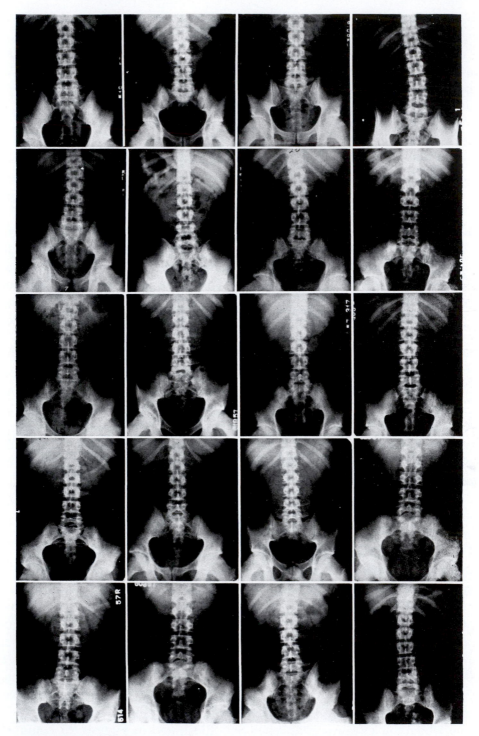

Figure 25-1. Radiographs of AP lumbar vertebrae of various patients made using a standardized technique chart.

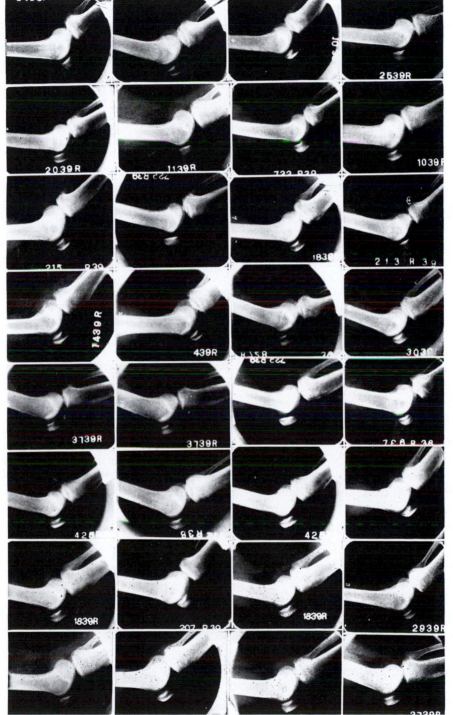

Figure 25-2. Radiographs of lateral knee of various patients made using a standardized technique chart.

within the average range. Note the uniformity in density and contrast manifested in each group.

An overview of the optimum kVp determined for each type of anatomical part and procedure is presented in Table 6-1, Chapter 6. Only in the most extreme cases of departure from the average would a kVp other than those listed in Table 6-1 be necessary. Variable mAs, primarily through the use of exposure time, should be used to adjust for most changes in thickness.

OPTIMUM MILLIAMPERAGE

There are only three considerations in selecting an mA station: How short exposure times it will allow the technologist to use to reduce the probability of patient motion, how small a focal spot it will allow the technologist to use to obtain the sharpest geometric detail, and the heat generated at the surface of the anode which may cause anode damage.

First, it must be determined whether the small focal spot size is necessary. If so, this will narrow the choices of mA stations to a range from 10 to 300 mA. At the large focal spot size, mA stations from 200 up to as much as 1200 may be available. Milliamperage stations in the small focal spot range do not usually present overheating problems at the anode, precisely because they are limited to 300 mA or less. An overload condition can occur at these stations if the small focal spot is imprudently used on procedures requiring high kVp levels. The more common problem with overheating occurs at the large focal spot when milliamperage stations above 600 mA are used. Therefore, the maximum mA stations for general use should be considered as 200 or 300 at the small focal spot (depending on the equipment) and 600 mA at the large focal spot.

For a given procedure, the mA station should be standardized at one of these maximum levels in order to achieve the shortest possible exposure times in obtaining the needed total mAs values. But, mA settings above 600 should not generally be used, except in special procedures where the time factor becomes critical. Having optimized both kVp and milliamperage, the short exposure times achieved will minimize the probability of motion unsharpness. This method also reduces the number of exposure variables changed during the procedure to one, which is simpler and narrows the probability of mathematical technique errors. The ability to obtain an exact mAs is not a serious problem, because any desired mAs can be very nearly obtained at any mA station with the times available, with few exceptions. As a rule, then, once it is decided which focal spot to use for a given procedure, the maximum mA station available at that focal spot size should be used so that minimum times can be achieved for "manual" technique.

Secondly, eliminating mA as a density control during a procedure reduces the number of factors that the technologist must consider when setting technique, making it easier to deal with and reducing the probability of error.

CONTROLLING DENSITY WITH EXPOSURE TIME

It is confusing indeed when a technologist looks up a technique on a chart for the second or third view in a procedure and finds a different kVp, a different mA station, and a different time setting from the previous view. It turns out that the smallest density adjustments practical can nearly always be achieved by a change in exposure time; thus, changing kVp or mA amounts to unnecessary work when done within a procedure from one view to the next.

SELECTION OF BASIC mAs

The mAs factor is the most reliable factor for regulating the *amount* of overall silver (density) in the image. There should be a satisfactory range of densities for interpretations of all portions of the image. The mAs can become a constant within certain limitations for a given projection. A *basic* mAs value can be established for any average thickness range of a part, provided it is established for an adult person.

Thickness Only a Guide

The thickness of any part serves only as a guide which the radiographer can use to expose the normal part and in determining what mAs will compensate for abnormal tissue changes. Obviously, if the part is normal and is in the average thickness range, the basic mAs can be employed. Knowledge of the structural makeup of the area is necessary when the kilovoltage has been fixed as a constant for the projection. The part should also be judged from a physiologic and pathologic standpoint as to whether it is reasonably normal. For the *small* part, the basic mAs value is halved; for the *average* part, the basic mAs value is employed; and for the *large* part, the basic mAs value is doubled. By means of these modifications, the radiographic density obtained will be approximately correct. If not, a slight increase or decrease in the mAs value in exposing a second film should provide the most desirable density. However, it will be found that a "remake" is seldom required.

OVEREXPOSURE

To the trained eye, the overexposed radiograph is easily identifiable. One type of overexposure exhibits an overall grayness with low contrast. Another type of overexposure produces such a great density of the thinner portions of the part radiographed that they are obliterated. Regardless of how it is developed, an overexposed film lacks the requisites of ideal radiographic quality—proper radiographic density and contrast—as one or the other is invariably sacrificed. If the kilovoltage is correct, overexposure due to the mAs factor may usually be corrected by making another radiograph with one-half the original mAs ($^1/_2$X). Very frequently, the density of this second radiograph is satisfactory or is so near in quality that if a third radiograph is made, only a minor adjustment of the mAs is needed to secure the most desirable quality.

Example. Two anteroposterior screen-grid radiographs of the lumbar vertebrae, Figure 25-3, were made with 70 kVp and a 36-inch SID. The first radiograph (A) was made with a trial exposure of 200 mAs. The density was excessive. Applying the rule of thumb for density, the second radiograph (B) was made with 100 mAs. The density was reduced, which yielded a satisfactory image density.

UNDEREXPOSURE

A radiograph is underexposed when important details are lacking because of inadequate radiographic density. Details of thin structures may be visible but those representing the heavier parts will be absent. When the kilovoltage is of a value to secure proper penetration of the part yet the mAs is insufficient to secure proper density, the radiograph will reveal very faint detail in image areas corresponding to the greater tissue densities. It may be presumed, therefore, that the kilovoltage is satisfactory for the part and that detail may be better visualized if more silver were

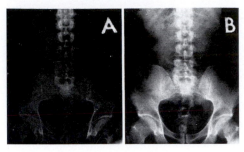

Figure 25-3. Screen radiographs of lumbar vertebrae demonstrating the effect of halving the mAs in correcting for a very dark image.

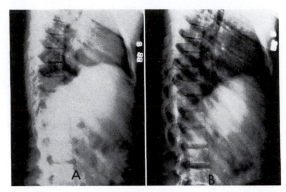

Figure 25-4. Screen radiographs of the lateral thoracolumbar vertebrae demonstrating the effect of doubling the mAs in correcting for a very light image.

deposited on the film. To achieve this result, the first step in correction is to *double* the mAs. Usually the density will then be satisfactory. However, a further small adjustment in the mAs may be made, if necessary, to provide a more satisfactory image.

Example. Two lateral screen-grid radiographs of the thoracolumbar vertebrae, Figure 25-4, were made employing 85 kVp, 36-inch SID; 100 mAs and 200 mAs; thickness 32 cm. The first radiograph (A) made with 100 mAs was obviously underexposed. By doubling the mAs value to 200 in making the second radiograph (B), a satisfactory overall density was obtained.

VARIABLE KILOVOLTAGE TECHNIQUE

Technique systems using various approaches to varying the kVp have been developed over the years. Many of these are actually hybrid systems, using both variable mAs and variable kVp, a practice difficult to rationalize. A few have proven to work with good reliability in controlling image density, and will be discussed briefly.

Probably the most common variable kVp system consists of using a "base" kVp of 40, to which an additional value equal to two times the measured part thickness is added. For example, for a cervical spine measuring 14 centimeters in thickness, the kVp would be:

$$40 + (2 \times 14) = 68 \text{ kVp}$$

A proper mAs value must still be established for each general body area, such as lower extremity, upper extremity, abdomen, chest and head. Let us suppose that the determined mAs value for chest radiographs is 10 mAs. The average chest measures 22 centimeters in PA projection and 30 centimeters in lateral projection. The derived techniques would then be:

PA: $40 + (2 \times 22) = 84$ kVp at 10 mAs
LAT: $40 + (2 \times 30) = 100$ kVp at 10 mAs

Varying the kVp in this manner would cause a change in image contrast between the two views, with the lateral view presenting lower contrast than the PA view. For many procedures, the changes in kVp from one view to another would not be extreme enough to appreciably alter image contrast, but as the above example shows, this is not always the case, since a change of 16 kVp will result in a visible difference in image contrast. Typically, this discrepancy is adjusted for by using a new mAs value, resulting in a hybrid approach to technique.

Variable kVp systems are workable from the standpoint of controlling image density, and are indeed impressive in their accuracy for this. But they fundamentally ignore the fact that kVp affects other image qualities. Worse, the use of variable kVp may frequently lead to reductions in kVp for thinner patients that result in inadequate penetration for the tissue. Optimum kVp is essential for proper penetration and radiographic demonstration of each body part, in accordance with the proportions of different types of tissue that create subject contrast for the image. While kVp can be safely increased above the optimum level to a certain extent, reductions in kVp can prove disastrous to image quality. The use of fixed kVp and variable mAs, on the other hand, has the following advantages:

1. Changes in mAs made within the reasonable ranges of daily practice, affect *only* image density.

2. mAs is *directly* proportional to image density, while kVp is not. This allows more accurate prediction of densities that will result from adjustments made in technique.

3. Because mAs is directly proportional to image density, the entire proportional anatomy system presented in Chapter 26 can be applied with ease. Variable mAs is compatible with the proportional anatomy approach.

4. Since variable mAs is predicated upon fixed, optimum kVp, adequate penetration of anatomy is assured with high reliability.

5. Because mAs adjustments are easier to calculate than kVp changes in their effect on image density, less errors are likely to be made, and less repeats taken.

For all of these reasons, *a fixed kVp approach, using optimum kVp techniques, is recommended.*

SUMMARY

1. *Uniformity* and *consistency* in image qualities between the radiographs of a given procedure are essential to accurate diagnosis.

2. The use of an *optimum kilovoltage* level for each procedure will eliminate variations in image contrast and make technique manipulation more accurate and simple.

3. The use of *optimum milliamperage* for a given focal spot size within a procedure will improve the accuracy of density control, simplify technique, and reduce the probability of patient motion.

4. In most cases, a *halving* of the *mAs* will correct for a dark exposure, and a *doubling of the mAs* will correct for a light exposure.

5. Three factors should be standardized in a radiology department: (1) exposure factors, (2) projection routines, and (3) processing procedures.

REVIEW QUESTIONS

1. Define "optimum mA":
2. Name two advantages to standardizing an optimum kVp on all techniques used within a procedure:
3. Name the three areas in which radiographic procedures should be standardized within a radiology department:

4. If an x-ray machine is properly calibrated, the most accurate and reliable technique factor to vary in compensating for different thicknesses of patients is:
5. In most cases, a very light or dark radiograph can be corrected by adjusting the mAs by a factor of _____.

Chapter 26

TECHNIQUE BY PROPORTIONAL ANATOMY

MANY WORKABLE TIPS or "tricks of the trade" regarding technique are passed from one radiographer to another, whereby a technique for a certain body part may be derived from a known technique for another body part. A central pattern emerges from these which is based on the logical premise that the body parts can indeed be proportionately related for the average body habitus. A close examination of any good technique chart will reveal the same pattern of *total techniques* (that is, mA-time-kVp combinations) when the 15 percent rule is used to adjust for kVp differences and total resulting mAs values are compared. For example, the techniques listed below from a typical technique chart are all roughly equal in terms of *total technique*:

AP Lumbar Spine = 300 mA, $^1/_5$ sec., 80 kVp
AP Abdomen = 200 mA, $^3/_{10}$ sec., 78 kVp
AP Pelvis = 300 mA, $^1/_{10}$ sec., 92 kVp
Townes Skull = 200 mA, $^1/_5$ sec., 86 kVp

To become comfortable with the concept of "total technique" as the above example illustrates, the student must completely familiarize himself with the 15 percent rule. The exercises in Chapter 6 are recommended for this purpose. In the tables that follow, *total technique* levels and adjustments are stated according to the proportional change they would normally cause in the final density of the image. *These tables do not recommend whether to change kVp or mAs specifically; they only list the desired end result in overall technique.*

The radiographer must then decide whether to use kVp or mAs to make the adjustment. If kVp is used, it must be done according to the 15 percent rule. Some examples are given in the following table:

To change total technique by a factor of	Adjust the kVp up or down by
2	15%
3	22%
4	30%
50% up or $^1/_2$ up	8%
30% down or $^1/_3$ down	5%

In making this decision, *the rules of optimum kVp for each body part must not be broken. The kVp used should never be less than the optimum amount listed for each body part as given in Table 6-1, Chapter 6.* For example, Table 26-2 states that a knee technique may be derived by doubling an ankle technique. However, simply doubling the mAs to accomplish this might violate the optimum kVp recommendation in Table 6-1, which lists 70 kVp as optimum for the knee, and 64 kVp for the ankle. By the 15 percent rule, one can surmise that a 6-kVp increase in this range will increase density by about one-half or 50 percent, and thus takes us half-way to the desired total doubling. An increase in mAs of 50 percent, added to the 6-kVp increase, will result in an overall doubling of *total technique*.

The entire proportional anatomy system can be adapted to the variable kVp approach by applying the 15 percent rule.

Many technologists increase about 8 kVp when changing from an AP foot technique to a lateral foot technique, leaving the original mAs. This agrees perfectly with Table 26-2, which recommends a doubling of the AP foot technique to derive a lateral foot technique. Fifteen percent of 60 kVp is 9 kVp. Hence, the popular 8-kVp increase approximates an overall doubling of *total technique.*

A second important consideration is the minimum change in overall technique required to see a visible difference in image density. It will be recalled that changes of less than 30 percent in *total technique* are unlikely to cause a visible difference in the image. When using kVp adjustments, any change of less than 5 percent will not be visible.

Finally, one must bear in mind that the following tables are applicable only to *average, adult patients.* In assessing a patient to derive an appropriate technique, the radiographer must consider the *shape* of the patient as well as his habitus and size. No amount of instruction can compensate for carelessness in doing so. Figure 26-1 illustrates how body torso shape, in cross-section, deviates from that of the average adult (c) for premature babies, healthy infants and fluid-distended hypersthenic patients.

The average adult torso is oval in shape, measuring 22 cm in AP by 30 cm laterally. Table 26-2 recommends 4 times the AP technique for lateral projections of all torso anatomy, including the chest and the abdomen. (Note that this also agrees with the 4-centimeter rule, since two doublings would be required where the anatomy is 8 centimeters thicker.) This very workable rule of thumb fails, however, for very young children or for fluid-distended abdomens.

Healthy newborn infants have a rounder torso, (Fig. 26-1B), so there is less difference in technique from the AP projection to the lateral projection. A good rule of thumb for infants (less than one year old) is to double the AP technique for the lateral view. An increase of about 8 kVp will accomplish the overall doubling. This will work for both chest and abdomen radiography. Experienced radiographers know that the same technique can be used for both the AP and the lateral views on premature babies in intensive care that are well below normal birth weight. These babies have torsos that are nearly circular in cross-section, so there is little difference in thickness from any angle (Fig. 26-1A).

Some hypersthenic patients, particularly those with fluid distention of the abdomen, have a very round torso shape (Fig. 26-1D). After increasing the AP technique from average for the added thickness, the radiographer may find himself using the same technique for a lateral projection. Radiographers who are observant of body shape as well as body habitus and thickness will have lower repeat rates and save unnecessary patient exposure.

USEFULNESS OF THE PROPORTIONAL ANATOMY SYSTEM

Having reviewed the foregoing considerations, Tables 26-1 and 26-2 can be applied to daily radiography practice in estimating techniques. It is recommended that both of these closely related tables be memorized. At a glance, this will seem overwhelming to the student, but rest assured that many of the factors listed are duplicated several times, and that the commitment of these rules of thumb to memory will be well worth the effort because they are so useful in daily practice.

Figure 26-2 demonstrates a series of radiographs which were taken using the proportional anatomy system to derive techniques. The AP lumbar spine projection (A) was exposed using 30 mAs and 80 kVp on a three-phase machine with 200-speed "medium" rare earth intensifying screens. This patient measured average dimensions, 22 cm in AP and 30 cm in lateral. The lateral lumbar spine (B) was taken with 120 mAs at 80 kVp, four times the mAs used for the AP projection in (A) and maintaining optimum kVp for the series. The lateral view of the lumbosacral junction (C) utilized the same 120 mAs as in (B), but with kilovoltage increased to 90 in order to penetrate the additional iliac bones which are superimposed over the spine at this level.

Radiograph (D) is a PA skull projection taken with 20 mAs at 80 kVp. Note that this technique is precisely 2/3 of the lumbar spine in (A). Derived by proportional anatomy using Table 26-2, the Townes view of the skull would be equivalent in technique to the average AP abdomen or lumbar spine, and the PA skull would be ²/₃ the mAs used for the Townes view, i.e., ²/₃ the AP lumbar spine technique.

Radiograph (E) is an AP projection of the cervical spine taken with 12 mAs and 76 kVp. By Table 26-2, this view would require one-half the technique for the PA skull in (D). Note that the mAs is cut almost to one-half, but that the kVp has also been reduced by 4, making an overall reduction in *total technique* of slightly less than one-half the PA skull.

Radiograph (F) is a PA wrist projection taken with 6.4 mAs at 58 kVp. Derived by proportional anatomy from the AP cervical spine in Table 26-2, this adjustment is made in several steps as follows:

Cervical Spine to Knee:
Minus 8 kVp = 10 mAs @ 68 kVp

Knee to Ankle:
¹/₂ (using 15% kVp) = 10 mAs @ 58 kVp
*200-Speed "Medium" Rare Earth Screen to
75-Speed "Extremity Cassette" (See Chapter 14):
Slightly less than 3 X technique = 28 mAs @ 58 kVp

Ankle to AP Foot or AP Elbow:
¹/₂ = 14 mAs @ 58 kVp

AP Elbow to PA Wrist:
¹/₂ = 7 mAs @ 58 kVp

Using the proportional anatomy system, the derived technique is only 14 percent off from the actual technique used. Remem-

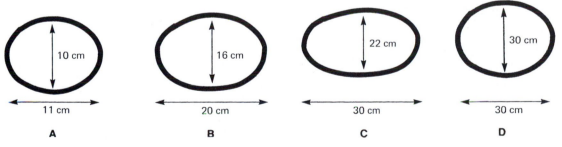

A 10 cm / 11 cm **B** 16 cm / 20 cm **C** 22 cm / 30 cm **D** 30 cm / 30 cm

Figure 26-1. Cross-sectional diagrams of body torso shapes and dimensions (not to scale) of (A) premature infant presenting an essentially round torso; (B) healthy baby with more oval shaped torso, requiring a doubling of the AP technique for lateral projections; (C) average adult measuring 8 cm more laterally than in AP projection, requiring almost two doublings of technique from AP to lateral; and (D) fluid-distended hypersthenic adult, with AP and lateral techniques roughly equal.

bering that a 30 percent change is required to see a visible difference, this calculation is close indeed.

The lateral wrist (G) was exposed using 13 mAs and 58 kVp, double the mAs from the PA projection as recommended by Table 26-2. All of these views were exposed using the same x-ray machine, and illustrate the practical value of the proportional anatomy system.

Technique derivation by proportional anatomy has proven to be extremely useful in at least three types of situations: (1) Complete technique charts and other radiographers are not always available when performing mobile radiography. If the radiographer does not have a written or memorized technique for a knee, for example, but does have one for an ankle, a good knee technique can be derived from the ankle technique. (2) When asking another radiographer for recommended techniques for a particular procedure, one would only have to ask for and remember a single technique. For example, having been given a technique for the PA view of the skull, one can then derive techniques for the remaining views. (3) In devising a new technique chart "from scratch," perhaps for a newly installed x-ray machine, many techniques can be derived from just a few proven exposures. In the next chapter, the derivation of an *entire technique chart* using this approach is demonstrated. If a handful of proven exposures are used to cross-check the development of the techniques, an entire chart can be derived with remarkable accuracy. Naturally, such a chart would need refinement in use, but the proportional anatomy system provides the radiographer a systematic starting point that is helpful indeed.

PROPORTIONAL ANATOMY GROUPINGS

Table 26-1 presents groupings of anatomy which share roughly equivalent technique requirements. Approximately the same technique can be used for all projections listed within a group. Groups 1 and 2 cover over fifteen projections that can be taken with just two memorized techniques! It is this simplification that makes the system worth memorizing.

For example, Group 1 shows that the same technique can be used for an AP abdomen, a lateral hip, an AP dorsal spine, and a Townes view of the skull *on a patient of average habitus*. The radiographer may wish to slightly decrease this technique for the AP dorsal spine, or slightly increase it for the lateral hip view, but for an average patient, these techniques are so close that one "rounded" technique will produce adequate density for all of them. Naturally, adjustments must be made for patients that are not average and situations that are not normal.

For each grouping, an actual technique is listed for the "reference" anatomy, assuming that three-phase equipment with 400 speed "rare earth regular" screens are used. If the machine is single-phase, *or* if the screens are 200-speed calcium tungstate, then the mAs must be doubled. All possible variations on technique cannot be listed here, but those two listed should cover the most common circumstances. Group 4 lists three subgroupings of extremities which share equivalent techniques. Again, two variations on technique are given for each group assuming the 75-speed "extremity cassettes" (or "slow-speed" calcium tungstate screens) are used.

Table 26-1
PROPORTIONAL ANATOMY GROUPINGS

Group 1: (Reference: AP Abdomen, Average 22 cm)

Technique: 3-phase equipment, 400-speed screens:
15 mAs, 80 kVp
If single-phase OR 200-speed screens:
30 mAs, 80 kVp

AP Abdomen
AP Pelvis
AP Lumbar Spine
AP Dorsal Spine
AP Hip
Lat Hip
Townes (Grashey) View, Skull

Group 2: (Reference: AP Cervical Spine, Average
13 cm)

Technique: 3-phase equipment, 400-speed screens:
5 mAs, 76 kVp
If single-phase OR 200-speed screens:
10 mAs, 76 kVp

AP Cervical Spine
All Cervical Spine Views (if at same distance
and grid)
Open-Mouth Odontoid (George View)
AP Shoulder
AP Clavicle
AP Femur
Lat Femur
AP or PA Chest (grid)
Lateral Skull
AP Sacrum/Coccyx

Group 3: Solid Column Barium Studies (Reference:
AP Views)

Technique: 3-phase equipment, 400-speed screens:
4 mAs, 110 kVp
If single-phase OR 200-speed screens: 8
mAs, 110 kVp

Upper G.I., AP
Barium Enema (solid column), AP

Group 4: Extremity Groupings, Using "Extremity"
Cassettes

Subgroup	*Technique using 75-speed screens*
1. AP Foot AP Elbow	} 3-phase: 5 mAs, 64 kVp 1-phase: 10 mAs, 64 kVp
2. Lat Foot AP Ankle Lat Ankle AP Humerus	} 3-phase: 10 mAs, 64 kVp 1-phase: 20 mAs, 64 kVp
3. AP Leg Lat Leg Lat Humerus	} 3-phase: 10 mAs, 68 kVp 1-phase: 20 mAs, 68 kVp

TECHNIQUE DERIVATIONS BY PROPORTIONAL ANATOMY

Table 26-2 lists a series of comparisons of total technique according to average body parts, so that a given technique may be derived from any one of several other known techniques. Of course, not every possible derivation can be listed, nor every projection. But, the list is quite comprehensive and unlisted techniques can be extrapolated from those listed in many cases.

Many of these rules of thumb can be proven out before actually trying them by simply observing good radiographs. For example, examine the cervical spine on a lateral view of the skull. You will see that the lateral skull technique is ideal for demonstrating the cervical spine. Examine the clavicles on a radiograph of the cervical spine, or the pelvis on an abdomen view.

Two precautions bear mention: First, Table 26-2 does *not* indicate adjustments for changes other than anatomy, such as changes in screens, grids, or distances.

These adjustments must be made *in addition* to the rules of thumb presented here. For example, a lateral cervical spine is equivalent in technique to the AP cervical spine. But since the lateral is normally taken upright using a 72-inch SID, the mAs must then be tripled as described in Chapter 18 to adjust for the increase in distance from the 40-inch AP projection. If the upright cassette holder has no grid, an additional compensation must be made.

Second, note that oblique projections of the torso are broken down into 30-degree and 45-degree obliques. There is great variation in the amount of obliquity used in practice. Very shallow obliques of torso anatomy require no increase in technique from the AP projections. Many oblique views are close to 30 degrees and require a 50 percent increase in technique. But, the oblique lumbar spine, for example, must be taken at a true 45-degree angle to properly demonstrate the anatomy of interest, and this steep oblique will require a doubling of the mAs when compared to the AP view.

Five *key derivation references* are listed, below. These might be thought of as the five most important derivations to memorize, because they allow one to "jump" between very different portions of the body and still arrive at an estimated technique. The first takes us from a distal lower extremity or an upper extremity to the knee, the second from the knee to the neck, the third and fourth from the neck to the skull, and the fifth from the skull to the torso:

KEY DERIVATION REFERENCES

1. AP Knee = 2 x AP Ankle OR 2 x AP Humerus
2. AP Cervical Spine = AP Knee + 8 kVp
3. Lat Skull = AP Cervical Spine
4. Townes (Grashey) Skull = 3 x Lat Skull
5. *Average* AP Abdomen = Townes (Grashey) Skull

Memorize these five relationships first, then review Table 26-2.

APPLYING THE SYSTEM

For practice, try the following EXERCISE 20 to help in your memorization of proportional anatomy relationships. Check your answers from the Appendix.

EXERCISE #20

Proportional Anatomy Practice

For each of the following relationships of anatomy, write the proportional change in *total* technique required:

1. PA Skull to Townes Skull: _____
2. Lateral Facial Bones to PA Facial Bones: _____
3. AP Cervical Spine to Oblique Cervical Spine: _____
4. Barium Enema AP View to Sigmoid (35-degree angled) View: _____
5. PA Chest to Lateral Chest: _____
6. Townes Skull to AP Abdomen: _____
7. PA Wrist to AP Elbow: _____
8. AP Knee to AP Shoulder: _____
9. AP Leg to AP Leg With Dry Plaster Cast: _____
10. PA Adult Skull to AP Infant (2-week-old) Skull: _____
11. AP Foot to Lateral Foot: _____
12. AP Ankle to Lateral Ankle: _____

Table 26-2
TECHNIQUE BY PROPORTIONAL ANATOMY

A. TRUNK:

AP Abdomen
AP Pelvis
AP Hip
Lat Hip
AP Lumbar Spine
AP Dorsal spine
} all are roughly equal to each other
and equivalent to a Townes (Grashey) Skull

30° Obliques on All Above = $1^1/_2$ x AP
45° Obliques on All Above = 2 x AP (average thickness increase is about 4 cm)
Laterals on All Above = 4 x AP (average thickness increase is about 8 cm)
All Barium Studies = about $1/_4$ mAs and up about 30 per cent kVp

B. SKULL:

PA/Caldwell = $2/_3$ Abdomen, = $2/_3$ Townes, = 2 x Lateral, = 2 x C-Spine
Lateral = $1/_2$ PA, = C-Spine, = Shoulder = Femur = PA or AP grid Chest
Lateral Sinus = $1/_3$ PA
Townes = $1^1/_2$ x PA, = 3 x Lateral, = AP Abdomen
Submentovertex = Townes ($1^1/_2$ x PA)
Waters = PA + 4-6 kVp
Mandibles, Mastoids, etc. = roughly $1/_3$ PA

C. CHEST:

PA CXR = AP Shoulder, = Cervical Spine, OR = AP Knee + 10 kVp IF BOTH are done non-grid
or both in the bucky (if one is grid and one non-grid, technique must be adjusted by a
factor of 4)

Lateral = 4 x PA (the common "double mAs and up 10 kVp" is equivalent to two doublings, or 4X)

D. PEDIATRICS:

Skull: Newborn = $1/_4$ Adult
              1 Year = $1/_2$ Adult
              5 Years = $3/_4$ Adult

Torso: Newborn = $1/_4$ Adult
              1 Year = $1/_2$ Adult
              5 Years = $3/_4$ Adult

Extremities: Newborn = $1/_6$ Adult
              2 Years = $1/_4$ Adult
              8 Years = $1/_2$ Adult
              12 Years = $3/_4$ Adult

E. EXTREMITIES, ETC.:

Cervical Spine: AP = AP Shoulder grid, = Lateral Skull, = $1/_2$ PA Skull, = Femur
                 Obliques
                 Lateral*   } all equal to AP
                 Odontoid
                 *If lateral is done at 72" FFD, but non-grid, technique will equal AP at 40" grid.
                 Otherwise, adjustment must be made for distance or grid changes.

Table 26-2 (Continued)

E. EXTREMITIES, ETC.: (Continued)

    Femur = $2/3$ AP Abdomen, = 2 x Knee grid, = Shoulder, = Cervical Spine
        Lateral = AP

    Knee = 2 x Ankle, = PA Chest - 10 kVp if BOTH are grid or both are non-grid,
        = AP Shoulder - 8 kVp or AP C-Spine - 8 kVp if grid
        Lateral = AP

    Leg = $1/2$-way between AP Ankle and AP Knee
        Lateral = AP

    Ankle = 2 x AP Foot, = $1/2$ AP Knee, = Lateral Foot
        Lateral = AP

    Foot = $1/2$ AP Ankle (usually down 8 kVp, NOT less mAs), = $1/4$ AP Knee, = AP Elbow
        Lateral Foot = 2 x AP, = Ankle

    Shoulder = C-Spine, = Knee + 8 kVp, = $1/2$ PA Skull, = PA Chest IF grid, = Lat Skull, = Femur

    Humerus = $1/2$ way between elbow and shoulder
        Lateral = AP + 6 kVp

    Elbow = 2 x Wrist, = $2/3$ Humerus, = AP Foot
        Lateral = AP + 4 kVp

    Forearm = $1/2$ way between wrist and elbow

    Wrist = $1/2$ Elbow, = $1/2$ Foot, = 1.5 x Hand (usually up 8 kVp, not mAs)
        Oblique = $1^1/2$ x PA
        Lateral = 2 x PA

    Hand = $1/3$ Elbow, = $2/3$ Wrist
        Oblique = $1^1/2$ x PA
        Lateral = 2 x PA

    Digit = PA Hand

F. CASTS AND SPLINTS:

    Plaster Casts: Dry plaster, small extremity = 2 x non-cast technique
                    Wet plaster, small extremity, OR   3 x non-cast
                    Dry plaster, large extremity (femur)
                    Wet plaster, large extremity (femur) = 4 x non-cast

    1" Wood Splint, two $1/2$-inch wood splints, or plaster half-cast = $1^1/2$ x non-cast technique
    Pure Fiberglass cast or Air Splint = No Change in Technique
    Fiberglass-Plaster Cast = $1^1/2$ x non-cast technique
    Wet Fiberglass Cast = $1^1/2$ x non-cast technique

SUMMARY

1. Using the proportional anatomy system, *groupings of anatomical parts* that require approximately the same *total radiographic technique* can be made, helping to simplify techniques.
2. Using the proportional anatomy system, *techniques can be derived* from one body part to another with fair accuracy.
3. *Optimum kVp* guidelines must never be neglected in deriving techniques by proportional anatomy. This means that the radiographer must be adept at using the 15 percent rule in making adjustments.
4. No system can compensate for neglecting proper *evaluation of patient shape and habitus*, the radiographer's responsibility.
5. The proportional anatomy system must be used in conjunction with all of the technique guidelines presented in this text for changes in *distance, screen speed, grids,* and other variables.

REVIEW QUESTIONS

1. Compared to average adults, the torso of an infant requires _____ (more, less, or equal) adjustment in technique from a frontal (AP) to a lateral view.
2. Changes in total technique for proportional anatomy adjustments may be made in mAs, kVp, or both?

For the following, what is the proportional change in *total technique* required:

3. AP Pelvis to AP Lumbar Spine: _____
4. Lumbar Spine Oblique View to Lateral View: _____
5. AP Ankle to AP Knee: _____
6. Upper G.I. AP View to Lateral View: _____
7. PA Wrist to Lateral Wrist: _____
8. AP Foot to AP Ankle: _____
9. Lateral Leg to Lateral Leg with One-Piece 3/4-inch Wood Splint: _____
10. AP Adult Humerus to Infant (2-week-old) AP Humerus: _____
11. PA Esophagus (with barium) to 15-degree Anterior Oblique: _____
12. AP Shoulder to AP Cervical Spine: _____
13. PA Skull to Lateral Skull: _____
14. Townes Skull to Submentovertex Skull: _____

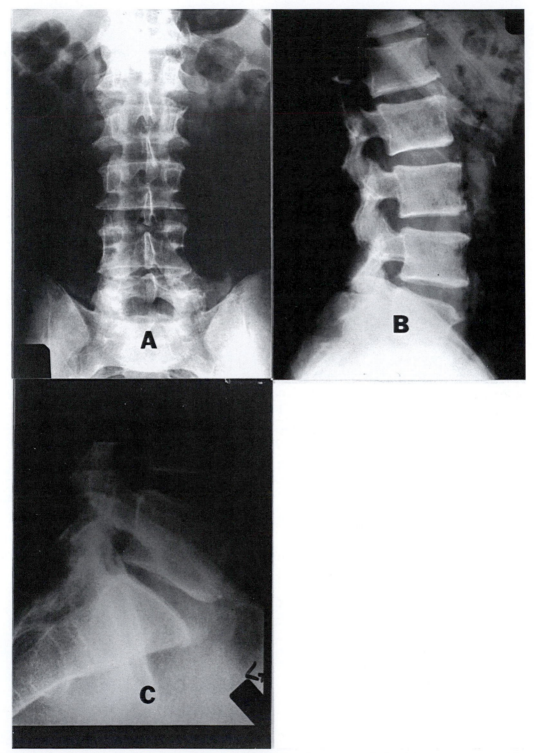

Figure 26-2. Demonstration of usefulness of proportional anatomy derivations on average patient in producing balanced densities. Techniques: (A) AP lumbar spine with 30 mAs at 80 kVp, (B) lateral lumbar spine with 120 mAs at 80 kVp (4 X AP), (C) lateral L5-S1 spot with 120 mAs at 90 kVp, (D) PA

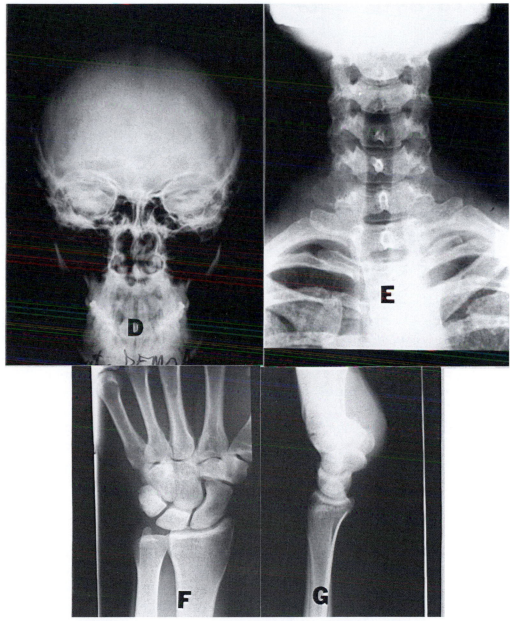

skull with 20 mAs at 80 kVp (^{2}/₃ the mAs in *A* for AP lumbar/abdomen or Townes skull), (E) AP cervical spine with 12 mAs at 76 kVp (approximately 1/2 the PA skull in D and equal to a lateral skull), (F) PA wrist with 6.4 mAs at 58 kVp using extremity cassette tabletop, and (G) lateral wrist with 13.2 mAs at 58 kVp (double the PA wrist).

Chapter 27

TECHNIQUE CHARTS

EVERY RADIOLOGY DEPARTMENT should develop technique charts for each machine. The use of technique charts has its limits. Whether using computer-generated charts, technique computers, the bit system, or homemade charts, no written device can replace the need for the technologist's assessment of each individual patient and situation. Nonetheless, the technique chart has been proven to reduce repeat rates considerably and to be indispensable as a starting point and a reference. Radiographers who are critical of the use of charts simply never learned how to construct and use them properly. It would be unprofessional to ignore something that has been scientifically, objectively demonstrated to reduce patient radiation exposure, as well as help control costs for the radiology department.

Table 10-1 in Chapter 10 presents the results of thousands of measurements taken on adult patients, and states the average range of thickness for each body part. For most distal extremities and skulls, more than 90 percent of adult patients fall within the average range of thickness. For these radiographic procedures, a single technique can be written on the technique chart. The radiographer must always be observant and capable of adjusting the "average" technique upward or downward for uncommon circumstances, but space on a written chart need not be committed to such rare adjustments. The "extremities" section of the technique chart in Table 27-1

demonstrates this format, with a single technique for each anatomical part.

Another look at Table 10-1 shows that the abdominal (lumbar) region is the most variable area of the body for thickness. Even for abdominal procedures, a single technique would work for more than two-thirds (69 percent) of adult patients. (This certainly remains a high enough factor of reliability to substantiate the value of a technique chart, even if only one technique were listed for each procedure.) To adapt for this level of variation, the torso section of a technique chart should be broken down into columns according to measured thickness as illustrated in Table 27-1. Note that the technique changes listed there follow the *four centimeter rule*, doubling for each increase in thickness of four centimeters, and cut to one-half for equal reductions in thickness.

The chart in Table 27-1 is written for three-phase equipment, using 10:1 grids, and 400-speed screens. Variations in equipment and calibration may require the entire chart to be adjusted up or down by a certain ratio for it to be useful. If the *entire* chart is adjusted consistently, it should be more than 85 percent accurate. Change ONLY mAs values, not kVp.

- For single-phase equipment, double all mAs values
- For "high"-speed calcium tungstate screens, double the techniques listed, (except those marked EXTREMITY

CAS).

- For other screen conversions, see Chapter 14, Tables 14-4 and 14-5.

This chart, while it may be of practical use, is primarily presented to illustrate the concepts taught in Chapters 25, 26, and 27. Take special note of the format: The torso section is organized according to variable part thicknesses, with an average cm measurement given for reference. The extremities section lists a single mAs value, with adjustments described at the top for patients which are smaller than average or larger than average. "Small," "Average," and "Large" mAs columns could be used as an alternative, but generally measurements are not needed here. The extremities section also has an additional column just to illustrate how both the mA and the exposure time can be listed in one column, as an option to listing the total mAs. Overall, it is concise and yet it covers nearly every procedure including pediatric procedures in just three pages.

This is a variable mAs, fixed kVp chart, as recommended in Chapters 6 and 25. Torso measurements are organized into 2-cm columns as discussed in this chapter. And, you will note that if you take both the kVp and the mAs values into consideration as a "total technique," it very closely follows the proportional anatomy rules of thumb presented in Chapter 26. Careful analysis of this chart in reference to the concepts in these chapters will prove a valuable learning experience.

The use of calipers as explained in Chapter 10 to measure the part thickness is a must for torso radiography and for pediatric radiography. Radiographers can become adept at estimating body part thicknesses after acquiring considerable experience, and only require calipers for exceptional cases. The student must not take this practice in the wrong vein—the less the experience, the greater the need for the calipers. One should only engage in such a practice *after fully establishing his or her accuracy over the course of many months.* This is done by persistent practice, by estimating the thickness of each patient and then checking *with the calipers* to see how accurate the estimate was. For more rare procedures, or whenever there is any doubt at all regarding patient thickness and appropriate technique, *calipers and technique charts should be used in conjunction.*

It should be noted that the foregoing is a philosophical statement, and not a legal one. Some states require the use of both calipers and technique charts *by law*. Such requirements are not unreasonable, since the objective data obtained from taking actual measurements will be more reliable than any estimation, assuming that the calipers are used properly. This practice should reduce repeat rates and enhance professionalism.

DEVELOPING CHARTS

The proper construction and use of technique charts *must* include the following:

1. A quality control program for calibration of machines and monitoring of processing conditions.

2. Input from all radiographers using a given machine as the chart is developed and corrected.

3. Strict enforcement by administrative technologists that no individual radiographer be allowed to alter the chart in any way once it has been developed and tested. Radiographers who continually cross out and rewrite techniques are usually radiographers who use incorrect distances, incorrect screens or film, or incorrect positioning. The next radiographer to use the room may use the right distance, screen, film, and

position, and have to repeat radiographs because of the rewritten techniques.

4. Encouragement by administrative technologists that all radiographers use the system.

5. Periodic checks and updates of all technique charts using the same system of input by which they were originally developed. *Periodic* here means perhaps every 6 months.

Suppose you are in charge of a newly constructed radiology department and must devise some charts from scratch. Using the rules of thumb and relationships discussed in Chapter 5, 6, 7, 10, 25, and 26, you can write a reasonably accurate preliminary technique chart completely from just one test film on a phantom (or patient, if necessary). To demonstrate, try the following Exercise #21. Answers and explanations for Exercise #21 are found in Appendix II.

Once the correct mAs is determined, it then becomes the basic value to be employed for all thicknesses in the average thickness range established for the projection.

Example 1. In posteroanterior adult chest screen radiography, the average thickness range may be considered to be 20 to 24 centimeters. As shown in Table 10-1, this range of measurements represents those of about 82 percent of patients. In this projection the basic mAs should be established for a normal healthy adult measuring 22 cm. (the middle thickness in the range). Projections that have relatively little variation from the average thickness range, such as a posteroanterior view of the chest, require refinement in application of the mAs values to those thicknesses in excess of or less than the average. A typical example of a standardized posteroanterior technique is shown in the unretouched radiographs, Figure 27-1. It is interesting to statistically evaluate in Table 27-2 the physical characteristics of the patient's whose radiographs are shown in Figure 27-1.

Radiation that completely penetrates the part and produces a consistently uniform density and contrast is most important in applying a standardized technique. It becomes readily apparent that the characteristics of height, weight, or sex cannot per se be employed to determine the x-ray absorbing properties of the tissues being exposed.

Thickness Greater than Average

When a chest measurement is slightly greater than average, the only change that need be made in the factors is in the mAs. The increased thickness of the 26- and 27-centimeter chest only requires *more* radiation of the quality as produced with 80 kVp on chests within the average range. The kilovoltage is held constant since it has been predetermined that 80 kVp provides the necessary quality of radiation to penetrate any size adult chest within a reasonable range in the posteroanterior direction, using *nongrid* exposure.

Smaller Thicknesses

To balance the densities for the 18- and 19-centimeter chests, $\frac{1}{2}$X mAs may be used. For chests that are 14 centimeters, $\frac{1}{4}$X mAs may be employed. For infants (less than 10 centimeters) $\frac{1}{4}$X mAs may be employed, but the kilovoltage should be reduced from 80 to 70 to provide the increase in contrast that may be needed for the chests of these young subjects. It should be pointed out that only *one exposure factor should be changed at a time* when any exposure technique is to be altered. Changing two factors at a time introduces too many variables that are difficult to control.

Table 27-1
TORSO/SKULL CHART

ABBREVIATIONS: GD = Grid
NG = Non-Grid

PROCEDURE	Notes	VIEW	kVp	Ave CM	Total MAS by PART SIZE								
					-6cm	-4cm	-2cm	AVE	+2cm	+4cm	+6cm	+8cm	+10cm
GRID	72"	PA/AP	106	22	1	1.3	2	2.5	3.7	5	7	10	14
CHEST		LAT	116	30	2	2.5	3.7	5	7	10	14	20	26
NON-GRID	72"	AP	80	22	1	1.3	2	2.5	3.7	5	7	10	14
CHEST		LAT	90	30	2	2.5	3.7	5	7	10	14	20	26
SUPINE CHEST 40" NG		AP	80	22	0.6	1	1.4	1.8	2.7	3.6	5.5	7	10
	72"	AP↓Diap	60	22	8	10	15	20	30	40	60	80	120
RIBS / Sternum		OBL↓Dia	64	24	11	15	22	30	45	60	90	120	170
	72"	AP↓Diap	76	22	22	30	45	60	90	120	180	240	340
ABDOMEN /	GD	AP/PA	80	22	6.2	8	11	15	22	30	45	60	90
IVP		30°OBL	80	24	8	11	15	22	30	45	66	90	130
PELVIS / HIP	GD	AP	80	22	6.2	8	11	15	22	30	45	60	90
HIP (Unil or Groin)	GRID	LAT	80	22	6.2	8	11	15	22	30	45	60	90
SACRUM	AP / Coccyx All		74	20	6.2	8	11	15	22	30	45	60	90
	GD	LAT	80	28	11	15	22	30	45	60	90	120	170
		AP	80	22	6.2	8	11	15	22	30	45	60	90
LUMBAR		45°OBL	80	26	11	15	22	30	45	60	90	120	170
SPINE	GD	LAT	80	30	22	30	45	60	90	120	180	240	340
		L5/S1 SP	^90	30	22	30	45	60	90	120	180	240	340
THORACIC	GD	AP	80	22	5	7	10	13	19	26	38	52	76
SPINE	Breathing LAT		64	30	25 mA / 2.5 s		25 mA / 4 sec			50 mA / 4 s		100 mA /4 s	
TWINING C/T	GD	LAT	76	28	10	14	20	28	38	56	78	108	150
CERVICAL	40" GD	AP/Odon	76	13	2	2.5	3.7	5	7	10	15	20	30
SPINE	72"GD	OBL/LAT	76	13	6.2	8	11	15	22	30	45	60	90
	72"NG	OBL/LAT	76	13	2	2.5	3.7	5	7	10	15	20	30
		PA/Cald	80	19	4	5	7	10	15	20	30	40	60
SKULL	GD	LAT	76	15	2	2.5	3.7	5	7	10	15	20	30
		Townes	80	22	6.2	8	11	15	22	30	45	60	90
SINUSES /		PA/Cald	75	19	4	5	7	10	15	20	30	40	60
FACIAL BONES	GD	Waters	80	20	4	5	7	10	15	20	30	40	60
		Lat	75	15	1.5	2	3	3.8	5.6	7.6	11	15	22
AIR CONTRAST		AP/PA	90	22	1.8	2.4	3.2	4	6	8	12	16	24
U.G.I. / B.E.	GD	OBL/SIG	90	24	3	4	5	6	10	14	20	28	40
		LAT	90	30	6	10	12	16	24	32	48	64	96
SOLID-COLUMN		AP/PA	110	22	1.8	2.4	3.2	4	6	8	12	16	24
U.G.I. / B.E.	GD	OBL/SIG	110	24	3	4	5	6	10	14	20	28	40
		LAT	110	30	6	10	12	16	24	32	48	64	96

Table 27-1 (Continued)

EXTREMITY CHART

PROCEDURE	Notes	VIEW	kVp	mAs
HAND		PA /All Fingers	54	2.2
	SFS	OBL	54	2.5
	EXTCAS	Fanned Lat	54	4.5
WRIST		PA	60	2.2
	SFS	OBL	60	3.3
	EXTCAS	LAT	60	4.5
FOREARM	SFS	AP	64	2.2
	EXTCAS	LAT	64	4.5
ELBOW		AP	64	3
	SFS	OBL	64	4
	EXTCAS	LAT	64	6
HUMERUS	SFS	AP	72	2.2
	EXTCAS	LAT	72	3.6
TOES	SFS/EXT	All	60	2.2
FOOT		AP	64	2.5
	SFS	OBL	64	3.3
	EXTCAS	LAT	64	5
CALCANEUS	SFS	PD	68	7
	EXTCAS	LAT	68	3.6
ANKLE	SFS	AP/OBL	64	5
	EXTCAS	LAT	64	5
LEG	SFS	AP	68	5
	EXTCAS	LAT	68	5
TABLETOP KNEE	EXTCAS	AP	70	5
		LAT	70	5
TBLTOP KNEE REG		All	70	0.8
BUCKY KNEE	GD	AP/OBL	70	5
		LAT	70	5
FEMUR	GD	AP / LAT	76	12
HIP	GRID	FRG/GROIN	80	14
SHOULDER	GD	AP/Transax	76	6
		Transthoracic	90	15
CLAVICLE	GD	AP/PA	74	6
SCAPULA	GD	AP	74	6
		LAT	74	10

ABBREVIATIONS: GD =Grid, NG =Non-Grid, SFS =Small Focal Spot, EXTCAS =Extremity Cassette, REG =Regular Cassette, PIGOST = Pig-O-Stat${}_{TM}$

FACIAL CHART

PROCEDURE	Notes	VIEW	kVp	mAs
MANDIBLE	GD	PA	76	8
		OBL LAT	66	8
	NON-GRID OBL LAT		60	5
ORBIT Rheese	GD	PA OBL	76	5
SINUSES	GD	SMV	80	15
ZYG. ARCH	EXTCAS	SMV	62	2
NASAL BONE	EXTCAS	LAT	54	2

PEDIATRIC CHART

PROCEDURE	Notes	VIEW	kVp	mAs
"PREMIE" CHEST	40" NG	AP	54	0.6
		LAT	54	0.6
INFANT CHEST	40" NG	AP	60	1
		LAT	68	1
2-YEAR CHEST	72" PIGOST	PA	66	1.5
		LAT	76	1.5
6-YEAR CHEST	72" NG	PA	70	2
		LAT	80	3
ABDOMEN / IVP / PELVIS SPINES	INFANT NG		62	1.5
	2-YEAR GD		68	4
	6-YEAR GD		74	8
CERVIC. SP	2-YEAR	All	64	2
SKULL (PA/AP)	INFANT NG		62	1.5
	2-YEAR GD		68	3.5
	6-YEAR GD		74	5
UPPER EXTREMITY	INFANT EXTCAS		54	0.5
	2-YEAR EXTCAS		58	0.7
	6-YEAR EXTCAS		62	2
LOWER EXTREMITY	INFANT EXTCAS		58	0.5
	2-YEAR EXTCAS		62	1
	6-YEAR EXTCAS		66	2

EXERCISE #21
Constructing a Manual Technique Chart

===

INSTRUCTIONS: Assuming that the listed technique was good, complete the rest of the chart using proportional anatomy and the 4 cm rule of thumb.

Procedure	Projection	kVp	Ave CM	MAS						
Lumbar Spine	AP	80	22	18 cm	20 cm	**22 cm** **16**	24 cm	26 cm	28 cm	30 cm
	Oblique	80	26	22 cm	24 cm	**26 cm**	28 cm	30 cm	32 cm	34 cm
	Lateral	80	30	26 cm	28 cm	**30 cm**	32 cm	34 cm	36 cm	38 cm
Skull	PA	76	19	15 cm	17 cm	**19 cm**	21 cm			
	Lateral	76	15	11 cm	13 cm	**15 cm**	17 cm			
Shoulder	AP	76	14	10 cm	12 cm	**14 cm**	16 cm			
Knee	AP	70	12	8 cm	10 cm	**12 cm**	14 cm			

Other Formats for Technique Charts: Referring to the completed mAs chart for a wrist series fill in the variable time chart and variable kVp chart:

Procedure	KVP	mAs for each view		
WRIST	60	PA	OBL	LAT
		5	7.5	10

VARIABLE KVP CHART

Procedure	mAs	kVp for each view		
WRIST	5	PA	OBL	LAT

VARIABLE TIME CHART

Procedure	KVP	mA	Time for ea. view		
WRIST	60	200	PA	OBL	LAT

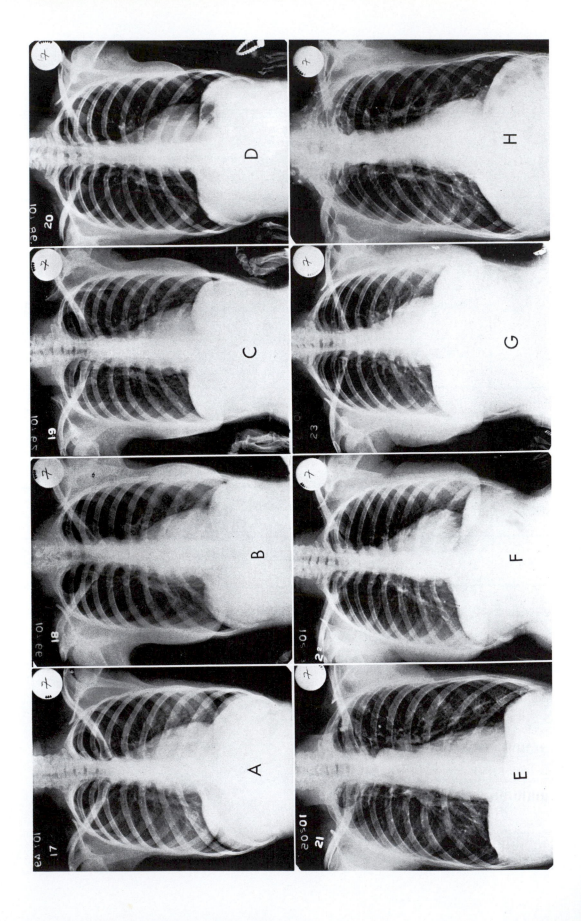

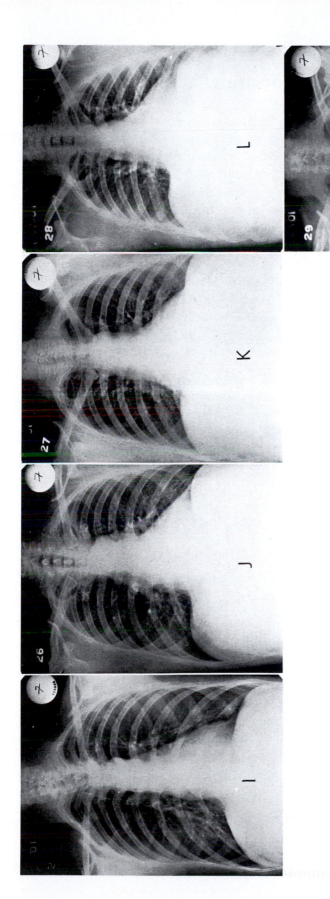

Figure 27-1. Standardized chest techniques for various patients using a technique chart. Note consistency of results.

FORMATS FOR TECHNIQUE CHARTS

Formats for making a technique chart are as varied as the individuals who use them. Charts can be made using index card boxes with a card for each procedure, using a drawing of the body in frontal and lateral views with the techniques written near each part indicated, using a loose-leaf "flip chart," or using a table or grid lined out on paper.

Some useful observations may be made, however, which apply to any chart: First, standardizing the optimum kVp and mA for a given procedure, as discussed in Chapter 25, is necessary for building a chart. A table only accommodates two variables, one for the rows, one for the columns. One of these variables must be body part thickness, usually listed at the tops of the columns. The rows can then be used for exposure time or total mAs, but not for all three technique factors (kVp, mA, and time). Second, optional notes must be condensed so that the chart does not become cumbersome. For example, use one column for notes such as "extremity cassette," "bucky," "small focal spot," etc. And third, the chart must be broken down for different body part thicknesses on *any torso anatomy*, such as lumbar spines, barium enemas and chests. It is suggested that a new column be made for every change of 2 *centimeters* in part thickness, as shown in Table 27-1.

Table 27-1 presents a sample completed technique chart using these concepts. Also examine this chart for comparison with the proportional anatomy rules of thumb listed in Chapter 26. A blank chart is found in Appendix I, which may be useful for you to copy.

Finally, note that no chart attached to a wall will help you on a *mobile* procedure! *Every radiographer should carry a "portable" technique reference* in the form of a telephone/address booklet or a similar pocket-sized book. Simply list procedures alphabetically, and make a note of techniques that work as you learn them from experience. Mobile equipment often requires techniques that are very different from those used in the department. If it works, write it down!

Table 27-2

LIST OF PHYSICAL CHARACTERISTICS OF THE PATIENTS WHOSE RADIOGRAPHS APPEAR IN FIGURE 28-6

Radio-graph	Thick-ness (CM)	Sex	Age (Years)	Height (Inches)	Weight (Lbs.)
A	17	F	20	65	105
B	18	F	24	63	110
C	19	F	29	60	101
D	20	F	22	63	107
E	21	M	61	67	135
F	22	F	21	58	132
G	23	F	24	60	123
H	24	M	60	68	165
I	25	M	34	63	130
J	26	M	60	67	173
K	27	M	55	67	199
L	28	M	36	70	206
M	29	M	60	69	193

AUTOMATIC EXPOSURE TECHNIQUE CHARTS

The use of automatic exposure controls (phototimers) does *not* preclude the need for technique charts! For each projection and anatomical part, optimum kVp must be listed for adequate penetration, the correct configuration of the photocells (which ones to activate) must be given, the density control setting must be specified, and the recommended back-up time stated. An optimum mA should also be stated, high enough to minimize motion, but not so high that exposure times are reduced beyond the response time for the detectors, as discussed in Chapter 28. Additional notes may needed.

Table 27-3 is a sample technique chart written for an automatic exposure unit. Note that in addition to the above mentioned factors, columns are also provided for focal spot size and distance. The *minimum* information for such a chart would included kVp, back-up time or back-up mAs, detector configuration, and density control setting for each projection. Measurement of the patient is not required for automatic exposures.

SUMMARY

1. *Technique charts* should be used in every radiology department. They have been scientifically proven to reduce *patient exposure.*
2. The *proper use* of charts includes initial and ongoing input from the staff radiographers as a group, strict enforcement by administrative technologists and quality control of equipment and processing.
3. A first draft of a complete technique chart may be developed from only one or two test exposures using the guidelines and methods found in preceding chapters. Only minor adjustments to such a chart would be needed in use.

The *development* of technique should be a *systematic* approach, not a trial-and-error approach.

4. *Calipers* must be used by radiographers to measure patients so that technique charts are utilized properly. This is required by law in some states.
5. Technique charts with *measurement columns* (for torso anatomy) should be organized with a technique listed for every change in part thickness of 2 cm.
6. Every radiographer should carry a *pocket-book technique chart* for personal reference.
7. Technique charts are also necessary for *automatic exposure controls.*

REVIEW QUESTIONS

1. Describe two reasons why a radiographer might claim that a certain technique chart "does not work" when in fact there is nothing wrong with the chart itself:
2. What is the *most important* reason for utilizing technique charts instead of relying on intuition or memory?
3. Describe three of the things that an administrative technologist must have done in a department in order to ensure the reliability and proper use of

Table 27-3
BUCKY AUTOMATIC EXPOSURE CONTROL GUIDE

Based on: Three Phase Generator (12:1 Grid: A 200 Speed Film/Screen Combinatoin)

ANATOMY	Projection	kVp	Dist	MILLIAMPERAGE Suggested	MILLIAMPERAGE Selected	Backup mAs	Detector Selection	Master Density Selection	Focal Spot Small	Focal Spot Large
SKULL	All	80	40"	200		100		(N) Normal	✓	
SKULL	Basilar (SMV)	86	40"	200		100		N	✓	
SINUSES	All (cone)	80	40"	200		160		N	✓	
SINUSES	SMV (cone)	86	40"	200		160		N	✓	
FACIAL BONES	All (cone)	80	40"	200		100		N	✓	
OPTIC FORAMEN	Rhese (cone)	80	40"	200		100		N	✓	
NASAL BONES	Waters (cone)	80	40"	200		100		N	✓	
NASAL BONES	PA Caldwell (cone)	80	40"	200		100		N	✓	
MANDIBLE	PA (cone)	80	40"	200		50		N	✓	
MANDIBLE	Lat (cone)	70	40"	200		50		N	✓	
MASTOIDS	All (cone)	76	40"	200		100		N	✓	
CERVICAL SPINE	AP	76	40"	200		50		N	✓	
CERVICAL SPINE	Odontoid	80	40"	200		50		N	✓	
CERVICAL SPINE	Lat - Obl	76	72"	200		50		N	✓	
THORACIC SPINE	AP	80	40"	500		100		N		✓
THORACIC SPINE	Lat - Obl	76	40"	50		100		N	✓	
LUMBAR SPINE	AP	80	40"	500		150		N		✓
LUMBAR SPINE	Lat - Obl	90	40"	500		150		N		✓
LUMBAR SPINE	Lat L5, S1 (cone)	100	40"	500		150		N		✓
PELVIS - HIP	AP	80	40"	500		100		N		✓
RIBS	AP AD	76	40"	600		100	or	N		✓
RIBS	Obl AD	76	40"	600		100		N		✓
RIBS	AP BD	80	40"	600		100		N		✓
RIBS	Obl BD	80	40"	600		100		N		✓
ABDOMEN - IVP	AP	80	40"	600		160		N		✓
KIDNEY	AP (cone)	80	40"	600		160		N		✓
ABDOMEN - IVP	Obl	80	40"	600		200		N		✓
ABDOMEN - IVP	Lat	90	40"	600		200		N		✓
IVP	AP	70	40"	600 to 1,000		200		N		✓
HIGH CONTRAST	Cone AP	70	40"			200		N		✓
GALL BLADDER	PA	80	40"	600		200		N		✓
GALL BLADDER	Obl	80	40"	600		200		N		✓
GALL BLADDER HIGH CONTRAST	PA	65	40"	600		200		N		✓
GALL BLADDER HIGH CONTRAST	Obl	65	40"	600		200		N		✓
GI — STOMACH COLON	PA - AP	120	40"	400		100		N		✓
GI — STOMACH COLON	Obl	120	40"	400		100		N		✓
GI — STOMACH COLON	Lat	120	40"	400		100		N		✓
ESOPHAGUS	AP	110	40"	400		100		N		✓
ESOPHAGUS	Lat	110	40"	400		100		N		✓
SHOULDER CLAVICLE SCAPULA HUMERUS	AP	76	40"	200		40		N	✓	
SHOULDER CLAVICLE SCAPULA HUMERUS	Trans Thoracic	90	40"	600		180		N		✓
FEMUR	AP	80	40"	100		40		N	✓	
FEMUR	Lat	80	40"	100		40		N	✓	
KNEE	All Views	70	40"	100		40		N	✓	
CHEST	PA	125	72"	400 to 500		50		N		✓
CHEST	Lat	125	72"			64		N		✓
HIGH KVP CHEST	PA	140	72"	400		20		N		✓
HIGH KVP CHEST	Lat	140	72"	400		50		N		✓
HIGH KVP CHEST	RAO	140	72"	400		50		N		✓
HIGH KVP CHEST	LAO	140	72"	400		50		N		✓

technique charts:

4. It is recommended that technique charts for torso anatomy be organized into columns for every _____-cm change in part thickness.

5. What device must be used by radiographers to measure patients so that technique charts are utilized properly.

6. Why should pocket-book charts be kept by radiographers?

7. What three items must an automatic exposure control technique chart include *which are different from manual technique charts?*

8. Below is an incomplete technique chart which has one average technique listed. Assuming that the listed technique is good, complete the rest of the chart:

PROCEDURE	PROJ	kVp	AVE CM				mAs			
				18cm	20cm	22cm	24cm	26cm	28cm	30cm
	AP/OBL	110	22			8				
Barium	35°			22cm	24cm	26cm	28cm	30cm	32cm	34cm
Enema	Sigmoid	110	26							
	Lateral			26cm	28cm	30cm	32cm	34cm	36cm	38cm
	Rectum	110	30							

9. Below is a variable mAs technique chart for a wrist series. In the second chart, given the set mAs as indicated, convert the chart into a variable vKp chart, listing the appropriate kVp for each view:

PROCEDURE	kVp	mAs FOR EACH VIEW		
		PA	OBL	LAT
Wrist	56	5	7.5	10

PROCEDURE	mAs	kVp FOR EACH VIEW		
		PA	OBL	LAT
Wrist	5			

10. Referring to the original variable mAs technique chart for the wrist in #9 above, complete the following exposure time chart *using fractions* (not decimals) which will result in the correct total mAs values:

PROCEDURE	kVp	mA	EXP. TIME FOR EACH VIEW		
			PA	OBL	LAT
Wrist	56	200			

Chapter 28

AUTOMATIC EXPOSURE CONTROLS

AUTOMATIC EXPOSURE CONTROLS or *phototimers* were developed for the purpose of achieving more consistent film densities, reducing repeat rates, and ultimately reducing patient dose. All automatic exposure control devices work on the same physical principles, based upon the ability of radiation detection devices to convert radiant energy into an electrical current.

The two most commonly used types of detectors are the ion chamber and the photomultiplier tube. The ion chamber induces an electrical current when gas atoms are ionized by the impinging radiation, freeing electrons from the gas atoms. These electrons are then attracted to and strike a positively charged anode plate. Continuing to be attracted toward the positive terminal within a circuit, the electrons flow out of the anode plate and down a wire, thus becoming an electrical current.

The photomultiplier tube is similar but adds an additional step in the process: It uses a fluorescent screen to convert impinging x-rays into light. The light then strikes a photocathode which induces an electrical current from the light energy. In either case, the induced electrical current can be used to charge an electromagnet which pulls the main exposure switch open and terminates the exposure.

As remnant radiation from the patient reaches the detectors, the electrical charge induced by them is stored in an electrical capacitor. A device called a *thyristor* sets a maximum charge which the capacitor may hold. When the charge on the capacitor reaches this maximum level, the thyristor allows it to be discharged through the circuit (Fig. 28-1) and the exposure is terminated. The thyristor is preset by a service specialist to always produce the desired density level on the radiographs taken according to the film-screen system being used. If film or screen type is changed, the thyristor must be readjusted.

When a patient is turned sideways, or when larger patients are radiographed, more radiation is absorbed in their bodies so that there is less remnant radiation per second striking the detectors. Hence, it takes a longer time for the capacitor to reach its maximum electrical charge and the exposure time is automatically lengthened until proper film density is achieved.

It should be emphasized that automatic exposure controls only control the *exposure time*, and consequently the total mAs. *Optimum kVp and optimum mA must be manually set by the radiographer when using the AEC*, in accordance with all of the principles discussed in Chapters 5 and 6. If the kVp used is less than optimum for the particular anatomy of interest, this anatomy will be underpenetrated. Assuming that the anatomy is properly positioned over the activated photocells, the sensors will detect a reduction in exposure rate, and the automatic control will allow a longer exposure time to try to compensate.

As explained in Chapter 6, *no amount of*

mAs will compensate for inadequate penetration. The radiograph will therefore come out slightly too light in spite of the automatic compensation. Even if the "density control" knob is adjusted to darken the overall image, with insufficient penetration the mAs required will be excessive, and result in unnecessary patient exposure. This is a particularly insidious problem, because the radiographer is not aware (at least until after the fact) of the final mAs value. Such a practice is both uninformed and unprofessional. The radiographer must know by memory and apply the *optimum kVp* for every procedure, phototimed or otherwise.

Optimum mA must also be set manually for automatic exposures. For "manual" technique, optimum mA was defined as the maximum mA available for a given focal spot size, which does not overload the x-ray tube heat capacity. Defining the optimum mA is actually a bit more complicated for automatic exposure control than it is for "manual" technique, because there is the additional consideration of *minimum response time.*

MINIMUM RESPONSE TIME

All electronic devices require a minimum amount of time and "signal" or input in order to operate. The automatic exposure control is no exception. It takes time, albeit thousandths of a second, for the circuit to detect and react to the radiation received.

Minimum response times vary greatly from one radiographic unit to another and between manufacturers. When a new unit is installed, it is a good idea for the quality

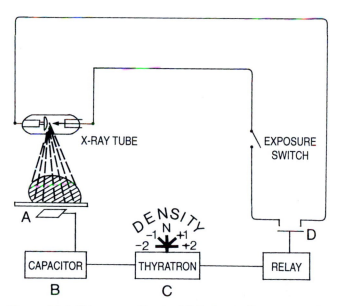

Figure 28-1. Diagram of basic AEC circuit. Remnant radiation penetrating through patient ionizes atoms within the detector cell (A), creating an electrical charge that is stored within the capacitor (B). The thyratron (C) releases the charge on the capacitor when a preset amount is reached, and can be adjusted by the density control. When the electrical charge is released, it flows to a relay which pulls a switch (D) open, thus terminating the exposure.

control technologist to ensure that staff radiographers are made aware of its minimum response time (MRT), especially if this unit will be frequently used for pediatric radiography. Perhaps the best way to ensure this over time is to post it in writing on or near the control panel of the unit. Typical MRTs range from 0.002 seconds for state-of-the-art equipment up to 0.02 seconds for older units.

With extremely high-speed screens, such as 800-speed rare earth screens, the exposure times required for proper radiographic density can be reduced to such an extent that they are too short for the AEC circuit to respond to. The delay caused by the circuit would result in a dark, overexposed image. In such a circumstance, the best alternative is to decrease the mA station used until sufficient exposure times are produced.

It is common for pediatric radiology departments to maximize the efficiency of the overall imaging system by using 3-phase or high-frequency generators and very high-speed screen-film combinations, in order to shorten exposure times as much as possible and thus control motion. Such situations are particularly vulnerable to the risk of overexposure due to the minimum response time. The following example will illustrate:

Let us assume an MRT of 0.005 seconds for a modern 3-phase machine, when using the AEC. To keep exposure times short, the radiographers are in the habit of using the 300 mA station. At the 300 mA station, the minimum total *mAs* this machine can produce would be:

$$300 \text{ mA} \times 0.005 \text{ sec.} = 1.5 \text{ mAs}$$

Suppose that the ideal technique for a PA chest on a child was 65 kVp and 1 mAs. If the radiographer "phototimes" the exposure on this child using the 300 mA station,

the radiograph will turn out dark: The AEC cannot shut off in less than 0.005 seconds—it cannot produce less than 1.5 mAs at this mA station.

Note that in this situation, *adjusting the density control knob to a "minus" setting will not help.* Regardless of the density that it is set to, the machine still cannot respond in less than 0.005 seconds. The solution is to *lower the mA station.* Reducing the mA to 200, the minimum achievable mAs would be:

$$200 \times 0.005 \text{ sec.} = 1.0 \text{ mAs}$$

This is right at the desired technique, and should work if the machine is calibrated accurately. Note that if 0.8 mAs were needed, a further reduction to the *100 mA* station would be necessary. Minimum response time is of concern whenever the following factors compound: High-speed receptor systems, high-power generators, high mA stations, and small anatomy.

Optimum mA for automatic exposure control, then, would be defined as high enough at a given focal spot size to minimize motion, but not so high that the needed exposure times are shorter than the AEC can handle.

BACK-UP TIME

Whenever the automatic exposure control circuit is activated, the main exposure time control, whether a knob or a set of buttons, becomes a "back-up timer" for the AEC. A back-up timer is crucial to prevent extreme overexposure to the patient if some electrical component of the AEC circuit should fail. In such an event, the exposure might otherwise continue until the radiographer realized that something was amiss and released the exposure button. Consider the implications of such an event for patient exposure: If the required time was one-half second, and it took the radiographer 4 seconds to realize, comprehend, and react to the situation, the patient would receive *8 times* the normal exposure. If the required time was $1/40$ second, and the reaction time for the radiographer was an unlikely 2 seconds, the patient would receive *80 times* the necessary exposure. Clearly, a safeguard must be built into the electronic systems.

Fortunately, many recently-manufactured x-ray machines now include circuitry which automatically sets an appropriate back-up time or back-up *mAs* for all AEC exposures. For older equipment, proper back-up times must be determined. The most recommended approach is for the quality control technologist to determine a specific back-up time for each view and have this written on an *AEC technique chart* posted in each room (see the preceding chapter). If it is left to individual staff radiographers in daily practice, they should at least employ some rules of thumb. Both types of information will be presented here.

It is a common practice to simply set the back-up time at 1 or 2 seconds on all procedures. For torso radiography on unusually large patients, the radiographer must be mindful to increase the back-up time to 3 or even 4 seconds. Otherwise, the back-up timer will shut off the exposure before the AEC would have, before an adequate density is produced. The result will be a light radiograph *and a repeated exposure to the patient.*

On the other hand, modern chest techniques, even on adult patients, often require only 2 or 3 mAs for a good image density. Note that using the 200 mA station, 2 mAs can be achieved with an *extremely short* exposure time of only a hundredth of a second (0.01 sec.). In chest radiography, it is not uncommon to find exposure times measured in *thousandths* of a second. Note the implications, then, of the common practice of setting the back-up time at 1 second. Suppose that the average chest radiograph requires $1/100$ second exposure. If the AEC fails to function properly, and the exposure continues to the back-up time of 1 second, the patient will receive 100 times the necessary exposure! *In effect, the patient received an exposure equivalent to 100 chest x-rays in order to obtain a single chest radiograph.* Clearly, when it comes to *chest* radiography, even one second is excessive as a back-up time. The same argument holds for proximal extremities that are "phototimed." A useful rule of thumb for these procedures is to generally set the back-up time at 0.2 ($1/5$) second. (This is 20 times the "average" and thus encompasses even large chests or single-phase equipment.)

Thus, radiographers must be conscious of the two extremes when setting back-up times: chests and extremities on the one hand, which require much less than one second, and torso procedures on very large patients on the other hand, which may require much more than one second. Since most radiographers are not likely to know from memory the specific manual exposure *times* for various procedures, some broad rules of thumb for setting back-up times are useful. These are presented in Table 28-1 and should be committed to memory.

It is better, still, for the quality control technologists to determine *specific* back-up times for *each view*, and write these onto AEC technique charts for each room. To calculate these, a workable rule is to approximately *double the expected manual exposure time* for that particular anatomy, *if the same mA station were used.* For example, if a typical manual technique for an AP abdomen projection were 15 mAs, what

Table 28-1
"RULE OF THUMB" AEC BACK-UP TIMES

All Chest and Proximal Extremities:	0.2 second ($1/5$ sec.)
Average Torso and Skull Procedures:	1 second
Very Large Torso Procedures:	2 to 4 seconds

would be an appropriate back-up time using AEC at 300 mA? The manual exposure time is:

$$15 \text{ mAs} / 300 \text{ mA} = 0.05 \text{ second}$$

An appropriate back-up time then would be $2 \times 0.05 = 0.1$ second. For very large or very thin patients, the 4 centimeter rule can be used to adjust: *Change technique by a factor of 2 for every 4 centimeters change in thickness.* For example, for a very large patient measuring 30 cm through the AP abdomen, double the average technique of 15 mAs in 4 cm steps as follows:

22 cm (average) = 15 mAs
22 cm to 26 cm = 30 mAs
26 cm to 30 cm = 60 mAs

Now find the exposure time required at 300 mA to obtain 60 mAs:

$$60 \text{ mAs} / 300 \text{ mA} = 0.2 \text{ sec}$$

Doubling this figure, an appropriate back-up time for this very large patient would be 0.4 second, or rounding it up, about $1/2$ second. This calculation only needs to be done once for each view, if these specific back-up times are then included on AEC technique charts in each radiographic room. In this way, on a daily basis staff radiographers and students need only follow the charts, rather than determining back-up times case by case.

A common error while using the AEC is to forget to activate the correct *bucky* mechanism, such as when doing a chest at the vertical chest board but leaving the table bucky on. The bucky selection button also activates the AEC detectors for that bucky. In this case, the exposure would continue at the chest board, while the detectors at the table are "waiting" to receive adequate exposure. The result is an overexposed chest radiograph, since the exposure will continue until the back-up timer stops it. Always check all stations at the console before making an AEC exposure, including the bucky selection and the density control to make sure it was not left on a *plus* or *minus* setting from the previous patient.

THE AEC DENSITY CONTROL

A knob or series of buttons labeled *Density* may be found on the console which applies to the AEC circuit. This control increases or decreases the preset sensitivity of the thyratron by specific percentages, so that the exposure time will automatically be extended or shortened by those amounts. There are various formats for this control: Some have only three settings, for small, average, and large patients. In this case the "small" setting will usually cut the exposure time to one-half, and the "large" setting will double it. Others are labeled as $1/2$, $3/4$, N, $1\frac{1}{2}$, and 2. The "N" represents "normal" or average, $3/4$ would be a 25 percent decrease, and $1\frac{1}{2}$ would represent a

50 percent increase as expected. The most common format is to have seven settings which may be labeled 1 through 7, or -3, -2, -1, N, +1, +2 and +3, or in some cases there is no labeling but symbols showing a bar or light that becomes wider to indicate an increase and narrower to indicate a decrease. In this format, each station usually represents a *25 percent increase or decrease* in technique. For example, the +2 setting would indicate a 50 percent increase in technique (two 25% sets), *not a doubling of technique.*

When using the density control, it is essential to remember rules of thumb used for manual technique change, especially the rule of thumb for *minimum density change* discussed in Chapter 5: *Technique must be changed at least to* $^3/_4$ *or to* $^4/_3$ *the original in order to see a visible difference image density. Always increase technique by at least one-third, or decrease it by at least* $^1/_4$. In this regard, note that if the AEC density control is formatted in steps of 25 percent, *the +1 station or 25 percent increase may not darken the film enough to even see a visible change.* This is illustrated in Figure 28-2: Note that the radiograph exposed using the +1 setting (B) is not visibly darker than the radiograph exposed with the "N" setting on this machine. On the other hand, the -1 setting (A) did result in a visibly lighter exposure.

In Chapter 5, it was recommended that one generally increase mAs by 50 percent to obtain a darker image. On AEC density controls that are formatted in 25 percent steps, this corresponds to the +2 setting. As with manual technique, so with AEC: Often additional repeats are caused by being too timid and not changing the technique enough. To obtain a darker film, it is recommended that you skip the +1 (or 1 $^1/_4$) station, and go straight to the +2 (or 1$^1/_2$) station. To obtain a lighter image, the

-1 or $^3/_4$ station will usually result in a visibly lighter radiograph. As with manual technique, when a radiograph is *substantially too light or too dark*, it is advisable to adjust technique by a *factor of 2*, doubling it or cutting it to one-half.

As long as the AEC circuit is functioning properly, the density control should only need to be used infrequently. Constant adjustments are indicative that the AEC is being misused by the technologist or that there is a calibration problem with the equipment. For example, always setting it to +1 for oblique positions and +2 for lateral positions most likely indicates poor positioning: The AEC should normally compensate for the differences in thickness between these views. However, if sloppy positioning on oblique L-Spines causes them to frequently be off-centered by just one inch, this error alone is enough to cause the radiograph to turn out too light. (Almost one-half of the center detector would lie under soft tissue rather than bone, and the density produced will be a compromise between these two tissues (Fig. 28-10). The solution is not to get into the habit of using the +1 density setting, but rather to improve one's centering skills for the oblique position. The density control should generally not be used for changes in part thickness, nor to compensate for adjustments in kVp.

It *is* appropriate to adjust the density control up or down when the position and configuration of the detector cells cannot be adapted to placement of the anatomy of interest. For example, on a unilateral "frog-leg" position of a hip, a problem is created by the fact that the acetabulum and head of the femur, which must be demonstrated dark enough on the film, are not near the center of the film. When the center detector cell is activated, it will produce a good density in the femoral neck area that lies

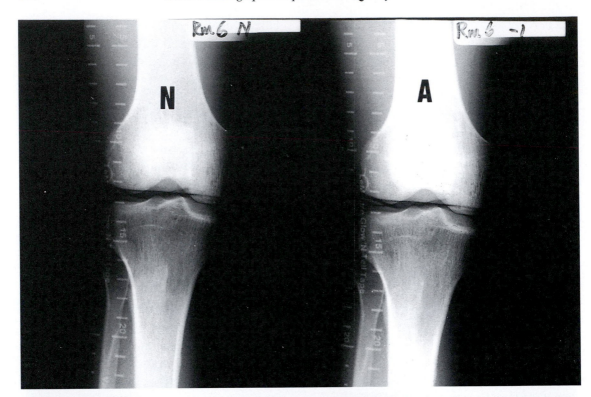

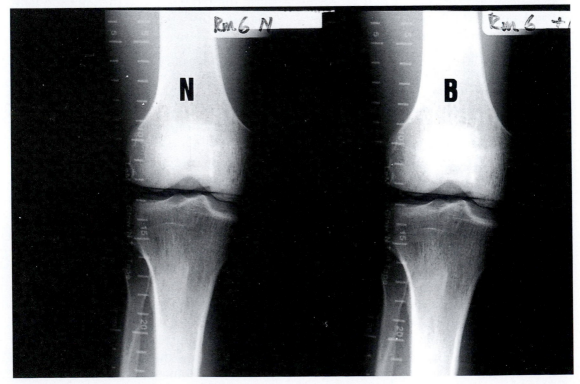

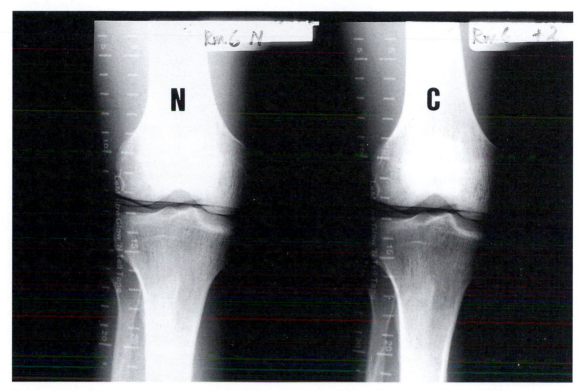

Figure 28-2. Demonstration that the minimum density change rule also applies to AEC exposures: Compare each set of radiographs by observing the middle of the upper tibia. Note that in radiograph A, using a density control setting of -1 (a 25% decrease in exposure), is just visibly lighter than radiograph N, but in the following set the +1 setting (a 25% increase in exposure) *did not produce a visibly darker image in* B. In the third set, radiograph C was produced at the +2 setting (a 50% increase in technique), and produced a visibly darker film. An increase of at least $^1/_3$ or 30% is required to ensure a visibly darker image.

over it, but frequently the acetabulum and femoral head area will turn out too light because this anatomy lies in a corner of the film rather than over the detector. When using manual technique, we generally settle for the neck area being a bit dark in order to have the acetabulum area dark enough. Selection of the +2 density setting (a 50% increase) will often darken up the acetabulum area enough without overexposing the neck area to an unacceptable degree.

Another example would be "phototiming" a smaller pediatric chest, perhaps on a six-year-old: If the two side detectors are used on this small a chest, there is often a risk that the upper portions of the cells might extend above the shoulders of the child, thus being exposed to the "raw" x-ray beam, and shutting the exposure off too early, resulting in an underexposed film. This problem is precluded by activating the center cell only, but since this cell lies over the heart and spine, the resulting image would likely be too dark in the lung fields. A minus-2 setting would correct this.

When equipment is out of calibration, the density control can provide a *temporary* coping tool while waiting for service. The density control *itself* can be out of calibration, and there is a simple way for a radiographer to check this: Most AEC units include a digital mAs indicator on the console which reads out the actual total mAs used *after* the exposure is completed. No film is required, but a knee, skull, or torso phantom, or some other absorber to simulate a body part, is needed. For a knee phantom, select the "knee" button or setting on a preprogrammed machine. Take an automatic exposure of the phantom part without any film in the bucky, with the density control set to "N." Immediately after the exposure, write down the digital mAs readout. Do the same for all density control settings, without changing any other variables. Now for each *plus* or *minus* setting, perform the following calculation:

$$\frac{N - A}{N} \times 100$$

where *N* is the mAs readout for the "N" setting, and *A* is the mAs readout for the plus or minus station. This calculation will yield the percentage by which the technique was changed up or down from "N."

Observe the following results for one modern machine tested by the author:

+1 = +17%	-1 = -14%
+2 = +42%	-2 = -51%
+3 = +75%	-3 = -67%

It seems clear that this machine was designed for each setting to be an increment of 25 percent; The -2 and the +3 settings fit almost exactly. The +2 setting falls 8 percent short of a 50 percent increase, and the -3 setting falls 8 percent short of a 75 percent decrease. Most interesting, though, are the +1 and -1 settings: The +1 setting is only increasing technique by 17

percent, only ²⁄₃ of the expected 25 percent. It has already been said that a 25 percent increase may not be visible—a 17 percent increase would certainly not be. The -1 setting is the most inaccurate; it is 44 percent off! This 14 percent reduction in technique may well not be visible either. Radiographers using this machine would do well to go right to the +2 or -2 settings when needed.

On another machine tested by the author, it was discovered that the -2 and -3 settings actually *increased* the mAs readouts to almost double! Radiographers using these stations would be guaranteed to have to take yet another repeat. This should serve as a wake-up call to radiographers and quality control technologists alike: Density controls can be and often are out of calibration. The procedure to check them is easy to do and well worth the short time it takes. Stations that are far out of calibration could be marked to avoid use until a service technician corrects the problem.

The AEC circuit is automatically engaged when the machine is set for spot-filming. Overhead radiographs may also be phototimed at the option of the radiographer. In many procedures, the use of the automatic exposure control will reduce repeat rates and improve radiographic quality and consistency. Nonetheless, there are many limitations to automatic exposure controls, and unknowledgeable use of them can actually cause higher repeat rates on some procedures.

LIMITATIONS OF AEC

Automatic Exposure Controls are used by some radiographers as an escape from the mental work needed to set manual techniques. Patient dose has indeed been reduced in many procedures. But AECs were not intended to be used on *all* procedures, and radiographers who use them inappropriately actually increase their repeat rate and overexpose patients. The major technique constraints on using AECs

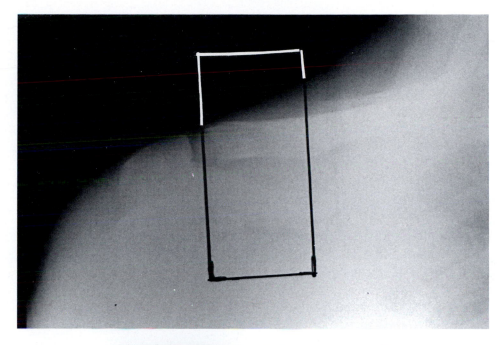

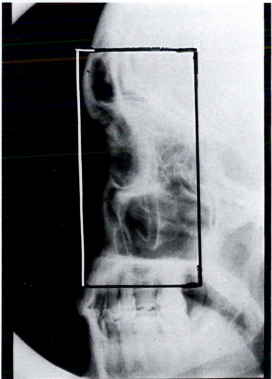

Figure 28-3. Automated exposure of (*top*) clavicle with upper portion of detector cell exposed to the raw x-ray beam, and (*bottom*) lateral sinus with portion of detector cell exposed to raw x-ray beam near bridge of nose, both resulting in underexposure.

are:

1. AECs should never be used on anatomy that is too small or narrow to completely cover the detector cell. This includes most distal extremities and extremities on small children. Detectors measure the average amount of radiation striking the area they cover. Portions of the detector cell not covered will receive too much radiation and the AEC will shut off too soon, resulting in a light, underexposed radiograph.

2. AECs should not be used on anatomy that is *peripheral* in relation to the x-ray beam, such as the clavicle, mandible or lateral projections of the scapula, sternum, or sinuses. In each of these situations the central ray is centered close to an edge surface of the body part, so that portions of the detector cell may extend beyond the part into the raw x-ray beam. As it averages the measured exposure, the detector cell will terminate the exposure early, resulting in a light radiograph (Fig. 28-3).

3. Even when automated exposure is used for proper applications, positioning and centering must be perfected within the limits of human ability. For the correct density level to be produced, *the detector(s) used must be covered with the anatomy of interest,* not just covered with any anatomy (Figs. 28-4 & 28-10). The *tissue of interest* must cover most of the collective detector area. For example, using the two side photocells for the PA chest radiograph, centering must not be so low that the cells overlap abdominal tissue below the diaphragm (Fig. 28-5), or a dark density will result.

Perhaps the single most common cause of repeated AEC exposures is *centering the bucky and film too low for PA chest projections.* This is especially common on short patients, and is probably due to the fact that so many radiographers center chests in terms of where the *top of the film and the top*

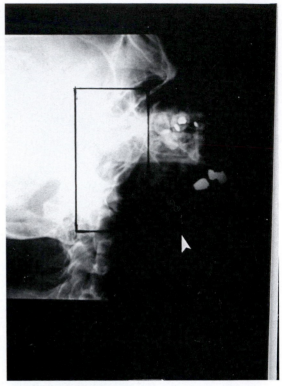

Figure 28-4. Automated exposure attempted for a lateral-oblique mandible. Detector cell is over thicker skull anatomy, so that mandible is grossly overexposed (arrow).

edge of the field light fall in relation to the patient's shoulder shadows, rather than in terms of the cross-hair indicator for the central ray. Suppose you form the habit of allowing one inch of field light above the shoulders: On a short or a small patient, the lung field will not be as long, and leaving the same amount of light above the shoulders will result in both the central ray and the detector cells effectively being centered lower in relation to the *diaphragms* (Fig. 28-5). If even the bottom one inch of the detector cells extends below the diaphragm, the cells will be recording abdominal tissue and will average the density between the abdominal tissue and the lung fields. This results in a longer exposure and an overexposed image. Figure 28-

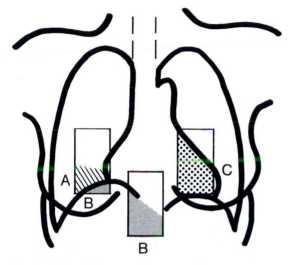

Figure 28-5. Diagram of the critical importance of superior-inferior centering during AEC chest radiography: Centering even an inch low may place the detector cells over (A) thicker breast tissue and (B) abdominal tissue below the diaphragm, and (C) more heart tissue, all of which darkens the radiograph. Simply by centering higher the radiograph will be significantly lightened, as shown in Figure 28-6.

6 demonstrates how much lighter the exposure will result solely by allowing more film above the shoulders so that the detector cells are completely over the lung/heart field. There was no adjustment in technique between these two radiographs, only the change in centering.

Centering *even one inch* low on a PA chest projection can make enough difference to cause a repeat. This is because there are *three* different tissue factors which all compound with low centering: First, the position of the diaphragm is critical. Centering low may place a portion of the detector cells over abdominal tissues below the diaphragm. There is such a great difference between abdominal tissue and lung tissue that even a small amount of abdominal tissue over the cells will significantly darken the exposure. Note also that if the patient takes poor inspiration, the diaphragms will be higher and worsen the situation. A good

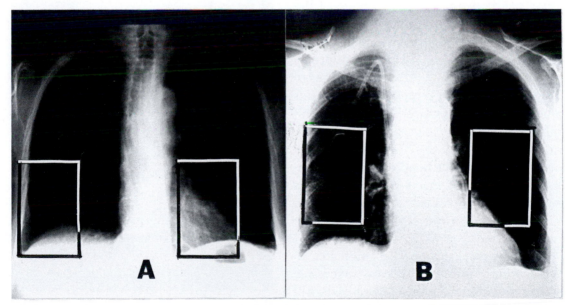

Figure 28-6. Automated PA chest exposures illustrating the significance of the density change caused by simply centering higher, as diagrammed in Figure 28-5. In (A) overexposure resulted from the detector cells lying partially over abdominal tissue below the diaphragm and over too much heart tissue. Note how much lighter the repeat (B) resulted, when the only correction made was to center about 1 $^1/_2$ inches higher (technique was not changed).

inspiration is essential.

Second, the amount of heart tissue over the left detector cell is a very significant factor. There is almost always some heart "shadow" over the left cell, but centering one inch low can result in one-half of this entire cell being covered with cardiac soft tissue. Note here that many patients have a condition of cardiomegaly which can place the upper border of the ventricles an inch higher than normal. If the patient has an enlarged heart, *and* the chest board is centered one inch low, the bulk of the left detector cell might fall under heart tissue. Third, on female patients, centering low places the detector cells under thicker portions of the breasts. For patients with pendulous breasts, centering even one inch low can make a significant difference in tissue thickness affecting *both* side cells. When using the AEC for chest radiography, technologists must constantly bear all three of these factors in mind: Breast tissue, the effect of the heart, and the location of the diaphragm, in respect to the detector cells.

4. As shown in Figure 28-10, demands of positioning for some phototimed procedures are *not* within the reasonable limits of human ability. Off-centering adjustments attempted for such procedures might result in an unacceptable projection of the anatomy (e.g., "closed joints," superimpositions or distortion), or in unacceptable collimation adjustments. *Proper positioning should never be compromised* for automated exposures. In such cases, manual technique must be employed.

5. The x-ray field must be collimated to the anatomy of interest, because excessive scatter radiation from the table or body will also cause the AEC to shut off prematurely.

6. The AEC should never be used when there is any type of radiopaque surgical apparatus, orthopedic corrective devices, orthodontic dental work, or other artifacts which cannot be readily removed from the area of interest. Figures 28-7 and 28-8 show two classic examples of this problem, both of which resulted in gross overexposures. In Figure 28-7, not only is there bridge work but also a metal tooth over the detector cell. As the AEC averages the exposure from the surrounding tissues with these areas where virtually no radiation is reaching the cell, it stays on too long and the odontoid anatomy is overexposed. In Figure 28-8, the AEC stays on for an extended time as it attempts to achieve some shade of gray under a radiopaque hip pin, resulting in an excessive exposure to the bones of the femur and pelvis.

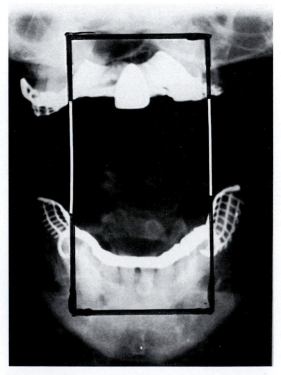

Figure 28-7. Automatic exposure of odontoid projection with dental hardware absorbing beam. The detector cell increased exposure time in an attempt to average the densities between the dental work and the anatomy, resulting in overexposure to the spine.

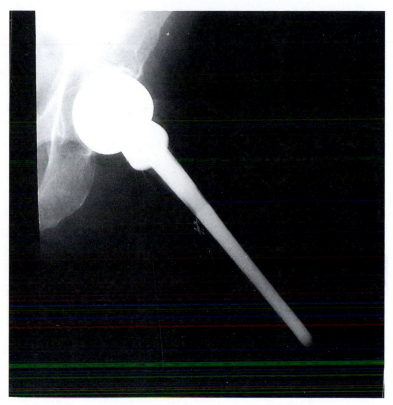

Figure 28-8. Automatic exposure of hip with surgical pin present. As the AEC attempts to produce a density under the pin, the surrounding anatomy is overexposed. Manual technique should be used on all patients with previous hip surgery.

Radiographers must be conscientious enough to screen patient's charts and x-ray requisitions, and to verbally communicate with the patient regarding the presence of any surgical, orthopedic or orthodontic hardware prior to radiographing the patient.

Given these various technical constraints on the employment of automatic exposure controls, it is recommended that they be used primarily for procedures in the trunk of the body, the femurs, neck and cranium. They should never be used for mastoids, mandibles, distal extremities or other complex, peripheral or small anatomy.

7. Automated exposure should never continue to be used when repeating a radiograph unless the radiographer fully understands the cause of the improper density on the first attempt and is confident in the adjustment needed. If there is any uncertainty in analyzing the initial radiograph, manual technique should be used for the repeated exposure. If further repeats are necessitated, the manual approach will assure predictability which automatic exposure control cannot provide.

DETECTOR CELL CONFIGURATION

The location of the detector cells is often demarcated by a triad of rectangles drawn on the radiographic tabletop or on a wall-mounted Bucky mechanism (Fig. 28-9). Sometimes it is demarcated by dark lines in the field light, projected from a plastic insert in the collimator. For this type, the indicated size of the cells will be accurate *only* at a specified distance (usually 72 inches for chest units).

Figure 28-9. Typical configuration of detector cells in Bucky mechanism, with center cell lower than two side cells. (*Left*) center cell activated for procedures such as skull or abdomen, (*right*) two side cells activated for typical PA chest, such that cells are covered with *tissue* of interest.

The actual detectors are located behind the tabletop. For older machines, photo-multiplier tubes were placed behind the bucky tray, so as to not cause any artifact on radiographs. To maximize efficiency, this placement required a large hole in the bucky tray and special phototiming cassettes that allowed more of the remnant beam to reach the detectors. The modern development of ionization chambers that are made of extremely thin aluminum allowed such detectors to be placed directly behind the tabletop, in front of the bucky tray and cassette. At extremely low kVp techniques, these chambers can show up as artifacts on the finished radiograph, but are not normally visible with most techniques.

Positioning of the patient for an automated exposure must be done in relation to the detector as well as to the film cassette, in order to assure a proper density out-

come. This means that the selection of the detector cell configuration to be used (e.g., middle cell only, side cells only, or all three), effectively becomes part of positioning.

It should be further pointed out that it is not adequate to position for automated exposures with an eye to simply covering the detector cell with *any* anatomy. *For proper density results, the detector cell must be fully covered with the tissue of interest.* It is frequently said that AEC technique requires good positioning, and this is generally true. But, in some cases the implied positioning skills are unrealistic, and automated exposure should not be attempted at all.

Let us assume, for example, that the lumbar spine is approximately 2 inches in width, and that the detector cells used are also 2 inches wide. Activating the middle cell only, it is easy to secure an AP projection with proper density, assuming that the field light center markings are accurate. For oblique views of the lumbar spine, however, estimating the exact alignment of the

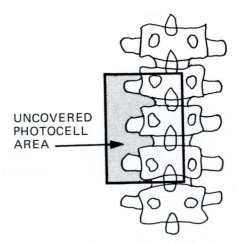

28-10. Diagram showing how off-centering of oblique spine by only 3/4 inch places one-fourth of detector cell outside of tissue of interest (bone). Underexposure will result.

spine with the detector is much more difficult. If the spine were off-centered by *only* *¹/₂ inch*, fully one-quarter of the detector would be under soft tissue rather than bone (Fig. 28-10).

In this soft tissue area, the detector will pick up additional radiation, "assume" that the bone image is darker than it really is, and shut off sooner than normal. A light image would result.

There is no question, then, that radiographers must be much more conscientious about centering of the anatomy of interest exactly over the detector cells used. This requires not only good positioning skills, but a better appreciation of all related anatomy and the relative densities of these tissues. With such an appreciation of the anatomy, there are several parts of the human body where an astute radiographer can become creative with the configuration of the detector cells used, and to great advantage. A classic example is the unilateral "frog" position or Lauenstein method for the hip. This position was discussed in the previous section on the density control. The problem encountered is that, as shown in Figure 28-11, the *anatomy of interest includes the head of the femur and acetabulum of the pelvis*, and that these structures are not normally positioned over the center of the film. Thus, when only the center detector cell is activated, a very nice density will result for the femoral neck area over that cell, but this will often be too light in the acetabulum area.

Observe Figure 28-11 and ask yourself if a *different* detector cell might have been used to achieve a darker image. There are two distinct possibilities: The "side" detector cell which lies more *medially* into the thicker portion of the pelvis could be activated alone, which should darken the image substantially. Or, this medial cell could be activated *in combination* with the center cell to obtain a slightly darker film, where the exposure is averaged between the femoral neck area and the pelvis area (Fig. 28-12). The author's experience is that such a combination does not adequately darken the image, and it is recommended that the medial cell be used alone. In fact, even though using the medial cell darkens the image significantly, it is often *still* not quite enough, and so it is recommended that this cell be used *along with a density control setting of +2.*

The lateral rectum view for a barium enema is another example where one of the side detector cells, the cell lying under the posterior half of the pelvis, might be used to advantage on some patients rather than the center cell. The radiographer must

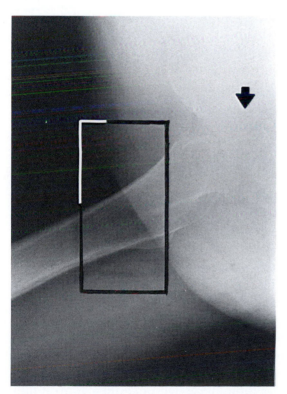

Figure 28-11. Automated exposure attempt for "frog" lateral hip. Anatomy over center detector cell is properly exposed, but anatomy of interest includes femoral head and acetabulum (arrow) which are underexposed.

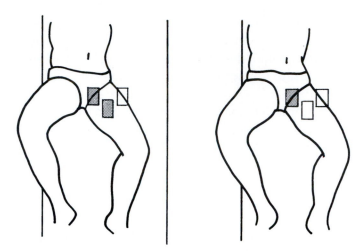

Figure 28-12. Options for resolving the problem demonstrated in Figure 28-11: The detector cell lying *medially* into the thicker anatomy should be activated either in combination with the center cell (*left*) or by itself (*right*). In addition, the density control should be set to +2.

be observant of the position of the cell in relation to the patient's pelvis and be sure that no portion of the cell would extend behind the patient's body. Certainly for most projections the center cell alone should be used. Some confusion may result when considering anatomy such as the stomach which lies predominantly to one side of the body. With proper centering even on a small film, the center cell will be over the barium filled stomach, and the left detector should *not* be used. The same logic applies to a coned-down view of the left ribs. On a lateral L-spine, it is *not* appropriate to use the posterior cell—if the position is centered correctly, the spine should lie directly over the center cell.

Screening chest radiography, which we do so much of, is in fact one area where radiographers can and should be much more creative about cell selection. Probably the most common practice on the PA chest is to activate both "side" cells without the middle cell. Use of *all three* cells results in an exposure averaged between the lungs and the heart tissue, with the

lungs getting "two-thirds of the vote." This provides a chest view that is slightly darker than if the two side cells are used. Do not be intimidated about trying this combination—it is not likely to overexpose the film, and is in fact the preferred configuration in some departments. To obtain views that are slightly lighter, the *right* cell (that is, the cell over the patient's right lung) may be selected by itself. This works well, because typically the left cell is partially covered with heart tissue, and by eliminating that input, the right cell will provide a density base solely upon lung tissue which is somewhat lighter. Again, do not hesitate to employ this method to obtain lighter films—it is not likely to overcompensate. For chest radiography, cell selection provides just the kind of flexibility to meet the individual preferences of radiologists. Without changing the mAs or kVp used, simply use all three cells for radiologists who like their films a little darker, and the right cell only for those who like their films a bit on the light side. For the lateral chest projection, the center cell should always be used, squarely centered within the heart shadow, to ensure that the image will be dark enough when penetrating laterally through two lungs and mediastinal structures.

Table 28-2 is a sample automatic exposure technique chart which includes suggested cell configurations for each anatomical part. Anatomical parts not listed on this chart are not recommended for AEC use—manual techniques should be used on these. For example, the humerus is not listed because the bone is too thin to cover the center cell with the *tissue* of interest. Upright abdomens are excluded as well—they should not be "phototimed." The centering of the upright abdomen is such that the diaphragm is close to the center of the film. Almost no matter which cells are selected, it becomes a guessing game as to which portions of these cells will lie over lung and which over abdomen, and so the resulting density will be unpredictable.

Manual technique skills are still very much needed and will continue to be, for tabletop "extremity" procedures, for decubitus views, mobile radiography, and for those anatomical areas that have been discussed in this chapter which are not amenable to the centering required for automatic exposure. Radiographers must use excellent judgment in deciding when to use the AEC and when to opt for manual technique.

AEC TECHNIQUE CHARTS

In the foregoing discussion, we have seen that the use of AEC does not obviate the need for the radiographer to set technique factors—the only the AEC sets automatically is the exposure time and the resulting total mAs. Optimum kVp must still be set "manually" to ensure adequate penetration and gray scale. An optimum mA station must be selected by considering the minimum response time for the machine, the associated focal spot size, the probability of motion and x-ray tube heat load. The small focal spot should be selected for extremity procedures. An intelligent choice from various options of detector cell configurations and density control settings must be made. An appropriate back-up must be selected for machines that do not do this automatically, such that the patient is protected from excessive exposure in the event of AEC circuit failure. For all these reasons, it makes good sense to construct and use *AEC Technique Charts* for all AEC units. An example of an AEC chart is presented in Table 28-2, showing columns for all of this information. Additional guidance such as the recommended SID or film/screen combination may also be included on charts like this. They are strongly recommended. Appendix II provides a blank AEC chart in identical format, which you may wish to copy for personal use.

TROUBLE-SHOOTING

Whenever an AEC exposure turns out too light or too dark, the radiographer should have a "mental checklist" of possible causes to run down. Table 28-3 presents a checklist of possible causes for overexposure, and Table 28-4 is a checklist for

Table 28-2
AEC TECHNIQUE CHART

PROCEDURE	VIEW	kVp	mA	BACKUP TIME(s)	DETECTOR SELECTION	DENSITY SETTING	NOTES
CHEST	PA/AP	106	200	0.1		N	72"
	LAT	116	200	0.2		N	72"
6-YR CHEST	PA	90	200	0.05		- 2	72"
RIBS ↑DIAPH	AP/OBL	60	400	0.2		-1	72"
RIBS ↓DIAPH	AP	76	400	1.0		N	**72"**
ABDOMEN	AP	80	400	0.2		N	
IVP	AP/OBL	80	400	0.2		N	
G.B. / Coned	AP/OBL	80	400	0.2		N	
PELVIS	AP	80	400	0.2		N	
HIP Unilateral	AP/LAT	80	400	0.2	*■	+2	*medial cell
LUMBAR SPINE	AP	80	400	0.2		N	
	OBL	80	400	0.4		N	
	LAT	80	400	1.0		N	
	L5/ S1	90	400	1.0		N	
THORACIC SPINE	AP	74	400	0.2		N	
	LAT	60	10	5		N	breathing
TWINING C/T	LAT	76	400	0.4		N	
CERVICAL SPINE	AP	76	200	0.2		N	40"
	Odontd	76	200	0.2		N	40"
	Lat/Obl	76	200	0.5		N	72"
SKULL (SINUS) (FACIAL)	PA/Cald	80	400	0.2		N	
	Waters	80	400	0.2		N	
	Townes	80	400	0.3		N	
	LAT	76	400	0.1		N	
Mastoid/Coned	LAT	76	400	0.1		N	
SHOULDER	AP	76	200	0.2		N	
FEMUR	AP/LAT	76	200	0.2		N	
KNEE / LEG	All	70	200	0.1		N	
U.G.I.-A.C.	All	90	400	0.2		N	air con
B.E.-A.C.	AP/OBL	90	400	0.2		N	air con
	Sigm/Lat	90	400	0.2		N	air con

Table 28-3
CAUSES OF DARK AEC EXPOSURES

-Wrong bucky activated

-Needed exposure time *less* than minimum response time (small anatomy, high mA, high screen speeds)

-Density control left on *plus* setting from previous patient

-Electronic malfunction of AEC, (back-up buzzer sounds)

-Incorrect detector cell configuration, such that activated cell(s) lie under tissue *denser* or *thicker* than tissue of interest

-Presence of radiopaque artifacts or appliances within the anatomy (hip or knee prostheses, orthopedic rods, pins, plates, or screws, dental appliances, pacemakers, bullets, etc.)

-Presence of external radiopaque artifacts such as lead sheets or sand bags over sensor

underexposure. When an unacceptable AEC exposure is produced, the radiographer should mentally go through the checklist, identify the probably cause, correct it, and repeat the exposure. If the second exposure is still too dark or too light, further repeats using the AEC *should not be attempted unless the radiographer has confidently identified the cause and corrected it.* If there is any uncertainty about the cause after two exposures have been attempted, the appropriate action is to *revert to manual technique at that time.* Even if a repeat is necessitated after changing to manual technique, only one such repeat should be required. This is better than continuing to "phototime" when there is no clear understanding of the exposure problem, which can lead to a multiplication of unnecessary exposures.

The use of automatic exposure control does not require any less knowledge on the part of the radiographer than does manual technique. Different types of information are needed, but the radiographer must be just as astute. Thus, the modern radiographer must learn *both AEC and manual tech-*

Table 28-4
CAUSES OF LIGHT AEC EXPOSURES

-Backup time shorter than needed exposure time (esp. on large patient)

-Density control left on minus setting from previous patient

-Inadequate collimation (excessive scatter radiation reaching cells)

-Incorrect detector cell configuration, such that activated cell(s) lie under tissue less dense or thinner than tissue of interest

-Detector cells not fully covered by tissue of interest:

　　-Anatomical part too small

　　-Anatomy too peripheral

　　-Specific tissue area too small

　　-Specific tissue area not centered over selected detector cell(s)

nique skills thoroughly, and maintain clinical proficiency in both. Because of the advent of AEC, there is *more* to learn about radiographic technique and exposure, not less, in our school curriculum and continuing education.

PROGRAMMED EXPOSURE CONTROLS

Some modern equipment has been designed to simplify technique manipulation for the radiographer by programming preselected technical factors into a computer-type memory for each anatomical procedure. The control buttons on the console are marked with anatomical drawings rather than numbers. The radiographer first selects the procedure button and then may make a programmed technique adjustment upward or downward by selecting a patient-size button. The patient-size selection available is usually limited to average, small and large. The anatomical programmer may also be overridden so that manual techniques may be selected if desired.

The benefit of programmed exposure controls is their simplicity. The inevitable disadvantage is their lack of flexibility. Just as technique charts cannot be universally applied to all patients without the radiographer's professional assessment of patient status and condition, preprogrammed techniques cannot take into account all of the many variations of habitus and condition that occur.

No amount of computerization or automation can ever totally replace the necessity for the professional judgment of a well trained radiographer.

SUMMARY

1. *Automatic exposure controls* can reduce repeat rates and *patient exposure* on many procedures, particularly in the trunk of the body. They cannot be used properly on all procedures, however, and should not become a *crutch* for radiographers trying to avoid mental work. Such a practice may actually increase repeat rates.

2. Automatic exposure controls should not be used on *complex*, peripheral or very *small anatomy*, as improper density levels will result.

3. When phototimers are used, *positioning* must be perfected, the x-ray field must be properly *collimated* to the anatomy of interest, and the correct combination of *photocells* must be used.

4. Activated photocell detectors must always be completely covered with the *tissue of interest*, not just any anatomy.

5. In unique situations, such as where hardware or prosthetic devices might interfere with the photocell measurements, it is more reliable to use *manual technique* rather than automatic exposure. Whenever there is any doubt regarding the cause of a poor quality automated exposure, manual technique should be used.

6. *Optimum kVp, optimum mA,* and *appropriate back-up time* must be manually set for automated exposures, along with the correct photocell configuration.

7. *Technique charts* are required for the proper use of automatic exposure controls, and should include the information in #6 above as a minimum, along

with photocell configuration, density setting, etc.

8. If excessive mA or receptor system speeds are used, the required exposure time may be less than the *response time* required by the AEC for accurate control.

9. *Density controls* on AECs should be checked periodically for accuracy by noting the readout mAs values at each setting. Most density controls are formatted in increments of 25 percent up or down from average.

10. The *density control* may be used whenever the detector cells cannot be configured so that the specific anatomy of interest is completely positioned over them for proper density, or temporarily when the AEC is out of calibration until it can be fixed.

11. When using high-power generators, high mA stations and high speed image receptors, radiographers must be aware of the *minimum response time* for the machine, especially on pediatric patients or small body parts. Optimum mA will be *low* enough to ensure that the needed exposure time is *longer* than the MRT.

12. When adjusting the *density control*, remember that a $^1/_3$ increase or $^1/_4$ decrease is the minimum change required to see a difference in density. The +1 station may not provide enough increase to be visible.

13. *Back-up time* should generally be set at about double the expected manual exposure time. Quality control technologists should include back-up times on AEC technique charts. As a rule of thumb, use 0.2 seconds for all chests and proximal extremities, 1 second for abdominal and skull projections, and 2 to 4 seconds for very large torso projections.

14. The most common cause of repeats on *PA chest* projections is *low centering* of the film. To avoid this, allow more film above the shoulders on smaller patients. Beware of placing any portion of the cells *below the diaphragm, or over excessive heart or breast tissue.*

15. *Programmed exposure controls* are simpler but less flexible than a standard technique console. They do not replace the need for the radiographer to evaluate each patient for habitue and condition.

REVIEW QUESTIONS

1. Programmed exposure controls were designed to simplify technique. What is their disadvantage?

2. Why does it take the AEC longer to shut off the exposure on a larger patient?

3. A radiographer uses AEC a 6-year-old pediatric chest using the two *side* photocells. Explain why the radiograph might come out light.

4. A radiographer uses AEC an AP thoracic spine using the middle photocell.

Why might inaccurate positioning result in a light radiograph?

5. A radiographer uses AEC an AP cervical spine on a wall-mounted bucky, and uses a 72-inch SID instead of the normal 40 inches. Why will the radiograph NOT come out light?

6. When changing to a new film/screen system, why must the AEC be completely recalibrated?

7. A radiographer uses AEC on a pediatric chest. The detector cells are cov-

ered completely but the field size is left uncollimated much larger than the patient size. Describe how the density of the radiograph will come out *and* why:

8. If any radiopaque prosthesis or hardware cannot be removed from the detector cell area during an automated exposure, how will the image density turn out?

9. How can extremely high speed image receptor systems lead to inaccurate automatic exposures?

10. As a rule, the back-up time should be set at _____ the expected exposure time required.

11. A radiographer repeats an automated exposure that came out too light, increasing the density control setting. The second image turns out light again. What should he/she do next?

12. List four items that an AEC technique chart should include information about:

13. Are there any procedures which should never be "phototimed," even though the positioning skills of the radiographers are high?

14. The needed total mAs for a particular procedure is 0.8 mAs. The minimum response time for the machine is 0.006 seconds. Using AEC at the 200 mA station, will the radiograph turn out light, dark, or correct density?

15. Why might it be a good idea *not* to use the +1 setting (+25%) in order to obtain a darker exposure?

16. How can the radiographer quickly check the accuracy of the density control settings without exposing any films?

17. What is the most common cause of overexposed PA chest radiographs using AEC?

Chapter 29

MINIMIZING PATIENT EXPOSURE

THE ENTIRE FOCUS *of radiographic technique is to produce the best diagnostic image quality at minimum risk to the patient.* The second part of this task is as important in professional practice as the first, and is in fact the greatest justification for the first, since high quality precludes repeated exposures to the patient. The properly educated radiographer has both the concern for the patient and the knowledge to practice good radiation protection.

The implications of technique factors for patient exposure have been discussed in detail in each of the foregoing chapters, so this chapter will only broadly review each of these variables as it relates directly to patient exposure.

MILLIAMPERE-SECONDS (mAs)

The *total* mAs used to produce a radiograph is *directly proportional* to patient exposure. Twice the mAs will deliver twice the skin entrance exposure to the patient. Other factors, such as kVp, distance and screen speeds must be optimized with an eye to keeping mAs levels as low as image quality will allow (for example, without quantum mottle).

It is appropriate to change mAs as needed, however, to obtain proper image quality for different views within a given procedure and for patient thicknesses that vary from average. The alteration of kVp for these two functions can cause inconsistencies in penetration, fog levels and image contrast that may necessitate repeated exposures. Generally, image quality should not be sacrificed as a means of lowering patient exposure, as it can defeat its own purpose. One example of an exception to this rule is in doing encephalo-pelvimetry or fetography, where the primary goal is to obtain a measurement rather than produce a pathological diagnosis: by using high kVp instead of increased mAs, the image will be overpenetrated and fogged, but the measurements can be made, and important fetal dose is saved in this manner. The radiographer should consult with the radiologist in making this decision.

KILOVOLTAGE-PEAK

All other factors equal, an increase in kilovoltage results in a net increase in patient exposure. The higher energy of the electrons striking the anode in the x-ray tube results in more x-rays being produced (see Chapter 6). Since these x-rays are collectively more penetrating, a lower percentage of the x-ray beam is absorbed within the patient, but this effect is not enough to cancel out the added numbers of x-rays produced in the tube. The net result is more exposure.

However, when higher kVp levels are compensated by reducing other factors in order to maintain image density, the net result is a *decrease* in patient exposure. For example, if the kVp is increased by 15 percent, approximately 25 percent more x-rays would normally be produced, having more penetrating power. If the mAs is then reduced by one-half to compensate, the net intensity of the x-ray beam would be about one-half of 125 percent, or 63 percent of the original. In addition to this net loss of x-rays, the increased penetration ability of the rays will further reduce internal dose to the patient. From the standpoint of maintaining image density, *high kVp techniques result in less net patient exposure than low kVp techniques.*

PHASE AND RECTIFICATION

A common misconception is that 3-phase, high-frequency or CPG equipment produces much lower patient exposure because lower mAs values can be used. These designs are more *electrically* efficient in producing x-rays, but compensatory techniques used in practice cancel out any difference in skin exposure. For example, 3-phase equipment produces almost twice the exposure rate of 1-phase for a given selected mAs, and thus requires only one-half the mAs. Exposure times are shorter for 3Φ because there are more x-rays *per second* at the same mAs value. A *slight* savings in patient dose is achieved because of higher average energy levels in the 3Φ beam.

A battery-powered mobile unit also achieves higher average kV levels, but it is common practice to use a set kVp on these machines that is much lower than one would use with a fixed unit, such as 70 kVp instead of 80 kVp for chest radiographs. In practice, the electrical efficiency of equipment has little effect on net patient exposure.

FILTRATION

Protective filtration is designed for the express purpose of reducing unnecessary patient exposure. It does so by eliminating low-energy x-rays that would not make it through the patient to the film, and are therefore diagnostically useless. When filtration levels increase enough to affect radiographic density in the image, such as with compensating filtration, technique must be adjusted upward to restore density, and the net change in patient exposure is nullified.

A minimum of 2.5 mm aluminum filtration is required on all x-ray equipment operating above 70 kVp.

FIELD SIZE LIMITATION

Although limitation of the field size contributes to image quality, it should be regarded by the radiographer as an essential component of good radiation protection practice. Even if mAs is increased by 30-50 percent to compensate for collimation, this is outweighed by the reduction of the amount of tissue irradiated. This is further supported by the fact that highly radiosensitive organs may be spared exposure by collimation. This reduction is on the order of *100 times* less when the exposure just outside the edge of the primary beam is compared to the exposure within the beam. Such a change eclipses any compensatory increase in technique.

Radiographers should therefore be ever-mindful of proper collimation. However, students will learn from experience that *overcollimation* is worse than insufficient collimation. If anatomy of interest is "clipped off" by collimating too tightly, the exposure must be repeated, doubling the exposure to the patient. Because, field lights are not always accurate, a very good rule of thumb is to *always allow at least ¹/₂-inch of light beyond each border of the anatomy of interest.*

Proper collimation is the most effective means for the individual radiographer to control patient exposure.

PATIENT STATUS

For thicker patients, higher mAs values are required to maintain image density, with a correspondingly higher exposure. Additive diseases, casts, and splints also require higher techniques and higher patient exposure. In most cases, these circumstances are outside of the radiographer's influence. *Compression* using a suitable device is one example of an exception where intervention by the radiologist or radiographer can reduce the required technique.

GRIDS AND CASSETTES

It has been traditionally taught that the use of grids results in higher patient exposure. This is generally true, since mAs may be increased to compensate density when a grid is introduced into the remnant beam. But, it should be remembered that the relationship of the grid is an *indirect* one–it is the change in mAs, not the grid itself, that increases patient exposure. The same can be stated for cassette materials which may be more or less radiolucent to the x-ray beam.

IMAGE RECEPTOR COMBINATIONS

Intensifying screens were developed for the purpose of reducing patient exposure. Like grids, screens *indirectly* affect patient dose by allowing a reduction in mAs which is very substantial at high speeds. The usable speeds are limited by mottling effects and loss of sharpness in recorded detail. Within these limitations, *the higher the screen speed, the lower the patient exposure required to produce radiographs.*

Radiographic films are also available in various speeds, and the highest speed should be generally be used *within* the limitations of the gray scale and detail levels required by the radiologist.

Screens must be properly matched with the films they are designed for, as discussed in Chapter 15. Any type of mismatching results in a loss of image density, and unnecessary increases in technique may ensue.

Conversion of a radiology department to "rare earth technology" does not guarantee any reduction in patient exposure levels. Many departments, in order to avoid the rewriting of technique charts, have adopted rare earth screen systems with the same speed index as their older screens. ("Medium" rare earth screens are about equal in speed to "high-plus" speed calcium tungstate screens.) These departments have no basis for advertising state-of-the-art practice. Any reduction in patient exposure hinges upon the actual mAs values used. If these are not reduced, there would seem to be little justification for making a change in screen technology.

Aside from establishing a quality control program, the selection of appropriate screen-film combinations is the most effective means for the technical manager to control patient exposure.

DISTANCES

In practice, distances have no direct bearing upon patient exposure. Any change in SID must be compensated with mAs in order to maintain image density. The compensated technique will always precisely cancel out the inverse square law effects of modified distance, and result in the same net patient exposure.

POSITIONING AND INSTRUCTIONS

Positioning considerations necessary to

proper diagnosis do not frequently lend themselves to modification for protective purposes. There are some exceptions: radiographing the skull with PA rather than AP projections reduces dose to the eye lenses by placing them behind the major volume of tissue, which acts as a natural filter. Male gonadal dose may be similarly reduced for some procedures.

Proper and clear instructions to the patient regarding breathing, swallowing, and holding the position are essential to avoiding repeated exposures. Timing of the exposure, particularly for chest radiographs on small children, is a crucial ability that comes only with supervised practice.

TECHNIQUE SELECTION

In selecting an appropriate technique, the guidelines for optimum kVp and mA and the concepts in Chapter 24 should be followed. Technique selection should be *systematic* and *scientific*. Radiographic technique is *not* an art in the sense of being a creative act of imagination, or a guessing game—it is an art only in the sense of a skill requiring specialized knowledge, and it is a science of estimation.

TECHNIQUE CHARTS

Studies have demonstrated that the proper use of technique charts reduces repeat rates by as much as 30 percent *even when no other quality control methods are used.* The implications for patient exposure reduction should be motivation enough for every radiographer to use charts. Technique charts are fully discussed in Chapter 26.

For the student, it is worth noting that many radiographers who *appear* to set techniques without the benefit of charts are indeed using a chart—they have simply memorized it by repeated use, so that they no longer have to look it up. You can be assured that the techniques they use did not originate in their imagination, but ultimately came from a chart. A chart is simply a written record of what works—why deprive others of this knowledge by refusing to write it down?

AUTOMATIC EXPOSURE CONTROLS

As described in the last chapter, the mere use of phototimers or automatic exposure controls does not guarantee any reduction in patient exposure, and the *abuse* of them can increase patient exposure. Optimum kVp, optimum mA, and an appropriate back-up time must be combined with proper collimation of the x-ray beam and knowledgeable positioning to minimize repeated exposures.

The AEC must be used only for those procedures which fall within its limitations to produce correct radiographic densities—those procedures involving relatively simple tissues, and thick enough, axially located anatomical parts that will properly cover the correctly chosen detector cell configuration. Technique charts should be provided for AEC units.

It cannot be overemphasized that, *when the radiographer is unsure of the cause of poor quality on phototimed radiographs, he or she should immediately revert to "manual" techniques, rather than continuing to attempt automated exposures.* Even if a manual technique results in an additional repeat, the needed adjustment can be predicted with confidence. This is not true of repeats using the AEC. Electrical malfunctions of the AEC are outside the expertise of the radiographer, and attempts to compensate for unfamiliar problems can lead to a string of repeated exposures. This is yet another reason why *every radiographer should be comfortable with manual technique.*

FLUOROSCOPY AND MOBILE PROCEDURES

Protection of the patient during fluoroscopy is discussed in Chapter 33, and only key points will be emphasized here. It must be remembered that true fluoroscopy and spotfilming are two distinct operations. Traditional cassette spotfilming is essentially identical to phototimed "overhead" radiography. Optimum kVp and mA should be used so that exposure time is minimized, and the back-up timer must be set as described in Chapter 27 for phototiming. The control marked "fluoro mA", listed in multiples of 100, is actually the spotfilming mA applied to the x-ray tube under the table. The overhead kVp control becomes the spotfilming kVp and must be set for adequate penetration of the anatomy and contrast agents employed.

For dynamic fluoroscopy, the "fluoro kVp" control should be set to correspond to the spot-filming kVp level. The true fluoro mA is not normally changed and not always accessible, *but the radiographer is responsible for being aware of the actual mA readout when Fluoroscopy is underway. This readout is obtained from the same mA meter that one watches during routine exposures to ensure that the exposure took place.* If this actual value ever exceeds 8 mA, the first reaction should be to increase fluoro kVp if possible. Fluoroscopic kilovoltage should always equal or exceed the optimum kVp for the procedure as listed in Table 6-1. For example, at least 110 kVp should be used for solid column barium studies, and at least 90 kVp for air contrast barium studies. The actual kVp can be much more than this, but should never be allowed to drop below the optimum amount.

Fluoroscopic exposure rates to the patient must never exceed 10 Roentgens per minute measured at the tabletop. This rate can be checked with an ion chamber as described in Chapter 30.

Fixed fluoroscopy units must have a 5-minute timer which sounds an audible signal when this amount of fluoroscopy exposure to the patient has been reached. While the time of fluoroscopy is under the control of the radiologist, *the radiographer is responsible for monitoring fluoro time and for communicating with the radiologist when the recommended limit of 5 minutes is exceeded.* It is strongly recommended for legal and professional reasons that the total accumulated fluoro time for each patient be noted on requisitions or patient records for future reference.

An understanding of this responsibility should discourage the practice of constantly resetting the timer without noting the reading in order to avoid annoyance of the physician. There are at least two reasonable options open to the radiographer: (1) Be sure to be in the control booth when the timer approaches zero, allow the audible signal to begin to sound, but immediately reset it, or (2) reset the timer each time it reaches, say, one minute remaining, *but note the accumulated time, and tell the physician when 5 minutes has been exceeded.* This second approach may be illegal in some states, so consult with administrative radiographers prior to engaging in such a practice.

When the radiographer fluoroscopes a patient, he must use good collimation and remember to bring the fluoro tower down in near-contact with the patient in order to minimize patient dose.

Mobile C-arm fluoroscopes often do not have fluoro timers. The distance from the C-arm x-ray tube and the surface of the patient must never be less than 12 inches.

QUALITY CONTROL

Quality control methods for equipment are discussed in Chapter 30 and those for processing conditions in Chapter 41. Quality control is the use of diagnostic tools to detect trends that will eventually cause repeated exposures to the patient, and correct them *before* such unnecessary exposures come about. By definition, then, *QC* plays a vital role in minimizing patient exposure.

Studies show that radiology departments employing comprehensive quality control programs, with technique charts, processor monitoring and repeat analysis can reduce the number of repeated exposures by 35-50 percent. The budgetary savings of such an achievement, combined with the reduction in patient exposure and increase in professionalism, would seem more than adequate incentive for any administrative radiographer to take heed.

SUMMARY

1. Screen speeds, grids, distances and many other variables only indirectly affect patient exposure, in that they alter the amount of total *mAs required* for proper density results. The mAs is *directly proportional* to patient exposure.

2. *High-kVp, low mAs* exposure techniques reduce patient exposure.

3. Higher *phase* or more electrically efficient equipment does NOT necessarily reduce patient exposure. While lower mAs values are used, the *exposure rate* is proportionately higher for the mAs.

4. At least 2.5 mm of total aluminum equivalency is required as *filtration* in all machines operating above 70 kVp.

5. The most effective way for the individual radiographer to minimize patient exposure is through proper *collimation. Overcollimation* can result in clipping the anatomy of interest and cause unnecessary repeats and patient exposure.

6. The two most effective ways for the technical manager of a radiology department to help reduce patient exposure for routine procedures is to select appropriate receptor systems and to establish a quality control program with technique charts, equipment checks and processor sensitometry.

7. Used improperly, automatic exposure controls can result in increased repeat rates and patient exposure.

8. To reduce patient exposure, fluoroscopy requires the use of optimum kVp just as overhead radiography does.

9. Fluoro timers should be allowed to run out and sound the audible signal when 5 minutes is accumulated.

10. Fluoroscopic exposure rates to the patient must never exceed 10 R/min. as measured at the tabletop.

REVIEW QUESTIONS

1. What effect do high-kVp, low mAs exposure techniques have upon patient exposure ?

2. How much total aluminum equivalency is required as filtration in all machines operating above 70 kVp?

3. The most effective way for the individual radiographer to minimize patient exposure is:

4. The two most effective ways for the technical manager of a radiology department to help reduce patient exposure for routine procedures is to select appropriate _____ and to establish a _____ program.

5. When available, does the use of automatic exposure controls always result in saving patient exposure?

6. To reduce patient exposure, fluoroscopy requires the use of optimum _____.

7. Generally, fluoro timers should be allowed to run out and sound the audible signal when 5 minutes is accumulated, but if the radiographer resets the timer prior to the sound, he/she should at least _____ when 5 minutes has lapsed.

8. The use of technique charts can generally reduce patient exposure by _____ percent.

9. Fluoroscopic exposure rates to the patient must never exceed _____ as measured at the tabletop.

Chapter 30

QUALITY CONTROL

THE REDUCTION of repeat rates in a radiology department has professional, ethical, biological and economical benefits. The objective of all quality control programs is to minimize the repeat rate through ensuring consistency in the quality of radiographs produced.

A complete quality control program has no less than six different components. They include radiation exposure monitoring, radiographic unit monitoring, sensitometry and darkroom monitoring, the use of technique charts, the analysis of repeat rates and continuing education.

RADIATION EXPOSURE MONITORING

All radiology departments should employ a system for monitoring the cumulative occupational exposure to employees who work with ionizing radiation. Thermoluminescent dosimeters or film badges should be provided to all such employees and the monthly dosages posted on a bulletin board.

In addition, many departments also monitor patient exposure to radiation through simple mechanisms as both a patient advisement tool and as a legal precaution. For example, the total fluoroscopy exposure time accumulated during a fluoroscopic procedure can be taken from the fluoro timer and *noted* on patient records. The number of overhead exposures taken for each procedure can also be noted on patient records. Radiation procedure record forms are available from the government which can be given to patients to maintain themselves.

RADIOGRAPHIC UNIT MONITORING

Most of the quality control and fundamental calibration checks for radiographic equipment can be performed by the radiographer. The importance of this kind of monitoring is illustrated in the fact that the radiation output per milliampere has been found to vary as much as 50 percent from one unit to the next within a radiology department and as much as 100 percent between units in different radiology departments.

Tests that are able to be carried out by radiographers such as mA linearity, kVp accuracy, timer accuracy, focal spot damage, alignment, collimation and distance checks should be done monthly or bimonthly. This does not preclude the need for professional backup and additional checks on fluoroscopes and other more complex equipment by certified radiation physicists. It is recommended that all equipment in a department be thoroughly checked by a radiation physicist at least once each six months.

SENSITOMETRY AND DARKROOM MONITORING

This aspect is described in Chapter 41. Most of these functions can be and should be performed by staff radiographers, with occasional backup from processor specialists. When no quality control program is in place, processing errors and conditions account for well over 35 percent of all repeats. All quality control programs should begin with the processor.

USE OF TECHNIQUE CHARTS

Radiology departments using a systematic approach to the development of techniques and enforcing their proper use often reduce repeat rates by as much as 25 percent. Seventy-three percent of all repeats are caused by radiographs coming out either too light or too dark. Part of this is from darkroom and processing variables; the rest is from improper selection of technique. When technique charts are used in combination with processing sensitometry, repeats can be literally cut in half. The con-

struction of technique charts is discussed in Chapter 27.

These tests will be explained in this chapter.

ANALYSIS OF REPEAT RATES

There would be little sense in implementing any other aspect of a quality control program without the benefit of repeat analysis. Table 30-1 graphically illustrates the effect that quality control programs can have on the accountability of both the medical imaging department and the individual radiographer.

The greatest value of repeat analysis lies in the identification of continuing education needs for the imaging staff. By addressing those needs through inservice education, repeat rates can be reduced and patient exposure spared. Education is an integral part of any quality control effort, but the *specific* educational needs of the staff must be identified if it is to be effective.

CONTINUING EDUCATION

There would be no sense at all to monitoring radiographic quality if no intention of acting upon the results existed. When the technological variables are all monitored and controlled, the greatest factor determining radiographic consistency and quality is the skill of the radiographer. The field of radiography is advancing so rapidly, with new image receptor systems, computerization, and whole new subspecialties in imaging techniques, that continued learning should be a matter of survival as well as professionalism.

Every radiology department should explore both traditional and nontraditional methods of encouraging and providing opportunities for the staff to update their knowledge and skills and to better appreci-

Table 30-1
NATIONWIDE RADIOGRAPH
REPEAT ANALYSIS*

Reason for Repeat Exposure	Per Cent of All Repeats for Department Without Quality Control Program	Per Cent of All Repeats for Department With Quality Control Program
Positioning Errors	13	41
Density Too Light	41	18
Density Too Dark	32	15
Blank Film	12	11
Motion	1	5
Other	1	10

*Taken from *Nationwide Evaluation of X-Ray Trends, United States Bureau of Radiological Health.*

ate the plight of the modern patient. Every radiographer must realize that there is no *arrival* at total competency or total knowledge, that certification is not the end but the beginning of growth and improvement, and that there is always somebody else who knows something we could use. Developing an attitude of continued learning leads not only to professionalism, it leads to greater enjoyment and fulfillment in a career.

REPEAT ANALYSIS

The national average repeat rate for all operators of x-ray equipment (registered and unregistered) is about 13 percent. More than one out of every ten radiographs must be retaken. Many radiology departments have succeeded in bringing their overall repeat rates down to 5-7 percent by employing complete quality control programs. Such departments represent the epitome of professionalism in radiography.

The analysis of repeat rates amounts to nothing less than accountability—accountability to employers, to the public, and to ourselves. Repeat rates can be analyzed in a fashion which is not threatening to each individual radiographer. At the end of each month, all of the repeats for the staff as a whole may be sorted according to cause: too light, too dark, positioning error, blank, motion, darkroom error, etc. The staff can then identify the need for in-service education or quality control programs dealing with *specific* areas for improvement. As another alternative, each individual radiographer may be asked to sort and analyze his own repeats for the month, after which the radiographs are discarded. There are several variations possible for a repeat analysis program. Whatever method is used, it provides accountability and a mechanism for continuing professional improvement.

Such analysis has been done on a nation-wide level by the government. The results for departments with quality control programs intact and for those without quality control programs are presented in Table 30-1. Note that where no QC program exists, most repeats are caused by poor technical quality of the radiograph, but where a QC program is used, 41 percent of all repeats (the greatest percentage) are from positioning errors. This places the burden of radiographic quality directly upon the shoulders of the staff radiographer, where it belongs. In a positive way, the staff of a radiology department may then turn their attention to continuing education and the further development of positioning skills by identifying those areas of need. No longer can poor radiographs be vaguely attributed to electrical line surges, unpredictable processors and the darkroom technician. The radiographer is clearly accountable for manipulating the equipment and working with the patient in producing radiographs of high quality.

DETERMINING REPEAT RATES

There are many methods of obtaining repeat rate figures, some more accurate, others easier to implement. There are also several ways of categorizing these figures according to the needs and interests of the department and its staff: The two most useful methods of categorizing repeat rates are (1) by *type of cause*, such as positioning errors versus technique errors; or (2) by *type of procedure*, such as head procedures versus spine procedures. This second method has been largely neglected by texts on quality control, perhaps because it can be threatening to staff radiographers if used by management to "point fingers." Yet, it can be extremely helpful to the *individual* radiographer as a self-analysis which does not have to be divulged to any one else, and thus is included in this discussion.

It should be pointed out as well that *repeat rate studies can and should be modified as needed to target specific problems.* For example, suppose a department doing a monthly repeat analysis by *cause* finds that repeats due to positioning errors are much higher than desired. An analysis *by procedure* is now in order to determine if there is a particular type of procedure with which the staff radiographers are having difficulty positioning. A higher rate in pediatric procedures would be expected, but an unusually high rate in head procedures might indicate a need for some inservice education or sharing of case studies in that area. Having identified a specific category of procedures, such as head positioning, still another modification might be to acquire data for one evaluation period categorizing all repeats due to head positioning errors into categories of improper rotation of the part, improper flexion/extension, improper tilt or abduction/adduction, improper centering or angling of the x-ray beam, improper collimation or artifacts such as markers superimposing the anatomy. Note that the categories used in Tables 30-2 and 30-3 can be exchanged between the two forms.

Departmental Repeat Analysis

To determine the overall repeat rate for a department, there must be a way of ascertaining (1) the total number of views taken during the evaluation period, and 2) the number of films used for repeated exposures during the period.

If an actual film count is not available, the total number of each type of radiographic procedure performed during the evaluation period (a statistic which most departments track) may be multiplied by the average number of overhead views taken for each procedure, as in Table 30-2. For the individual radiographer, or if a log of procedures is not already kept in the department, Table 30-3 may be used. The period of the study must be relatively long, at least one month, in order to provide reliable statistics.

Old rejects must be discarded and a new "throw-away" box or "reject bin" must be started at the beginning of the study period. Some departments keep individual boxes for each radiographer. At the end of the period, count the total number of films in the throw-away box. Subtract those which are green, blank or cannot be attributed to radiographer error, such as sensitometry films or dark room errors as in Table 30-4. Sort and count the remainder according to the desired categories. For example, if categorizing by *cause*, sort those which were *primarily* rejected because they were too light, those that were poorly positioned, and so forth. Many will present more than one problem, and the *primary* cause for the repeat, the most significant error, must be determined.

A "total waste" figure may be of economic interest to management and can be calculated by adding the number of all films in the throw-away box (including green and blank films) to the total number of "good" films used, and then dividing the number of throw-aways by this total of all films used, as shown in Table 30-4. Multiply the result by 100 to obtain a percentage.

For radiographic quality control, the total repeats (after subtracting the number

Table 30-2
REPEAT ANALYSIS: LOG OF TOTAL VIEWS

At the end of each working day, fill in the number of each *type of procedure* performed that day. At the end of the study period, fill in the routine number of views taken for each type of procedure. Multiply the number of views by the number of each procedure done to obtain a total.

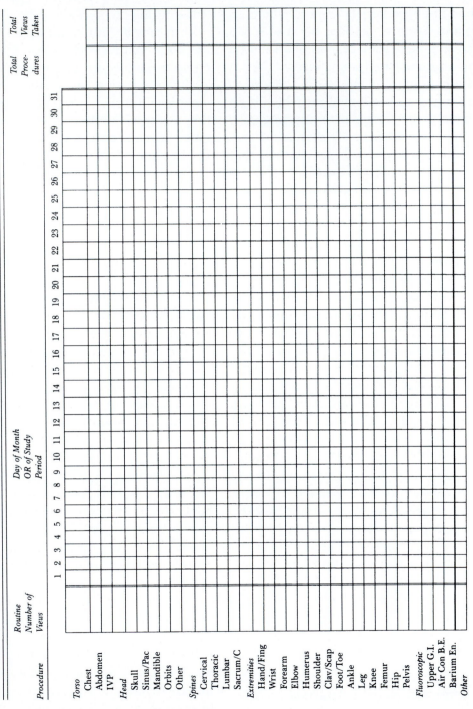

Procedure	Routine Number of Views	Day of Month OR of Study Period																															Total Proce-dures	Total Views Taken
		1	2	3	4	5	6	7	8	9	10	11	12	13	14	15	16	17	18	19	20	21	22	23	24	25	26	27	28	29	30	31		
Torso																																		
Chest																																		
Abdomen																																		
IVP																																		
Head																																		
Skull																																		
Sinus/Pac																																		
Mandible																																		
Orbits																																		
Other																																		
Spines																																		
Cervical																																		
Thoracic																																		
Lumbar																																		
Sacrum/C																																		
Extremities																																		
Hand/Fing																																		
Wrist																																		
Forearm																																		
Elbow																																		
Humerus																																		
Shoulder																																		
Clav/Scap																																		
Foot/Toe																																		
Ankle																																		
Leg																																		
Knee																																		
Femur																																		
Hip																																		
Pelvis																																		
Fluoroscopic																																		
Upper G.I.																																		
Air Con B.E.																																		
Barium En.																																		
Other																																		

Grand Total #
Views for Period

Table 30-3
REPEAT ANALYSIS: LOG OF REPEATED EXPOSURES
(BY TYPE OF PROCEDURE)

After *each procedure performed,* fill in the number of *repeated* exposures taken according to the categories of procedures below. Use more than one log sheet as needed for the evaluation period. At the end of the period, total the repeats in each category, then divide *each* category total by the grand total of all repeats to obtain percentages.

NOTE: "Torso" includes chest, abdomen, and IVP. "Extremity" includes pelvic and shoulder girdles. "Fluoroscopic" includes UGI, BE and air contrast BE.

Type of Procedure:	*Torso*	*Head*	*Spine*	*Extremity*	*Fluoroscopic*	*Other*	
Fill In Number Of Repeats Taken							
							B Grand Total # Repeats For Period (Add All Columns from **A**):
A Totals for Period:							
Percentage of All Repeats: (A/B × 100)							

Table 30-4
REPEAT ANALYSIS BY CAUSE

Name/Department:_____ Period–From:_____

To:_____

Cause	Number of Films	Percentage of All Repeats
1. Positioning Error		
2. Patient Motion		
3. Too Light		
4. Too Dark		
5. Artifacts (including fog, markers, static)		
6. Acceptable Films*		
7. Other		

A. Total Number of Views Taken for Period . . . .: _____
(from Log in Table 30-2, or film count)

B. Total Number of Repeats for Period . . . .: _____
(Sum 1-7 above, OR from Log in Table 30-3, OR total films in throw-away
box minus clear, green, and unrelated films)

C. **OVERALL REPEAT RATE:** . . . .**B/A x 100 =** _____

D. For each category, divide the number of repeats taken in that category by the total number of repeats for
the period (B) to obtain the percentage of all repeats in the last column.

E. Total Waste (total films in throw-away box divided by total films used OR
B + green and clear films divided by A + B + green and clear films) . . . .: _____

*Refers to films of good quality in the opinion of the quality control technologist, which may have been reject-
ed by radiologists or technologists for reasons other than image quality, or where there is disagreements
regarding the acceptability of the radiograph.

of green and blank films) should be divided by the sum of repeats and good films
used for the period. Again, multiply this
number by 100 to obtain the repeat percentage for each category of the analysis as
in Table 30-4.

Individual Repeat Analysis

Potentially one of the most beneficial
uses of repeat analysis is for each individual
radiographer to perform their own. A
department may encourage staff radiographers to do so, and provide the forms, yet
allow each radiographer to keep his/her
own results private. Every radiography student should have the experience of analyzing his/her own repeat rates for a period of
time as a part of their radiography education.

The Repeat Analysis Logs in Tables 30-
2 and 30-3 are particularly suited for indi-

vidual analysis. The log in Table 30-2 is filled in once each day to track the total number of views taken during the evaluation period. Table 30-3 should be filled in on a procedure-by-procedure basis to keep an accurate count of repeated views taken.

By using Table 30-3, the individual is then allowed to discard the rejected films in a collective throw-away box, and does not have to maintain an individual throw-away box, reducing obtrusiveness (threat) and embarrassment.

IMPLEMENTING A REPEAT ANALYSIS PROGRAM

Obtrusiveness refers to the effects of the radiography staff knowing that they are being evaluated upon their performance. When a repeat analysis program is started, obtrusive effects must be expected in the initial stages—repeat rates may increase due to a sense of higher standards, or suddenly decrease from various attempts to manipulate the rate downward. The results are therefore unreliable until the staff has accustomed itself to the program. Some authors recommend not informing staff that an analysis is underway, but suspicions of such activity will cause more severe obtrusive effects than knowledge of the study. To assure reliability:

1. The analysis program should be planned as an ongoing, regular study, not a one or two-time event, and the staff should be told this.
2. Staff must be assured that results of repeat analysis will be used to help meet departmental needs, and not in employment or advancement decisions.
3. The results of the first month should not be used to make any conclusions or decisions—rather, the first period of evaluation should be used as a "practice run". It may be wise to extend this "practice period" to two months. Staff should *not* be told that there is such a practice period, much less when results will begin to be used, or a new obtrusiveness effect will result.
4. After the practice period, baseline data should be accumulated over the next couple periods to which future trends can be

compared. Minor fluctuations must be expected, and only gross deviations from national norms or baseline data should be regarded as "problem areas."

GOALS AND RESULTS

Each department must determine its own goals, but realistically, an overall repeat rate of 5 percent or less should be considered as ideal. Repeat rates above 10 percent in *most* categories (excepting pediatrics, for example) should be considered as problem areas needing some kind of remedial action. Recall that *uncertified* radiographic technicians can achieve repeat rates as low as 13 percent. Certainly, properly trained equipment operators might be expected to achieve rates well below (e.g., one-half of) this amount.

The proper use of the information obtained by repeat analysis is to identify gross trends within the department which substantially deviate from either national norms or from the baseline data obtained for the department and determine corrective action needed for equipment and continuing education needs for staff.

The final column in Table 30-4 calculates the percentage of all repeated exposures attributed to each cause. It must be remembered that as some of these percentages are reduced due to corrective actions taken, other percentages in this column will increase, even though the actual number of repeated exposures for those causes has *not increased.* Such changes must not be misinterpreted as problem areas. The general goal would be for this column to appear roughly in line with column two in Table 30-1. Implementation of a quality control program primarily reduces repeats for technical causes, and is *expected* to increase percentages under the positioning category.

The emphasis should be upon reducing the overall repeat rate, and this last column should be interpreted only in relation to norms, and as a way of identifying trends.

RADIOGRAPHIC EQUIPMENT

TIMER QUALITY CONTROL

The precision of exposure timers has developed a great deal in the last several decades, from spring-wound timers to electronic impulse timers which can measure one pulse of electricity as short as $1/120$ second in duration. Nonetheless, modern exposure timers are found to be inaccurate and requiring adjustment quite often. In the worst situation, for example, the time knob may loosen and slip one notch, so that the actual time set is a whole step away from that actually achieved. Inaccurate exposure times lead to unpredictable technique and a loss of control over image density.

Guidelines for Accuracy

It is suggested that a workable range of accuracy for regular timers would be plus or minus 5 percent.

Test Procedures

SINGLE-PHASE TIMER. Single-phase timers may be checked with a simple manual spinning top (Fig. 30-1). The moving hole in the top records each separate pulse of x-rays from the tube in a different location on the film. Since electrical current flows at 120 pulses per second, simply divide 120 into the number of dots you count on the film to get the exposure time. For example, $1/4$ second should produce 30 dots $(30/120 = 1/4)$ (Fig. 30-2). If the dots are not fully separated, you spun the top too slowly; if the dots complete a circle and begin to overlap each other, you spun the top too fast. (Note: If you should get exactly one-half of the dots you expected, this indicates the failure of a rectifier, not the timer.)

THREE-PHASE TIMER. For a three-phase machine, you cannot use a manual spinning top because the electrical pulses over-

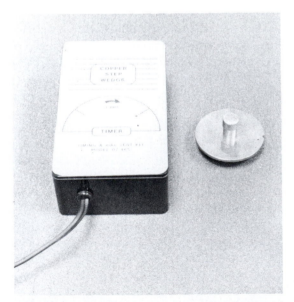

Figure 30-1. Photograph of electric and manual spinning tops used for quality control checks of the exposure timer.

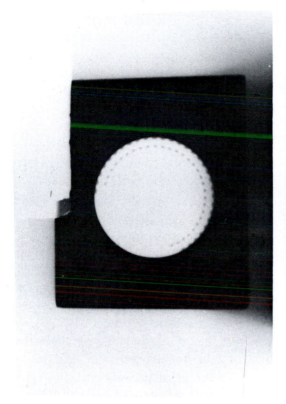

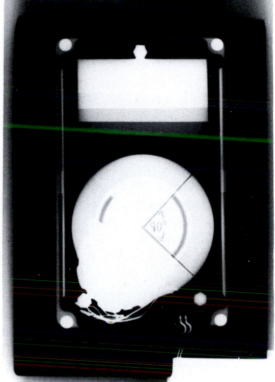

Figure 30-2. Radiograph of manual spinning top test for single-phase machine showing an accurate ¹/₄-second time. Thirty dots equals ¹/₄ of the 120 x-ray impulses per second emitted by the tube.

Figure 30-3. Radiograph of electrical spinning top test for three-phase machine showing an accurate ¹/₄-second time. At a speed of one revolution per second, a 90-degree arc equals ¹/₄ of the 360 degree cycle.

lap. You must use an electrical spinning top (Fig. 30-1) (which can also be used for a single-phase machine). Most electrical spinning tops revolve consistently at 360 degrees (one revolution) per second. A slit in the top records a black arc on the x-ray film. To find the true time, carefully measure the degrees of the arc with a protractor centered to the center of the image of the top. Divide 360 degrees into your measured degrees to obtain the time. For example, ¹/₄ second should produce a 90-degree arc (90/360 = ¹/₄) (Fig. 30-3).

MILLIAMPERAGE QUALITY CONTROL

Milliamperage is an electrical function.

There are normal statistical variations in the generation of electrical current, which may be added to fluctuating demands on electricity throughout the hospital, and to wear, aging, and abuse of the x-ray equipment itself, which may cause inconsistencies in the actual mA obtained at a given setting over time. Such fluctuations in milliamperage output can cause significant changes in the density recorded on radiographs.

The direct relationship between milliamperage and image density remains true, but control over density is totally lost when the actual milliamperage obtained is different than the milliamperage set at the machine console. The technologist must be able to trust the accuracy of the mA controls. When they are out of calibration, radiographic technique becomes unpredictable.

Guidelines for Accuracy

Linearity refers to the proportionate accuracy of the output of one mA station in relation to another station. In other words, the 200-mA station should put out twice as great an intensity of x-rays as the 100-mA station, the 400-mA station should emit four times more, etc.

Federal standards require that each mA station be linear to within plus or minus 10 percent of each *adjacent* mA station. On step wedge images, this translates to an acceptable *density* deviation of plus or minus 0.1 as measured on a densitometer.

Reproducibility is the consistency with which a given mA station emits the set output from one exposure to the next. The set output should not vary up and down significantly between uses. Such fluctuation would result in unpredictable techniques and a loss of control, just as poor linearity would. Federal standards require that a given exposure setting be reproducible to within plus or minus 5 percent, or a density deviation of 0.05, when repeated 10 or more times. Although this repeatability generally applies to a total technique setting, including the set kVp and exposure time, these two factors do not tend to fluctuate significantly from one exposure to the next in comparison with milliamperage. Milliamperage, in fact, is somewhat notorious for fluctuating. Further, separate tests allow the kVp and timer to be calibrated, so that reproducibility tests may be considered to be primarily applicable to the mA stations.

Output between different rooms of the same phase within a radiology department

may also be measured in mR/mAs and should fall within 10 percent of each other, or 0.1 density, at the same mA and kVp settings.

Test Procedures for Linearity

The most accurate way to check the calibration of the mA stations is to use a good ionization chamber with digital readout. The intensity rate of the radiation in mR/second, or the total intensity in mR for a given exposure time, should double when the mA station is doubled and vice versa.

A less accurate but very practical and useful method which may be employed by radiographers is to expose a *penetrometer* step-wedge and measure the recorded densities with a *densitometer*, two devices likely to be found in most radiography departments (Fig. 30-4).

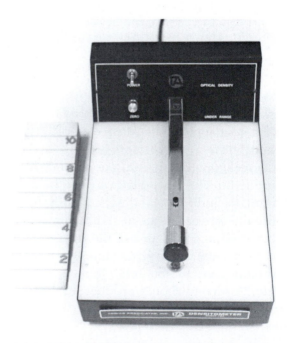

Figure 30-4. Photograph of a step wedge penetrometer and a densitometer (*right*) used to produce and measure densities on test films.

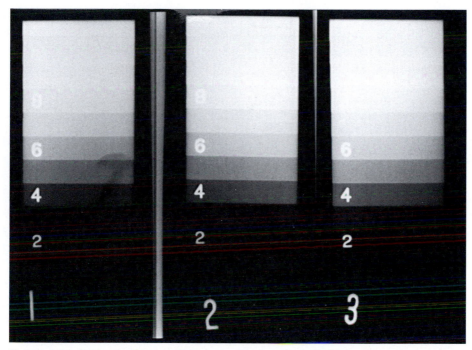

Figure 30-5. Radiograph of milliamperage linearity test using apenetrometer. Factors left to right: 100 mA at 1 second, 200 mA at $^1/_{20}$ second, and 300 mA at $^1/_{30}$ second. Observing medium- density step 4 or 5, it is apparent that the 100 mA station is slightly darker than the other two, but within acceptable limits as measured on a densitometer.

METHOD A. If there are only three or four mA stations to check and you begin with a radiograph with a relatively light, (0.3-0.4) density level, you can simply increase the mA station from one exposure to the next and take densitometer measurements off of one of the middle steps of the penetrometer. You must be sure to use the same step for each measurement. All other variables (screens used, processing, distances, field size, etc.) must be maintained equal throughout the experiment. To ensure equal processing factors, make all of the exposures on one 14 x 17-inch film, so that they are all developed at the same time. Within the accuracy ranges described, each change in mA station should produce a proportionate change in film density. Density measurements above 2.5 are unreliable using this method, and should not be used.

METHOD B. If several mA stations are to be checked for calibration, you must use an equal mAs approach, reducing the exposure time by an inverse proportion to each increase in milliamperage. For example, 100 mA at $^1/_{10}$ second, 200 mA at $^1/_{20}$ second, and 300 mA at $^1/_{30}$ second might be used. The measured density from each exposure should then be equal to the others within plus or minus 0.1 (Fig. 30-5). Although this approach allows several stations to be checked, it is dependent upon the assumption that the exposure timer is accurate. Therefore, this method should always be performed in conjunction with a timer accuracy test. If a particular time is found to be inaccurate, the percentage of inaccuracy may be calculated and subtracted from subsequent inaccuracies measured during the mA test to find the actual mA accuracy. Again, the same middle step should be used on the penetrometer image for each measurement and all other variables must be carefully stabilized.

Test Procedure for Reproducibility

To check for reproducibility of exposure, simply repeat the same exposure eight or ten times, using a penetrometer on one 14 x 17-inch film, for all exposures so that processing will be equal and measure a middle step with the densitometer to determine if it varies significantly from an average. To find the average, divide the sum total of all of the density measurements by the number of measurements taken; then compare each individual measurement to this average. *No single measurement* should deviate by more than 5 percent, or 0.05 density, from this average.

Test Procedure for mR/mAs Output

The unit mR/mAs is useful in comparing different machines *of the same phase and type of generation* to see if they are linear from one room to another. This is important to know because if these machines are within the recommended limits, then the same technique chart should be able to be used in all of the different rooms. Single-phase machines must *only* be compared to other single-phase machines, $3\Phi^{12}$ machines to other $3\Phi^{12}$, and $3\Phi^6$ to other $3\Phi^6$.

The actual output from the x-ray tube can be measured using an ion chamber. All compared measurements must be done at the same kVp, since kVp can affect the output of the tube. It is recommended that at least three series for comparison be done, one at 60 kVp, one at 80 kVp and another at 100 kVp. Comparisons can also

be done for each mA station. At a given mA, a relatively long exposure time (at least 0.5 seconds) should be used for the ion chamber to obtain an accurate measurement in mR (set for the "integrated dose" mode). This total mR is then divided by the mAs used (mA station multiplied by the exposure time) to find the mR/mAs. For most accurate results, three or more exposures should be repeated at each setting and an average taken, by adding the amounts and dividing by the number of exposures. The result should not vary by more than 10 percent from one room or machine to another of the same phase.

A practical quick check can be made by radiographers using a penetrometer and densitometer. Simply expose the step wedge penetrometer using identical techniques in the different rooms. It is best to use the same film for all exposures so that processing consistency will be assured. Collimation, distances, and all other variables must be kept constant. On the resulting radiograph, the measured density on a selected medium-density step should not vary by more than plus or minus 0.1 from one machine to another of the same phase.

KILOVOLTAGE QUALITY CONTROL

Penetration is the single most important quality of an x-ray beam. It is directly dependent upon the energy spectrum of the beam, which is controlled by the electrical kilovoltage applied across the x-ray tube. Since the energies of the x-rays in the beam vary across a heterogeneous spectrum, beam energy cannot be directly measured as a discrete quantity. However, the penetration ability of the beam may be directly measured and, because of its direct relationship with beam energy, the energy may then be extrapolated from the penetration data. It is essential to the radiogra-

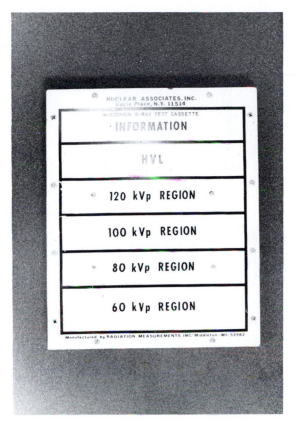

Figure 30-6. Photograph of a Wisconsin kVp test cassette showing demarcated exposure areas.

pher that such monitoring of the obtained energy take place, so that the selected kVp setting on the equipment may be trusted to produce the desired kVp.

The *Wisconsin kVp Test Cassette* (Fig. 30-6) was developed to derive the actual peak energy of the x-ray beam from its penetration characteristics. Inside the cassette, each exposure passes through two devices: on one side is a copper step-wedge; on the other is an intensifying screen with an *optical attenuator*–a simple light filter designed to always attenuate or stop exactly one-half of the light which the screen emits (Fig. 30-7). Both sides are covered by a lead mask with round holes in it so that two columns of round spots are recorded on the film.

After exposure and development, each kVp area on the radiograph will show two columns of density spots (Fig. 30-8). In the column which was under the optical attenuator, all of the spots will be of the same density. This density represents an exposure to exactly one-half the light emitted from the intensifying screen. The opposite column will consist of spots with a graduation of different densities, representing the exposure under each of the steps on the copper step-wedge, the lighter spots being under the thicker steps. By comparing these spots with the optical attenuator column and finding a *match*, it may be determined what thickness of copper was required to attenuate one-half of the x-rays. The thicknesses of copper required to absorb one-half of the beam are known for the various kVp levels, with greater thicknesses being required for higher kVp levels. So, once the half-value thickness is measured, a chart may be consulted to find the corresponding actual kVp of the beam.

Guidelines for Accuracy

It is suggested that actual kVp values should fall within plus or minus 4 kVp of the indicated kVp setting. If they are not within this range, a serviceman should be called to make electrical adjustments.

Test Procedure

The Wisconsin kVp Test Cassette must be used to determine actual kVp accuracy. Four exposures are made on one film, collimating to a marked area for each, in steps of 20 kVp from 60 to 120 kVp, using the following techniques, respectively, for a single-phase machine: 150 mAs at 20 inches SID, 20 mAs, 5 mAs and 3 mAs at 40 inches SID. For a three-phase machine, the mAs values must be cut in half.

To determine the kVp, first you must identify the two dots which most closely

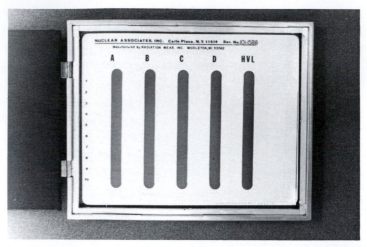

Figure 30-7. Photograph of opened Wisconsin kVp test cassette showing optical attenuator light filters (dark areas).

match in density. You may do this either visually or using a densitometer for accuracy. The column under the optical attenuator will have spots of all the same density, representing one-half the original exposure. The other column under the step-wedge will have spots of increasing density. The spot in this column which matches the other column represents the *half-value layer* (Chapter 8) in copper for the beam. Half-value layer is a measurement of

the penetration or energy of the beam, and kVp can be directly extrapolated from it. Graphs of the kVp/HVL relationship are provided with the cassette. To find the kVp, you simply locate the matching step number on the graph (which may fall between two spots on the film) and read across to the graph line and then down to the kVp axis.

Table 30-5 lists the typical matching step numbers for each kVp setting tested with

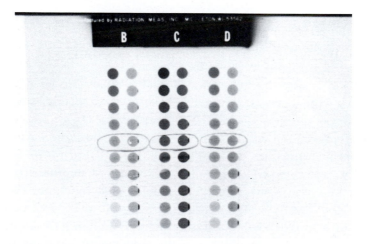

Figure 30-8. Radiograph produced with Wisconsin kVp test cassette showing matching density spots (circled) used to find the actual kVp output of the x-ray machine.

Table 30-5
WISCONSIN kVp TEST CASETTE;
MATCHING STEP NUMBERS FOR
ACCURATE kVp SETTINGS

kVp	Single-Phase Step Number	Three-Phase Step Number
60	5.0	5.6
80	5.2	6.0
100	5.1	6.1
120	5.0	5.75

the Wisconsin kVp Test Cassette when the kVp is accurate. If the actual matching step number you measure is above this number, the actual kVp is greater than the kVp station indicates. If the measured step number is lower, the actual kVp obtained is less than indicated.

HALF-VALUE LAYER AND FILTRATION

The most important quality of the x-ray beam is its ability to penetrate through a substance. Protective filtration is used to remove low-energy x-rays from the beam because they cannot penetrate through the patient. Optimum kVp levels are necessary to assure adequate penetration through the anatomy. Beam penetration may be raised in two distinct ways: (1) by increasing the *minimum* energies present in the beam through the use of filtration and (2) by increasing the *maximum* energies present in the beam through the use of higher peak kilovoltages. Either of these methods results in an increase in the *average* energy of the beam and in higher penetration.

Since kilovoltage does not tend to vary much from that value set at the control panel and can often be checked and adjusted by the service representative, any meas-

ured inadequacies in beam penetration usually reflect upon the amount of protective filtration placed in the collimator. If the kVp is found to be accurate but the penetration of the beam is too low, more protective filtration should be added to the collimator. Radiographers must be aware of any such need as a matter of professionalism and patient safety.

The only true measure of beam penetration is the *half-value layer*, abbreviated *HVL*. Half-value layer is defined as that thickness of absorber (usually aluminum) needed to reduce the intensity of the beam mR) to one-half of the original intensity. The higher the HVL, the more penetrating the beam.

Guidelines for Accuracy

Although NCRP regulations require a minimum of 2.5 mm aluminum equivalency in total filtration (inherent plus added) for most diagnostic x-ray machines, more filtration is required when the half-value layer does not exceed HVL recommendations at each kVp level. HVL is the direct measurement of actual beam penetration and indicates whether filtration levels are adequate.

At 80 kVp, the HVL must be at least 2.34 mm of aluminum equivalency. Required HVL values at other kVp levels may be found in governmental regulations, but one simple test at 80 kVp will often suffice.

Test Procedures

The Wisconsin kVp Test Cassette has an area on it for finding the beam HVL directly, using the same process of matching the resulting columns of spots as discussed in the last section. A technique of 4 mAs for single-phase or 2 mAs for three-phase must be used in this area at 60 kVp.

HVL can also be found by using pocket ion chambers with sleeve filters or large ion chambers and several thin sheets of aluminum filtration. First, for a given technique of average kVp level, a reading is taken of the beam intensity (mR) without using the sleeve filters or aluminum sheets. Then, readings are taken with increasing thicknesses of the filters added until less than one-half of the original reading is obtained. The readings may be plotted against the thicknesses of absorber on graph paper to form an absorption curve. To find the HVL in aluminum, simply find the dose which is one-half or 50 percent of the original dose, read across to the curve and down to the absorber thickness–this is the HVL.

COLLIMATOR QUALITY CONTROL

When the actual size of the x-ray field is greater than that indicated on the collimator control knobs, unnecessary patient exposure and additional scatter fogging of the radiograph occur. When the actual field size is less than that indicated, anatomy of interest may be cut off from the field of view, necessitating repeat exposures. It is essential to the radiographer, therefore, that both the field size control knobs on the collimator and the projected visual light field accurately indicate the size and location of the actual x-ray beam.

It is important to understand that the projected light field may not accurately represent the actual x-ray field location. Further, recall that the tabletop is at a different distance from the x-ray tube than the Bucky tray. For these two reasons, the practice of simply measuring the light field on the table to determine field size can lead to several errors. X-ray field size should be determined by directly measuring the exposed area on a radiographic film.

Inaccuracies in the field size indicator on

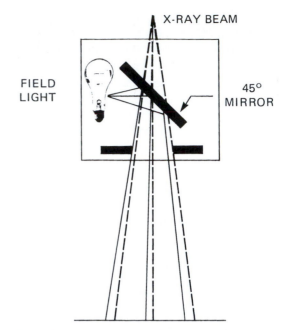

Figure 30-9. Diagram of collimator mirror responsible for alignment of the light field with the actual x-ray beam.

the collimator may be caused by slippage of the collimator shutters. These shutters are usually turned by gears and can occasionally slip, especially on older collimators.

Guidelines for Accuracy

It is recommended that each dimension (length and width) of the actual field size measure within plus or minus 2 percent of the SID being used (2 centimeters at 40 inches SID) from the size indicated on the collimator control knobs for that distance. It is suggested that each half of the field be symmetrical to within 1 centimeter of the opposite half.

It should be noted that light field edges are frequently as much as one-half inch off of alignment from the actual edges of the x-ray beam (Fig. 30-9). Where the actual beam edge is inside the light field edge, anatomy of interest may be cut off when tight collimation is used.

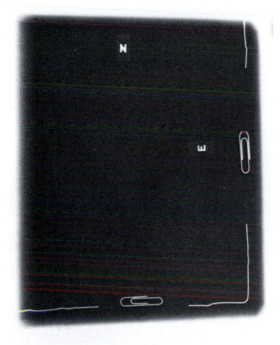 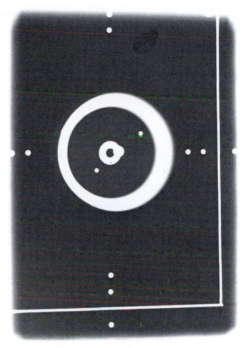

Figure 30-10. Radiographs of light field alignment checks using paper clips to demarcate light beam edges (*left*) and using the Wisconsin beam alignment device (*right*). Both examples demonstrate the light field misaligned to the *north* and *west* of the actual x-ray beam, so that the corresponding markers are not within the darkened area. The tool to the right also shows a true central ray angle out of vertical toward the *east* since the screw in the center is projected outside the outer edge of the washer, indicating an angle greater than 2 degrees.

Test Procedures

Collimate to any size smaller than the film you are using and make a very low mAs exposure without anything in the beam. Process the film and simply measure the exposed rectangle in both axes with a ruler to compare it with the collimator indicator. If there is a measured discrepancy, a collimator shutter has slipped and the collimator needs service. Proper alignment of the collimator shutters may be determined by measuring with a ruler the light field on the table from the midline to each edge and checking for symmetry. If one edge measures farther from the midline than the opposite edge, the shutter has slipped.

This test for field size accuracy is usually done in conjunction with the light field alignment test and vertical beam alignment test which follow. All three tests can be made with one exposure, as shown in Figure 30-10.

LIGHT FIELD ALIGNMENT QUALITY CONTROL

Inside modern collimators there is a light bulb and a mirror aligned in such a manner as to project a field of light in the same path as the x-ray beam. The light bulb cannot be placed in the path of the x-ray beam or it will appear as an artifact on radiographs, so it is set to the side at right angles to the x-ray beam central ray. Its light is then reflected by the mirror into the path of the x-ray beam. The mirror, although it acts as added filtration in the x-ray beam, does not create any artifacts on the film because of its even thickness and homogeneous composition. Normally, the mirror should be placed at exactly 45 degrees from the central ray, so that the light field will be projected precisely where the x-ray field is. When the mirror or the light bulb is misaligned, the center and edges of the light field will not accurately represent where the actual x-ray beam is directed (Fig. 30-9).

It should be noted by every radiography student that it is not uncommon for the light field to be misaligned by as much as one centimeter or one-half inch at the usual 40-inch SID. To avoid cutoff of anatomy, which could lead to repeat exposures, therefore, it is advisable to use the following rule of thumb: *Always allow yourself one-half inch of light beyond each border of the anatomy of interest.* Although collimating the beam down as closely as possible to the size of the anatomy of interest is a commendable professional practice, it must be remembered that to risk cutting off any portion of that anatomy is to risk a repeat exposure and therefore additional patient exposure. This rule of thumb will prevent many of the cutoff problems arising from the use of different x-ray machines with different degrees of alignment accuracy.

The accuracy of the light field alignment is an essential component of patient protection. Some machines are as far as one full inch off of alignment and cause frequent repeat exposures. Once the misalignment is detected, it can often be remedied by a simple adjustment of a screw in the collimator which controls the mirror angle (Fig. 9-3 in Chapter 9). If not, a service specialist should be called in.

Guidelines for Accuracy

Each edge of the actual x-ray beam must be within plus or minus 2 percent of the SID from the edge of the light field. The central ray of the x-ray beam must also be within 2 percent of the SID from the center of the light field. At the typical 40-inch SID, then, each of these should be within 2-cm accuracy.

Test Procedures

The edges of the light beam must be demarcated with radiopaque markers. Unfolded paper clips or wire serve well enough for a homemade check. Test plates may be purchased which indicate the exact percentage or amount by which the beam is off of align. Also, be sure that there is a marker in one corner of the light field so that you can orient the exposed film in the proper direction to match the collimator.

Make an exposure with one of the devices explained above marking the edges of a light field which is well less than the film size being used. Process the film. The exposed black rectangle on the film is the actual x-ray field, whereas the markers outline the light field (Fig. 30-10). Be sure to orient the film to North-South and East-West so that it matches the collimator you are checking. If the black area is one inch to the West of the markers, then the *light field* must be adjusted toward the West one inch. The center of the beam may be checked against the center of the light field by drawing diagonal lines from the corners of the film and from the corners of the exposed area. Where the diagonals cross in each case marks the central ray, light versus x-ray beam.

If the light field central ray is found to be one-quarter inch off from the x-ray field central ray, while the edges of the light field are found to be one-half inch off, or perhaps off in a different direction, then the indication is for *two* distinct problems: light field misalignment and possible shutter slippage. The central ray location should be used as the criterion for adjusting the light field alignment first. Vertical beam alignment should also be checked (see next section). Finally, collimator shutters should be checked for conformity of edges.

VERTICAL BEAM ALIGNMENT QUALITY CONTROL

Occasionally, a light field which appears to be off-centered to the x-ray table transversely is not, in fact, off-centered but misangled. This can occur when the transverse tube angle lock has been used for some procedure by a radiographer who did not take special care to restore it to an exact vertical position afterwards. Normally, this transverse angle lock should not be used for any procedure. It is possible to achieve the same results by first swivelling the tube on its axis and then utilizing the usual longitudinal angle lock.

It is critical to radiographic procedures that the central ray of the actual x-ray beam be exactly perpendicular to the planes of the tabletop and Bucky mechanism. This should be checked in combination with field light alignment and field size tests, so that one problem will not be misconstrued with another.

Guidelines of Accuracy

The x-ray beam must be within two degrees of perfect vertical alignment.

Test Procedures

To check vertical alignment of the beam, you need two radiopaque objects fixed in perfect vertical alignment. Six-inch Plexiglass™ test cylinders may be purchased

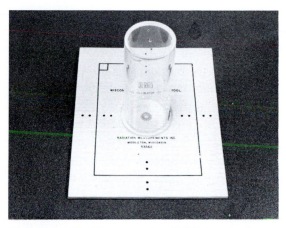

Figure 30-11. Photograph of Wisconsin beam alignment test tool.

(many come with the light field test plates mentioned previously) which have a small screw embedded in perfect center on the top and a washer embedded similarly on the bottom (Fig. 30-11). An exposure is made centering the light field to the screw, and the film is processed. On observing the radiograph, if the edge of the screw lies outside of the *outer* edge of the washer (Fig. 30-10, *right*), then the beam is off of vertical more than two degrees and must be adjusted by using the locks on the tube head or, if the tube is fixed in position, by a service specialist.

DISTANCE INDICATORS

Newly installed distance indicators rarely present inaccuracies, but older equipment or reinstalled equipment should be checked for slippage.

Guidelines for Accuracy

It is recommended that SID indicators be accurate to within plus or minus one-half inch or two centimeters.

Test Procedures

Distance indicators on the x-ray machine may be checked for accuracy by simply using a tape ruler. The measurement must be taken from the exact location of the focal spot within the cylindrical tube housing (*not* from the collimator). Most anodes are 3-4 inches in diameter, placing the focal spot about $1^1/2$ inches toward the collimator from the middle of the cylindrical tube housing.

FOCAL SPOT QUALITY CONTROL

It is important to understand that the *nominal* focal spot size quoted by tube manufacturers is a measurement obtained under the most ideal conditions with a low mA setting. The actual size may be as much as 50 percent larger than the nominal size for several reasons. To estimate how small a thrombus or embolism may be resolved during an angiogram, you must know the true size of the focal spot at the mA stations normally used for the procedure. The most significant reason for this problem is *blooming* of the focal spot. At high mA settings, many electrons are boiled off of the cathode to form the *space charge* or electron cloud. Being of the same electrical charge, they repel each other so that the size of the cloud *blooms* or expands beyond the normal diameter. When they are propelled across the tube, they strike a larger area on the anode, creating a larger actual focal spot. Although manufacturers of x-ray tubes generally consider a 30 percent margin of error as allowable, and government regulations allow for 50 percent deviation, special procedures technologists will want to know more accurately the real focal spot sizes they are using.

Still more important is the simple monitoring of the x-ray tube over time for possi-ble damage to the focal spot on the anode. Small cracks in the surface of the anode focal track, called *etching*, occur over time with the thermal shock produced from bombardment of high-speed electrons. Abusive use of the x-ray tube can cause acute problems such as fractures or melted pits on the anode surface. Since any of these conditions cause an uneven surface to the focal spot, changing its apparent projected size or configuration, they can be detected by sudden changes in the resolution or sharpness of detail in an image.

Test Procedures

STAR PATTERN TEMPLATE METHOD. The most accurate and practical method of obtaining an actual measurement of the focal spot size is to use a *star*-type test template (Fig. 30-12). The template should be placed at an object-film distance equal to one-half of the SID. Recommended distances are 12 inches from the film to the template and 24 inches SID. It is important that the middle axes passing through the line pairs of the pattern be aligned with the length and width of the x-ray tube (hence,

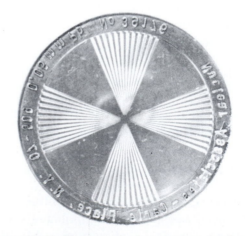

Figure 30-12. Photograph of star pattern focal spot test template used to obtain accurate measurements of focal spot size.

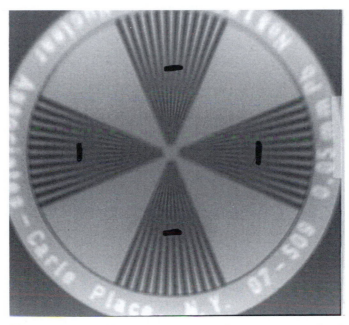

Figure 30-13. Radiograph of star template to measure focal spot size. Diameter measurements taken between the marked *first* blur points are multiplied by a constant to obtain the actual size.

the focal spot) and that they not be placed diagonally. A light exposure is made and the radiograph processed.

A blur pattern will result on the finished radiograph. The radiographer should scan from the periphery of the pattern *inward* until the *first* point where the line pairs are not distinguishable is located. A mark should be made at this point of blur (Fig. 30-13). It may be seen that further inward the line pairs seem to resolve again and then blur again. This phenomenon is *false resolution* and occurs from the overlapping of blurred line images. Thus, it is essential to measure only the outermost points of blur. A mark should be made at these points for each of the four arms of the star.

Using a millimeter ruler, record the measurements between the two *pairs* of marks across the pattern—length and width. If the template has the typical two degrees of arc per line, then these two measurements may simply be multiplied by the fac-

tor 0.035 to obtain the actual size, length and width, of the focal spot.

PINHOLE CAMERA METHOD. A second method for measuring focal spot size is with a pinhole camera. The pin-sized hole in a metal plate is placed one-half way between the tube target and the film, resulting in a magnification factor of one, so that the size of the density spot projected on the film represents the actual size of the focal spot itself (Fig. 30-14). (The geometry of the pinhole camera method is completely different from the geometry of normal image magnification discussed in Chapter 20. The two must not be confused.)

The pinhole camera method is less accurate than the star pattern template method because the shadow being measured has penumbral edges. It is also much less practical because excessively high exposures are required to record a density through the pinhole, which may lead to tube anode damage.

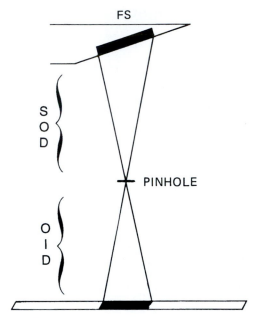

Figure 30-14. Geometry of pinhole camera focal spot test, showing the SOD and OID as similar triangles. With the pinhole at the mid-point, the projected image will measure precisely the same as the actual focal spot size.

WISCONSIN FOCAL SPOT TEST TOOL. The Wisconsin Test Tool consists of a metal template with groups of vertical and horizontal line pairs cut into it (Fig. 30-15). This template is placed six inches off of the film

and a light exposure is made with a SID of 24 inches. In similar fashion to the star pattern template method, the radiographer should scan the finished radiograph from the thickest line-pair groups down to locate the *first* group which is blurred enough to make the individual lines indistinguishable. The last group resolved *before* this blur point indicates the maximum resolution (Fig. 30-16). There should not be more than three lines resolved in this group–four lines would be caused by false resolution when blurred lines overlap. Since the resolution of sharpness is a direct function of focal spot size at given distances, a chart may be consulted to find the effective focal spot size from the smallest line-pair group resolved. With the listed distances, the chart should be one adjusted for $^4/_3$ magnification.

Like the star pattern template, a measurement is taken for each dimension of the focal spot–length and width. The template must be positioned so that the line pairs run with the length and width of the x-ray tube (hence, the focal spot). Each line-pair group is indicative of the focal spot measurement lying *perpendicular* to the lines in that group. That is, lines running cross wise

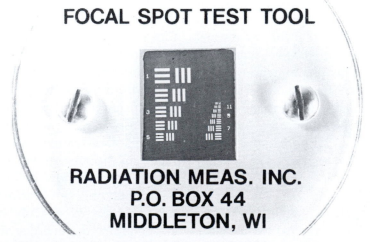

Figure 30-15. Photograph of Wisconsin focal spot test tool using line-pair groupings for both length and width measurements.

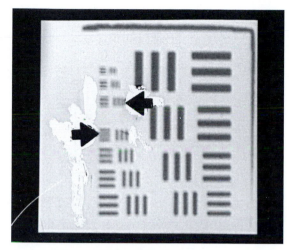

Figure 30-16. Radiograph of focal spot check using Wisconsin tool. Note that blur points (arrows) indicating focal spot size are different for width and for length.

are used to find the length of the focal spot, while lines running lengthwise indicate the width of the focal spot (Fig. 30-16).

The Wisconsin method is particularly useful in an ongoing program of checking for focal spot damage within a radiology department: An initial check is made in which the line-group number resolved is recorded. Without the necessity of consulting a chart to translate the line-group number into an actual measurement, a monthly check may be made to simply detect any sudden change in the line-group number resolved. Such a sudden change would be indicative of damage to the focal spot.

This method is not as accurate in taking actual measurements as is the star pattern template method. Since the line pairs are in *discrete* groupings, the actual point of blur lies somewhere between the last group resolved and the first group blurred. This means that the measurement taken is an estimate which may be more than 10 percent inaccurate. The star pattern template, on the other hand, has *gradient* line pairs, gradually thinning toward the center of the pattern, so that an exact point of blur may be found and

an exact measurement obtained.

IMAGE RECEPTOR SYSTEM QUALITY CONTROL

For the purposes of quality control, or of selecting appropriate recording media for a particular radiology department, radiographic film, intensifying screens and cassettes should always be considered in combination as a system. Some film/screen combinations are incompatible, and their characteristics must be carefully matched to obtain the optimum image quality. In determining resolution (the capacity to record sharp detail), speed, contrast or the proclivity to produce quantum mottle, one complete film/screen/cassette system should always be compared to another complete system.

By far, the intensifying screens are the most important component of the receptor system in controlling resolution, speed and contrast. That is, changing from one speed or type of screen to another has a much more dramatic effect upon these image qualities than a change in film type does. Therefore, when these qualities are measured, they primarily reflect the characteristics of the intensifying screens used, even though the film also has some bearing on them.

Regardless of the system used, it is critical to radiographic quality that the intensifying screens be in direct contact with the film across its entire surface. Poor screen contact results in a severe blurring of recorded detail in that area of the radiograph, along with a slight loss of density. The felt and metal backings provided by the cassette are responsible for proper screen/film contact, so that poor contact is always indicative of cassette damage. Hence, the condition of the cassette itself is essential as a component of the receptor system.

Guidelines for Accuracy

No specific standards are set for evaluating receptor performance or screen contact. Screen contact should be perfect across the entire surface. Measurements of resolution, speed and contrast in the system are valuable only from the standpoint of comparing them to other systems. Naturally, the most desirable system is that combination of film, screens and cassette which produces the highest resolution, greatest speed, optimal contrast and least mottling. In reality, some of these must be traded off for each other (for example, higher speeds often lead to excessive mottling) and some may only be evaluated arbitrarily by the individual radiologist, such as *optimal* contrast. Therefore, the selection of a specific system and the assessment of its performance depends upon the values and needs of a particular radiology department.

Test Procedure

To check for proper *screen contact*, place a fine wire mesh on top of the cassette and expose it to a light technique. Laminated wire meshes avoid the problem of the wire itself being bent in spots. When observing the processed radiograph, it is often difficult to distinguish areas where the edges of the wire are slightly blurred. It is much easier to step back away from the illuminator and observe the film from a five- or six-foot distance, from which the blurred areas will stand out clearly as areas of *darker density* on the film (Fig. 30-17). If there is a blurred area, it indicates that the screen is warped in that area, usually from physical damage to the cassette. The cassette must be repaired or discarded.

To compare different kinds of screens for resolution of detail, place a straightline res-

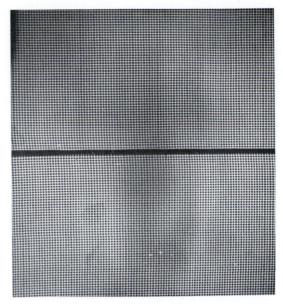

Figure 30-17. Radiograph of wire mesh test for screen-film contact showing areas of poor contact. From a distance, the blurring of the white lines of the mesh causes an appearance of increased density in these areas.

olution test pattern directly on the cassettes and expose lightly. On the exposed films, scan with the eye from the thicker lines toward the thinner ones until you find the first point where the line pairs are blurred into each other. You can simply compare this point on each film visually or you may find the actual line pairs per millimeter resolved (LP/mm) by looking up the blur point line-pair numbers on a table. It may be desirable, in addition, to expose anatomical phantoms and evaluate the sharpness of detail visually.

To compare different kinds of screen/film combinations for speed and contrast, simple exposures of a penetrometer step-wedge are made and measurements taken off of a densitometer. For speed, simply compare the same step between both films. For contrast, a lighter density step should be divided into a darker one, using the same two steps on both films.

VIEWING CONDITIONS

A radiograph is only as good as its illumination. The manner in which radiographs are viewed is as important to the radiographer as it is to the radiologist. Radiographs are made with translucent densities of varying tone value and details only become visible when they are transilluminated by light of conventional color and intensity.

THE ILLUMINATOR

The modern illuminator is designed for viewing radiographs up to 14 x 17-inches in size and consists of two fluorescent tubes suitably mounted in a reflecting box and behind opal diffusing glass. The quality and quantity of light transmitted through the radiograph by the illuminator determines the diagnostic worth of the image. The radiographer should provide a standard level of density that is translucent when the radiograph is viewed on the illuminator. The radiologist should view the radiographs on an illuminator that provides comparable color and intensity. To maintain the same quality and intensity of light, the illuminator should be cleaned regularly and old fluorescent tubes should be replaced with new, 15-watt bulbs.

To obtain the best transmission of illuminator light through a radiograph, all light that might pass *around* the radiograph should be blocked out. For example, when small CT or MRI films are viewed on a 14 x 17-inch illuminator, a mask may be used with an aperture cut to suit the size of the film being viewed. If this is not done, the density of the radiograph appears greater than it actually is.

AMBIENT LIGHTING

When radiographs are being read, the level of general illumination in the viewing room should be sufficiently low so that extraneous light is not reflected from the surfaces of the radiographs, thus lessening the brightness of image details.

AUTOMATIC EXPOSURE CONTROLS

Several electronic and radiographic checks can be made for automatic exposure controls, most of which should properly be done by a qualified physicist. Tests for reproducibility, kVp, and other parameters common to regular radiographic units are essentially identical to those described in preceding sections of this chapter. AEC exposures must be repeatable within an accuracy range of plus or minus 10 percent. To check repeatability, five exposures should be taken using a step-wedge penetrometer, and a densitometer should be used to measure and compare the densities obtained. AECs should also be linear to within 20 percent between different rooms. Three basic tests can be done by the radiographer to determine proper functioning of the unit:

Density Control

As described fully in Chapter 28, the density control settings can be checked for accuracy without using any film, by exposing a phantom knee, skull or abdomen to a series of exposures and simply reading off the digital mAs readouts. Make the first exposure with the density control set to "N" or "O." Immediately after the exposure, write down the readout on the mAs indicator. Do the same for each *plus* or *minus* station on the density control. For each readout, perform the following calculation:

$$\frac{\text{N-A}}{\text{N}} \times 100$$

where *N* is the mAs readout for the "N" station and *A* is the readout for the *plus* or *minus* density setting being checked. This will yield the percentage of increase or decrease in technique from the normal or average setting. These percentages can then simply be compared with what the buttons or knob on the density control indicate. These stations should not be more than 10 percent off from the indicated increase or decrease in technique.

Linearity

Place thick sheets of plexiglass or a plastic pail of water so that the detector cells activated are completely covered. Each detector chamber can be checked individually if all three cannot be covered at once. Make two exposures at the same kVp and with all other factors constant. For the first exposure, fill the pail with at least 3 inches (8 cm) of water or use a 3-4 inch thickness of plexiglass sheets. For the second exposure, fill the pail with 6 inches (16 cm) of water or double the amount of plexiglass thickness. Resulting densities should fall within 10 percent of each other as measured on a densitometer. For a more complete check, repeat the experiment at different kVp settings.

Back-Up Timer

Cover the activated photocell(s) with three sheets of leaded rubber. Set the back-up timer at 1 or 2 seconds, and expose. The exposure should automatically terminate at the set back-up time, or before the accumulated mAs readout exceeds 600 mAs.

TOMOGRAPHIC UNITS

Tomographic units must comply with the same linearity, reproducibility, kVp, and other radiographic parameters as other equipment. Special checks on exposure angle, section thickness, and resolution can be performed by a qualified physicist. A simple test can be done by the radiographer to determine the level of the section as indicated on the unit.

The test tool is a simple radiolucent wedge with wires and a set of numbers to indicate the height of each wire with respect to the maximum height of the wedge (25cm). Or, an aluminum step wedge with lead numbers placed on each step will do for a less complete check.

When linear movement is to be evaluated, the wedge must be positioned so that it is 45 degrees to the tube and film motion. Having placed the central ray to the center of the inclined part of the wedge, a section level on the unit (say 9cm) is set to correspond to that on the wedge (9cm). The wedge is subsequently exposed using appropriate technique factors.

When the film is processed, it should show a sharp image of the wire located at the 9cm mark if the indicator on the machine is correct. The section level should be within plus or minus 5 mm of the setting on the machine indicator.

FLUOROSCOPY

Testing and maintaining the fluorography unit for quality control is the job of a physicist, checking to assure that the following are present and/or operational and meet NCRP recommendations: Source-to-table distance (15" for the stationary unit and 12" for the mobile unit), primary barrier of 2mm of lead in the intensifier housing, filtration of no less than 2.5mm of aluminum equivalence, proper collimation to allow for an unexposed border on the monitor, bucky slot cover and protective curtain present, cumulative timer checked, and the x-ray output intensity should be checked yearly or more often as required by state regulations.

It should also be noted that in some states the technologist is required to record the amount of fluoro-on-time the patient was exposed to and compute the estimated total exposure by multiplying the intensity output rate by the number of minutes. As an example, if the physicist has determined the output intensity to be 2.1 R/min and the fluoro on time was 3.5 minutes, then the total estimated exposure would be computed as follows:

$$2.1 \times 3.5 = 7.35 \text{ R}$$

Furthermore in some cases the number of overhead and spot radiographs taken, including repeats, must also be recorded.

SUMMARY

1. A complete *quality control* program includes radiation exposure monitoring, radiographic unit monitoring, sensitometry, the use of technique charts, analysis of repeat rates and continuing education.

2. The proper construction and use of *technique charts* can reduce repeat rates by as much as 25 percent.

3. The *analysis of repeat rates*, especially in a department which employs a quality control program, can be used to identify the *continuing education* needs within a radiology department.

4. Exposure *timers* should be accurate to within 5 percent of the indicated time and may be checked with manual or electrical spinning tops.

5. *Adjacent milliamperage stations* should be linear to each other within 10 percent. The same mA stations between two machines of identical phase and rectification should be within 10 percent of each other in output. A given exposure should be reproducible to within 5 percent. All of these may be checked by exposing step wedge penetrometers or by using ion chambers for higher accuracy.

6. Kilovoltage settings should be within 2 kV of the actual peak beam kilovoltage. This can be *checked* by using the Wisconsin kVp Test Cassette.

7. Half-value layer *tests*, using the Wisconsin kVp Test Cassette or ion chambers and filters, can be used to determine the actual penetration quality of the x-ray beam. When the HVL is inadequate, it is more likely to be from insufficient protective filtration in the collimator than from inaccurate kVp stations. Although 2.5 mm of aluminum is the required minimum protective filtration for machines, more filtration may be needed if the HVL falls below 2.34 mm Al.

8. Field size indicators should be accurate to within $^1/_2$-inch (2% of the SID) and can be *checked* with a simple ruler measurement of the exposed black field on the film. The edges of the light field should be within $^1/_2$-inch of the edges of the actual x-ray field, and both should be within 2 degrees of vertical. These can be *checked* with field edge markers and an alignment test cylinder.

9. SID should be within $^1/_2$-inch of that indicated and can be *checked* with a tape ruler.

10. The actual focal spot size must be within 50 percent of the size listed by the tube manufacturer. It is important to know the actual size, because objects smaller than it may not be reliably recorded on radiographs. Damage to the focal spot may be detected by the use of the Wisconsin line-pair focal spot test tool. Accurate measurements may be made by using a *star* focal spot test template. The pinhole camera may also be used but is not recommended because of the high exposure required and possible tube damage.

11. A laminated wire mesh may be used to *check* proper screen/film contact. Resolution patterns may be used to compare the sharpness of detail obtained between different types of screens.

12. *Illuminators* must be kept clean and functional, and peripheral and ambient lighting must be reduced to optimize the viewing of radiographs.

13. Phototimed exposures should be *repeatable* within a 10 percent accuracy, using a densitometer. Density control stations should also be within 10 percent accuracy of the indicated increases and decreases in technique. These can be easily checked by the radiographer simply using the mAs readouts at the different stations.

REVIEW QUESTIONS

1. What is the acceptable range of deviation for the linearity of adjacent mA stations?

2. What is the acceptable range of deviation for exposure timers?

3. An electric spinning top revolves at a rate of 1 rps. For a three-phase timer test, what should the arc produced by an exposure time of one-half second measure in degrees?

4. Define "reproducibility" as it relates to mAs:

5. Why is it important for reliability on mA quality checks, to take all exposures on one film?

6. What is the acceptable range of inaccuracy for kVp settings?

7. What is the purpose of the optical attenuator in the Wisconsin kVp test cassette?

8. What is Half Value Layer and what does it measure?

9. At 80 kVp, the HVL for a particular x-ray machine is found to be 1.9 mm. Al. If the kVp control is accurate, what does this HVL indicate needs to be changed?

10. The borders of the light field must be within plus-or-minus _____-inch (or _____-cm) of the actual borders of the x-ray field.

11. What device in the collimator is responsible for alignment of the light field with the x-ray beam?

12. The intersection of two diagonal lines drawn from the opposite corners of the

black area on a light field alignment test radiograph will locate the center of the:

13. In a light field/x-ray field alignment test radiograph, the borders of the black area overlap the paper clips used on the east and south sides by 1 inch, and cut off those on the north and west sides by 1 inch. In which directions is the light field misaligned from the x-ray beam? Is this an acceptable amount of misalignment?

14. The x-ray beam must be vertical within plus-or-minus _____ degrees.

15. What is the purpose of putting black masks around radiographs?

16. Old plastic covers on illuminators can cause _____ on the apparent image.

17. It is determined that a given time setting lasts about 10 percent too long. During a film density test to check the mA stations, this time was used with the mA station in question, but was not used for the original reference technique. The exposure on the mA station in question produced 23 percent more density than the reference exposure. What is the actual accuracy of the mA station in question?

18. In repeat analysis, what is "obtrusiveness"?

19. A radiographer used 120 films and made 110 exposures to obtain 80 diagnostic quality radiographs of the skull during a one-month period. What is her repeat rate for skull work?

20. Automatic Exposures must be reproducible within what percent?

21. An AEC density control check is done by exposing a knee phantom and yields the following mAs readouts:

$$N = 10.5 \text{ mAs}$$
$$+1 = 12.1 \text{ mAs}$$
$$+2 = 17.3 \text{ mAs}$$
$$-1 = 7.9 \text{mAs}$$
$$-2 = 5.3 \text{ mAs}$$

Which station is much too *low* for the indicated change? Which station is much too *high*?

Chapter 31

SOLVING MULTIPLE TECHNIQUE PROBLEMS

MULTIPLE TECHNIQUE PROBLEMS like those about to follow are valuable, not only in preparation for similar problems on certifying examinations, but also as a concise review of the most basic and important relationships in radiographic technique. The problems presented here will seem overwhelming at a glance, but the whole point of this exercise is to demonstrate that, *taken one step at a time*, even the most complex problems can be solved (see Table 31-1).

Although you may wish to attempt solving them "on your own" first, this is not necessary. The discussion following the table of problems takes you step-by-step through their solution. At each point where you are unsure, refer to the discussion for guidance.

There are several approaches to solving the kind of multiple technique problems that are presented on certification examinations. The author has used and taught four different types, including the *function* system, and the method presented below is recommended highly because of its simplicity. All of the various methods are workable and accurate enough, but many are unnecessarily complex. It is asserted that the easiest approach will also be least likely to result in errors.

Regardless of the method used, the student must begin with a thorough understanding of the principles in each section of this book. Screen and grid factors for density must be thoroughly memorized. Also,

an appreciation for which factors have a greater or a lesser effect upon image qualities such as contrast or sharpness of detail must be developed.

Remember that for each type of problem, you must first select only those columns of variables which directly affect the image quality. For example, if you are solving for image contrast, cross out any columns for mAs, phase, SID, tube angles, or focal spot size–these variables either are not related to contrast at all, or they make too little difference to consider. After eliminating unrelated variables, take the remaining columns one step at a time, following the directions.

1. SOLVING FOR DENSITY

Most multiple technique problems encountered on certifying examinations are for solving the net resulting density of the radiograph. In solving for density, use the following rules:

For mA, time or mAs:	*Direct proportion*
For machine phase:	*3Φ or CPG = 2 x 1Φ*
For kVp:	*The 15 percent rule*
For SID:	*The inverse square law*
For OID:	*Estimate + or -*
For Screen Speed:	*See Tables 14-4 and 14-5*
For Grid Ratio:	*See Table 13-3*
For Filtration:	*Estimate slight + or−*

Always determine the total mAs first by multiplying the mA and time. Then, for each column, simply multiply the mAs value by the appropriate factor to obtain a *density value* number. For example, if A has 15 percent more kVp than the other choices, double the density value for A and then cross off that column and do not go back to it; if A has a 400-speed rare earth screen, multiply the density value by four times; if A has a 15:1 ratio grid, divide the density value by 5, and so on. The *density value* becomes, as you adjust it, a number representing the relative density that will result from the technique and must not be confused with actual mAs. The density value simply tells you relatively how dark the film will be. When you finish, the greatest density value is the darkest film.

2. SOLVING FOR PATIENT SKIN DOSE

These may be solved in exactly the same method as the density problems as discussed above. However, different factors will be considered—filtration becomes a significant column to evaluate, while screen speeds and grid ratios should be completely ignored (since they are behind the patient and after the fact) if the mA and time are already given. *Exposure values* will replace density values.

For machine phase, recall that 3Φ equipment is about 70 percent more efficient in actual mA output than single-phase. For the purpose of these problems, this amount can be rounded upward to roughly a doubling. Consider 3Φ equipment to produce roughly twice the patient skin dose as 1Φ equipment for the same mAs setting. For kVp: Skin dose increases about *25 percent* for each increase of 15 percent in kVp, and decreases 25 percent for a 15 percent reduction in kVp.

Thicker patients absorb more radiation in accordance with the 4-centimeter rule used for technique. However, when estimating *skin dose*, the only significance in patient thickness is that the larger patient's surface will be slightly closer to the x-ray tube, reducing the effective SOD. This is usually a small percentage of the overall distance and may be ignored for these problems.

3. SOLVING FOR CONTRAST

The effect of the variables upon image contrast cannot be accurately quantified. Hence, you are reduced to using a system of *pluses* and *minuses* to solve for which film is the most contrasty or the least contrasty. It is essential that you develop a sense of the relative magnitude with which each variable affects contrast from the units in this book. For variables that have a great effect, use larger, bolder, or more pluses and minuses. A review of which variables affect contrast to a greater or lesser degree follows:

1. Grids have a dramatic effect.
2. Patient thickness has a considerable effect.
3. OID has a considerable effect.
4. Changing from direct exposure film holders to intensifying screens or vice versa has a dramatic effect; however, the difference in contrast from one speed of screen to the next is very minimal.
5. Changes of 6 or 10 kVp are not significant in their effect upon contrast when compared to the effects of grids or OID; but, kVp changes of 30 kVp or more have a considerable effect.
6. No other factors have a noticeable effect on image contrast.

4. SOLVING FOR SHARPNESS OF RECORDED DETAIL

The effects of SOD/OID ratio and focal spot size upon image sharpness of detail can be *quantified* as follows:

To find the SOD, subtract the OID from the SID. Insert the proper values into the sharpness formula:

$$S = \frac{SOD}{OID \times FS}$$

The resulting number gives you a relative measure of sharpness–the greater the number, the sharper the detail.

However, the effects of screen speed and film speed upon image sharpness cannot be easily quantified. Here, you must use a *plus-and-minus* system combined with the number obtained from the distance ratio and focal spot. Bear in mind that the effects of screen and film speeds are very minimal compared to the geometrical factors of distance and focal spots.

Using the two lists of variables that follow, five sample multiple technique problems are presented in Table 31-1. The solutions follow.

Table 31-1
SAMPLE MULTIPLE TECHNIQUE PROBLEMS

#1. Which of the following produces the greatest density? _____

	mAs	Machine Phase	kVp	SID	OID	Patient Thickness	Screen	Grid	Filter
A.	400	1Φ	72	40"	2"	22cm	Rare Earth Reg.	16:1	2.5mm
B.	200	1Φ	82	40"	2"	14cm	Extremity	12:1	2.5mm
C.	100	3Φ	94	80"	2"	30cm	High	6:1	1.5mm
D.	200	3Φ	72	80"	4"	24cm	Dir. Exp.	None	2.5mm

#2. Which of the following produces the greatest density? _____
#3. Which of the following produces the greatest contrast? _____
#4. Which of the following produces the greatest sharpness of detail? _____
#5. Which of the following produces the greatest patient skin dose? _____

	mA	Time	kVp	Screen	Grid	SID	OID	Focal Spot	Filter
A.	400	3/5	82	High	12:1	40"	2"	0.6mm	2.5mm
B.	300	4/5	94	Par	6:1	60"	6"	1.2mm	2.5mm
C.	600	0.4	72	Rare Earth Reg.	None	80"	2"	1.2mm	1.5mm
D.	200	1.2	80	High-Plus	16:1	30"	2"	1.2mm	2.5mm
E.	300	0.4	82	Slow	None	80"	2"	0.6mm	2.5mm
F.	800	0.6	94	Dir. Exp.	None	20"	2"	1.2mm	2.5mm

SOLUTIONS TO PROBLEMS IN TABLE 31-1

Solution to # 1: A is the densest radiograph.

Method:

1. In phase column, double mAs value for C & D. Write this to the side.
2. In kVp column, double B, double C twice (two sets of 15 percent increase).
3. In SID column, cut C & D to ¼ density value.
4. In OID column, you may place a minus by D or ignore it entirely if the final density values are not close to each other.
5. In patient thickness column, double the

density value for B twice (two sets of 4 cm thinner), cut C in half twice, and ignore D because it is too close to 22.

6. In screen column, multiply the density value of A by 4 times, divide that of B by 1.5, multiply that of C by 2 times, and divide D by 50.

7. In grid column, divide the density value for A by 5, that of B by 4, that of C by 3, and leave D as it is.

8. In filter column, you may place a plus by C or ignore it if the final density values are not close to each other. The final density values you should arrive at are:

A = 320   C = 33+
B = 267   D = about 2-

Solution to #2: D is the densest radiograph.

Method

1. Multiply all of the mA's and times to get the total mAs for each.

2. In the kVp column, use the two 82's and the 80 (essentially the same) as standards, thus leaving A, D & E as they are, double the mAs value for B & F, and cut the mAs value for C to ½.

3. In the screen column, par will be the standard so leave B as it is, double the density value for A, multiply the density value for C by 4 times and that of D by 3 times; divide that of E by 2, and divide that of F by 50.

4. In the grid column, use non-grid as the standard so leave C, E & F as they are, divide the density value for A by 4, that of B by 3, and that of D by 5.

5. In the SID column, use 40 inches as the standard because all the rest are rounded out fractions of it (1½X, ¾, ½, etc.) so leave A as it is, divide the density value of B by 2 and that of C & E by 4, multiply the density value of D by 2 times and that of F by 4 times.

6. In the OID column, place a minus by B or ignore it if the final density values are not close to each other.

7. In the focal spot column, do nothing– this factor does not directly relate to film density.

8. In the filter column, place a small plus by C or ignore it if the final density values are not close. The final density values you should arrive at are:

A = 120   C = 120+   E =15
B = 80-   D = 288   F = 76.8

NOTE: If you choose different *standards* in some of the columns which you compare the others to, your actual density value numbers may come out different than these, but they will be proportionately related in the same way and you will still get the right answer as long as you do not err in making comparisons in each column. When two answers come out very close numerically, then you must go back and carefully consider the pluses and minuses, the less significant factors.

Solution to #3: D has the highest contrast.

Method:

1. The mA, time, SID, focal spot, and filter columns should be ignored, as they are not directly related to contrast. (If two answers come out very close to tying, you may go back to the time column and consider it as a *potential* effect on motion and contrast.)

2. In the kVp column, the two 82's and the 80 should be used as the standard to save time, a small minus should be placed next to the two 94 kVp's listed, and a small plus placed by the 72.

3. In the screen column, simply use an additional plus or minus for each screen speed increase, except that three or four minuses should be used for the direct-exposure technique because it is

dramatically grayer than even the slowest speed of screen. Thus, you should put a small plus next to the high, nothing next to the par, three pluses next to the rare earth, two by the high-plus, one minus by the slow, and four minuses by the direct exposure. All of these should be relatively small.

4. In the grid column you should use large pluses and minuses. The three, non-grid techniques should have nothing by them, as they are standard. Using a similar approach to the screens above, there should be three large pluses by the 12:1, one large plus by the 6:1, and four large pluses by the 16:1.

5. In the OID column, a large plus should be placed by the 6-inch OID (this is *air gap technique*). Tallying everything up, you should arrive at something similar to this:
   A = 1 small plus & 3 large pluses
   B = 1 small minus & 2 large pluses
   C = 1 small plus & 3 large pluses
   D = 6 large pluses
   E = 1 small minus
   F = 5 or 6 minuses

Solution to #4: E has the sharpest recorded detail.

Method:
1. Eliminate the mA, time, kVp, grid, and filter columns, as these are not directly related to sharpness of recorded detail. (If you get two results that are close, you may go back to the time column and consider it as a *potential* for reducing sharpness.)
2. Subtract each OID from the SID to get the following SOD's: A = 38, B = 54, C = 78, D = 28, E = 78, F = 18.
3. Using the sharpness formula, SOD/ OID x FS, you should get the following relative sharpness values: A = 31.7, B =

7.5, C = 32.5, D = 11.7, E = 65, F = 7.5.
4. In the screen column, place a small minus by the high speed, nothing by the par, two small minuses by the rare-earth and the high-plus speeds, one small plus by the slow, and four pluses by the direct exposure. Your final result should be:
   A = 31.7+   B = 7.5   C = 32.5- -
   D = 11.7- -   E = 65++   F = 7.5++++

Solution to #5: F produces the highest dose to the patient's skin.

Method
1. Since the technique used is stated, screens and grids which are behind the patient have no bearing on surface skin dose, and may be ignored. Focal spots may also be ignored.
2. Calculate the total mAs value from the mA and time columns for each technique just as you would for a density problem. These numbers will then be considered as *exposure values.*
3. For the kVp column, recall that the 15 percent rule must not be used for skin dose, but only for radiograph density. For skin dose, we must know the actual change in radiation output from the x-ray tube when kVp is changed. This output is proportional to the square of the change in kVp, but as a rule of thumb, *it changes by about 25 percent for every 15 percent increase or decrease in kVp.* For example, if kVp is increased from 80 to 92, the skin dose would increase by approximately 25 percent or one quarter, and vice versa.
   Since there are three techniques close to 80 in the kVp column, select A, D and F as standards and leave their exposure values (mAs) unchanged. The new *exposure values* should be:
   A. 240

B. 240 mAs × 25% (0.25) = 60; 240 + 60 = 300

C. 240 mAs × 0.25 = 60; 240 - 60 = 180

D. 240

E. 120

F. 480 mAs × 0.25 = 120; 480 + 120 = 600

4. On the SID and OID columns, although it would be more accurate to subtract the OID from the SID to obtain the SOD (from the tube to the patient's surface), it is easier to ignore the 2-inch OIDs, in effect, *rounding out* the SOD's to equal the SID's, and only consider the 6-inch OID. Leaving the 40-inch exposure value at 240 as the standard, the 60-inch exposure value is roughly cut in half to 150, the 80-inch one in one quarter to 45, the 30-inch doubles to 480, the 80-inch one on E cuts to one quarter at 30, and the 20-inch one quadruples to 2400. Re-

garding the OID on B, you may estimate that moving the patient 6 inches closer to the tube would increase patient skin dose by roughly one-fourth or 25 percent, making the exposure value about 190, or you may plug the numbers into the inverse square law to get an exact value of 185 (set up as $X(54)^2 = 150(60)^2$).

5. On the filtration column, the 1-mm less filter that C has will cause a significant increase in skin dose, probably between 50 and 100 percent. To take the extreme case, you may double the exposure value for C to roughly 90. The final results are:

A = 240   C = about 90   E = 30

B = about 190   D = 480   F = 2400

Try the following review questions for practice. (An answer key is available in the Appendix.)

REVIEW QUESTIONS

1. Which of the following produces the greatest density:
   a. b. c. d.

	mA	Sec	Phase	Patient Thickness	kVp	SID	OID	Ratio Grid	Screen	Focal Spot Size	m.m. Filter
a.	150	1/2	3Φ	25 cm	48	60"	2"	12:1	400	1.0	2.5
b.	200	1/5	1Φ	25 cm	48	40"	2"	8:1	300	1.0	3.5
c.	400	1/10	3Φ	29 cm	56	30"	4"	none	Direct Exposure	1.0	2.5
d.	300	1/4	1Φ	20 cm	40	40"	4"	16:1	200	0.5	2.5

2. Which of the following produces the highest patient skin dose:
   a. b. c. d.

3. Which of the following produces the highest contrast:
   a. b. c. d.

4. Which of the following produces the sharpest detail:
   a. b. c. d.

	mA	Sec	Phase	Patient Thickness	kVp	SID	OID	Ratio Grid	Screen	Focal Spot Size	m.m. Filter
a.	150	1/2	3Φ	25 cm	48	60"	2"	12:1	400	1.0	2.5
b.	200	1/5	1Φ	25 cm	48	40"	2"	8:1	300	1.0	3.5
c.	400	1/10	3Φ	29 cm	56	30"	4"	none	Direct Exposure	1.0	2.5
d.	300	1/4	1Φ	20 cm	40	40"	4"	16:1	200	0.5	2.5

Part V

SPECIAL IMAGING METHODS

Chapter 32

MOBILE RADIOGRAPHY

BECAUSE OF THE MANY additional variables involved in mobile radiography, such as other equipment and furniture being in the way, limited space, and immobility of the patient, mobile or "portable" radiography frequently presents the greatest challenges faced by radiographers in securing quality images. The adaptability and creativity required to maintain all radiographic variables at the optimum level possible for mobile and trauma procedures is what sets the most skillful radiographers apart. Following are special technique considerations that will help enhance image quality.

MOBILE GENERATORS

Generators for mobile units are of two common types: battery-powered units and capacitor-discharge units. The battery-powered units are the state of the art, producing a very efficient current similar to a 3-phase, 12-pulse machine. Comparing techniques with the most common type of stationary unit, *a modern battery-powered mobile unit typically requires approximately 6 kVp less than the 3-phase, 6-pulse machine* to produce the same density for any given procedure.

Modern capacitor-discharge mobile units use precharged batteries to charge a capacitor to a preset voltage level selected at the console. Older CD units must be plugged into an electrical outlet during each use in order to charge the capacitor. In either case, the stored electrical charge is released and discharges across the x-ray tube when the exposure button is depressed. As the exposure progresses, the electrical charge drains off of the capacitor, and the remaining voltage drops. Therefore, the average voltage is much less than the starting kV peak. For this reason, capacitor-discharge units require roughly twice the total technique than battery-powered units to produce the same density on a radiograph.

Exposure on the battery-powered unit is initiated identically to stationary machines—rotor and expose. The capacitor-discharge unit, however, requires a special protocol: the total mAs value and kVp must be selected prior to charging the capacitor. A charge button is then depressed and held down until the preset technique is indicated on a meter (Fig. 32-1). At this point, the charge button is released and rotoring may begin with exposure shortly following. If exposure is delayed for more than a few seconds, the charging button must be pressed again to recharge the capacitor. This is due to the fact that capacitors quickly lose their stored charge through electron "leakage." (Since electrons repel each other, it is difficult to keep them concentrated on a single small device.)

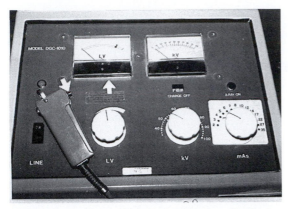

Figure 32-1. Console of a capacitor discharge mobile unit, showing line voltage meter at upper left (arrow) with line voltage compensator knob directly below. Charging button is on exposure switch (*left*, arrow). Controls to preset kVp and mAs, and kVp meter are also visible.

Both types of mobile units must be plugged into an electrical outlet between uses in order to recharge their batteries. Some older portable units are half-rectified, and require twice the mAs of a single-phase unit, or four times the mAs of a three-phase unit. Such equipment requires twice the mAs values as the capacitor discharge unit, or four times the mAs of a modern battery-powered unit. Generators are more fully discussed in Chapter 7.

mAs SELECTION

Most mobile units have a single "mAs" control, rather than mA and exposure time being selected separately (Fig. 32-1). The units are usually designed to operate at a high, fixed mA value, so that exposure time becomes the main variable. For capacitor-discharge units, the mAs selected should not exceed about one-third of the kVp selected, or the actual mAs produced becomes unreliable. Any mAs value available may be selected for battery-powered units.

KVP AND LINE VOLTAGE COMPENSATION

Modern battery-powered units require about 6-8 kVp *less* than typical three-phase equipment. Capacitor discharge units are comparable to single-phase equipment, which produces an *average* keV at about one-third of the kV peak.

Optimum kilovoltage is essential for proper penetration of the anatomy and for sufficient gray scale in the radiograph, and the radiographer must be able to rely on the equipment to produce the kVp selected. Capacitor discharge units which must be plugged in during each use have a *line voltage meter* and a *line voltage compensator* control (Fig. 32-1). This meter indicates whether the incoming voltage from the wall receptacle is sufficient. Variations in the supply voltage can easily occur in a hospital environment, where renal dialysis, radiology, and other departments make high demands on electricity. If the meter indicates that the line voltage is not adequate, the line voltage compensator must be turned up until the meter reads sufficient voltage. This adjustment actuates a capacitor circuit that stores additional charge to "boost" the electrical supply to the x-ray tube.

GEOMETRICAL FACTORS

Radiographers must often perform "cross-table" projections during mobile procedures, and in working around other equipment and the patient with all attached devices it seems that every conceivable angle of tube and cassette can be encountered. In this process, all proper distances and alignment must be preserved to the extent possible to maximize image sharpness, and to minimize magnification and distortion.

DISTANCE CONSIDERATIONS

The SID must often be estimated during mobile procedures. If a measuring tape is attached to the tube or collimator, it should be used, or the radiographer may wish to carry a compact tape measure in a pocket. *To estimate 40 inches,* the *average* person may extend one arm, and *measure from the contrary side of the body to the fingertip. To estimate 72 inches, measure from fingertip to fingertip with both arms extended.*

For angled projections, the *one inch for every 5 degrees* rule should be used to maintain SID. These rules of thumb are more fully discussed in Chapter 18.

The radiographer must remember to make every effort to place the film in contact with the part during mobile procedures. If this is not possible, the minimum OID possible should be achieved, and an increased SID should be considered as compensation. Changes in SID can be compensated with mAs to maintain density, according to the following rules of thumb:

Changing from 40 inches to:	*Increase mAs by:*
50 Inches	50 percent
60 Inches	2 x
72 Inches	3 x

These factors can be inverted to compensate for distance reductions. For example, use one-third the 72-inch technique for a 40-inch chest radiograph. For a 60-inch chest radiograph, use $2/3$ the 72-inch technique. *Any distance change of more than 20 percent will require technique compensation to maintain density.* All of the concepts in Chapters

18 through 20 should be fully appreciated and applied in mobile radiography.

Distance Rule of Thumb

Given the typical intervals between available steps on the mAs settings for most mobile radiography units, an extremely useful rule of thumb can be stated that allows one to work around emergency room and intensive care equipment and be able to compensate technique for various distances with confidence. The rule is, *change one step in mAs for every 10 inches change in SID.*

For example, it is wise to always maximize the SID when performing a "cross-table" horizontal beam projection of the lateral cervical spine, as this assists in precluding the shoulders from obscuring C-7. If you have a technique for a 40-inch distance, but 50 inches can be achieved in a particular situation, just increase the mAs to the next step for the 50-inch SID. For 60 inches, increase another step. If you have a good 72-inch technique, but because of equipment and tight spaces you can only achieve a 60-inch SID, reduce the mAs by one step from your 72-inch technique. This rule is not perfectly accurate, but works well enough to be of great utility in mobile radiography, and should be committed to memory.

ALIGNMENT AND POSITIONING CONSIDERATIONS

The radiographer must become adept at visually estimating the alignment of the x-ray beam with the patient and film cassette. This skill is necessary to minimize shape distortion and avoid superimposition of unwanted anatomy over the anatomy of interest. While the light field provides an easy approach to centering, it does *not* give

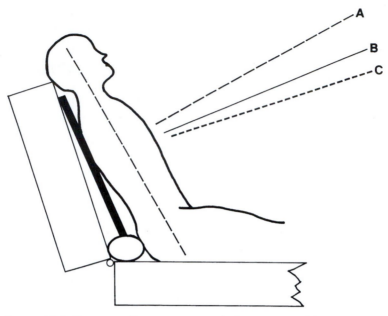

Figure 32-2. Diagram illustrating typical alignment problems encountered in mobile AP chest radiography, when the axis of the body (dashed line) is not parallel with the film or bed. The proper x-ray beam angle is A, perpendicular to the patient, rather than the film B or the bed C. For demonstration of fluid levels, patient should be raised up as much as possible.

an obvious indication of off-angling unless it is very severe. The radiographer must always carefully observe the angle of the x-ray tube in relation to the patient, from *two perspectives.* (1) side-to-side angle as observed from behind the x-ray tube, and (2) cephalic/caudal angulation as observed from the side of the patient and the x-ray beam.

A rule that is very helpful to accurately determine the angulation of the x-ray beam in relation to the film and patient is to *stand back as far as you can* away from the machine and patient. *Alignment is always easier to see from a distance.*

The caudal angulation of the x-ray tube for sitting mobile chest radiographs provides a classic example of the awareness needed for proper alignment. As illustrated in Figure 32-2, in spite of all positioning efforts, the lower back of the sitting patient

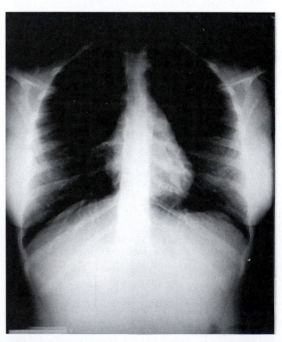

Figure 32-3. Lordotic mobile AP chest radiograph taken at angle **C** in Figure 32-2. Note straightened, linear appearance of ribs.

is frequently not in contact with the film cassette. This means that the long axis of the patient's body and the cassette are at different angles. Should the x-ray beam be angled perpendicular to the cassette or perpendicular to the patient's body? Without thinking, a radiographers may angle perpendicular to the cassette (and the bed), resulting in the common "lordotic chest" radiograph, with straightened ribs and diaphragm (Fig. 32-3). In this case the central ray should be angled caudally until it is truly perpendicular to the axis of the *body*.

When long bones or extremities cannot be positioned parallel to the film, *Ceiszynski's law of isometry* should be used, as explained in Chapter 21, splitting the difference between the angles. However, many projections are designed to "open" joint spaces or demonstrate anatomical relationships. For these, as with the mobile chest in Figure 32-2, *it is always more important for the central ray to be perpendicular to the anatomy than it is to be perpendicular to the film,* if one must choose.

If the purpose of the procedure is to rule out possible fluid levels, the central ray must be horizontal, regardless of part or film angulation.

OTHER CONSIDERATIONS

Some radiology departments prefer to use wide exposure latitude receptor systems for mobile radiography in order to reduce the probability of repeated exposures. These would include slightly slower screen speeds, wide-latitude films, and low ratio grids. Low ratio grids (5:1 or 6:1 ratios) can be especially helpful because their low selectivity allows a much wider margin for error in angulation, centering and especially distance variations. As described in Chapter 13, any grid must be carefully aligned with the x-ray beam to avoid grid cut-off. The mobile radiographer must watch for off-centering or off-angling of the beam, tilt of the grid/cas-sette, SID within the grid radius, and even upright placement for focused grids: It is not uncommon in surgery, for example, for the radiographer to place a grid-cassette into a sterile cover held by a nurse, and for the nurse to then place the covered cassette upside-down, or for a "wafer" grid to be taped onto a cassette upside-down.

Many portable units have added filters that can easily be removed from the collimator (see Fig. 8-2 in Chapter 8). The radiographer should ensure that proper filtration is in place at all times to protect the patient from unnecessary exposure to useless, low-energy radiation.

MANUAL VERSUS AUTOMATED TECHNIQUE

Automatic exposure controls have been available for use with mobile units in the form of phototiming "paddles" which are placed behind the cassette during portable exposures. These have been recalled by manufacturers because the placement of the photocell detectors in relation to the anatomy of interest has proven too unreliable for consistent results. They may lead to more repeated exposures than manual technique, and are not recommended for use. Most technologists continue to prefer manual technique for mobile procedures.

When manual technique is used for

mobile radiography, a *systematic approach* is as important as ever. Using the concepts from Chapters 25-27, *concise technique charts should be developed for mobile units.* There are many workable approaches to this need, but these charts must be compact and *permanently attached* to the mobile machine. They can be laminated or covered with clear x-ray film for protection, and chained or taped to the unit (Fig. 32-4).

Although mobile radiography can test one's skills and knowledge, the same high standards of image quality that apply to general radiography should be sought after for mobile procedures.

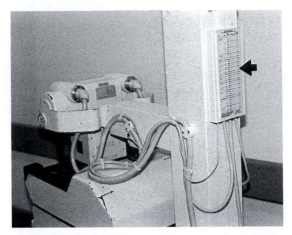

Figure 32-4. Modern mobile unit showing attached manual technique chart on back of tube stand (arrow).

SUMMARY

1. Battery-powered mobile units require slightly less *technique* (6 kVp less) than 3Φ equipment. Capacitor discharge units require about twice the technique of battery-powered units.

2. With *capacitor discharge* mobile units, one must always check the kVp meter immediately prior to exposure to ensure adequate charge. Recharging may be necessary if more than a few minutes have passed. Insufficient incoming line voltage is indicated and may be compensated on these machines.

3. Skill in estimating various *distances* and knowledge of the technique adjustments required for changes in distance are essential in mobile radiography.

4. Skill in visually aligning the x-ray beam

to the anatomy of interest is also essential for mobile radiography. *Alignment* can always be better seen by positioning oneself at a distance from the equipment.

5. If the anatomy and the film cannot be placed parallel, it is essential to *align the x-ray beam properly to the anatomy* rather than to the film.

6. Manual technique is recommended for mobile radiography. *Technique charts* should be provided for all mobile units.

7. Several *rules of thumb for distance* adjustments during mobile procedures are useful: Generally, increase mAs by one step for every 10" increase in SID. A 72" SID requires 3 times the technique of a 40" SID.

REVIEW QUESTIONS

1. How do techniques for battery-powered mobile units compare to those for 3Φ equipment?

2. For a capacitor discharge unit, what

must the radiographer do if more than a few minutes have passed between charging and exposure?

3. Inbetween uses, what should be done with most mobile machines?

4. Before making an exposure with a capacitor-discharge unit, what two meters must both be checked?

5. If a 72-inch technique is used with a 60-inch actual SID, will density be altered enough to require a repeated exposure?

6. How can the radiographer best position himself to assess proper alignment of the x-ray beam during mobile procedures?

7. For a projection of a joint space, if you have to choose between placing the x-ray beam perpendicular to the anatomy or perpendicular to the film, which would be best?

8. Is it practical to require technique charts for mobile units?

9. For every increase in SID of 10", increase the mAs setting on a mobile unit by _____.

Chapter 33

SPECIAL IMAGING TECHNIQUES

QUINN B. CARROLL AND EUCLID SEERAM

PARALLACTIC IMAGING METHODS

DEPTH PERCEPTION is created in an image by simulating the double vision of the human eyes. The brain is able to perceive depth or distance in an image because of the *parallactic shift* of the image which occurs between the two eyes. Parallactic shift or *parallax* is the apparent change in position of an object against a background reference point when seen from two different points of view. To demonstrate parallax, hold a pencil close to your nose and alternate closing one eye and then the other. The pencil appears to shift position in relation to the background you see. Although you are not consciously aware of this shift as you go about your daily business, your brain automatically and continually compares the parallax of objects seen by each eye to provide a sense of depth. When one eye is lost, there can be no more depth perception.

When the observer is moving, parallax can be thought of as the amount of apparent shift of objects against the background, or the speed at which they seem to pass by. For example, when driving, telephone poles or other objects that are near to the road seem to pass by quickly, while objects that are at some distance from the road seem to pass by more slowly. The speed or amount of shift is related to the distance from the object to the viewer. These principles are taken advantage of in radiograph-

ic imaging in the areas of foreign body localization, stereoradiography, and tomography.

FOREIGN BODY LOCALIZATION

There are several approaches to maximizing the detection of foreign bodies including soft tissue technique (Chapter 11), routine fluoroscopy, and positioning methods such as tangential projections. Parallactic shift is utilized in the single-film triangulation method and the fluoroscopic parallax method.

Single-Film Triangulation

The single-film triangulation method is especially useful when the exact depth of the object must be determined without moving the patient. A double-exposure is made on one film using one-half the normal technique for each exposure. For the first exposure, the x-ray beam is centered to the suspected location of the foreign body. For the second exposure, the x-ray tube is shifted in a direction perpendicular to the long axis of the foreign object. It is recommended that the tube be off-centered from the first exposure by about ten percent of the SID (4 or 5 inches for a 40-inch SID). The film is not moved. The collimator must be opened up so that the field does not cut off anatomy of interest when shifted. This produces a double-image of the foreign body on the radiograph.

Exact measurements must be taken and recorded for the following:

SFD: The skin-to-film distance, measured from the uppermost surface of the body part to the film.

SID: The source-image distance.

TSD: The tube shift distance.

ISD: The image shift distance, measured from the radiograph.

With the above data, the following formula will yield the *foreign body-film distance*, (FBFD):

$$\frac{SID \times ISD}{TSD + ISD} = FBFD$$

The FBFD is now subtracted from the SFD (the skin-to-film distance) to obtain the depth of the foreign object from the surface of the patient:

$$SFD - FBFD = \text{Foreign Body Depth}$$

Because of parallax, the deeper the object is from the surface of the body, the less its image will shift on the radiograph.

Fluoroscopic Parallax

A metallic object at the end of a stick may be held to the side of the patient's body during fluoroscopy. If the fluoro tower is then shifted side to side, both the foreign body and the metal indicator to the patient's side will appear to shift across the image. As this occurs, the indicator may be moved vertically up and down. When the image of the metal indicator shifts at exactly the same apparent speed and distance as the foreign body, the indicator is at the level of the foreign body. The level of the indicator may then be measured from the tabletop or from the surface of the body as a direct measurement of the depth of the foreign object.

TOMOGRAPHY

Some anatomical objects are not visible on routine radiographs because of overlapping, more contrasty anatomical structures such as bones which superimpose and obscure them. Tomography refers to the use of *motion* to blur out such overlying structures so that the anatomy of interest can be seen through them. The purpose of tomography is the *desuperimposition* of obstructing images (the reduction of noise). Tomography is known by a variety of names, including *laminography, planigraphy,* and *body-section radiography.*

The desuperimposition process achieved with tomography may be further divided

into two specific objectives: *Analysis* is the dividing of complex anatomy into small parts, so that each part may be diagnosed individually. Typical tomograms use large movements of the x-ray tube to focus in on very thin sections of anatomy for analysis. An example of analysis is tomography of the inner ear, where the ossicles, the cochlea, the vestibular area and the auditory nerve canal are each individually focused upon for diagnosis. *Localization* is the purpose of *zonography*–a type of tomography which employs only very small movements of the tube. These small movements result in thick sections of anatomy being in focus on the zonogram, so that a part of the body may be scanned through with a limited number of exposures in search of suspected pathology. An example of zonographic localization is the pinpointing of pulmonary lesions of low contrast, which may be highly suspected but difficult to visualize on a routine chest radiograph. Using zonography, the lungs may be scanned in sections from front to back, employing only 8-12 exposures.

Although most tomography is performed by moving the x-ray tube and the film in concert during the exposure, it is also possible to obtain tomographic images by having the patient move a body part during the exposure, while the x-ray tube and film remain stationary. This method is called *autotomography* and is commonly used in such procedures as the thoracic spine (breathing technique) and the upper cervical spine (wagging-jaw technique).

The way that tomography works is illustrated in Figure 33-1. The central ray of the x-ray beam is centered through the anatomy of interest to the film. As the x-ray tube moves in one direction, it also rotates on its axis so that the central ray remains centered through the anatomy of interest, forming a *fulcrum point.* The film moves in the opposite direction to maintain its centering to the CR. Note in Figure 33-1 that in doing so, the anatomy of interest (the circle) is always projected to the center of the film and is therefore not blurred. However, anatomy above and below the part of interest is projected by changing peripheral rays throughout the exposure, so that its image moves across the film and is blurred. Note in Figure 33-1 that the triangle and the square exchange places on the film from one extreme of the tube movement to the

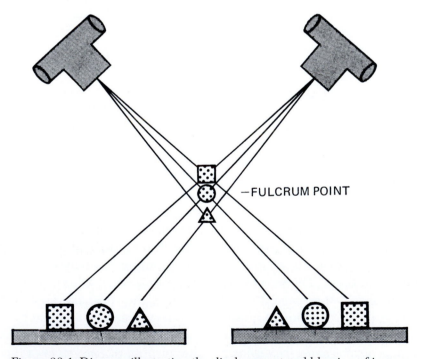

Figure 33-1. Diagram illustrating the displacement and blurring of images of objects above and below the fulcrum point of a tomographic tube movement. Note that during the course of the tube movement, the images of the triangle and square have moved across the film surface.

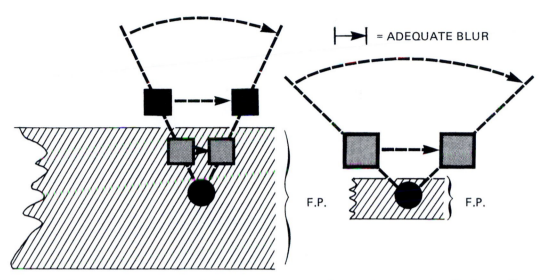

Figure 33-2. Diagram illustrating the definition of a tomographic focal plane as that thickness of tissue within which objects are not displaced enough to be visibly blurred. (*Left*) the gray box is not visibly blurred, will appear sharp in the image and is considered to lie within the focal plane. (*Right*) Increased tube movement now visibly blurs the gray box, and it is considered to lie outside the thinner focal plane.

other. They have both been blurred across the length of the film. The circle will be visibly in focus on the resulting radiograph, while the objects above and below it will be blurred out of visibility.

THE FOCAL PLANE

The further an object is above or below the fulcrum point, the more distance it will be blurred across on the film. Actually, everything is blurred on the tomogram to a greater or lesser degree. But there is a limit to the capacity of the human eye to see microscopic levels of blurring, so that an object must be blurred by a certain minimum amount before the blurring becomes visible to the eye. The practical effect of this is that a *focal plane*, a layer of anatomy with a distinct thickness which will be visibly recorded on the film, is produced during tomography (Fig. 33-2). Within the focal plane thickness, no anatomy has been blurred enough for the eye to detect the blur, so it all appears reasonably focused.

Anatomy which has been visibly blurred is considered to be outside the focal plane. In Figure 33-2, an imaginary minimum distance to cause visible blurring is diagrammed. This distance represents the limit of the human eye to detect blur. On the *left* side of the diagram, note that the solid box has been blurred across a distance greater than this minimum. It will be blurred on the image and not considered to be within the focal plane. The hollow box, however, is close enough to the plane of the fulcrum point that it has not been blurred across the minimum distance. It will appear focused on the image and is considered to be within the focal plane. To blur out this hollow box, the distance of the x-ray tube movement must be increased. As shown on the *right* side of Figure 33-2, where the tube movement is increased, the hollow box would no longer be considered to be within the focal plane since it is now blurred from visibility. In effect, the focal plane has been made *thinner*. That is, there is a thinner layer of tissue which is shown

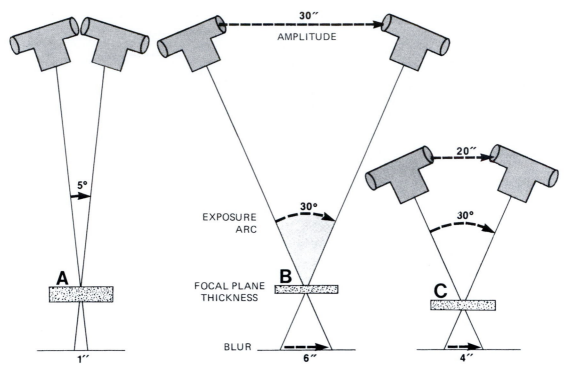

Figure 33-3. Diagram of two methods of obtaining thinner tomographic focal planes. Plane B is thinner than plane A because of increased exposure arc (30 degrees versus 5 degrees). Plane B is thinner than plane C because, even though the exposure arcs are equal, amplitude is greater for B (30 inches versus 20 inches) due to the longer SID.

in focus on the resulting radiograph.

Greater blurring effectiveness obtained through the tube movement always results in thinner focal planes. Two aspects of the tube movement bear upon its blurring effectiveness: the exposure arc and the amplitude (Fig. 33-3). *Exposure arc* refers to the angle between the extremes of the tube movement formed by the central ray, measured in degrees. The greater the exposure arc, the thinner the focal plane and the more effective the blurring. *Amplitude* refers to the actual distance traversed by the x-ray tube during the tomographic movement. The amplitude may be increased without changing the exposure arc by changing the pattern which the tube makes in moving. For example, the tube may trace out a 30-degree circle (15 degrees to each side of vertical) rather than

a 30-degree line. In doing so, it travels more than three times the total amplitude distance. The blurring of unwanted structures in the image is slightly more effective for circular movements than for linear ones of the same exposure arc for this reason.

MOVEMENT PATTERNS

In an attempt to obtain greater amplitudes, a number of different tomographic movement patterns have been developed over the years. Since all of the variations involve changing direction during the exposure, they are collectively referred to as pluridirectional movements. Pluridirectional tomography equipment is much more expensive than the unidirectional, linear tomograph, but *pluridirectional* movements have two distinct advantages over linear movements. The first advantage is the increased blurring effectiveness, or *selectivity*, by which thinner focal planes may be obtained for detailed analysis. The second is the elimination of *false images.*

False Images

False images are images *created* by the geometrical relationship between the tomographic tube movement and the anatomical structures within the patient. These images must not be considered to represent any real objects in the patient. They are *not* a form of distortion (a common misconception) but rather a form of *noise.* A distorted image, although it is changed in shape, still represents a real object within the patient. A false image, however, is an illusion created by movement. False images are a form of noise because they are completely useless and they obscure the desirable image.

The most common type of false image is *streaking* (Fig. 33-4). Streaks of density are produced on linear tomographs when long structures lying roughly parallel to the tube movement are not sufficiently blurred (Fig. 33-5). An area is left on the film over which some portion of the object was projected throughout the exposure. Nonetheless, since the portion of the object over that area was constantly changing during the exposure, its appearance does not accurately represent any real anatomy. To reduce streaking artifacts, it is recommended that whenever possible the anatomy to be blurred (not necessarily the anatomy of interest) be placed perpendicular to the long axis of the tube movement, so that the blurring distance required to completely blur out its image is reduced to its own width (Fig. 33-5). For example, most linear and elliptical movements are oriented with

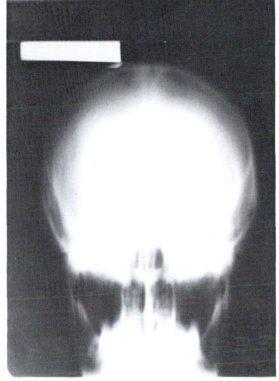

Figure 33-4. Linear tomograph (30 degrees) of skull exhibiting linear streaks.

their long axis along the length of the x-ray table. During lung tomography, the ribs lie perpendicular to this movement and are well blurred. During an IVP, however, the ureters which lie parallel to the tube movements are likely to produce streaking artifacts.

Annular (circular) artifacts may also be created when a circular x-ray tube movement cuts through a tube or vessel at a semi-axial angle. In order to eliminate linear and circular false images, more complex tube movements in which the pattern crosses over itself (the circle-eight, the cruciate and the hypocycloidal movements), and the spiral movement, were developed. By far, the spiral and the hypocycloidal tube movements are the most effective and produce the thinnest focal planes available.

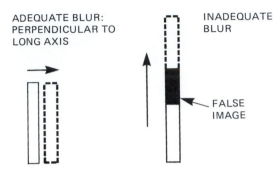

Figure 33-5. Diagram showing how streaking is produced when tomographic movement is insufficient to completely displace an image lengthwise. Placing obstructing anatomy to be blurred width-wise to the direction of tube movement is effective in eliminating streaking.

APPLICATIONS

Table 33-1 lists the various tube movement patterns with degrees of exposure arc, the typical thicknesses of focal planes obtained with those movements and the anatomy for which each movement type is recommended.

For the tube movement to be effective, the exposure must be *spread out* across the entire tube movement. If the exposure terminates before the movement is completed, the full effect of the blurring will not be obtained. Table 33-1 also presents the typical minimum times required for each type of movement to complete its cycle. The exposure time used in setting the electrical technique must be exactly as the manufacturer of the equipment recommends for each tube movement. The milliamperage will then need to be decreased substantially to maintain the proper total mAs.

To avoid creating double images and uneven density, the x-ray tube must be moving at a constant rate of speed throughout the exposure. It cannot be accelerating or stopped during the exposure. Therefore, the tube must be in motion before and after the exposure to allow for acceleration and deceleration. As an example, for a 30-degree linear tomogram, the tube would be angled more than 15 degrees to one side of vertical before starting. When the exposure button is

Table 33-1
TOMOGRAPHIC TUBE MOVEMENTS: RESULTING FOCAL PLANE THICKNESSES,
TYPICAL EXPOSURE TIMES, AND RECOMMENDED APPLICATIONS

Tube Movement	Focal Plane Thickness	Exposure Times	Recommended Applications
10-degree Linear Zonography	1cm	1 sec.	Biliary, Urinary, Pulmonary, and Mediastinal Localization
30-degree Linear Tomography	4 mm	2 sec.	Biliary, Urinary, Pulmonary, and Mediastinal Analysis
25-degree Elliptical or Circular	3 mm	3 sec.	Extremities (including casts), Spines, Brain Ventricles
Hypocycloidal, Spiral or Circle-Eight	1-1.5 mm	6 sec.	Inner Ear, Petrous, Facial, Orbital, Sella Turcica, Lymph Nodes, Cervical, and Vertebral Analysis
Autotomography			C1-C2 (wagging jaw), Brain Ventricles (head rotation), and T-Spine (breathing)
Pantomography			Dental

depressed, the tube accelerates. The exposure itself does not start until the tube reaches the 15-degree mark. When the tube reaches 15 degrees to the opposite side of vertical, the exposure terminates and the tube begins to slow down to a halt. The exposure switch must be kept depressed until the entire exposure is completed.

TECHNIQUE

In addition to the reduction of the mA station to compensate for the longer exposure time previously described, there is one other important technique consideration. Most tomographs move the tube and film in a plane parallel to the tabletop. On these machines, the *average* target-film distance during the movement is increased above the usual 40 inches, with 40 inches at vertical being the minimum and the extremes being as much as 55-60 inches. A loss of density results. A practical rule of thumb for such machines is to roughly double the total technique from a standard technique chart to maintain image density.

To reiterate the necessary technique adjustments for tomography, first find the technique on a routine chart for that anatomy and double the listed mAs. Set the exposure timer as required by the manufacturer for the tube movement being used. At that time, reduce the mA station as needed to achieve the desired (doubled) mAs. On occasion, this mAs value will not be obtainable and a reduction in kVp will be necessary, using the 15 percent rule.

FOCAL DEPTH, INTERVALS AND SCOUT FILMS

The *focal depth* refers to the location of the focal plane in centimeters from the *back* or *down-side* of the patient *upward*. Usually several exposures are taken at different lev-

els within the patient, commonly called cuts or *sections*. The focal depth is the location of the focal plane for each cut. It is determined by the location of the fulcrum point in the patient. Different tomographs will automatically move the table, the entire tube—Bucky linkage arm assembly, or the rotational axis of the tube to change the level of the fulcrum point within the patient. It is important to remember that the focal depth indicated by the machine is measured upward from the *tabletop*. Therefore, if a sponge or pad is placed under the patient, the thickness of that object must be subtracted from the indicated focal depth to obtain the actual focal depth from the patient's down-side. Tomographic films must be marked accurately as measured with reference to the patient and not to the tabletop for focal depth.

Before proceeding, the radiographer must determine the interval of distance to be used between the cuts that will be taken. This interval should be based directly upon the thickness of cut obtained by the tube movement as listed in Table 33-1. If the intervals between the focal depths of the cuts taken are too small, unnecessary patient dose results. If they are too great, then important anatomy or pathology may be actually missed between cuts and lead to a misdiagnosis. As a rule, the interval used should be slightly less than the thickness of the focal plane obtained. Consulting Table 33-1, for example, hypocycloidal cuts should be taken about every millimeter of depth, whereas 30-degree linear cuts may be taken every 3 millimeters.

Having determined the intervals to be used, *two* scout films should be taken for a tomographic procedure at two different but adjacent focal depths. Providing the radiologist with two scouts allows him to be certain of how many cuts to take in each direction, because he is able to see which scout is approaching the middle of the anatomy of interest. This procedure will spare much unnecessary patient dose, which results from taking the same number of cuts in both directions from one scout, only to find that several to one side were completely out of the anatomy of interest. The radiographer can also save patient dose by having a thorough knowledge of anatomy to localize a starting depth for scout films. For example, the kidneys typically lie about one-third of the way from the patient's back to his front. Thus, a good starting point on a 22-cm patient would be to take one scout radiograph at 7 cm and one at 8 cm. Because of all of the additional considerations and thorough knowledge of anatomy required of tomographic radiographers, this area may be considered as an advanced subspecialty of radiography.

SUMMARY

1. *Tomography* desuperimposes obstructing structures from the anatomy of interest by blurring all objects which lie above or below the focal plane. The greater the amplitude or exposure arc, the thinner the *focal plane.*

2. More complex tomographic tube movements help eliminate *false images* such as streaking, which are created by the geometrical relationship of the movement to the anatomy. Movements with a long axis are best used when aligned perpendicular to the long axis of the anatomy to be blurred.

3. On most tomographs, the total *technique* used should be roughly double that for the same anatomy in conventional radiography. Exposure times must be long enough for the tube movement to complete its cycle.

4. Two tomographic *scout films* at different focal depths should be taken so that the radiologist can orient himself. *Intervals* between cuts should be slightly less than the focal plane thickness being obtained, so that no anatomy is missed and patient dose is minimized.

5. Single-film triangulation and the fluoroscopic parallax method for foreign body localization use the apparent shift of images when the observer's viewpoint is changed to determine the depth of foreign bodies.

REVIEW QUESTIONS

1. Define parallax:
2. Explain the two diagnostic purposes for the use of tomography to desuperimpose anatomical parts:
3. Define autotomography and give an example of a procedure which uses it:
4. Define focal plane:
5. Define tomographic amplitude:
6. The longer the exposure arc, the _____ the focal plane produced.
7. Define false image and give an example:
8. Describe the advantage of pluridirectional tube movements over unidirectional (linear) ones in regard to image qualities:
9. For inner ear anatomy, which tomographic tube movements would be rec-

ommended:

10. What is the typical focal plane thickness obtained with 30-degree linear tomography?

11. Most tomographs use movements which result in varying tube-film distances throughout the sweep of the tube. As a rule of thumb, to compensate for this, the mAs value from a routine chart must be _____.

12. If a hypocycloidal movement produces focal planes 1.2 mm thick, the proper interval to change each focal depth (cut) is:

13. For a 25 cm-thick patient, at what focal depths should the first two "cuts" be taken for an IVP series:

14. List the four measurements that must be known in order to calculate the depth of a foreign body using the single-film triangulation method:

Chapter 34

FLUOROSCOPIC IMAGE INTENSIFICATION

ROBERT J. PARELLI

FLUOROSCOPY IS the production of *dynamic* radiographic images, in effect, moving pictures. Fluoroscopic images are obtained in *realtime* or immediately as they occur. Because fluoroscopy usually involves active diagnosis during the examination, it is usually performed by the radiologist, while the radiographer acts as assistant and follows up with regular overhead views.

The great inventor, Thomas Edison, is credited with introducing the first fluoroscope in 1896, the year after Roentgen discovered x-rays. His device was a light-tight, hand-held metal cone with a fluorescent screen in the bottom and a viewing window in the top–with the x-ray tube operating from the opposite side of the patient, this cone would be held over the patient so that the remnant x-ray beam struck the fluorescent screen, making it glow and producing an image that could be viewed through the window. Edison's fluoroscope evolved by attaching the x-ray tube mechanically to the intensifying screen in a single, movable carriage system. The operator would lean over the screen while the x-ray tube was energized to view the fluoroscopic image. This system had two major disadvantages. First, the image on the screen was extremely dim and required all of the extraneous light to be turned off in order to view the fluoroscopic image. Second, it required very high radiation exposure to the patient and the operator.

In the late 1940s, the first electronic image intensification tube was introduced. The image intensifier improved image visibility, lowered patient and operator dose, and brought with it the ability to add multiple devices for recording permanent images. Fluoroscopic image intensification provides dynamic real-time imaging in which the physiological function of organs may be observed. Various gastrointestinal organs can be observed with the use of contrast media. Image intensification allows the operator to position the patient to demonstrate anatomy and pathology of interest. Static images can be performed with the use of various recording devices such as a film/screen spot film device, 105 mm spot film camera, magnetic tape or disc, or cine (motion picture) camera.

Fluoroscopic image intensification examinations can require several hours with a total beam-on time up to an hour. During the fluoroscopic procedure, when the x-ray beam is on, the patient is being irradiated. To keep the radiation dose to the patient from becoming a health hazard, the exposure rate in fluoroscopic image intensification is several orders of magnitude lower than in radiography. For example, a typical overhead abdominal technique, using 250 film/screen speed system, for an adult male is 75 kVp, 600 mA, 0.1 second (60 mAs) would result in a skin entrance exposure of about 1.0 Roentgen to the patient. If 600 mA of tube current were used for 10 minutes of fluoroscopic beam-on time, the patient skin entrance exposure would be about 5, 900 Roentgen and would result in serious radiation injury to the patient. An actual fluoroscopic image intensification examination of this adult male would require only about 3 mA of tube current. Therefore, 10 minutes of fluoroscopic beam-on time would result in about 30 R to the patient. The exposure *rate* in fluoroscopy is much less than in radiography; however, the *total* x-ray exposure is usually more because of the amount of time the fluoroscopic beam is on.

Relatively few x-ray photons are used in forming a single fluoroscopic image; therefore, fluoroscopic images are statistically inferior to radiographic images. The radiographic image would be formed with 600 times more photons, over a shorter period of time, than the fluoroscopic image. The fluoroscopic system needs to produce an image bright enough for the operator to see with less x-ray photons penetrating the patient. Therefore, fluoroscopic image intensification units must have a very high brightness.

The modern fluoroscopic imaging system consists of any x-ray system capable of continuous low mA output, an image intensification tube, a closed-circuit video camera with monitor, and a tandem lens apparatus. Other components are often found attached to this basic system for added flexibility. Systems with the x-ray tube above the patient and the image intensifier under the patient are also common. The collimator that limits the size of the x-ray beam is automatically adjusted to the proper field of view. When the source-to-detector distance is charged, as it often is when panning over anatomical regions of variable patient thickness, the collimator opens and closes to accommodate the differing height of the image intensifier. The x-ray generator requires additional circuitry to operate in the fluoroscopic mode. In many systems, a three-phase radiographic system may have single-phase fluoroscopic circuitry. An additional electronic circuit, known as the automatic brightness stabilization control or the automatic exposure control, will alter the kVp or the mA (tube current) or both with changes in anatomic part thickness, tissue density differences, and atomic number differences.

The fluoroscopic system accommodates a wide variety of modifications and is the central component of many modalities, such as photospot filming, spot film acquisition, digital subtraction angiography, endoscopic examinations, lithotripsy, and cineradiography. It is important to understand how these systems function and what parameters influence image quality to perform fluoroscopic examinations with expertise and confidence.

IMAGE INTENSIFICATION DEVICE

Modern image intensifiers, though they are complicated devices, operate in a simple way. An x-ray tube, under the table, exposes the patient. The x-ray beam passes through the patient and is intercepted by the image intensification tube. The objective of the image intensification tube is to convert the remnant radiation coming out of the patient to a light image.

The image intensifier tube is an evacuated glass envelop, a vacuum tube that contains four basic parts: (a) input phosphor and photocathode; (b) electrostatic lens; (c) accelerating anode; and (d) output phosphor. The image intensifier tube design can vary in size. The input diameter size can vary from 6 inches to 9 inches, 12 inches, and 16 inches. The output diameter size will always be one inch. The difference in size of the input diameter to output diameter causes the light image produced at the input phosphor to be thousands of times brighter at the output phosphor. *An increase in the input diameter size will increase image resolution.*

Input Phosphor and Photocathode

The input phosphor of a modern image intensifier has cesium iodide fluorescent phosphors which transform the remnant radiation coming out of the patient to light. The light emitted is in the yellow-green wavelength. The photocathode is a photoemissive metal, which is a combination of antimony and cesium compounds, that will receive the light emitted by the input screen phosphors and convert the light energy to electrons. This is similar to the familiar photoelectric effect, except that many light photons are required to cause a single electron to be emitted from the photocathode. Thus, a beam of millions of

electrons is produced (Fig. 34-1).

Electrostatic Focusing Lens

The electrostatic focusing lens is a series of bands or rings of metal, which have varying positive voltage, through which the electron beam must pass. They have the capacity of pulling the electrons at the input side toward the output phosphor. The focusing rings have varying degrees of positive electrical charge and are so arranged that they will cause the electrons produced at the photocathode to be focused onto the much smaller output screen (Fig. 34-1). Electron focusing inverts the light image at the output screen. The light image at the output screen is reduced in size, which is the principle reason why the light image is brighter at the output screen. That is, the electrons are *concentrated* onto the much smaller screen, so it glows more brightly.

Accelerating Anode

Located at the neck of the image intensifier tube, the function of the accelerating anode is to attract the electrons from the photocathode and accelerate them toward

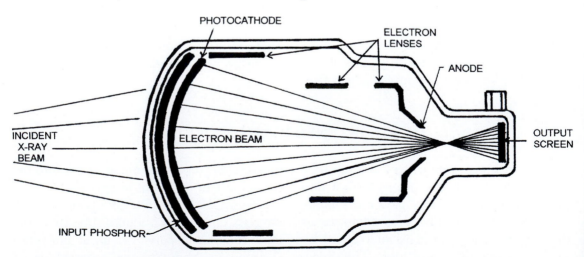

Figure 34-1. Image Instensification Tube Components.

the output screen. The accelerating anode is a small ring of metal, which has a positive charge of 25,000 volts. With this tremendous positive attraction to the anode, the electrons strike the output phosphor with much more kinetic energy, all of which will be transformed into light. This acceleration of the electrons is often called *flux gain* (an increase in the "flow" or intensity rate of the electron beam).

Output Phosphor

The output phosphor of the image intensifier tube (Fig. 34-1) is made of cesium iodide. When the electrons interact with the cesium iodide phosphor their kinetic energy is transformed into light. Since the output phosphor is typically only 1 inch in diameter, the light emitted from it is very concentrated and bright. This light then passes to the television camera or other recording device.

The focusing of the electron beam onto the smaller output phosphor is called *minification*. Minification gain can be easily estimated by forming a simple ratio from the areas of the input phosphor and the output phosphor. For example, the area of a 9-inch circular input phosphor, using the formula πr^2 is $3.14(4.5)^2 = 63.6$ square inches, that of the 1-inch circular output phosphor is 0.8 inches. These numbers round up to 64 and 1, respectively. If the entire 9-inch input phosphor is used, the minification gain will be approximately $64/1 = 64$. That is, the brightness of the light emitted from the image intensifier will be 64 times greater than the light originally emitted from the input phosphor, *from the minification process alone.*

Brightness Gain

Note from the above discussion that

there are actually *two* distinct processes which both contribute to image intensification: flux gain, and minification. It is the combination of these two processes that results in the final brightness achieved in the light image emitted from the image intensifier tube toward the television camera and other recording devices.

Conversion Factor

The result of the conversion of x-rays to light and amplification of the image results in an increase in light levels by as much as 20,000 times. This dramatic increase in the brightness of the image, termed brightness gain, is the prime factor in reducing the patient exposure and improving the visibility of the image. The International Commission on Radiologic Units and Measurements (ICRU) recommends evaluating the brightness gain of image intensifiers based upon the *conversion factor.* The conversion factor is defined as the ratio of the luminance of the output phosphor to the input *x-ray* exposure rate:

$$\text{Conversion Factor} = \frac{\text{Candela/Meter}^2}{\text{Milliroentgen/Second}}$$

Since radiation quantity and output luminance are explicitly defined, the method is accurate and reproducible unlike the older "total brightness gain."

Once the image is intensified it can be reflected through a series of mirrors to be received by a television camera or it can produce static images using the spot film camera (Fig. 34-3).

DUAL FIELD IMAGE INTENSIFIER TUBES/MAGNIFICATION MODES

The field of view (FOV) is a specification of the size of the input phosphor of the

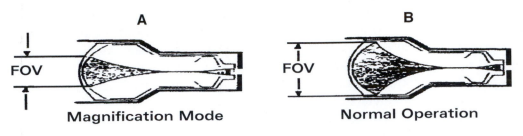

FOV – Field of view.

Figure 34-2. Field of View (FOV: In magnification mode, *A*, the field of view at the imput phosphor is reduced.

image intensifier. Large FOV image intensifier tubes are very useful for examinations in which a large area of the patient's anatomy must be viewed, for instance in lower gastrointestinal studies. A large FOV image intensifier allows more of the anatomy to be imaged simultaneously, resulting in less panning and potentially shorter studies. However, it may be necessary to focus in and magnify a selected region of the patient's anatomy. This can be accomplished on most image intensifiers by changing the electric field in the electrostatic lens system so that a smaller region of the input phosphor is projected to the output phosphor (Fig. 34-2). The magnified mode is selected by pushing a button. Image intensifier tubes with dual mode or trimode magnification are very common. For example, a trimode 9 inch (23 cm) input diameter tube usually has a 5 inch (12 cm) and 7 inch (18 cm) magnification modes.

When the size of the fluoroscopic image is unimportant, the magnified mode can be used for better spatial resolution: The number of pixels (picture elements) available in the final output image (the TV monitor) is the same, yet the area of anatomy being inputed to the image intensifier is smaller, so there are more pixels per area of anatomy. Just as with digital imaging, more pixels means smaller pixels per anatomical area, thus smaller, finer details can be made

out. However, for the same reason, the image will be much dimmer. That is, due to the short field of view being inputed, there is less input light per output pixel. To compensate for the dim image, the mA (tube current) must be increased. Therefore, the patient skin entrance dose is increased.

BEAM SPLITTER

In order to record the fluoroscopic image with spot film cameras and cine film, the image intensifier must be able to divide the light coming from the output screen and direct it in two separate paths. This system of reflecting light in two directions is called *beam splitting*. A semitransparent mirror is placed between the image intensifier and the television camera tube (Fig. 34-3). Ninety percent of the light is reflected to the recording system while the remaining light passes through the mirrors and is received by the television camera tube. Sufficient light is transmitted through the beam splitter mirror to the television camera to allow the operator to view an image on the monitor during the recording of the image.

Figure 34-3 shows an overview of the process: In the intensifier tube, the input phosphor and the photocathode convert the signal into a beam of electrons, which can be accelerated and focused (minified) onto the output phosphor. Options for pro-

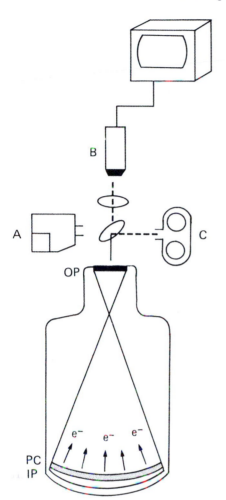

Figure 34-3. Image intensifier and fluoroscopic imaging options. Options for processing the image include the photospot camera, the television camera, and the cine camera. The beam splitter lens/mirror above the ouptut phosphor allows two of these options to be used simultaneously. As pictured here, the TV and the cine cameras receive the light image. If the beam splitter mirror is rotated 90 degrees, the photospot camera and TV camera would both receive the light beam.

cessing the image include the photospot camera, the television camera, and the cine camera. The beam splitter lens/mirror above the output phosphor allows two of these options to be used simultaneously. The television and the cine camera receive the light image. If the beam splitter mirror were rotated 90 degrees, the photospot camera and the television camera would both receive the light beam.

AUTOMATIC BRIGHTNESS STABILIZATION CONTROL VERSUS AUTOMATIC GAIN CONTROL

In image intensification, the brightness of the fluoroscopic screen or television monitor must be maintained at an acceptable level throughout the entire procedure. Two separate systems are available to compensate for part thickness changes as the patient moves onto his or her side, or as the physical density of the part changes during the procedure.

The first system is the *automatic brightness stabilization control (ABS)*. A properly designed ABS system must accomplish the following objectives:

1. It must hold the image brightness constant for variations of patient thickness and attenuation.
2. It must ignore information at the image margins.
3. It must operate to preserve image contrast and minimize image noise.
4. It must keep the operation within the ratings of the x-ray tube not to exceed 10 R/min.
5. It must effect a reasonable compromise between patient exposure and image quality.
6. It must keep the patient exposure within the radiation control regulations of 10 R/min, except when the operator selects an override mode of operation.
7. It must respond fast enough to track during an examination but slowly enough to avoid hunting between bright and dark portions of the image.
8. It must compensate for system vari-

ables, such as the magnification of the image, the intensifier, and the use of disc recorders.

9. It must be capable of being disabled or "held" at a particular equilibrium value prior to injection of contrast media.

10. It must be capable of being shut off to permit the manual control of factors.

11. It must display the operating factors and modes of operation to the operator.

Brightness Sensing

Fluoroscopic image intensifier systems use many methods of sensing light output from the image intensifier tube:

1. *Image Intensifier Photocathode Current.* The photocathode of the image intensifier is normally connected to the ground, while the accelerating anode is connected to a source of 25 to 35 kilovolts. The ground connection can be removed and fed to a current amplifier so that the amplifier output is proportional to the radiation input.

2. *Television Camera Signal Sensing.* Most television cameras have automatic gain control (AGC) circuits for controlling the camera tube target voltage or the gain in video amplifiers in order to provide a constant output signal over variations of image brightness. The AGC can be used to control the generator as well.

3. *Lens-Coupled Photo Tube Sensing.* This method uses a lens often combined with a prism or mirror so that the collimated light from the image intensifier is sampled and the image of the output phosphor is formed over an aperture plate in front of a photomul-

tiplier tube. This system will compensate for coning effects, field size changes, and mode changes of the image intensifier tube and will ignore bright flashes at the margin. The gain of the photomultiplier tube or photodiode can be controlled by adjustment of its power supply voltage so that it may be shared between the fluoroscopic ABS circuits and the various filming systems.

Types of Automatic Brightness Stabilization Circuits

Brightness stabilizers can be classified in terms of the variable controlled by the brightness sensor. There are four common types of brightness stabilization circuits.

1. *Variable mA, preset kVp.* This system allows the operator to set the kVp value and the brightness sensor will control the tube current (mA) over a range of 20 to 1. The operator can set this system to the required kVp for a particular examination and the brightness sensor will automatically adjust the mA to yield an image of sufficient contrast brightness.

2. *Variable mA with kVp following.* This system will vary the mA as a function of the brightness sensor, but it has an additional circuit that senses if an upper or lower boundary of mA has been exceeded and then controls the adjustment of kVp through a motor-driven variable transformer. Therefore, if the mA rises above a certain preset value, then the motor will drive the kVp value higher.

3. *Variable kVp with selected mA.* With this system, the brightness sensor controls the kVp. The operator will have previously selected the value of mA

required. If a motor-driven variable transformer is used to select kVp, the system has the additional advantage of remembering the last operating point as the operator energizes the system with the exposure switch. Therefore, restabilization of the system between scenes is very rapid. The operator can select a low mA that will force the brightness stabilizer to operate at a higher kVp for gastrointestinal examinations, or a high mA which will force the kVp of the system downward for best contrast when viewing iodine-based contrast media.

4. *Variable kVp, Variable mA.* With this system, the output of the brightness sensor controls both the kVp and the mA in order to maintain either constant image noise or constant image contrast. Unfortunately, such systems make it difficult for the operator to select the mode of operation best suited for the particular examination.

A second type of system is the *Automatic Gain Control (AGC)*. With this system the amplification of the *electronic* signal is increased or decreased as needed. The radiographic exposure factors remain unchanged. This system does not increase patient exposure; however, this system may not provide the best possible fluoroscopic image. *If an insufficient number of x-ray photons are reaching the image intensifier, no amount of increased electronic amplification can overcome the mottle or increased noise that is produced.* A brightness control switch or knob is sometimes found on the fluoroscopic image intensification tower, which can be adjusted by the operator as needed.

FLUOROSCOPIC TECHNIQUE/ VARIATIONS OF X-RAY EXPOSURE FACTORS

Operation of the fluoroscopic image intensifier at higher kVp values will result in increased transmission of the x-ray beam by the patient so that less radiation will be required. *The brightness of the fluoroscopic image varies directly to the mA used and roughly to the fifth power of kVp.* Therefore, as the kVp would vary from 80 to 88 kVp, a 10 percent change, there would be more than a 50 percent change in brightness. Table 34-1 lists the recommended kVp ranges for fluoroscopic imaging of various anatomical areas.

The fluoroscopic technique strategy is to use high kVp and low mA (tube current). Therefore, the automatic brightness stabilization control (ABS) should operate at high kVp values for reduced patient exposure and at low kVp values for higher image contrast. When viewing low-contrast objects using fluoroscopic image intensification, the system should operate at lower kVp values. This is particularly true when using iodine-based contrast media such as for arteriography, arthrography, hysterosalpingography, etc. More specifically, when examining the gastrointestinal tract using barium-based contrast media, operation at high kVp is better. The images are

Table 34-1

Optimum Fluoroscopic kVp Values	
Chest/Lung	60-65 kVp
Mediastinum	65-70 kVp
Gastrointestinal/Barium	110-120 kVp
Abdomen	70-80 kVp
Abdomen/Iodine Contrast	70-80 kVp
Pelvis/Hip	70-75 kVp
Lower Extremities	60-65 kVp
Shoulder	60-65 kVp
Upper Extremities	60 kVp

of fairly high contrast and the patient skin entrance exposure is reduced.

The kVp values mentioned are acceptable for use with the automatic brightness stabilization control and for manual fluoroscopic control. There are some manufactured ABS control units that need to have the kVp values set for the specific fluoroscopic procedure. For example, gastrointestinal studies require 120 kVp. However, other manufactured ABS units only adjust the fluoroscopic kVp up to plus or minus 10 kVp. If the fluoroscopic kVp is too high, the image on the monitor may be too bright to view the anatomic part. *Do not adjust the television brightness or contrast control on the monitor.* Increasing the brightness electronically also increases image noise. Turn the ABS control off and manually adjust the kVp down 10 percent adjustment until the optimum brightness is viewed on the television monitor; then turn the ABS control back on. This "10 percent rule" can be applied if the image on the television monitor is too dim or dark. The fluoroscopic 10 percent rule can also be applied for manual fluoroscopic technique, without ABS.

FLUOROSCOPIC EXPOSURE TIME

Operators of fluoroscopic image intensification equipment must restrict the x-ray beam "on time" to a minimum. Doubling the exposure time also doubles the skin entrance exposure to the patient. The x-ray beam need not be operated continuously. Image intensification can be accomplished with a series of short bursts of x-radiation. Five visual checks, assuming 12 seconds each, approximates one minute of exposure time. This translates, assuming 5 R/min exposure, to approximately 400 mR skin entrance exposure to the patient per visual check. Regulations require that the exposure switch activate a cumulative manual reset timer, which may produce an audible signal or temporarily interrupt the x-ray beam. This device is designed to make the operator aware of the relative beam "on" time during each fluoroscopic procedure.

IMAGE QUALITIES

The number of x-ray photons absorbed by the image intensifier determines the statistical quality of a fluoroscopic imaging system. No form of intensification can improve the image above the statistical level of the absorbed photons. Image quality of the image intensification system is defined by scintillation, resolution, contrast, and distortion.

Scintillation

Scintillation is known by many names, including *quantum mottle* or *quantum noise.* Viewed in the final fluoroscopic display, which is the television monitor, the effect will be that of a random noise pattern superimposed on the fluoroscopic image. This noise pattern, since it is random in nature, has the tendency to appear to be moving, giving rise to the colloquial expression of "crawling ants" or "snow." This effect occurs when an insufficient number of x-rays per unit of time are absorbed at the input screen. Quantum noise can be improved by high x-ray-to-light conversion efficiency. However, image quality can never be raised above that of the absorbed photons. *Therefore, the usual method employed to eliminate quantum noise is to raise the x-ray tube current (mA) to generate more x-ray quanta in a given period of time.* Once this threshold is reached, the noise may disappear and the fluoroscopic display takes on a much more pleasing appearance and is generally easier to interpret.

Contrast

One of the areas in which the image intensifier tube does not perform well is in the area of contrast. The contrast in the final image at the output phosphor screen is lowered or degraded by various effects. Any x-ray photon incident on the input screen of the image intensifier, which is *not* absorbed by the input phosphor, may pass through the intensifier tube and, if close to the intensifier tube axis, will strike the output phosphor screen. Since the x-ray photon has the property of exciting the output phosphor elements if it is absorbed, it will cause the output phosphor to fluoresce or emit light and produce an overall masking effect or a kind of inverse fog (brightness) on the output screen itself.

Another effect that would degrade the intensifier image would be any light emitted at the output phosphor screen moving backward, through the tube axis, which strikes the photocathode at the input side causing the photocathode to emit additional electrons. These electrons are in a random pattern and are not part of the original image, but are focused and accelerated back to the output phosphor screen just as those which originated from the primary x-ray beam. Contrast tends to deteriorate as an image intensifier ages. The deterioration rate can proceed at a rate of 10 percent per year; therefore, a periodic check of the image intensifier brightness is critical.

Distortion

PINCUSHION DISTORTION. This is a form of spatial distortion that warps the appearance of the image formed on a curved surface input phosphor to a flat output phosphor screen. Pincushion distortion results in slightly higher magnification of the input image toward the edge of the image. The amount of pincushion distortion is usually determined by an imaging grid or screen with regular spacing. Pincushion distortion can be reduced when magnification modes are utilized.

VEILING GLARE. Veiling glare is mainly the consequence of light scatter onto the output screen window of the image intensifier. The scattered light, just like scattered radiation, adds to the background signal and degrades the contrast in the fluoroscopic image. Therefore, there is not much that can be done to eliminate the presence of veiling glare.

VIGNETTING. The brightness measured at the output phosphor will vary from the center to the periphery of the image, even when a homogeneous x-ray field is incident upon the image intensifier. The brightness will be the greatest toward the center of the image and will fall off at the edges. One source of vignetting is a consequence of pincushion distortion. With pincushion distortion, the image is magnified to a greater extent toward the periphery. This means the minifying, electron-concentrating effect of the electron optics is reduced at the periphery, causing less brightness there. Vignetting also occurs in the optical coupling between the image intensifier and recording devices, because of scattered light effects.

IMAGE RECORDING SYSTEMS

Photospot Cameras

A photospot camera can be used to generate film images, taken from the output screen of the image intensifier. The most common formats are 100-mm cut film, or 105-mm roll film. Spot film cameras are convenient; if the physician wants to archive an image during the fluoroscopic examination, stepping on the floor pedal will activate the camera. The mirror in the optical distributor swings into the optical path, redirecting light rays toward the spot film camera. The x-ray generator produces a radiographic pulse of x-rays, and the image is recorded on film. The film is advanced and stored in a take-up magazine. Figures 34-4 and 34-5 show the typical loading of a photospot camera. Photospot images are made directly from the output phosphor of the image intensifi-

er, through lenses, and therefore enjoy the full resolution of the image intensifier systems, unencumbered by the video system. The aperture setting on the photospot camera itself determines the speed of the photospot images. A skin entrance exposure to the image intensifier of 75 to 100 microroentgen/frame is typically required for an image intensifier operating with a 9-inch (23-cm) FOV.

Digital Photospot

Digital photospot cameras (Fig. 34-6) are high-resolution, slow-scan television cameras in which the television signal is digitized and stored in computer memory. The contents of the computer memory can be instantly displayed on a television monitor, and therefore can be viewed without the time delay caused by film processing

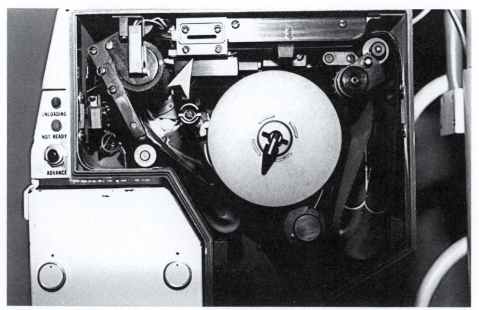

Figure 34-4. Photograph of photospot camera with cover removed. The aperture or shutter where the film is exposed is at the top of the camera (white arrowhead), and various rollers for film threading are shown (compare to Figure 34-5.)

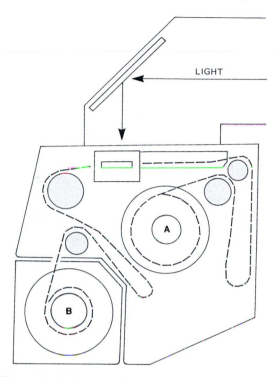

LIGHT

Figure 34-5. Diagram showing proper film threading path through rollers of the photospot camera in Figure 34-4, from supply spool (A) through shutter at top to take-up spool in receiver magazine (B). Light from the beam splitter is reflected down to the aperture by a mirror.

required in conventional photospot acquisition. Digital photospot cameras are typically 1023 scan-line television cameras. The television target is exposed to light emitted from the image intensifier, produced from a short radiographic pulse of x-rays, in the same manner and with the same exposure that conventional photospot images are acquired. The electron beam scans the television target slowly, often using four conventional frame times, for a total of 0.133 seconds.

An analog-to-digital convertor converts the voltage signal into a series of digital numbers stored in computer memory, and the contents of the computer memory can be displayed on the television monitor. Hard-copy images can be produced using

multiformat cameras or laser imagers, which are commonly used to produce film images from computerized sources such as CT, MRI, and DSA. Although the spatial resolution is less than 100-mm film, the rapid display and image processing capabilities enable a flexibility that is worth the slightly inferior spatial resolution.

Cineradiography

A cine camera (Fig. 34-7) is a simple strip-film motion picture camera that attaches to a port on the optical distributor of the image intensifier and can record a very rapid sequence of images on 35-mm film. Cine is used frequently in cardiac studies, where a very high frame rate is needed to capture the rapid motion of the heart. The frame rates of cine cameras operate from 30 frames/second to 120 frames/second or higher. Cine radiography uses very short radiographic pulses, and therefore special generators are needed. The x-ray tube loading is usually quite high, and so large anode, high heat capacity x-ray tubes usually accompany the other necessary cine hardware. A skin entrance exposure to the input phosphor of approximately 10 to 15 microroentgen/frame (9-inch diameter) is expected for cineradiography studies.

Spot-Film Devices

A spot-film device (Fig. 34-8) is an apparatus that attaches to the front end of the image intensifier and can automatically acquire images on a radiographic screen-film cassette by a simple press of a button. There is a small control panel on the attachment that enables the physician or operator to acquire a radiographic image using the spot-film device. The spot-film device has a transport mechanism which, when an

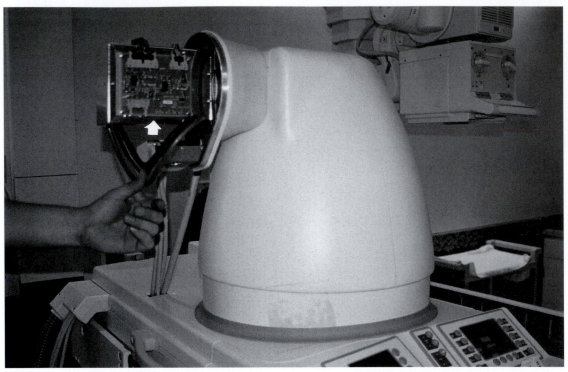

Figure 34-6. Digital photospot television camera assembly (arrow) attached to a modern digital fluoroscopy image intensifier.

image is called for, moves a screen-film cassette from the parked position to a position directly in front of the image intensifier tube. Newer systems automatically collimate to a variety of formats. For example, one 30-cm x 30-cm cassette can be exposed with four different 15-cm x 15-cm radiographic images. Although quite heavy and cumbersome, spot-film devices are convenient when large FOV images are routinely required as in gastrointestinal studies. The spot-film device allows the acquisition of radiographic screen film images. The fluoroscopic system participates in the positioning for the radiograph, but the image intensifier is not used to acquire the image. Since the screen-film systems deliver substantially more spatial resolution than an image intensifier, there is an important distinction between photospot cameras, which do use the image intensifier, and spot-film devices, which do not.

SPOT-FILMING TECHNIQUE

Inserting the spot film cassette into the fluoroscopic tower and selecting the imaging format, along with changing the spot film cassette during the fluoroscopic procedure, is the responsibility of the radiographer. The format selection knob or buttons are located on the image intensification tower.

It is important that radiographers familiarize themselves with all the different image intensification units in their department. Each unit may have different spot

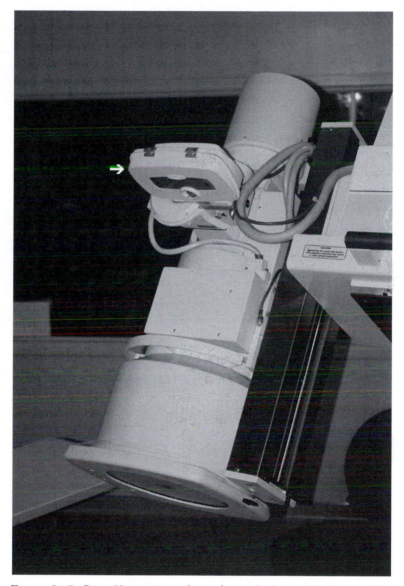

Figure 34-7. Cine film camera (arrow) attached to side of a cardiac catheterization lab image intensifier. (Television camera is in cylinder at top.)

film mechanisms, one that inserts the cassette from the front, and one that inserts the cassette from the rear or behind the image intensifier tower. The spot film cassette is held in reserve in the park position until the physician or operator depresses the spot film exposure switch. If the spot film cassette does not automatically come to the unload position after the spot film has been exposed the selected number of times, an unload button or release must be activated. Once the spot film cassette has moved into the unload position, there is a release button that must be triggered to release the spot film cassette from its carriage. Spot films are phototimed or automatically exposed radiographs. The fluoroscopic x-ray tube current will adjust from 1 to 5 mil-

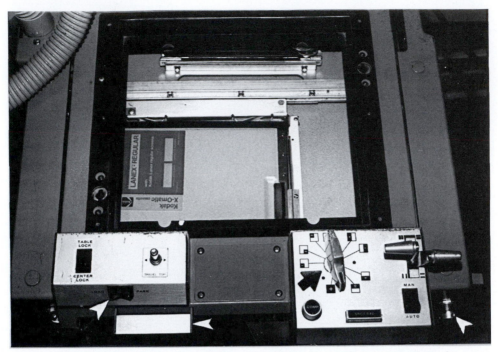

Figure 34-8. Traditional spot film changer with image intensifier removed so that spot film can be seen in position for exposure to one corner.

liamperes to a few hundred milliamperes. The radiographic phototimer or automatic exposure control must be activated to the spot film mode and the center or ion chamber must be initiated.

Milliamperage Selection

The fluoroscopic mA control on the generator controls the x-ray tube filament. The fluoroscopic mA is usually set at 200, 300, or 400, which will provide the quantity of x-radiation need for both the fluoroscopic and/or radiographic modes of operation. Selecting an appropriate mA station will allow the phototimer or automatic exposure control to operate.

Kilovoltage

Radiographic kVp must be set for operating in the phototiming or automatic

exposure control. Optimum radiographic kVp values must be assigned based on the anatomic part thickness, anatomic tissue density, and the atomic number of the anatomic part that will be imaged. Optimum kVp values should be the same as in the fluoroscopic mode (see Table 34-1).

Automatic Exposure Control

When the spot film cassette device is activated for radiographic images, the automatic exposure control (AEC) or phototimer will automatically terminate the radiographic exposure when the spot film cassette has received a predetermined x-ray exposure. AEC switches use radiation detectors that measure the radiation reaching the film/screen system. The signal from the radiation detector is integrated and when the integrated signal reaches a preset level, the exposure is terminated. Three types of AEC detectors are used: ion chambers, solid-state diodes, and scintillators coupled to photomultiplier tubes (PMTs). The flat, parallel-plate ionization chamber is the most commonly used and is mounted between the patient and the film. The ion chamber is radiolucent and does not leave a shadow on the radiographic image. The ionization generated in air within the chamber is collected as a signal, which is proportional to the intensity of the x-rays transmitted through the patient.

A radiographic density adjustment control is present on the generator console. The control is generally set on NORMAL density to produce the optimum radiographic density on the spot film. Changes in density should occur when the MINUS or PLUS density stations are used. On most equipment, each station represents a 25 percent increase or decrease in technique from the normal setting.

Back-up Time

The back-up time represents the maximum exposure that an AEC will permit for a given mA and kVp value. The manufacturer generally sets the back-up time within the instantaneous load capacity of the x-ray tube. On some units, the radiographer can manually select the back-up time on the control panel. The settings, either manual or automatic, must fall within the tube manufacturer's recommendations for instantaneous load.

The back-up time settings help to avoid additional x-ray exposure to the patient as well as damage to the x-ray tube. The back-up time can be set for 1 to 6 seconds. The AEC eliminates the need to measure part thickness or to calculate milliampere-second values.

MOBILE IMAGE INTENSIFICATION (C-ARM)

Mobile fluoroscopic image intensification units can be used in the emergency room, intensive care unit, coronary care unit, operating room, or fracture rooms. A "C" arm fluoroscopic image intensifier with closed circuit television attachment enables a physician to view the fluoroscopic image in "real time." An x-ray tube is mounted at one end of the "C" frame in alignment with an image intensifier and can be rotated around a fixed axis in many directions to avoid moving the patient. Fracture reduction, needle biopsy, catheter placement, or hip pinning studies are often performed using the mobile image intensifier. Once the initial set up is complete, it is important for the radiographer to test the unit to be sure of its operation and to orient the screen so it is automatically correct. An easy way to orientate the screen is to use a right or left lead markers during the test image. A coin or paper clip taped to the intensifier tube will also work. The radiographer can use the screen rotation buttons and the screen reverse button to properly display the image.

During the fluoroscopic procedure the radiographer may be called upon to manipulate the intensifier to follow the position of the pacemaker wire or catheter. It is important to know how to manipulate the arm and overhead tube locks. There are four basic locks on a C-arm: transverse, longitudinal, 360-degree circular rotation, and 180-degree AP to lateral rotation. These are illustrated on a typical C-arm unit in Figures 34-9 and 34-10. The transverse lock allows the C-arm to be extended

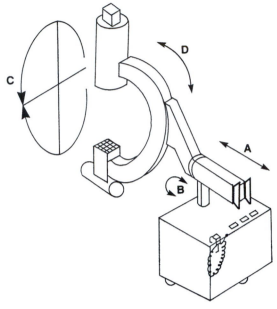

and retracted across the table or patient. For example, it could be used to follow a guide wire from the shoulder to the midline of a patient. The longitudinal lock allows the entire C-arm to swivel to the right or left. In situations such as a pacemaker or catheter placement, it may be easier for the radiographer to unlock both the transverse and longitudinal locks, giving the intensification tube nearly free movement in any direction whenever it is needed. The 360-degree lock rotates the C-arm so that the intensifier tube is above or below the patient. The 180-degree lock allows the x-ray tube and image intensifier to move between AP and lateral projections. The C-arm will move either over or under the patient, depending on where the image intensifier is positioned. If the intensifier is over the patient, the lateral movement will be below or under the patient. If the image intensifier is under the patient, the lateral

Figure 34-9. Diagram of C-Arm mobile fluoroscopy unit, showing transverse movement of entire arm (A), longitudinal swivel (B), 360-degree rotation (C), and 180-degree AP to lateral sliding movement (D).

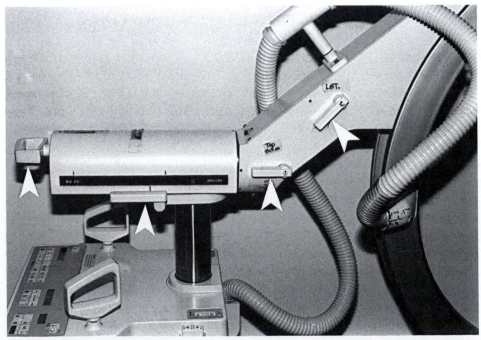

Figure 34-10. Close-up of typical locks on a modern C-Arm unit. Arrowheads left to right: Transverse lock, longitudinal swivel lock, 360-degree rotation lock, and 180-degree AP to lateral lock. Compare with Figure 34-9.

movement will be over the patient. Care must be used when changing from the AP to the lateral position. The C-arm should be raised or lowered while rotating the arm over or under the patient.

It is important to note that in many surgical, intensive care, and emergency room procedures, a special table extension or dedicated intensifier table must be used. The metal frames of the surgical tables, beds, and gurneys are not designed for use with the C-arm. A carbon-filter type table, having a low absorption rate, will significantly reduce patient exposure.

When observation of actual motion or real time imaging is not needed, such as with most orthopedic or urological examinations and parts of some surgical and cardiac procedures, operators of mobile image intensification equipment may incorporate an image storage, videodisc recorder with electronic radiography. This type of electronic imaging will significantly reduce the patient skin entrance dose.

MINIMIZING PATIENT AND OPERATOR EXPOSURE

Fluoroscopic image intensification represents a very large portion of the dose delivered in diagnostic imaging because of continuous x-ray production and real time image output. While the exposure techniques are quite modest, such as 1 to 3 mA of tube current at 75 to 85 kVp for most fluoroscopic studies, an exam usually takes several minutes and, in some difficult cases, can exceed hours of "beam on" time. For example, a single-phase generator system delivering 1 mA of tube current at 80 kVp for 10 minutes of fluoroscopy "beam on" time may produce a tabletop skin entrance exposure of 22 R/minute. Regulations require that the tabletop skin entrance exposure cannot exceed 2.2 R/min per mA of tube current when operated at 80 kVp.

Reduction of fluoroscopic exposure is achieved in several ways. The most important method is to limit the "beam on" time. The operator can significantly reduce fluoroscopic time by using only short bursts of on time instead of staring at an unchanging continuous display. A five-minute cumulative manual reset timer is required on all fluoroscopic units to remind the operator audibly of each 5-minute time interval and to allow the radiographer to keep track of the total amount of fluoroscopic "beam on" time for the examination. Last-image-hold devices using digital image memory are commonplace; one of these devices provides a continuous output image that can be examined by the fluoroscopist after a short burst of x-rays. The last-image-hold device can reduce the fluoroscopic on time by 50 percent to 80 percent in many situations. Videotape recording and playback are also helpful in the endeavor. *Pulsed fluoroscopy* can reduce doses: lower frame rates than real time, such as 15 or 7.5 frames/second, are used in conjunction with a digital image memory to provide a continuous output video signal with reduced x-ray pulsing and update rates of the displayed information. A pulsed fluoroscopic unit allows the x-ray tube to pulsate the x-ray beam at the same frequency as the power supply, which is 60 Hz. Therefore, the fluoroscopic image can be viewed at much lower framing rates than the common television frame rate of 30 frames/second.

The use of an optimal image intensification system with appropriate conversion gain, high contrast ratio, and acceptable spatial resolution and contrast sensitivity also reduce the patient dose. Restriction of the field size with collimation will help keep the integral dose to the patient ALARA (as low as reasonably achieved). Image quality will improve as the size of the x-ray beam is reduced because there is a reduction in the amount of scattered radiation reaching the image intensifier tube. More specifically, utilizing proper collimation will reduce quantum mottle/noise.

Filtration is any material placed in the useful/primary x-ray beam to absorb less penetrating radiations and "harden" the beam. When using 85 kVp and with a 0.5-mm aluminum filter, a typical exposure at 50-cm (19-inches) target to panel or table-top distance is 3.5m R/mAs. At 85 kVp and 2.0-mm aluminum filter, the table top/panel exposure is 1.2 mR/mAs.

Regulations require that the minimum amount of total filtration used for the fluoroscopic x-ray tube is 2.5-mm of aluminum equivalent. Therefore, the intensity of the x-ray beam at the tabletop should not exceed 2.2 R/min for each mA of operating tube current at 80 kVp.

SUMMARY

1. The fluoroscopic image is generated by a series of subcomponents, and the term *imaging chain* is descriptive of the image intensifier/television camera system. The image intensifier can either be over or under the table. The image intensifier electronically amplifies the information it receives to produce an image that is up to 20,000 times brighter. A spot film device or photospot camera may be used to record the fluoroscopic image.

2. The fluoroscopic image chain allows for the adjustment of the exposure rate used in producing the images. The *automatic brightness stabilization* system (ABS) will automatically control the fluoroscopic kVp and/or tube current in mA. The ABS control can be turned off and the selection of kVp and mA can be accomplished manually.

3. The *quality* of the fluoroscopic image is defined by scintillation, resolution, contrast, and distortion. The number of absorbed x-ray photons determines the highest possible statistical quality of the imaging system. Therefore, applying the proper amounts of fluoroscopic kVp and tube current in mA is important in producing the appropriate number of x-rays and quality of energy to produce a quality image.

4. *Image recording systems* are used to archive the fluoroscopic image. The various types of recording systems are the photospot camera, digital photospot camera, cineradiography camera, and the film/screen spot film device. The film/screen spot film device provides the highest resolution and the highest patient exposure of all the recording systems.

5. The *maximum exposure rate* to the patient permitted in the United States is governed by federal regulations. The maximal legal entrance exposure rate for normal fluoroscopy to the patient is 10 R/min. Most State health departments have identical regulations that are imposed on hospitals and private office. The tabletop skin entrance exposure cannot exceed 2.2 R/min per mA of tube current when operated at 80 kVp. Fluoroscopic image intensification examinations are the largest contributor of medical radiation expo-

sure to the general population, far exceeding the exposure due to radiog-raphy or computed tomography.

REVIEW QUESTIONS

1. What are the four basic parts of the image intensifier tube?
2. Focusing the electrons in the image intensification is accomplished by the _____.
3. The ICRU has recommended the _____ as the best method of evaluating brightness gain for image intensifiers.
4. How does the field of view (FOV) affect the spatial resolution of the output phosphor image when the image intensifier tube is operated in the magnified mode?
5. How does the field of view (FOV) affect the brightness level of the output phosphor image when the image intensifier tube is operated in the magnified mode?
6. The brightness of the fluoroscopic image varies directly with the mA and roughly to the fifth power of the kVp. Therefore, as the kVp is increased from 80 to 88 kVp, a 10 percent change, there will be more than a _____ percent increase in brightness.
7. What is the usual method to help eliminate quantum noise?
8. Contrast deterioration rate can proceed at _____ percent per year.
9. How does pincushion distortion affect the fluoroscopic image?
10. Dimness around the periphery of the fluoroscopic image is called _____.
11. A single-phase generator delivering 1 mA of tube current at 80 kVp for 10 minutes of fluoroscopic time may produce a tabletop skin entrance exposure rate of _____.
12. Which fluoroscopy tabletop has a low absorption rate that will significantly reduce patient skin entrance exposure?
13. Name the device that divides the light off the output phosphor between ancillary recording devices and the television camera.
14. Name the four major locks on a mobile C-arm:
15. List the three different ways of sensing the amount of light output from the image intensifier tube:
16. List the four different types of brightness stabilization circuits:
17. What term describes the loss of contrast from scattered light at the output phosphor of an image intensifier?

Chapter 35

DIGITAL IMAGING

EUCLID SEERAM

THE APPLICATION of computer processing of images (digital image processing) in the Radiology department has come to be known as *Digital Imaging.*

Digital image processing has its roots in the space program where various techniques were used not only to enhance images sent back from space but to restore them as well. Today the space program continues to utilize digital image processing and it has become the field which generates and uses the largest amount of digital data.

The success of image processing in the space program has had significant impact on applications in other fields. In radiology, for example, digital imaging techniques are the basis for computed tomography,

magnetic resonance imaging and digital radiography and fluoroscopy. In fact, radiology has become the field which generates and uses the second largest amount of digital data.

THE NATURE OF IMAGES

Images can be represented in several ways. In photography for example, images are formed by focusing light onto photographic film. In conventional radiography, images are projected onto x-ray film. In addition, images can be paintings, drawings, or they can be formed by photo-electronic means as well as be represented as mathematical functions. These images are

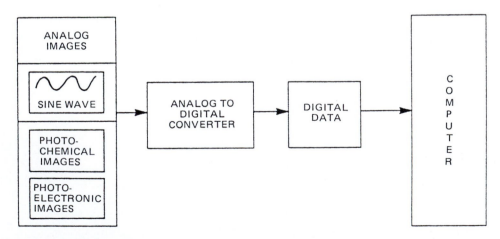

Figure 35-1. Block diagram showing the conversion of analog data into digital data for input into a digital computer. (From Seeram, E. *X-Ray Imaging Equipment–An Introduction.* Charles C Thomas., 1985. Reproduced by permission.)

referred to as *analog images*, which means that the information they represent is changing continuously with time, compared to information available in discrete units. The sine wave is a popular representation of an analog signal.

Images obtained in the conventional radiographic mode are analog images. In digital imaging these analog images must be changed into digital data so that they can be processed by a digital computer. In effect, the analog information is "rounded out" to discrete numbers so the computer can handle it (Fig. 35-1). Once the computer processes this information, it produces an output image in digital form as shown in Figure 35-2.

0	0	0	0	0	0	0	0	0	0
0	0	0	11	11	11	11	0	0	0
0	0	11	11	11	11	11	11	0	0
0	11	11	11	555	555	11	11	11	0
0	11	11	555	555	555	555	11	11	0
0	11	11	555	555	555	555	11	11	0
0	11	11	11	555	555	11	11	11	0
0	0	11	11	11	11	11	11	0	0
0	0	0	11	11	11	11	0	0	0
0	0	0	0	0	0	0	0	0	0

Figure 35-2. Computer processing of digital input data results in information which can be displayed in digital form. In this oversimplified example, the background is assigned a numerical value of zero, soft tissue has a pixel value of 11, and the bone in the middle is assigned a value of 555.

THE DIGITAL COMPUTER

Digital imaging requires a digital computer. It is mandatory that the technologist understand the fundamentals of the computer in order to fully appreciate digital imaging applications in radiology.

Hardware

The hardware refers to the physical units of the computer: the input devices, the processing system, the storage devices, and the output devices connected as shown in Figure 35-3. Input devices are physical devices such as keyboards, for example, which are used to send information to the processing system. The processing system is usually referred to as they *central processing unit (CPU)* and it serves to convert the input data through a series of processing operations, into output data.

The CPU consists of two major units, the *arithmetic/logic unit (ALU)* and the *control unit.* While the ALU performs arithmetic and logical operations on data, the control unit directs the flow of data between what is referred to as *primary memory*, and the ALU as well as between the CPU and the input/output devices.

Primary memory is also referred to as *main memory, internal memory* and *random access memory (RAM).* These are used to store the programs and data on which the computer is presently executing. These programs and data are erasable and RAM is said to be *volatile*, which means that the information in memory is lost when the computer is turned off. In contrast to this, the computer has memory chips which contain nonerasable programs. These chips are referred to as *read only memory (ROM).*

Once the data has been processed it is now ready to be sent to an output device so that it can be of use to people. Output devices generate either *hard copy* or *soft copy* of the data. While hard copy implies that the data has been recorded in a permanent form on film, soft copy refers to a temporary display of the information on a moni-

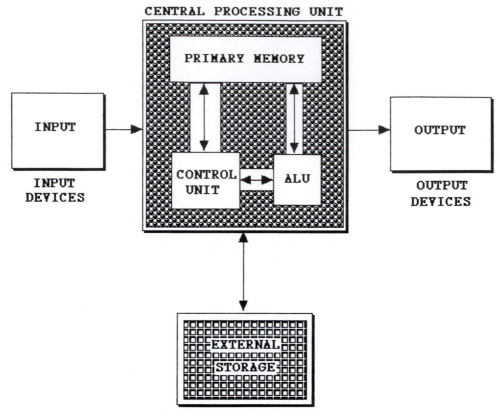

Figure 35-3. The functional organization of the four components which make up a computer.

tor, for example. Output devices include magnetic tapes, disks and optical disks, as well as printers, plotters, and the cathode ray tube (TV monitor).

It is clear from Figure 35-3 that there is a flow of information from input/output devices (I/O devices) and memory to the CPU. Such flow of data is facilitated through the use of a multiwire line called a *bus.*

The final component of hardware is that of storage of information external to the computer. Such storage is referred to as *secondary storage.* Secondary storage is intended to hold large quantities of programs and data on line to the CPU. This is accomplished through the use of such devices as magnetic tapes and disks. An emerging technology to store information in radiolo-gy is the optical disk which uses a laser beam to write and read data. *Optical disks* make use of either a compact disk read-only memory (CD ROM), WORM (write once, read many) or fully erasable technology.

The digital computer is based on the *binary system.* This system is a two-state system; a 0-state and a 1-state. A zero or a one is referred to as *bit* (binary digit). Computers therefore use a variety of binary-based codes to represent data and programs. A series of 8-bits is referred to as a *byte* and this is used to express the storage capacity of the computer. The size of the storage is often expressed in kilobytes (thousands of bytes), megabytes (millions of bytes), gigabytes (billions of bytes), or in terabytes (trillions of bytes).

Software

Software refers to computer programs. These are not physical devices but rather instructions which make the hardware components perform specific functions. There are two categories of software, *system software* and *applications software.*

In general, systems software refers to the *operating systems* which are a primary set of computer programs that coordinate the activities of the computer system. These programs perform the background tasks for people who are not only using the computer but those who are programming it as well. Popular operating systems are MS-DOS, PC-DOS, UNIX, OS/2, and Macintosh System Software. These enable applications software to be executed.

Applications software are programs that do useful work, such as scheduling, payroll and accounting, inventory control, preparing bills and budgets, managing files and databases, and playing games, of course. Out of applications software has come *productivity software* which are easy-to-use program packages such as word processing, spreadsheets, graphics, database management, and communications packages.

DIGITAL IMAGE PROCESSING CONCEPTS

The processing of the digital information by the computer which performs specific operations on the data to produce images which may serve a more useful purpose is called *digital image processing.* The computer-processed information can be manipulated in a number of ways to provide benefits such as image enhancement and restoration.

DIGITIZING IMAGES

How can analog images be converted into digital information? In Figure 35-4 the steps in digitizing an image are shown. In the first step the image is divided up into an array of small regions by a process known as *scanning.* Each small region is referred to as a *pixel* or picture element. Scanning results in a *matrix* of numbers consisting of rows and columns. In Figure 35-4, the matrix formed as a result of scanning is a 9 x 11 matrix which contains 99 pixels.

The next step involves a process called *sampling.* In sampling, the brightness of each pixel is measured by using special devices such as a photomultiplier tube (PM Tube) to detect the transmitted light and convert it into an electrical signal (analog signal).

The final step in digitizing an image is *quantization.* The analog signals obtained from sampling must be converted into digital information before they can be sent to the computer. In quantization, each brightness value is assigned a discrete number (0, a positive or a negative number) called a *gray level.* An image would therefore be made up of a range of numbers or gray levels. The total number of gray levels is called the *gray scale.* Figure 35-4 shows a four-level gray scale as a result of quantization. An image can thus be represented in 2, 4, 8, 16, 32, 64, 128, 256, 512, or 1024 gray levels. This range of numbers is referred to as the *dynamic range* and relates to the range of numbers that each pixel can represent. For example, if a pixel can represent four shades of gray, its (pixel) dynamic range is 2-bits deep ($2^2 = 4$).

Another concept which is important to digital image processing is the conversion

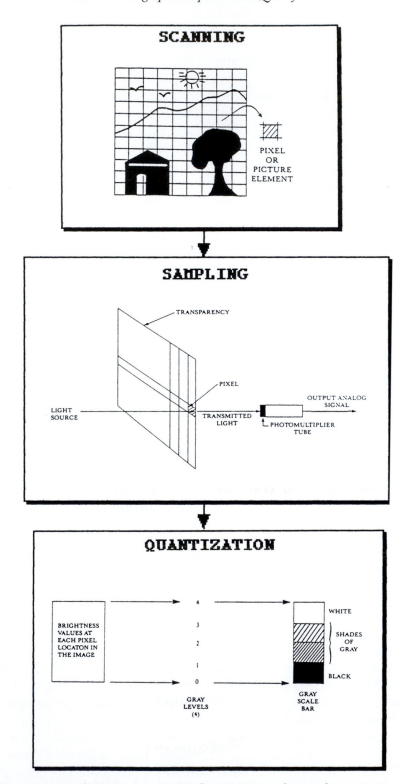

Figure 35-4. Three steps in digitizing any image: Scanning, sampling and quantization. (From Seeram, E. *X-Ray Imaging Equipment–An Introduction.* Charles C Thomas., (1985). Reproduced by permission.)

of analog data to digital data. This is achieved through the use of an *analog-to-digital converter (ADC)*. An important characteristic of the ADC is *accuracy* which refers to how close the digital data represents the analog signal. The range of the signal is divided up in to a number of parts of which the unit is the *bit* (binary digit). The more bits, the more accurate is the conversion. For example, a 1-bit ADC divides up the analog signal into two equal parts; a 2-bit ADC will generate four equal parts (2^2); and 8-bit ADC will result in 256 parts (2^8) or 256 numbers ranging from 0-255 and representing 256 shades of gray.

Now that the computer has digital data to work with, it performs certain operations on the data to generate a numerical image. This image can be recorded on tape or disc or it can be displayed on a television monitor for viewing. For it to be displayed on the monitor, the digital image must be converted to an analog signal since the monitor works only with these signals and not digital data. For this conversion, a *digital-to-analog (DAC)* converter is required. The arrangement of the ADC and DAC are shown in Figure 35-5.

IMAGE PROCESSING OPERATIONS

The major advantage of digital imaging is that the computer provides the opportunity to manipulate images and convert them into a more useful form by operating on the pixel array of data (which is already in digital form). Various computer programs are available for image processing operations such as *manipulation, restoration, enhancement,* and *analysis.*

In image manipulation, the digital data can be magnified and the range of numerical data allows one to roam up and down with a display window (windowing) to change the picture brightness and contrast. In image restoration, noise and blurring can be corrected, while image enhancement improves the visual appearance of the image. Finally, image analysis allows the operator to perform measurements and other quantitative analysis on the data.

These four fundamental processes are made possible by the following image processing operations.

1. *Point Processing Operations*—These work on individual pixels in the input image to change the identical gray scale pixel in the output image. These operations make use of the histogram of the input image. A *histogram* is a bar graph plot of the number of pixels in the image that have the same gray level. By scaling the histogram appropriately, the appearance of the output image can be changed.

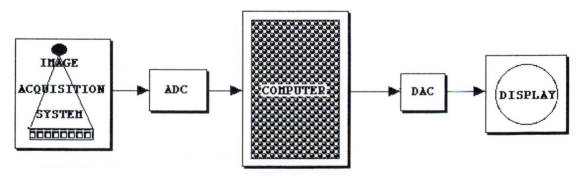

Figure 35-5. The general positions of the ADC and DAC in a digital imaging system.

Changing the window level (brightness) and window width (contrast) are point processing operations because *all* pixels in the image are acted upon by the computer logarithm (formula).

2. *Area Processing Operations*—These work on a selected group of pixels in the input image rather than individual pixels, to generate an individual pixel in the output image. These processing operations are also referred to as spatial processing operations. *Convolution* is the most common form of spatial processing.

    These operations can also be referred to as *digital spatial filtering*, since an image can also be represented as frequencies (number of cycles per second). These frequencies can be changed to modify the output image. Two common filtering techniques are *low-pass filtering* and *high-pass filtering*.

While low-pass filtering operates on low frequencies to change them to alter the appearance of the output image (one such low-pass filter results in smoothing the image as shown in Figure 36-9 in the next chapter), high-pass filtering operates on high frequencies (one such filter results in *edge enhancement*).

3. *Geometric Processing Operations*—These allow the operator to magnify, minify, rotate, translate and wrap the image. Pixel-shifting, shown in Figure 35-13, is an example of a geometric operation.

4. *Information extraction*—These allow the operator to perform quantitative analysis on the image, edge detection and image segmentation techniques.

COMPONENTS OF AN IMAGE PROCESSING SYSTEM

An image processing system consists of a minimum of three components arranged as shown in Figure 35-6. In a radiology image processing system, *image acquisition* consists of several different methods whereby data can be collected from the patient. Once this data is collected, it is then sent to the *image processing system.* In a digital imaging system, the processing is accomplished by computers. After processing, the output from the computer can be:

a. *displayed* on to a monitor for viewing by the technologist and radiologist

b. *stored* onto magnetic tapes, disk and/or optical disks

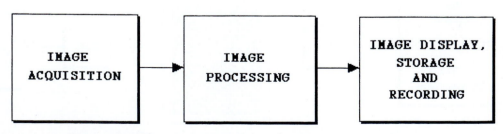

Figure 35-6. The major components of an image processing system.

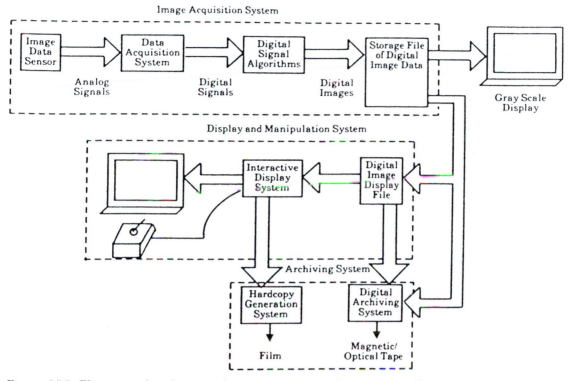

Figure 35-7. Elements of a digital radiography system. (From MacMillan et al. (1989) Digital Radiography. *Investigative Radiology*, 24:735-741. Reproduced by permission.)

c. *recorded* onto film for subsequent reading by the radiologist

In some instances, images can be sent to a remote location through the marvels of communications technology. In this case, *picture archiving and communications systems (PACS)* play a vital role in transmitting images. These components will be described in the remainder of this chapter.

A DIGITAL RADIOGRAPHY SYSTEM

While Figure 35-6 shows a generalized image processing of system, Figure 35-7 illustrates a digital radiography system. The major components include the image acquisition system, display and manipulation system and the archiving system. Each of these will be described subsequently.

DIGITAL IMAGING APPLICATIONS IN RADIOLOGY

In imaging, the computer is used to generate images based on data collected from the patient. These applications range from digitizing film radiographs, Digital Radiography and Fluoroscopy, Computed Radiography (CR), Computed Tomography (CT) and Magnetic Resonance Imaging (MRI) to three dimensional imaging and PACS.

DIGITIZING FILM RADIOGRAPHS

Digitizing film radiographs is the conversion of radiographic films into digital images. The process is shown in Figure 35-8. A laser beam scans the film to be digitized. The light intensity passing through the film is detected and the signal is sent to the ADC and subsequently to the computer which generates a digital image.

These images can be stored on magnetic tapes and disks and they can be enhanced and transmitted over networks. The advantages of this technology are obvious and include assisting the radiologist in making a diagnosis because the images can be digitally manipulated and they can be easily stored, handled, and transferred.

Even after the commitment to a filmless environment has been made, the problem of how to deal with all of those old important x-ray images stored in the file rooms must be addressed. Though these older images will need to be retained, the use of computed radiographic and digital radiographic systems will reduce space require-

ments for any new images. As older film images are retired, the personnel and space needed for this activity will decline steadily. Though it may not be cost effective to transfer all of the old images into to the picture archiving system, it is essential that means for converting older images into a digital format are acquired.

The device most often used to accomplish this process is called a digitalizer (Fig. 36-8). A digitalizer has about the same size and cost of a desk copy machine. Images fed into this device are scanned and converted into digital data in just a few seconds. Once the image has been scanned, information contained can be input into the picture archiving system (PACS).

DIGITAL RADIOGRAPHY

A digital radiography (DR) system implies that the x-ray beam passes through the patient to project the anatomy onto some form of radiation detector which converts the energy from x-rays into an *electronic* signal. The detector array is perma-

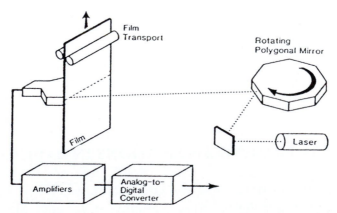

Figure 35-8. Digitalizer used to convert film radiographs into digitized images for more efficient storage and retrieval. (From Cook et al. (1989) Digitized Film Radiography. *Investigative Radiology,* 24:910-916. Reproduced by permission.)

nently mounted in a unit that replaces the Bucky tray of a conventional radiographic table. The electronic signal generated from the detectors is then converted into to digital data for its display on a CRT monitor. Several forms of digital projection systems have been implemented. These include spot-beam imaging, slot-beam imaging, and area-beam imaging systems.

Figure 35-9 shows a spot-beam configuration. These scanners utilize a point- or a pencil-shaped beam to scan the patient. The detector must repeatedly process the radiation energy it receives into an electrical signal, send the signal to the computer, and reset itself for another measurement. The detector must also be indexed back and forth across the scan as it moves down each row collecting data. Because of this cumbersome repetitious process, the time required to produce a single image is excessive and impractical, as much as 4 seconds. In Figure 35-10, a slot-beam or fan-beam system is illustrated. In this system a mechanical bar holds an linear array of detectors arranged in one row or a few rows. The fan-shaped beam produces an entire row or column of collected data from each exposure burst as the detector bar indexes across or down the scan area.

Both the spot-beam and slot-beam methods result in very little scattered radiation because the beams are tightly collimated. Signal-to-noise ratio is very high, but the spatial resolution (sharpness) tends to be low. Area-beam systems use a full rectangular beam of x-rays just as conventional radiography does. This shortens the exposure time and improves spatial resolution; however, it requires hundreds of detectors so that both the practical construction and the expense of the detector array are prohibitive. With an area beam, scatter radiation becomes significant and degrades the image. Of these three approaches to digital radiography, the obvious choice is the slot-beam or fan-beam method which strikes a reasonable compromise between scan time and image quality.

The ability to enhance the contrast to provide improved detectability of low-contrast structures is the digital image's most

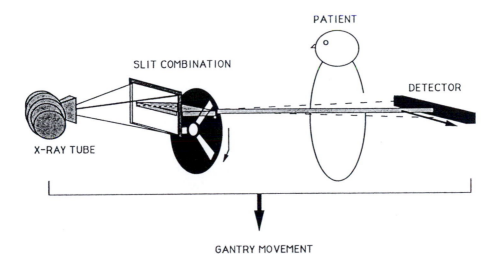

Figure 35-9. A "spot" beam or "pencil" beam scanner configuration. (From Greene, RE & Oestmann, JW (1992). *Computed Digital Radiography in Clinical Practice.* Thieme Medical Publishers, Inc. Reproduced by permission.)

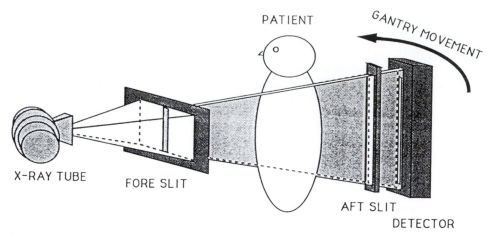

Figure 35-10. A "slot" beam or "fan" beam scanner configuration. (From Greene, RE and Oestmann, JW (1992). *Computed Digital Radiography in Clinical Practice.* Thieme Medical Publishers, Inc. Reproduced by permission.)

beneficial characteristic. It is this same property that enables the CT scanner to display the tissues of the brain as separate from the collections of blood or cerebral fluids. Without this ability, these tissues are indistinguishable from their surroundings and are virtually invisible on conventional radiographic (analog) images. Improvements in both software and hardware components have now made it possible to produce digitally acquired images that are virtually indistinguishable from their radiographic counterparts. Though this type of imaging system provides for the instant retrieval of images, at the present state of technology, the inability to obtain the table top and mobile radiographic images appears to be limiting its widespread acceptance.

DIGITAL FLUOROSCOPY

The ideas relating to digital fluoroscopy may be traced back to the 1970s when image intensifiers were used in a technique called *digital subtraction angiography (DSA)* which will not be discussed in this chapter. Later, with refinements in video digitizer technology, systems using image intensifiers were developed for routine use in the radiology department.

A typical digital fluoroscopy system for use in gastrointestinal and genitourinary work is shown in Figure 35-11 The essential components include the imaging system (x-ray tube, image intensifier, light coupling optics, and the TV camera tube) data acquisition electronics (video preamplifier and A/D converter), TV digitizer, and image display and recording.

The imaging system captures the data from the patient. The TV camera tube is a high resolution tube (1023 scan lines at 60 Hz) which can operate in the interlaced and progressive scanning modes; however, the progressive scanning mode provides a higher signal-to-noise ratio which means that the image is a much sharper image compared to the image produced by interlaced scanning.

The signal leaving the TV camera is the video analog signal and it is this signal that is sent to the TV digitizer which converts it into a digital image. This digital image can be stored in the image memory and by using a computer system the image can be

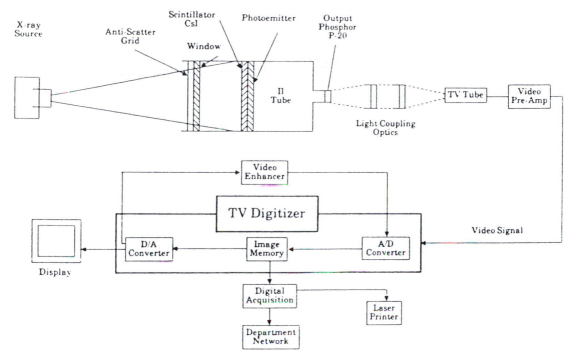

Figure 35-11. A digital fluoroscopic imaging system. See text for further explanation. (From MacMillan et al. (1989) Digital Radiography. *Investigative Radiology*, 24:735-741. Reproduced by permission.)

manipulated further. The digital data is then converted into analog signals by the D/A converter for display on a high resolution TV monitor. In addition, the digital data is then sent to a laser printer to be recorded onto x-ray film, or it can be transmitted to another location through a picture archiving system (PACS).

COMPUTED RADIOGRAPHY

Computed radiography, originally called *Photostimulable Storage Phosphor Digital Radiography (PSPDR), Scanning Laser-Stimulated Luminescence, or Storage Phosphor-Based Digital Radiography*, was introduced as a means of replacing film/screen imaging. CR is also referred to as "filmless radiography."

A Computed Radiography system is illustrated in Figure 35-12. There are four essential components:

1. X-ray detection by an Imaging Plate (IP)
2. Laser scanning of the IP
3. Computer processing of the data from the laser scanner
4. Image recording by a laser printer and storage of the information.

The imaging plate is a flexible plate less than 1 mm in thickness and is coated with a *barium fluorohalide* phosphor which is photostimulable, that is, during exposure electrons in the phosphor crystals are raised to a higher energy state and there they remain trapped. The plate is then scanned by a helium-neon laser which causes the trapped electrons to return to their stable state and in the process emit light. The light is converted into electrical signals which are subsequently converted into digital data fed into the computer for processing.

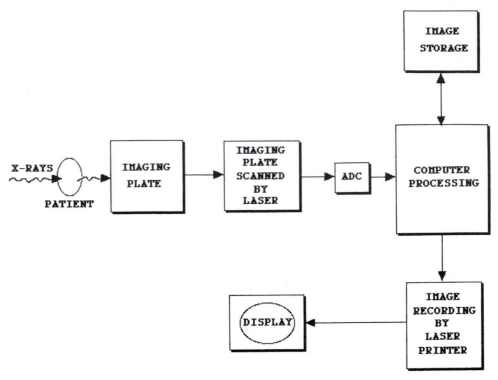

Figure 35-12. The general configuration of a scanning laser-stimulated luminescence x-ray system (Computed Radiography or CR).

After processing, the digital output image can be laser-printed onto film and subsequently displayed on a gray scale display device, or it can be stored in a large volume memory such as optical disks.

Storage phosphor-based systems are becoming commonplace and they are gaining widespread use in several areas in radiology including chest and extremity imaging, mobile radiography, excretory urography and GI tract imaging. Computed Radiography is discussed in detail in the next chapter.

DIGITAL IMAGE RECONSTRUCTION FROM MULTIPLE PROJECTIONS

The idea of collecting a set of x-ray transmission (attenuation) measurements from a patient and using special mathematical techniques (Fourier transformation, for example) to build up an image of a selected slice in the patient is referred to as *image reconstruction from multiple projections*. A computer is central to this process for it is used to reconstruct the image and therefore the technique is digital in nature.

Two techniques to reconstruct an image from a set of projection data are *Computed Tomography (CT)* and *Magnetic Resonance Imaging (MRI)*.

Computed Tomography

CT involves at least three processes: *data collection, data processing* and *image display, recording* and *storage*.

First data is collected from the patient. This involves a very systematic way of having the x-ray tube scan the patient. The tube is coupled to a set of detectors which measure the relative transmission of x-rays.

The analog signals from the detectors and are sent to ADCs where they are sampled and digitized.

The data is then sent to a computer which performs a mathematical technique for reconstructing the image. The image can be displayed on to a television monitor or it can be stored on magnetic tapes, disks, or optical disks. It can also be sent to a video or laser multiformat camera to be recorded on film.

The transmission measurements are converted into attenuation and thickness data and are used to calculate *CT numbers* or *Hounsfield numbers* (after the inventor).

The computed CT numbers are arranged to form an image *matrix* usually a 512 x 512 x 12-bits in which the numbers in each pixel correspond to the voxel (volume element) of the anatomy of interest in the original (scanned) slice. Each number is assigned a gray level and hence a gray scale image can be generated. The range of the CT numbers is referred to as the *window width (WW)* and the center of the range is called the *window level (WL)*. Window width and level can both be manipulated by the operator to alter the contrast and brightness or "density" of the image.

Magnetic Resonance Imaging

Magnetic Resonance Imaging (MRI) is a digital imaging technique based on Image Reconstruction principles similar to those used in CT.

Magnetic resonance (MR) is based on the fact that when protons (magnetic dipoles) are placed in a strong magnetic field, they move from their normal random distribution and align with the magnetic field. At the same time, because they are spinning on their own axes, they begin to wobble (like a spinning top wobbles) or

precess at a particular frequency because of the influence of the magnetic field.

This precessional frequency is the *Larmor frequency*. When exposed to radiowaves (RF) of the same frequency, the Larmor frequency, the protons absorb energy. When the the RF is turned off, the protons emit radiowaves which can be collected by a detector (antenna) and used by a computer to produce an image of the distribution of the protons in the body. Because the body is made up of mostly water, the principles of MR are used to produce images of the hydrogen nuclei (protons) in the water. This technique is Magnetic Resonance Imaging (MRI). The imaging process is as follows:

1. The patient is placed in the magnet. The coils in the magnet surrounds the patient.
2. The patient becomes magnetized (protons align with the magnetic field).
3. The patient is exposed to radio waves generated by the radio frequency transmitter for a short period of time.
4. The radio waves are turned off.
5. The patient emits radio waves which are detected by the receiver.
6. The receiver sends the analog signals to the ADC. Digital data is sent to the computer for processing.
7. The output from the computer is the MR image which can be stored magnetically or optically, recorded on film or displayed on a TV monitor for viewing.

Image qualities, manipulation and terminology are similar to those of CT, with *window width* representing gray scale and *window level* representing the average density or brightness. A full discussion of CT and

MRI is outside the scope of this text, and may be found in most radiologic physics books.

IMAGE TERMINOLOGY

Perhaps the most confusing aspect of computerized imaging methods for a radiographer to learn is the difference in terms used to describe the image and the equipment functions. It is particularly useful to be able to translate the terms used to describe computerized images into the more common terms used in radiography—density, contrast, noise, etc.

The primary reason that different terms are used in these computerized modalities is that these image qualities are not final but are able to be manipulated, so that there are controls on the machine to change them if desired after the image is displayed on the CRT screen, (TV). After one exposure is made, several different images may be derived, observed and permanently recorded by adjusting the center of the gray scale up or down and by adjusting the range of densities displayed to broaden or restrict it.

In digital fluoroscopy, the *center* refers to the mid-point of the gray scale displayed in the image. It might be considered as the *average* brightness level or density level and is therefore the equivalent of *density* in radiography. In computerized tomography, the same mid-density level is referred to as *window level.* Moving the center or window level adjusts all of the densities displayed up or down by an equal amount, just as changing mAs does in radiography.

The total number of different brightness levels or density levels may also be broadened or restricted, which in turn changes the ratio of difference from one density to the next. This range of brightness levels is equivalent to *gray scale* in radiography (the opposite of *contrast*). In digital fluoroscopy, it is referred to as the *window.* In computerized tomography, it is called *window width.*

APPLICATION OF TECHNIQUE

Technologists specializing in any of these areas must become familiar with the typical computer keyboard and the basic language used on computer terminals, which has several variations from a typing keyboard. To initiate a procedure, a new frame or file must be acquired from the computer, into which the technologist enters all of the pertinent demographic patient data as well as basic format and technique data for the procedure.

Electrical technique factors are entered into the computer on CT scanners but are usually set at the regular x-ray generator console for digital imaging. Digital imaging techniques are typically equal to normal radiographic techniques for the generator used. For a given anatomical part, an overhead radiographic technique may be taken from the routine technique chart for use in digital fluoroscopy rapid sequence spot exposures. All of the guidelines for optimum kilovoltage, adequate penetration for the anatomy and intensity control by milliampere-seconds discussed in Chapters 4-6 apply to digital imaging. Occasionally, higher kVp levels are required to ensure adequate flux or intensity at the detectors, in which case mAs may be adjusted downward by the 15 percent rule, so that the *total* technique is still roughly equivalent to that of an overhead exposure. Computerized tomography scanners use equivalent techniques to radiography also but typically employ much higher kVp levels with the mAs adjusted downward according to the 15 percent rule.

In addition to electrical technique factors, several other image variables may be predetermined in computerized imaging. The *matrix size* refers to the number of pixels, lengthwise and crosswise, which will be displayed on the CRT screen. Matrix size bears primarily upon the resolution or sharpness in the image. The greater the number of pixels to be displayed, the smaller the pixels must be to fit into the display field of view. Smaller pixels result in sharper image edges, just as smaller crystals in intensifying screens and film lead to sharper edges. Each pixel is *filled* with one density level. A small matrix size with large pixels will result in a checkerboard image with very poor resolution. Therefore, the largest feasible matrix sizes, with the smallest pixels, are always the most desirable.

Magnification modes may also be selected in order to focus in on specific regions of anatomy. These usually work by changing the effective size of the input phosphor on the image intensifier tube. In other words, the useful beam is effectively collimated to the specific anatomical region, but, since the image will be displayed on the same CRT screen, it will appear magnified to fill that screen.

For digital subtraction angiography, the camera time or *C-time* must be set to include the exposure time being used, *in addition* to a 33-millisecond lag time which the camera needs to interrogate the next frame before the next sequential exposure begins.

After the patient has been positioned for digital subtraction angiography, a scout frame must be taken to evaluate the adequacy of the electrical technique factors. With the *window* (gray scale) set at 1.0, an exposure is acquired into the computer memory. The *center* knob is then adjusted up and down to determine the point at which the image becomes completely blacked out. Image *blackout* should occur close to a center number specified by the

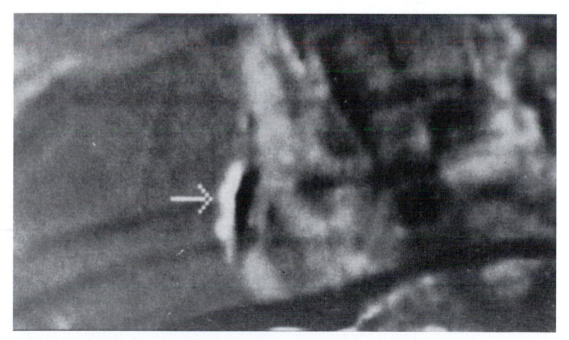

Figure 35-13. Misregistration artifact on a digital subtraction image of a blood clot (arrow) caused by lateral motion. This artifact can be corrected digitally by *pixel-shifting* the two superimposed images.

equipment manufacturer. If blackout occurs at a center above this number, an increase in electrical technique is needed. If blackout occurs below this number, the kVp or mAs must be reduced. A recommended center for *whiteout* is also specified by the manufacturer and may be checked.

Having evaluated the scout frame and made any necessary adjustments, the machine may be set for rapid serial framing and any injection readied. The exposure switch (many machines have a foot switch) is depressed first and then the *begin* button on the computer console is depressed to initiate the procedure. The exposure switch must be kept depressed until the exposure sequence is completed and the end button pressed. *Cine forward* or *cine reverse* buttons are used to review the exposures.

At this point, each image may be manipulated by further adjustments to the center, window, orientation (inverting or rotating), or the subtraction of any other chosen frame. Subtraction images may be *pixel-shifted* to align the two images if slight motion has occurred (Fig. 35-13). The computer can then be directed to save any of these manipulated images onto computer disks for permanent storage.

THREE-DIMENSIONAL IMAGING (3-D IMAGING)

Another exciting avenue of digital imaging techniques such as CT and MRI is that of 3-D imaging. Figure 36-9 in the next chapter demonstrates a 3-D CT image. At the heart of 3-D imaging is the computer. 3-D imaging involves the use of computer programs to transform the conventional CT or MR transaxial slice data into simulated 3-D images. This is referred to as *rendering techniques.*

There are two classes of 3-D Rendering Techniques. These are:

1. Surface-based Rendering Techniques
2. Volume-based Rendering Techniques

Essentially 3-D imaging consists of:

a. *Volume formation,* where initially-acquired images are stacked to form a volume.
b. *Classification,* which determines the various tissue types present in individual voxels.
c. *Image projection.* This is the last step and it involves projecting the classified data into a 2-D or 3-D image.

A brief description of the two classes of rendering techniques is in order. In *surface-based rendering,* only the surface of the patient or object is demonstrated. For example, the computer program is such that given a set of numbers (digital image) it takes only the numbers corresponding to the anatomy intended to be displayed and then it carries out the 3-D reconstruction. Subsequent shading of specific pixels is done to give the illusion of depth. This perception of depth allows the image to appear in 3-D. In *volume-based rendering techniques* not only is the surface of objects displayed but also other portions of a specified volume within the patient or object. The computer programs must also look at the numbers (values) for the other parts of the anatomy to be displayed such as bone and muscles. This volume is then classified and the pixels are displayed as though they are translucent, so that it is now possible to see in front and behind various tissues. 3-D imaging has found applications in radiation therapy, cranio-facial surgery, and orthopedics.

LASER IMAGING SYSTEMS

The word "laser" is not a new word since it has become commonplace in several facets of human activity. For example, lasers are now used the military, communications, surveying, industry, space studies and in medicine. In medicine, lasers are used in surgery (as a scalpel) gastroenterology, dermatology, otolaryngology, urology, pulmonary medicine, and finally in radiology.

WHAT IS A LASER?

The term *Laser* is an acronym for *Light Amplification by Stimulated Emission of Radiation.* It was invented in 1960 by T.H. Maiman, who worked on what was called a Ruby Laser as shown in Figure 35-14. Three essential components comprise the laser:

1. The *medium,* which in this case is the Ruby rod, which gives rise to the laser beam and also indicates the operating wavelength of the laser.
2. A *source of power* which provides energy to the medium. This is also referred to as the *pumping source.*
3. A *resonant cavity* which may assume a cylindrical shape or that of a prism.

The production of a laser beam is such that when atoms in the medium (solid, liquid or gas) are excited by a certain amount of energy (supplied by the power source). Their electrons are raised to an excited energy state and this process results in the emission of light. This light is confined to the cavity which begins to resonate at one of the emission frequencies. As a result, the light energy is amplified at this specific frequency resulting in the production of a coherent beam of light (light in which the waves are in phase and have the same frequency). This is the laser beam.

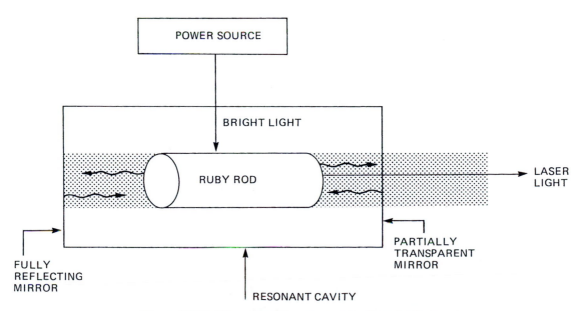

Figure 35-14. The essential components of a ruby laser.

TYPES OF LASERS

Lasers differ according to the medium which is used to produce the laser beam. This medium can be a solid, liquid or gas. The ruby laser described earlier is an example of a laser which used a solid. Other types of lasers include semiconductor lasers as well as those which use gas, such as the argon ion laser, the nitrogen, carbon dioxide and helium laser, and the helium-neon laser, one which is commonly used in radiology.

The helium-neon laser emits red light with an output power of 10 to 100 milliwatts (mW).

LASERS IN RADIOLOGY

There are four ways in which lasers are presently being used in the radiology department:

1. In digitizing x-ray films. These are referred to as Laser Film Digitizers.
2. In Scanning Laser-Stimulated Luminescence X-Ray Imaging Systems.
3. In Laser Film Printers.
4. In Laser Optical Disk Storage.

Laser Film Digitizers

A laser film digitizer converts x-ray films into digital images. This process is referred to as *Digitized Film Radiography*. Such a system is illustrated in Figure 35-15. The film to be digitized is scanned line by line by the laser beam. The laser light which is transmitted through the film is detected by special detectors which generate an output signal. These detector signals are then digitized and subsequently fed into a digital computer for processing and storage.

Digitized film radiography is used not only for archival storage of digitized x-ray

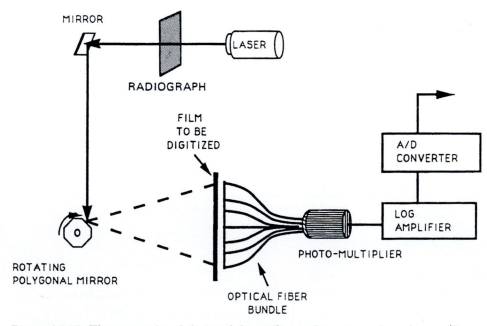

Figure 35-15. The principle of digitized fim radiography using a laser beam. (From Greene, RE & Oestmann, JW (1992). *Computed Digital Radiography in Clinical Practice.* Thieme Medical Publishers, Inc. Reproduced by permission.)

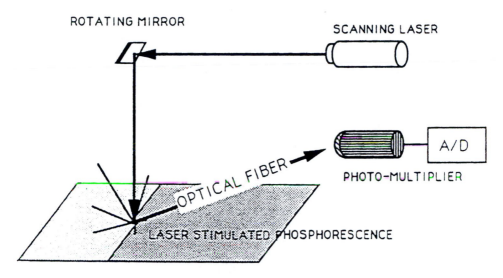

ROTATING MIRROR   SCANNING LASER

A/D

PHOTO-MULTIPLIER

OPTICAL FIBER

LASER STIMULATED PHOSPHORESCENCE

STORAGE PHOSPHOR IMAGING PLATE

Figure 35-16. The basic principle of storage phosphor imaging. A laser beam is used to read the storage phosphor imaging plate which holds the latent x-ray image. The image data from the plate are detected with a photomultiplier tube and the data is subsequently digitized for input into the computer. (From Greene, RE & Oestmann, JW (1992). *Computed Digital Radiography in Clinical Practice.* Thieme Medical Publishers, Inc. Reproduced by permission.)

films but also for transmission of images from the radiology department to other parts of the hospital such as intensive care and cardiac care units. In addition, not only is the image sent but also a copy of the radiologist's report is transmitted as well.

Scanning Laser-Stimulated Luminescence X-Ray Imaging Systems

These systems make use of a special *storage phosphor imaging plate* which is *photostimulable*. When the plate is exposed to x-rays, the phosphor electrons are raised to a higher energy level and remain trapped there until the plate is scanned by a laser beam. As the beam scans the plate, it luminesces and this light is detected and converted into electrical signals which are then converted into digital data. These data are processed by the computer which generates images that can be recorded on film or stored on magnetic tapes and disks as well as on optical disks. This process is shown in Figure 35-16. This technique will be described further in the next chapter.

Laser Film Printers

Laser Film Printers are becoming commonplace in radiology departments which have digital imaging equipment such as CT, MRI, and Digital Fluoroscopy and Radiography.

These printers typically use a helium-neon (or solid state diode) laser to write digital data onto special film. The digital data from the computer is sent to the printer, which, through a series of operations convert the data into a signal which is sent to the laser. The laser then scans the film to produce the image as can be seen in Figure 35-17. Heat from the laser develops an image in a carbon-based emulsion. This

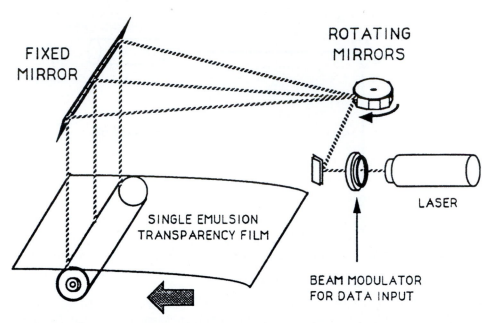

Figure 35-17. The fundamental principle of a laser printer. (From Greene, RE & Oestmann, JW (1992). *Computed Digital Radiography in Clinical Practice.* Thieme Medical Publishers, Inc. Reproduced by permission.)

technology eliminates the need for *chemical* processing.

Even with a totally filmless department, there are likely to be few instances where hard copy images will need to be transferred out of the network. For these situations, all departments will need to maintain at least one laser printer capable of producing high quality transparent hard copies of the stored images. Laser printers can be directly networked to the image processor or PACS to print the small number of hard copy images that will be required in special situations.

Optical Disk Storage

Another way lasers are used in radiology is in the storage of information, particularly image data. The storage device is the optical disk. The optical disk makes use of a high intensity laser beam to write data onto the disk and a low intensity laser to read the information from the disk.

Optical disks are now being used in conjunction with CT units. A 5.25-inch optical disk can store about 1 gigabyte of data.

PICTURE ARCHIVING AND COMMUNICATIONS SYSTEMS (PACS)

In this chapter, several digital imaging techniques were described. The images produced by these systems can be stored on magnetic tapes and disks as well as on optical disks. This means that a system could be developed to retrieve these stored images, display them for viewing and interpretation on a television monitor, transmit them to remote locations as well as provide archival storage. Such a system is a *Picture*

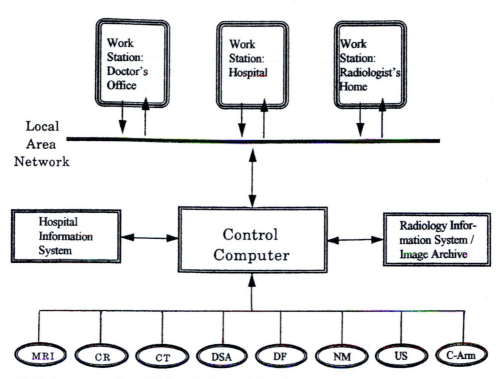

Figure 35-18. Diagram of a PACS. All digitized imaging equipment within the department feeds acquired images and patient information into the control computer, which then allows universal access through the hospital information system (HIS), radiology information system (RIS), and work stations and display stations throughout the hospital, affiliated centers and offices, and even the radiologists' homes. All input and output points of the system are called *nodes* of the *network*.

Archiving and Communications System (PACS).

The major components of a PACS is shown in Figure 35-18. These include image acquisition systems, the hospital information system (HIS), the radiology information system (RIS) including the image archive, the image display and work stations, a control computer, and a local area network (LAN).

First, the *image acquisition devices* (MR Scanner, CT Scanner, Computed Radiographic Unit, etc.) send their images to a *control computer* which stores the images (for later retrieval) onto magnetic disks, tapes and optical disks, several of which (about 100 or more) can be found stacked together in a device called an *optical jukebox*. These images can also be printed onto

film by a laser printer, for example.

The important point about the control computer is that it should interface with both the Radiology Information System, (RIS) as well as the Hospital Information System (HIS).

In addition to interfacing is another important component of PACS, that is, the *image display work station*. These work stations feature a keyboard, a pointing device (mouse or trackball) and one or more display devices such as monitors. A vital function of a display monitor is that it must be a high resolution monitor (2048 x 2048 is the minimum matrix size) which would enable a radiologist to make a diagnosis. A PACS should also allow the operator/viewer to manipulate these images using such image processing operations as edge enhancement, windowing, highlighting, scrolling, zooming, and so on.

A PACS can also facilitate the transmission of images to various parts of the Hospital or within the Radiology Department. Such transmission is accomplished using *local area networks (LANS)* in which case, work stations are connected by a cable. New technologies employ fiber optic LANS. If the data is to be transferred to another building or a remote facility located in another city, for example, then *wide area networks (WANS)* will be used.

At the current state of technology, a modern PACS can store the equivalent of about 1,000,000 radiographic-type images. It may be surprising to discover that the rate of permanently lost, misfiled, and temporarily lost images and documents is estimated at between 5-20 percent. There have been a number of reported incidents where these losses have led to multimillion-dollar judgments and out-of-court settlements against doctors and medical institutions. The improved storage and reporting aspects of a PACS is deemed by many to be the greatest advantage of a filmless system for the radiology department.

One of the most beneficial aspects of a PACS involves the placement of display stations in key locations in a medical facility, which allows clinicians' ready access to medical information and reports at the touch of a keyboard. By placing these display terminals in the ER, OR, ICU, CCU,

etc., the doctors have nearly instant access to images and information that could otherwise take critical minutes or hours to obtain without the system. Whether these display nodes are connected by cables (internal) or by telephone lines (external), it is possible for a health care provider to directly access the images and/or reports that are stored in PACS more quickly. When doctors' offices are networked into the system, delays in obtaining images are all but eliminated. Radiologists with display stations in their homes can quickly relay readings in emergency care situations to local or distant institutions.

Many institutions have found a display station rarely requires the same quality as the workstation; it is often possible to use lower cost 1000 x 1000 CRT monitors and a keypad, thereby replacing the costs of the system.

All display stations need to be located in an area in which the control of ambient light is possible. Too much ambient room light has been shown to be detrimental to the amount of contrast that can be perceived on the image. In order to help reduce the effect of extraneous light from the room, all display monitors should be provided with anti-reflection coatings. After the examination of all of the pertinent information, there is a growing body of evidence that indicates appropriate soft-copy imaging does not compromise but often enhances the diagnosis of images.

DIGITAL TELERADIOLOGY

The transmission of images at a distance has been referred to as *teleradiology*. The technology dates back to 1954 in Montreal, Canada, where two hospitals were linked together with a coaxial cable.

A typical teleradiology system is shown

in Figure 35-19. The major components include equipment to transmit (send) images and equipment to receive and display these images. The transmission components include a film illuminator box with film, a video camera to capture the image

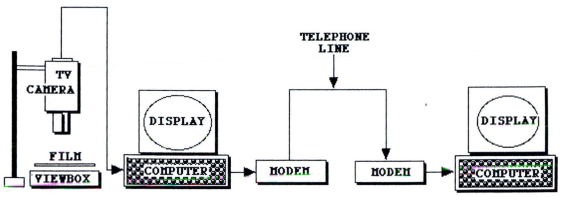

Figure 35-19. The major components of a digital teleradiology system.

on the box and a personal computer with a modem which is used to send the images through a phone line. The analog signal from the camera tube is digitized using an ADC and the digital image is stored in the computer.

The stored image is then sent to the modem (modulator-demodulator) and subsequently through the phone line at a certain speed (bits per second).

The signal from the phone line is received by another modem located at the remote site. This modem then sends the information to a microcomputer which is coupled to a monitor. The image is now ready for viewing.

Teleradiology systems have become affordable and more and more departments are beginning to acquire these systems.

Although teleradiography requires that the user have a display station in the home or office, it provides immediate access to any medical images that are stored in the PACS. As an example, if a CR chest image that was just taken has a questionable finding, this image can be transmitted to an on-call radiologist at his home for a definitive reading. Acting as an electronic file room, a PACS can store, retrieve, and display images on any number of display workstations that have been networked to the main storage device. Since a PACS also can vastly reduce storage space required to maintain the old images, the growth of filmless storage systems is likely to become universal in the foreseeable future.

CONCLUSION

Digital imaging is becoming commonplace in radiology. Already conventional radiographic equipment is being converted to digital equipment. This is evident in areas such as chest, genitourinary, gastrointestinal and even breast imaging and including CT, MRI and Digital Angiography.

The technologist must therefore make every effort now to understand these principles which will become increasingly important in the near future.

SUMMARY

1. All digitized images are processed through a *computer*. The main components of every computer are the central processing unit, input/output devices, and memory storage. The CPU is composed of the control unit, the arithmetic/logic unit, and primary memory.

2. Systems and applications *software* are computer programs that can be stored as RAM or ROM memory in primary or secondary storage. All computer languages are ultimately based on the *binary* number system.

3. All digital images are formed by *scanning*, which divides the image into a *matrix* of picture elements or *pixels*. In *sampling*, the intensity of radiation (light or x-rays) for each pixel is measured. Each pixel is assigned a gray level or brightness level for later display on a CRT display monitor. This is called *quantization*.

4. In the quantization process, *analog* (continuous spectrum) measurements in the form of x-rays, light, or electrical current must be rounded into *digital* (discrete spectrum) numbers which the computer can assimilate. This is done by the analog-to-digital converter or *ADC*. The range of these digitized brightness or gray level values which the computer can store is called the *dynamic range*. The dynamic ranges of a computer and all of its peripheral input and output devices must match in order for them to be compatible.

5. *Postprocessing* manipulation of the image consists of point processing operations which act on all pixels, area processing operations which act on selected pixels such as the edges of an image, geometric processing which reorients the image matrix, and information extrac-

tion which allows quantitative analysis.

6. *Digitizing film radiographs* uses scanners called digitalizers to convert conventional radiographs into digital images.

7. *Digital radiography* uses dozens of x-ray detection devices, usually a slot-beam or fan-beam scanning process (SPR), to convert the x-ray beam attenuation values directly into electrical current which is then digitized by the ADC.

8. *Computed radiography* uses a phosphor-coated plate in a cassette which allows a typical area x-ray beam to be used at much shorter exposure times than DR allows. The *photostimulable phosphor plate* stores the energy from the x-ray beam as trapped electrical charges. Later, upon scanning the plate with a red laser beam, these trapped electrons are induced to fall back into their respective atoms, causing blue-violet light to be emitted by the plate. Photomultiplier tubes convert this light into electrical current and amplified the signal before digitized by the ADC.

9. *Digital fluoroscopy* utilizes a conventional image intensifier but picks up the light signal from the output phosphor with a special high-resolution television camera. The camera converts the light image into an electrical signal which is then digitized by the ADC.

10. *Digital image reconstruction from multiple projections* is a complicated process upon which both CT and MRI are founded: While CT measures the attenuation of the x-ray beam through each *voxel* of tissue, and MRI measures the intensity and frequency of radio waves induced from each voxel of tissue, both do so repeatedly from multiple directions in order to compile this information and obtain a "slice" image of

defined thickness in axial, coronal, or sagittal planes.

11. While terminology varies somewhat between digital subtraction angiography, CT, MRI, DR, and CR, all of these modalities allow postprocessing adjustments to brightness (window level), contrast (window width), edge-enhancement processes, magnification, and other reorientation of the image.

12. Rendering techniques for *3D images* are surface-based or volume-based.

13. A *laser* consists of a source of power, a ruby medium, and a resonant cavity to produce light that has a homogeneous wavelengths which are also synchronized together. This refined light beam is used in scanning for digitizing films and computed radiography, for laser film printers and for optical disc recording and reading.

14. Picture archiving and communication systems, *PACS*, greatly enhance the accessibility and storage capabilities of medical images and thus improve and expedite patient care. The PAC system utilizes a central control computer in which all digitally-acquired images throughout the imaging department may be stored and managed along with patient information in the hospital or radiology information systems. All of these images and information are accessible through workstations and display stations at various sites through a *local area network (LAN)*.

15. *Teleradiology* allows images to be scanned, digitalized, and sent over phone lines or cable networks to distant sites with great speed and preservation of image quality.

REVIEW QUESTIONS

1. What is meant by the term "digital imaging"?

2. What is an analog image?

3. Identify four devices which make up a digital computer:

4. Define the term "digital image processing":

5. What are the three steps involved in digitizing images?

6. What is the radiographic equivalent of window level?

7. What is the radiographic equivalent of window width?

8. What is the difference between the ADC and the DAC?

9. Digitizing the image in a computer allows us to manipulate the image qualities _____ recording the image

   (before or after)

   permanently.

10. In digital fluoroscopy, the gray scale (contrast) range is called the:

11. In computerized tomography, the average density level is called the:

12. An image displayed on a CRT (TV) using a *small* matrix size will have _____ resolution of details.

13. Cine forward and cine reverse buttons are used to:

14. Is it possible on CT scanners to produce radiographs from different viewpoints *without* further radiation exposure, once an original series of "cuts" has been obtained?

15. How many gray levels would be generated by a 10-bit ADC?

16. Identify four image processing operations:

17. Explain the meaning of the term "digital spatial filtering":

18. How does high pass digital filtering affect the appearance of the image?
19. What are the three major components of a digital image processing system?
20. Why are films digitized in radiology?
21. List the steps involved in digitizing images in fluoroscopy.
22. What is meant by image reconstruction from projections? List two applications in the radiology department.
23. Identify two three-dimensional techniques used in radiology:
24. Explain the difference between surface-based 3-D and volume-based 3-D techniques:
25. What is PACS? Describe the major components of a PACS in radiology:
26. Define "teleradiology":

27. A digital imaging system with a dynamic range that is 4 bits deep can produce how many different shades of gray?
28. What is the meaning of the acronym LASER?
29. List three components of a laser:
30. List four ways in which lasers are used in radiology:
31. What type of laser is commonly used in radiology?
32. What is the purpose of a laser film digitizer?
33. How is a laser used in storage phosphor plate imaging?
34. A laser film printer writes digital data onto what recording medium?
35. What is a laser optical disk used for in radiology?

Chapter 36

COMPUTED RADIOGRAPHY

ROBERT DEANGELIS

DIGITAL IMAGING is the general name given to any imaging technique that creates computer-generated images providing an accurate representation of the anatomic structures of the body. Images are computer-processed in nuclear medicine and sonography, and they are *reconstructed* as "slices" from multiple projections in CT and MRI. But, two main methods of producing digitized images that appear like a conventional radiograph and are acquired directly from the remnant x-ray beam are *digital radiography* (DR) and *computed radiography* (CR). Of these two, computed radiography is becoming predominant.

Ironically, the actual quality of most directly acquired digital images is only slightly improved, mainly in the area of enhancing the detectability of low subject-contrast anatomy. Perhaps the most often asked and poorly understood questions concerning digital imaging systems is why would an imaging center spend millions of dollars on a "new" imaging system that will have only slight impact on the overall quality of the images? A large part of the answer comes from looking at not only the costs but also some of the inherent problems of the hard copy or film-based process. The greatest overall benefit of a digital imaging system often has more to do with the retrieval and display of the images than it has with an improvement in the diagnostic quality of the images them-selves. This apparent inconsistency can only be understood by looking beyond our images to one of conventional radiography's greatest deficiencies:

The purpose of medical imaging is to provide physicians and patients with the appropriate diagnostic information in the shortest possible time. The steps in this process can be summarized as follows: image production, reading/reporting, and image archival. Problems in any of these areas can lead to the failure to communicate critical information to a physician in a timely fashion. The three requirements of the medical imaging process may be summarized as:

1. Image production: The process by which medical images are produced that accurately represent the anatomic structures of the body
2. Reading/reporting: The process that makes medical images available to the physician in a timely manner
3. Image archival: The process by which maintains images for their further reference

All diagnostic images must possess the desired quality to provide the physicians with the information to make an accurate diagnosis. Presently, both soft copy digital and hard copy film images possess sufficient quality to meet this requirement.

The second requirement is the need to provide these images in a timely manner so that an effective care plan can be established. A medical image is only useful when the information it provides is obtained in time to identify a life-threatening condition or improve the diagnosis or treatment plan. The last requirement is the need to provide a report of findings and the ability to examine images for medical changes. Though these conditions are met by conventional imaging techniques, there are a number of well-documented problems with the turn-around time of medical images and the inability to always be able to find stored images.

Because a well-designed digital imaging system can significantly improve on these functions, the most important benefit of the transition to filmless digital imaging system is likely to be an improvement to the care of the patient. The development of digital imaging is intended to improve the reading/reporting and image archival portions of this process. Interestingly, it is the way digital images are stored or archived that provides the greatest potential benefits and cost savings in the filmless imaging process. The role of the picture archival and communications system (PACS) in this process will also be outlined later in this chapter.

The digital imaging landscape changes with each new generation of computers or about every three years. In the near future, radiography will complete its transition from the film-based (hard copy) imaging format to a soft-copy (filmless) computer-based imaging format. This transition has been made possible by ever more affordable and more powerful computers, recent advances that have been made in high-resolution cathode ray tube monitors, optical (laser) printing systems, teleradiographic communication devices, and computerized information storage systems (PACS).

COMPUTED RADIOGRAPHY

In the 1970s, Fuji began the development of a digital imaging system that was able to acquire static images using the area type beam employed in conventional radiography. Because an area beam spreads out in all directions from the x-ray, it is able to encompass the entire region of interest enabling the acquisition of image data in just a few milliseconds. The main advancement that made this possible was the development of a new type of imaging plate called a photostimulable phosphor (PSP). (In digital radiography, hundreds of individual detectors have to be used to accommodate such an area beam; otherwise, a scanning projection system has to be used which requires relatively long exposure times.) Following its exposure to radiation the imaging plate retains the image in an electronic form that can be scanned by a laser beam to release the information for its conversion into digital form.

One of the main advantages of this imaging system is in its ability to house the image plate in a cassette that is similar to those used in conventional radiography. The term computed radiography (CR) is commonly applied to this type of cassette-based digital imaging system. After an exposure is completed, the digital or CR cassette is imprinted with patient identification information and placed in the reader section where the image is scanned and converted into a digital format which is displayed on a CRT (cathode ray tube or "TV") monitor of the workstation. At the present, the majority of departments converting over to digital imaging systems in radiography seem to prefer the familiarity and flexibility of the cassette-based computed radiographic (CR) system over the digital radiographic (DR) systems. Even with advances in technology, the scanned projection systems used for DR were not able to reduce the long acquisition times, making this technique impractical in performing the chest and abdominal images they were designed to acquire.

The Matrix and Pixel Size

The numerous picture elements or pixels that make up the digital image matrix play an important role in all of the visual properties associated with the image. A 6 x 6 image matrix appears as a square field that is 6 pixels in height and 6 pixels in width. A multiplication of the two dimensions (height x width) will determine the total number of pixels in the matrix. The diagram in Figure 36-1 shows the effect of the size of the matrix to both the number and relative size of the pixels that make up the image. Figure 36-1A represents a small 6 x 6 image matrix that is made up from 36 individual pixels. Figure 36-1B represents a larger 12 x 12 image matrix consisting of 144 individual pixels.

Most of the early digital imaging systems had an image matrix of 256 x 256 pixels.

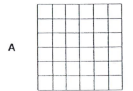 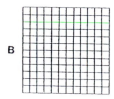

Figure 36-1. A shows a 6 x 6 image matrix, which is made up by 36 individual picture elements or pixels. The number of pixels in the matrix is found as the sum of the number of pixels on the two axes (height, width) of the matrix. Note that the relative size of the pixels in the A matrix is considerably larger than in B matrix, which shows a larger 12 x 12 matrix. In the 12 x 12 matrix the number of pixels will increase to 144. Since both matrices have the same linear dimensions the main difference in the B matrix is the reduced size of the pixels.

By current standards these images would be considered poor quality. Even the 512 x 512 matrix that was used in many of the first and second generation computer tomographic scanners has been upgraded to the 1024 x 1024 matrix size in recent years. In less than 20 years, the number of pixels in digital images has risen from 65,536 pixels in the 256 x 256 matrix to 1,048,576 in the 1024 x 1024 matrix.

The size of the individual picture elements or pixels in a digital image is the most important factor in the production of images that appear sharp or have what is termed a high spatial resolution. Images composed of a large number of pixels with small dimensions will more accurately represent the tissues of interest than an image composed of a small number of larger pixels.

Field of View and Pixel Size

In modern digital imaging systems, the size of the pixel is related not only to the size of the matrix, but also to the field of view (FOV). The field of view (FOV) is often defined as the size of the relevant image displayed on the cathode ray tube monitor. (In CT scanning, the matrix size is often called the *scan field of view* or SFOV, and is defined as all of the voxels of information acquired from the original scan, whereas the *display field of view* or DFOV is only that portion of the matrix selected for display on the CRT monitor. In computed radiography, the term *field of view* normally refers to the *display* field of view.) In a conventional radiographic system, the field of view is the collimated portion of the radiograph image containing the anatomic structures of interest.

In a computed radiographic system, the field of view is the portion of the imaging (photostimulable) plate that contains relevant anatomic information. For example, the field of view for an adult hand would be considerably smaller than for an image of an adult chest. Since digital images of both the chest and hand are displayed using the same image matrix (the same display screen), the smaller field will have more pixels in a given area than the larger field used for the chest. Because of the size of the field depends on a number of patient related factors, the size of the pixels will normally vary between .1 mm and .4 mm in size.

The relationship of the pixel size to the size of the matrix and display field of view is expressed by the relationship below:

$$\text{Pixel size} = \frac{\text{Display Field of view (DFOV)}}{\text{Size of the matrix}}$$

This formula shows that the size of the pixel is directly related to the display field of view and is inversely related to the size of the matrix.

Question 1: In a digital imaging system having a 1024 x 1024 pixel matrix, calculate the pixel size for a 23 cm x 23 cm field used for a computed radiographic image of a hand.

Answer:

$$\frac{230 \text{ mm FOV}}{1024 \text{ matrix}} = .22 \text{ mm}$$

Using the information above, the pixel size will measure .22mm by .22 mm.

Question 2: In a digital imaging system having a 1024 x 1024 pixel matrix, calculate the pixel size for a 42 cm x 42 cm field used for a computed radiographic image of the chest:

Answer:

$$\frac{420 \text{ mm FOV}}{1024 \text{ matrix}} = .41 \text{ mm}$$

Using the information above each pixel will measure .41 mm height and width.

Because the pixel size of the computer radiographic image of the chest is greater than the pixel size of the hand, the smaller field of view provides an image that has a higher degree of sharpness than that of a chest. Figure 36-2 is a CT scan of the head provided to show the appearance of digitally acquired images taken using different size pixels. The upper half of this scan was reconstructed with 7-millimeter pixels: Note the blockness or step-stair appearance of the edges of the frontal bone, left arrow. The lower half of this same image was reconstructed using a pixel size of only 3 millimeters. As shown by the right arrow, the see-saw or step-stair appearance is still present but very much diminished so that the spatial resolution of the occipital bone is greatly improved.

One might question why a company doesn't simply manufacture digital units with 2048 x 2048 matrix or a 4098 x 4098 matrix to further improve the image quality of the digital image. The answer has to do with some important limitations of the imaging system components. At the current state of technology, the power and speed of the computer and the limitations in the CRT monitor are two main limiting factors that restrict the size of the matrix and pixels. In any digital imaging system, both the size of the matrix and pixels are a function of amount of digital data that must be acquired and processed. In order to improve the image quality, the amount of digital data that is processed must be increased. Because the relationship between the size of the matrix and the required digital data is not linear, it will take the acquisition of four times more digital data to accomplish a doubling in the size of the image matrix. Until recently, this was one of the greatest limitations preventing the use of larger image matrices. This factor underscores the reason why computed radiographic systems have only recently become part of radiology's imaging services.

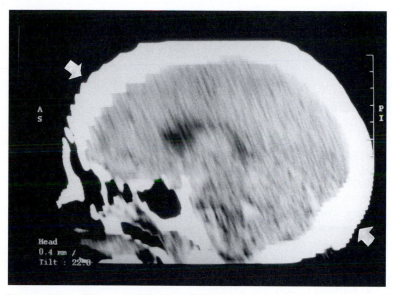

Figure 36-2. CT scan of the head showing the relationship between pixel size and spatial resolution. The upper half of the image was reconstructed with 7 mm pixels and shows a gross step-stair appearance to the frontal bone, left arrow. The lower half of the image used 3 mm pixels and shows much improved resolution of the occipital bone, right arrow.

A second and even more important limitation is the ability of the digital image display device or cathode ray tube monitor to provide the high spatial resolution that is necessary for a larger matrix. It is now the limitation of the various types of display device systems, such as the cathode ray tube monitors and the laser printers that are likely to slow improvements in the digital imaging process in the near future.

Pixel Brightness and Attenuation Coefficient

In a film-screen imaging system, the optical density seen on radiographic images is based on the amount of radiation exiting from the object or the degree to which the radiation has been attenuated. In tissues that have a greater thickness or a higher physical density, a smaller portion of the incident radiation reaches the image receptor, resulting in a lower optical densi-

ty on the film. Therefore, it can be said that the optical density on the radiographic image represents the attenuation properties of the entire plane of tissues from the front to the back of the patient.

In the digital imaging system, the shading (gray shade) assigned to each pixel in a digital image is also a function of the relative attenuation of the tissues, from the front to the back of the patient. In order to maintain the proper location of the attenuation values, the data is acquired from a three-dimensional area called a voxel. Since the attenuation properties of the tissues included in the voxel are not recorded on a film, the term optical density cannot be employed. In a digital imaging procedure, the different shades associated with the attenuation values are displayed as gray shades or gray scale values. Figure 36-3 shows the relationship between the displayed brightness of each pixel and the attenuation coefficient of each voxel in the

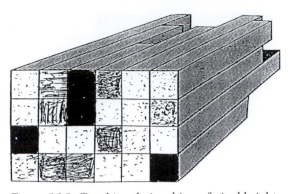

Figure 36-3. Graphic relationshipo of pixel brightness to the attenuation coefficient of the voxel from the front to the back of the patient. Bright pixels result from a high attenuation coefficient (longer bars), while darker pixels result from a low attenuation or low absorption of the x-ray beam from front to back as it passes through the patient.

patient. Note that, whereas in CT a voxel would be considered a small cube of tissue contained within the projected "slice," in computed radiography a voxel is a very elongated square "tube" which extends all the way from the front to the back of the patient. This is because the x-ray beam in CR passes clear through the whole thickness of the patient and records an attenuation coefficient for that entire thickness for each pixel.

During the acquisition of a digital image, the absorption properties of the tissues in the voxel are recorded as numerical values called the attenuation coefficients. Using the attenuation coefficients of the tissues, the computer is able to assign each pixel a gray scale value (digital density) for the tissues in the corresponding voxel. Once the brightness level or gray shade is selected for the voxel, it can be displayed on the cathode ray tube (monitor) as the gray shade for the pixel. In other words, the gray scale values of the pixels that form the individual segments of the digital image are derived from the attenuation coefficients of the voxel. The number of gray shades that are associated or can be assigned to a pixel

is a function of the capabilities of the computer to process digital information. In most modern systems, the ability to assign gray scale values can be approximated by the code values of the analog-to-digital converter (ADC).

In the early digital imaging systems, the use of an 8-bit ADC permitted 256 (2^8) individual shades of gray for each of the pixels within the matrix. Today, a typical computed radiographic system is more likely to use a 10-bit ADC allowing for up to 1024 (2^{10}) shades, or a 12-bit ADC permitting as many as 4096 shades for each individual pixel.

Acquisition Time

In order to provide a radiograph-like static image, the image data must be collected in a short period of time to help limit the amount of motion that is apparent on the acquired image. Again, this is largely a function of the power and speed of the computer. For a computer to acquire and process the image data for a 1024 x 1024 matrix, the solution of over a million equations is required. If this cannot be accomplished in a reasonable amount of time, the process would be impractical. Fortunately, modern computers used in the imaging fields have the ability to acquire and process the staggering amount of data required to produce a diagnostic quality in a timely manner. Though this is true today, computers with this capacity have only been available for a little more than a decade. In fact, the long acquisition times were the last of the major obstacles that needed to be overcome in the development of a practical computed radiographic system. This deficiency was resolved through the steady progress that continues to be made in the power and speed of computers used to process digital images. At the present state of technology, the speed of digital computers enables the use of acquisition times that rival those of conventional film-screen radiography.

Image Gray Scale Enhancement

One of the main advantages of a digital system is in its ability to manipulate the gray scale values of the pixels. The use of special software or processing functions enables the selection and assignment of different gray scale values to tissues based on the assumption that this can improve the visualization of selected low subject-contrast tissues. Figure 36-4A shows a portion of a pixel matrix and its four corresponding voxels.

Through the application of software programs it is possible to assign pixels different gray scale values based on the differences in the attenuation values. Figure 36-4B shows the same pixel matrix after three of the pixels have been assigned lighter gray values mathematically by the computer. In

this way, the contrast of these structures is enhanced.

When the computer assigns pixels gray scale values that are similar to the optical densities seen on a radiographic image, the reconstructed digital image will share many of the same image characteristics as an x-ray film. The clear or lighter regions of the image will represent those tissues that attenuate the greatest amount of radiation such as bone or contrast agents. The darker regions will represent gasses or fatty tissues that have a low attenuation to x-rays. The main advantage of the digitally acquired image is that the technologist has the ability to enhance the image characteristics through the adjustment of the processing controls after the image has been acquired.

Spatial Resolution

The ability of an image to display two or more closely spaced objects as separate images is termed spatial resolution. In

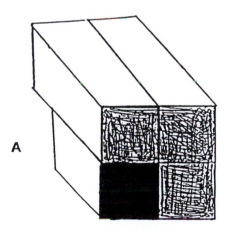
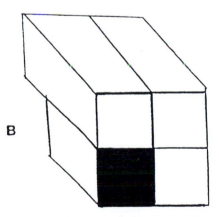

Figure 36-4. The relative gray scale values for four different pixels shown in A were obtained from the true attenuation coefficients of the tissues. Because there are only small differences in these values the corresponding pixels have similar gray scale values. The result is an image with a low amount of image contrast or a poor low contrast detectability, and it is difficult to see the darker pixel in the lower left-hand corner. After the three other pixels have been assigned a different gray scale level (B), the ability to demonstrate this pixel is greatly enhanced. The result is an image that has a greater image contrast or a higher detectability of low subject-contrast structures.

modern systems, the spatial resolution is normally determined by the use of a high-contrast (line pair) resolution phantom that can record the limit of resolution for the imaging system in line pairs/mm. Until recently, the greatest restriction associated with the formation of the digital image was the inability of the system to provide the necessary spatial resolution required to accurately represent the minute differences in the structural anatomy of the body. As mentioned earlier, the ability to perceive structural detail is a function of the size or number of pixels in the image matrix, the speed and power of the computer, and the ability of the CRT monitor to display the image.

For the computer, the ability to obtain a high spatial resolution is a function of the size of the pixels in the matrix. It has been found that with pixels measuring .4 mm, no more than 2 line pairs per millimeter can be resolved on a standard resolution phantom. When pixel values are reduced to below .1 mm, the spatial resolution increases to about 6-8 lp/mm on the line pair phantom.

In the 1970s, the early digital units such as computed tomographic (CT) scanner had a spatial resolution of less than 1 lp/mm; in the 1980s the spatial resolution of the computer tomographic scanners and the first digital subtraction angiographic (DSA) units had improve to about 2-4 lp/mm. By the 1990s, improvements in both the computers and cathode ray tube monitors had improved the spatial resolution of modern digital systems to around 6-8 lp/mm. Though slower-speed film-screen imaging systems can achieve a higher spatial resolution of between 10-12 lp/mm, this small difference is not considered significant for most imaging situations. Since the resolution provided by a modern digital system does not significantly degrade the ability to make a proper diagnosis, this is no longer a major limitation of a digital imaging system. In fact, it appears that the higher consistency and ability to manipulate or post-process the acquired images may in some situations actually improve the visualization of many pathologic conditions. Most present-day radiographic images can be acquired at a resolution that is comparable to the 6-10 lp/mm resolution of a conventional 400-speed film-screen imaging system. Though the spatial resolution in a digital imaging system is not likely to improve much beyond these current values in the near future, this is not longer considered an important limitation.

IMAGE DISPLAY

Cathode Ray Tube (CRT) Monitors

Nearly all digital images are displayed on a cathode ray type (CRT) system such as that used in a standard television or a computer monitor. The ability to provide and maintain the high spatial resolution of a state-of-the-art digital image is a function of two independent factors: the vertical resolution controlled by the number of lines in the video display, and the horizontal resolution controlled by the frequency or bandpass.

Vertical Resolution

The vertical resolution of the cathode ray tube is controlled by the number of scan lines or the total number of lines that make up the image displayed on the CRT monitor. In a standard broadcast television, each frame of the image consists of 525 scan lines that run from the top to the bottom of the screen. The actual resolution of the standard (525 line) television image is considered poor, providing a maximum spatial resolution of only .5-1 mm lp/mm. Since this is far below the resolution needed for a proper display of the high-quality diagnostic image, a more sophisticated 1000 or 2000 scan line system is required for use in all diagnostic-imaging applications. The greater number of scan lines in these new CRTs are able to resolve images approaching the 6-10 lp/mm resolution of a 400-speed film-screen imaging system.

Horizontal Resolution

The second factor that affects the display of a cathode ray tube monitor is the horizontal resolution of the system. The horizontal resolution is the amount of information that can be carried in a particular scan line. The amount of information that can be stored on a given line is dependent on the frequency at which the electrons in the scanning beam of the television camera are modulated during a scan line. Most standard broadcast televisions operate at a frequency or bandpass of about 4.5 MHz. This frequency is far below what is normally required for most diagnostic imaging applications. In order to provide the desired horizontal resolution with a 1000 or 2000 scan line system, a frequency or bandpass of 20 MHz-40 MHz is required. at this frequency, it is possible to display a horizontal resolution nearly equal to that of the vertical resolution of the higher scan line systems.

In order to enable the radiologist to view images in the familiar size format, digital radiographic or computed radiographic images are displayed on full-sized screens that are similar in size to the field of view of a 14"-17" film.

IMAGE QUALITY

Contrast Resolution (Detectability of Low Subject-Contrast Structures)

Though at the present time digital images cannot quite match the higher spatial resolution of a film-screen imaging system, digital images are capable of displaying much smaller differences in subject contrast of the tissues. This factor is known as *contrast resolution*, and it is the digital imaging system's greatest advantage. Due to the limitations of the human eye, a film-screen imaging system requires a contrast difference of at least 10 percent between adjacent tissues to enable the perception of adjacent structures.

The ability of a digital imaging system to assign different gray scale values to tissues with similar attenuation coefficient values allows the perception of tissue contrast differences of as small as 1 percent. The improved contrast resolution possible with the digital imaging technique provides increases the ability to distinguish between cerebral spinal fluid, blood, and brain tissue, far better than with an analog (film-screen) imaging system. The relationship between the ability to detect contrast and display fine structural details in analog and digital imaging systems is demonstrated in Figure 36-5. Table 36-1 summarizes the comparisons between analog and digital imaging systems.

Dynamic Range

In digital radiography, the range of number of shades of gray that are assigned to the pixels is referred to as the dynamic range. Since the human eye is only capable

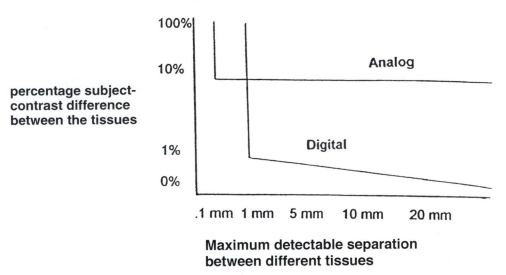

Figure 36-5. The graph shows the ability of an analog and digital imaging system to display structural details as a function of difference in the subject contrast between the structures. The graph clearly shows the higher spatial resolution that is possible when a significant (10% or more) contrast is provided in a radiographic (analog) image. Just as dramatic is the near complete loss of image perception as the subject contrast falls below a value of 10%. For a digital image, the enhanced detectability of low contrast structures enables perception of structures with nearly the same physical density.

of distinguishing about 32 shades of gray, from black to white, most of the 500-1000 gray scales produced in a digital system and the infinite number of optical densities on a radiographic image are undetectable.

To help narrow this range in a film-screen radiographic system, the radiographer selects a set of exposure factors that limits the range of optical densities appearing on the radiograph. For example, on a chest radiograph, the selection of the proper exposure factors helps to produce a range of optical densities best suited to

imaging the air in the lungs and the fluid densities of the heart and soft tissues. A different set of exposure factors would be needed to better visualize the thoracic vertebrae when these are the structures of primary interest.

Therefore, a radiographer must learn to select the appropriate exposure and technical factors that will provide the optimal densities and maximum contrast range in the image and eliminate the appearance of tissues that transmit too much or too little radiation. In a digital radiographic system,

Table 36-1

Imaging System	Low Subject-Contrast Detectability	Maximum Subject-Contrast Detectability	Spatial Resolution lp/mm
Analog (film-screen)	Fair	10%	10-12 lp/mm
Analog (fluoroscopy)	Fair	10%	4-8 lp/mm
Digital Fluoroscopy (DSA)	Excellent	1%	4-5 lp/mm
Computer Radiography	Excellent	1%	6-8 lp/mm

the maximum contrast sensitivity is obtained through the control of the appropriate dynamic range. In order to help simplify this process, all digital radiographic systems are designed with pre-selected the dynamic range settings to optimize the visualization of a specific anatomic region.

These instructions or protocols are programmed into the operating system of all digital imaging systems. Because a digital system can precisely detect and assign gray scale values to the tissues, it is possible to assign values that enable the perception tissues with a similar physical density. On conventional radiographs, tissues such as blood and cerebral spinal fluid are perceived as having the same optical density and are therefore not visible as separate tissues. By re-assigning gray scale values to these tissues, they can be perceived by the eye. It is this ability that provides the improved contrast perception of digital images.

Quantum Mottle

In addition to the three geometric factors (matrix size, pixel size, field of view) that relate to the spatial resolution of electronically acquired images, an additional property known as noise must also be considered. One of the greatest limitations in a modern electronic circuit is the loss of image quality caused by the presence of the random variations in the number of photons striking an image receptor, called quantum mottle. Though all x-ray imaging systems are associated with a random fluctuation of the x-ray photons striking the image receptor, quantum mottle is rarely observed in a 400-speed film-screen imaging system. Quantum mottle is an effect that only becomes noticeable in extremely high (800) speed imaging systems when a small amount of radiation is used to record

the image. Images showing this effect will demonstrate regions having small areas of increased or decreased optical or digital densities. This effect creates a blotchy appearance on the image, most often referred to as *grain*.

Electronic Noise

All electronic imaging system components, such as the television cameras, image intensifier and cathode ray tube monitors, are associated with the aberrant movement of electrons resulting in an artifact called electronic noise. Like quantum mottle, electronic noise is also a random effect that produces regions of increase image brightness that appear on image displays as flashes of light or "snow." The snow-like pattern seen on television monitor tuned to a weak station or the background static (white noise) in audio system are two examples of electronic noise.

Since electronic noise does not contribute any useful information to the image, it serves only to degrade its quality. When high noise levels are present they can significantly compromise or obscure a digital image. The high sensitivity of the digital radiographic system makes it extremely susceptible to all types of image noise.

Signal-to-Noise Ratio

A standard means has been developed to express noise in comparison to the strength of the signal, called the signal-to-noise (S/N) ratio. This value is used to indicate an acceptable noise level for a given signal strength. In an analog imaging system the signal strength is directly related to the amount of mAs used in the production of the images. Because the mAs values used in conventional radiography are relatively large, noise is rarely a problem in film-

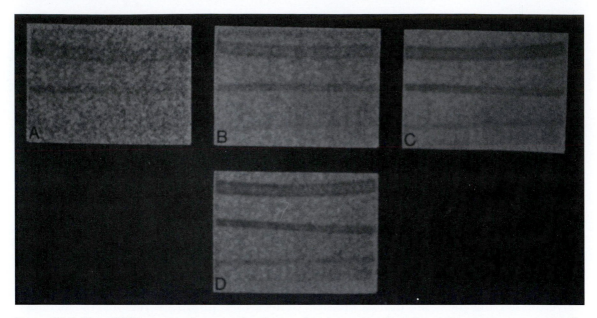

Figure 36-6. Four CRT monitor images of catheters demonstrating the effects of image noise or scintillation: As the signal is increased from A to D by increasing the intensity of the original x-ray beam, signal-to-noise ratio is improved and the image becomes more visible. *Reprinted with permission of Lea & Febiger, Christensen's Physics of Diagnostic Radiology.*

screen images.

The same cannot be said for other types of electronic imaging systems. A signal-to-noise ratio of less than 200:1, though relatively low, is acceptable for the poor quality of a standard broadcast television set. A S/N ratio value of 500:1 is normally considered acceptable for a modern televised fluoroscopic chain. A signal-to-noise ratio of 1000/1 is normally required for cathode ray tube monitors used with most digital imaging systems. Figure 36-6 shows four digital images taken at different signal-to-noise levels.

Many departments have found that a doubling of the recommended mAs values during digital imaging techniques may be required to avoid the appearance of grain when computed radiographic images are acquired.

COMPUTED RADIOGRAPHY

Though both computed radiographic and digital radiographic systems are competing for their share of the static digital imaging market, the practical advantages associated with computed radiography (CR) are guiding more departments to choose these systems when the conversion to digital imaging system is desired. One of the reasons for this is the high degree of compatibility the system has with standard or existing radiographic units. Radiographers find the conversion to a CR system is extremely easy because the only change required to acquire images is the use of a new type of cassette. Though the processing of the images is very different, the actual way in which images are obtained is virtually identical to the way images are obtained with a film-screen imaging system.

THE COMPUTED RADIOGRAPHIC (CR) CASSETTE

The computed radiographic or CR cassette is designed to look and in most respects act to perform many of the functions of a standard cassette. CR cassettes come in many of the same sizes and can be used for all mobile tabletop or Bucky applications. Like its analog counterpart, the images can be acquired with tabletop or Bucky tray using manual or automatic exposure techniques. The main difference in the system is in how the image is processed and stored. Since there is no film, the image must be processed in a different manner. In a totally filmless system, no hard copy image is produced. The completed image will be displayed on a CRT monitor and can be stored as a soft copy on a storage system called a PACS or printed on a transparent medium by a laser printer or other hard copy production system.

Radiographers do need to be aware that the image plate housed in the cassette does have only a single emulsion surface and must be placed facing forward in the CR cassette.

Stimulated Luminescence (PSP) Imaging Plate

A major breakthrough in the search for a practical replacement for the film/screen imaging system came about from the development of special imaging plate called a photostimulable phosphor (PSP). This imaging plate has the ability to store and release image data without an appreciable amount of lost information over time. It was found that a small number of barium-fluorohalide compounds, i.e., barium fluorobromide and barium fluorochloride, possess a unique property called stimulated luminescence. When a pure crystal of barium-fluorobromide is "doped" or activated with small amounts of europium, the crystal develops a series of tiny defects called meta-stable sites or **F** centers throughout its crystal lattice. These **F** centers act like small "electronic holes" in the crystal that can capture or trap electrons that are released when the exit radiation of the beam strikes the photostimulable phosphor (PSP) imaging plate. In a process that is somewhat similar to the formation of the latent image in a sensitized silver bromide crystal, the imaging plate stores the energy of the exit x-ray beam in the form of a latent electrical image within the **F** centers of the crystal lattice.

Because the energy retained by these latent electrons in the **F** centers is stable for relatively long periods of time, the image can be retrieved without any appreciable loss of information (fading) for many hours. It has been estimated that the standard PSP imaging plate will retain up to 75 percent of the original latent image for as long as 8 hours after the exposure. Unlike the processing solutions necessary to convert the latent film image into the black metallic image, the latent image of the photostimulable phosphor needs to be excited by an optical laser to release this trapped energy. When the image carrying electrons in the **F** centers of the image plate are stimulated by a red light helium-neon laser (see Fig. 35-16 in the previous chapter), the retained electronic (latent) image of the crystals releases its "trapped" energy in the form of blue-violet phosphorescence. The intensity of the blue-violet light is directly proportional to the amount of radiation that reached the imaging plate from the various tissues.

Unlike an intensifying screen that rapidly converts the energy of the x-ray beam into visible light (fluorescence), a photostimulable phosphor stores the energy of the x-ray beam within the crystal lattice of the compound as an electronic latent image. The electrons preserving the image will release this stored information as a visible light pattern only after the crystals in the plate have been activated or stimulated by a coherent light source or laser beam.

READING OF THE STIMULATED LUMINESCENCE (PSP) IMAGING PLATE

Photomultiplier (PM) Tube

The conversion of this phosphorescent light into digital data is a two-step process that is accomplished by changing a light into an electronic signal and converting this into digital data that can be understood by a computer. The first step in this process is accomplished by a special tube known as a photomultiplier (PM) tube. The photomultiplier is a small electronic tube that converts visible light into an electronic signal.

The visible emitted light from the excited PSP imaging plate is directed through a light-channeling guide onto a photocathode layer on the input side of the PM tube. This layer serves to convert the visible light from the PSP imaging plate into a low intensity electronic signal. Since this signal is too small to be detected by most other types of electronic devices, it needs to be amplified. This is accomplished in the dynode section of the PM tube. The electrons emerging from the photocathode layer are directed towards a series of positively charged plates called dynodes that attract the electrons. As the electrons are accelerated toward the first charged plate (dynode), they collide with the dynode to release about five electrons for each of the incident electrons produced in the photo-

cathode layer. By having the electron beam pass through 10-12 of these dynodes in succession, the electronic signal can be amplified by more than a million times.

Analog-to-Digital Converter

In order for the computer to use the amplified signal from the photomultiplier, it must first be converted in to a digital form or digitized. This is accomplished by a device called an analog-to-digital converter (ADC). In typical computed radiographic system it is likely to be accomplished 12-bit ADC that converts the information contained in image signal into the desired gray scale value for each individual pixel of the image matrix.

PROCESSING OF THE COMPUTED RADIOGRAPHIC (CR) IMAGE

In a traditional analog system, once the image is acquired, there is little that can be done to improve the visualization of the structures appearing on the radiographic or the fluoroscopic monitor. An image that is too light or too dark cannot be modified to any great extent and must be repeated if an improved image quality is desired. One of the important advantages of the digital imaging technique is in its ability to permit the enhancement of the images both before and after the original acquisition of the image data. All of the digital imaging techniques include processing or preprocessing systems that can be used to manipulate the image data before images are presented in a final form.

Processing of Digital Images

Unlike the conventional film-screen imaging system process that is completed after the film has emerged from the processor, in a computed radiographic system, the reading of the image represents only the first of four steps that are needed to complete the imaging process that will eventually provide a form that is suitable for the interpretation by the physician. Though various manufacturers of computed radiographic equipment use different names for their components, the four processing steps are similar in all systems:

1. Image identification (ID tablet)
2. CR reader (digitizer)
3. Digital workstation
4. Image display (hard and/or soft copy) (laser printer)

Image Identification (ID Tablet)

In computed radiographic systems, after the PSP imaging plate contained within the computed radiographic cassette is exposed, it must be imprinted or marked with the appropriate patient information before the image is "read." This is accomplished in the identification unit (ID tablet). Not unlike an ID flasher, this device uses a light source to affix the patient name, ID number, exam date, institutional ID, patient position, and other pertinent information to the image before it is scanned or processed. The required information is typed from a keyboard or electronically transferred into the ID tablet from a bar code scanner. Once the patient information has been entered, it should be checked to insure that each image is imprinted with the correct data. Each cassette needs to be placed into the ID tablet prior to being placed in the CR reader.

CR Reader (Image Processor)

After the CR image has been identified, it is placed in the CR reader or digitizer to convert the analog image on the PSP image plate into a digital form. The reading of the image plate is accomplished by an automated system that begins with the removal of the PSP plate from the cassette by the image processor. Following its removal from the CR cassette, the imaging plate is moved by a series of rollers into the area where a mirror deflects the laser beam to move rapidly across the plate, causing the release of the stored latent image. The crosswise direction in which the laser beam scans across the plate is called the *fast scan direction*, whereas the direction of the plate itself is moving through the reader is called the *slow scan* or *subscan direction*. The visible emitted light from the excited PSP imaging plate is directed through a light-channeling guide onto a photomultiplier (PM) tube that records and amplifies the relative intensity of the light. Following the digitization of the signal by the analog-to-digital convertor, the data enters the digital processing section of the computer that compiles the data into a series of gray scales that mimic a radiographic image.

Once the image plate has been scanned, it continues to move in the sub-scan direction toward the "eraser" section of the image processor. In this section, the PSP plate is exposed to a bright white light to remove any remaining information from the plate so it can be reused. The "clean" image plate is now reloaded back into the original CR cassette. After the PSP plate is reinserted to the CR cassette, it passes on to the output tray of the processor and is ready to be re-exposed. The entire reading and erasure process will normally take about 90 seconds to complete. Unlike the radiographic film that can be used only once, the PSP imaging plate, when properly erased, can be used thousands of times.

Since all PSP imaging plates are extremely sensitive to even small amounts of background radiation, a plate that has not been used for 24-

72 hours may have collected a sufficient exposure from background radiation to cause the appearance of noise in the image. For this reason, all manufacturers recommend that imaging plates that have not be used for more than 24 hours should be erased before they are used to acquire additional images.

DIGITAL WORK STATION

Unlike a radiographic image that can no longer be altered once the chemical processing steps have been completed, the computed radiographic can be manipulated in a number of important ways. Though each company that manufactures CR units will provide different names for these functions, all units will provide controls that enable:

1. Windowing
2. Frequency processing
3. Dual energy subtraction
4. Dynamic range controls

Each of these functions enables the operator of the equipment to correct for factors that have created images that are less than optimal.

WINDOWING

The contrast processing or rescaling programs provide the operator a simple means for maximizing the image contrast and gray scale of the image. They are used mainly to enhance the appearance of clinical features that cannot be well visualized on "raw" images. These controls are driven by a number of complex linear and non-linear transforms to alter the window level and window width parameters on the display.

Window Level Controls

The window level control is provided to help select the set of factors that will provide the desired attenuation coefficient values for the tissues in a given anatomic region. By focusing in on a particular attenuation coefficient and the narrow range of values around selected tissues, a more desirable image quality can be achieved. Just as the mAs controls the overall optical density of a conventional radiograph, the window level controls the brightness of the display in the CR image. Since the brightness is most closely related to the overall optical density in an analog system, the correct setting of the window controls is essential for maintaining CR images that are not too dark or light. Just as you would not use the same technical factors on a chest and thoracic spine on radiographic images, the same window levels cannot be used on the chest and thoracic spine images in a computed radiographic or digital imaging system.

*Increasing the window level makes the image on the CRT **darker***, as shown in Figure 36-7C and D. Normally window levels range from -1000 to +1000. With zero being a mid-range gray shade, minus numbers yield a brighter image and plus numbers yield a darker image. Relative contrast between tissues in unchanged except at very extreme window levels.

Window Width Controls

The window width controls change the gray scale values of the individuals pixels to expand or compress the range of image values that are visible to the human eye. In other words, the window width alters the

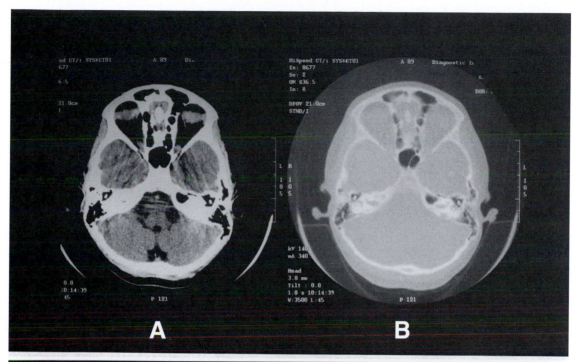

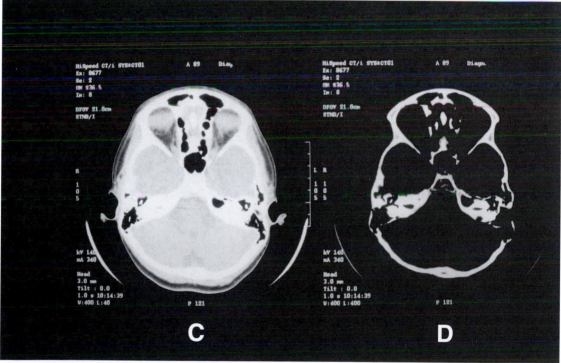

Figure 36-7. Window width vs. window level. *A* and *B* are two axial CT scans of the cranium which demonstrate equal overall brightness with the window level set at 45, but a much longer gray scale in *B* due to increasing the *window width* from 97 to 3500. Compare this pair of images to the pair C and D, in which only the *window level* was altered, showing a dramatic change in overall brightness. For both *C* and *D*, window width was fixed at 400, window level for *C* was 40, and for *D*, 400. (Courtesy of Jason Swopes, RT.)

number of gray shades included at a particular window level. When the window width is reduced, there is a greater difference between the individual shades of gray providing the appearance of a higher image contrast. When the window width is increased, an expanded number of gray shades are included in the image display resulting in an image with a lower image contrast.

An increase in the window width is somewhat analogous to an increase in the kVp setting in radiography. When a higher contrast in a computed or digital image is desired, the width of the window should be reduced. *Increasing the window width gives the image on the CRT* **longer gray scale**.

Figure 36-7 is provided to emphasize the difference between window width and window level. Note that the two CT images *A* and *B* demonstrate equal overall brightness, but vastly difference gray scales. Only the window width was changed on these two images. In *C* and *D*, only the window level was changed, and the apparent difference is primarily brightness.

By first setting the **window width** *to obtain the desired range of gray scale for the particular tissues to be demonstrated, then optimizing the window level or brightness, the image can be manipulated to demonstrate air-filled tissues, soft tissues and organs, or bones with optimal visualization.* Figure 36-8 shows two CR images of the chest taken at different window levels and window width settings adjusted in this manner. Radiograph *A* was taken with a low window width for high contrast to demonstrate any fluid in the lungs—note that the cervical vertebrae are also well-visualized. For radiograph *B*, window width was increased for a long gray scale, then the window level was reduced to -500 in order to brighten the image overall: This combination of high window width and low window level shows the soft tissues of the lungs and neck much better.

FREQUENCY PROCESSING: SMOOTHING AND EDGE ENHANCEMENT

When images are acquired with only small amounts of raw data, the display may appear to have an excessive amount of contrast due to the presence of high-frequency noise. The use of frequency processing techniques has been developed to help overcome these limitations. Some of the most commonly used terms for these functions include edge enhancement, unsharp masking, and smoothing functions. All of these techniques are used to accentuate or suppress portions of the raw data to increase or decrease the differences between the pixels in the display matrix.

In some cases, the quality of the image can be improved through a process called low-pass filtering that electronically amplifies the lower frequencies in the data and reduces the presence of high frequency noise in the image. When this function is applied, the difference between adjacent pixels is reduced, resulting in a reduction in the contrast and a "smoothing" of the image. Figure 36-9 shows how a smoothing algorithm removes noise both from the background (white arrow) and from the anatomy (black arrow) of a high contrast 3D CT image of the elbow. In some of the state-of-the-art systems, a subtracted image containing only low spatial frequencies can be generated and amplified before being added back to the original high frequency image.

In images that do not have the desired amount of image contrast, a process called high-pass filtering can be applied that amplifies the higher frequency portions of the image data. This tends to enhance the difference between the pixels, improving

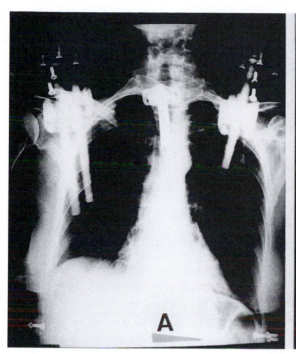
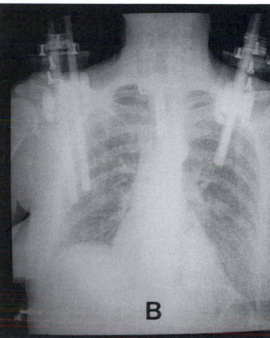

Figure 36-8. Effects of windowing: *A* shows a CR of the chest at a window level of 50 (used for fluids) and at a window width of 500. *B* shows the same view at a brighter window level of -500 (used for the lungs) but with an increased window width of 1600. The second image taken at a wider window width is used to improve the visualization of the air filled soft tissues of the lung by using a longer gray scale.

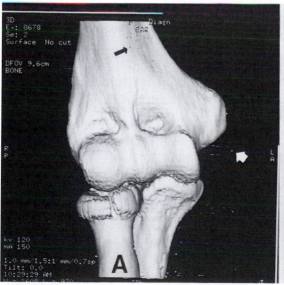
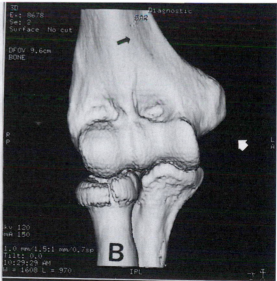

Figure 36-9. Smoothing from low-pass filtering of a 3D CT image of the elbow. Note that in this high-contrast image (A), high-frequency noise artifacts appear in both the background (white arrow) and over the anatomy (black arrow). A smoothing alogrithm was employed to remove these artifacts in *B*. (Courtesy of Jason Swopes, RT.)

visibility of the edges or borders between different tissues. This process, sometimes called "sharpening," produces an image with a higher contrast but a more grainy appearance due to the increased visualization of noise within the image.

The operator must be aware that excessive modification of images using any of the frequency control functions may introduce unwanted artifacts or "non-patient" data into the image.

DUAL ENERGY SUBTRACTION CONTROLS

One of the more interesting functions of a computed radiographic system is its ability to subtract two images of the same region using different attenuation factors. In this mode, two images of the same anatomic region are obtained at different kVp settings. When these images are reconstructed, an energy subtraction program can eliminate selected structures based on the differences of the attenuation coefficients of the tissues. Though the actual programming to accomplish this is quite complex, the result is a so-called "tissue-only" subtracted image that can display soft-tissue structures of the chest cavity without the images associated with the ribs or spine. Using different settings can produce "bone-only" images that eliminate a vast majority of the soft tissue structures (lung, heart) for an image of the thorax.

DYNAMIC RANGE CONTROLS (DRC)

The dynamic range control is used by some manufacturers as an adjunct to the frequency processing controls. Rather than modifying the image by a manipulation of the high or low frequency data, the DRC controls modify the contrast in the image as a function of the gray scale. For example, the reduced signal produced from the mediastinum or sub-diaphragmatic regions of the chest can be selectively enhanced based on their low density or gray scale values. The result is a portion of an image that is enhanced without adversely affecting the remaining areas of the image. This technique has proved most useful for images of the chest and studies of the cervical and thoracic spines.

EXPOSURE TECHNIQUES IN COMPUTED RADIOGRAPHY

Exposure Estimation (Normalization)

At the present time, most of the photostimulable phosphors used in CR systems have a sensitivity that is nearly equal to that of a 200-speed, film-screen image receptor. Because of this, patient exposures during a CR examination are likely to be somewhat higher than those obtained from conventional radiographic procedures.

Though the spatial resolution of these CR systems is still somewhat below the 10 lp/mm resolution of a 400-speed, film-screen imaging system, the vastly improved contrast resolution (detectability of low subject-contrast anatomy) and post-processing abilities make CR a highly desirable option for nearly all diagnostic radiographic procedures.

One other important advantage of a CR system is its ability to provide images having an acceptable image quality throughout a greater range of exposures (exposure latitude). For example, in most analog techniques the exposure factor that will provide an acceptable range of optical densities is about plus or minus 40 percent of the optimal technical settings. Because of this relatively narrow range, a radiographer must be highly skilled at choosing the desired factors and/or selecting the proper imaging parameters of the automatic exposure device to produce images with the proper optical density and contrast. The exposure latitude in most CR systems is such that overexposures as high as +120 percent and underexposures as low as -60 percent can be corrected at the workstation. Because of this increased latitude, CR techniques can be expected to considerably reduce the repeat rate due to over- and underexposure.

Though digital imaging systems can provide a wide range of acceptable exposures, *manipulation of large under- and overexposures will not provide optimum image quality.* During a CR exposure, the operator is provided with an indication of how much enhancement is required to correct for over- and underexposure to produce an image with the desired quality. In practice, this process, which is often referred to as *normalization,* should be kept at a minimum to insure the highest image quality and reasonable patient dose. The amount of normalization can be estimated through the relative exposure paradigm (Agfa), the exposure index (Kodak), or the sensitivity number (Fuji) controls of a computed radiographic system.

AEC and Digital Image Acquisition

Since the production of images using photostimulable phosphor plates may require different amounts of radiation than with conventional film/screen imaging systems, some modifications to exposure factors may be required. When automatic exposure control devices are used for exposures on a CR cassette, it may be necessary to make adjustments to insure that the optimal the exposure index or sensitivity numbers can be obtained. Though CR systems have the ability to adjust for a wide range of exposure deficiencies, these do not correct for, but merely mask inappropriate exposure settings. For this reason, it is still important for the radiographer to select optimal exposure settings for an anatomic region and not rely on the processing controls to adjust for improper exposure settings. *The high exposure latitude of CR does **not** preclude the need for the radiographer to set techniques that will provide sufficient penetration through the part and sufficient signal in the remnant x-ray beam to the image receptor, just as in conventional radiography.*

IMAGE RETRIEVAL AND STORAGE

The Beginnings of Filmless Radiography

According to Dr. Reuben Mezrich of the Hospital of the University of Pennsylvania, the framework for the design of the first filmless radiology department was developed in the late 1970s. Though the blueprint was in place, it would take more than two decades before the state of the technology reached the point where a completely filmless radiology department was possible. Interestingly, it would not be the American companies who dominated the conventional radiographic field and many of the other digital imaging fields, such as CT, MRI, and sonography. Instead it would be a Japanese company, Fuji, and a German company, Agfa, who would embrace digital radiographic imaging and market the first successful computed radiographic systems and digital information storage systems (PACS).

At the present time, as many as 90 percent of all medical images are read from film-type media. In the coming decades the conversion to soft-copy reading is expected to increase dramatically. Presently, it has been estimated there are fewer than 200 radiology departments nationwide that have completed the changeover to an entirely filmless environment. This number is expected to grow rapidly throughout the next two decades. An interesting paradox is that digital imaging storage systems (PACS) and computed radiographic systems now appear to be succeeding from the bottom up. Unlike other technologies that inevitably appear at larger institutions first, filmless imaging systems are now appearing more frequently in smaller 50-200 bed hospitals than in the larger medical institutions. The reason appears to be due in part to the lower overall costs that smaller institutions need to incur to accomplish this change and the inability of current network systems to provide the extensive connections that are needed in the larger medical centers to make the system practical.

Workstation (Digital Processing Station)

Because digital images are acquired in a soft copy format, a special computer terminal, called a *workstation* or *digital processing unit*, is required for the manipulation of the image. Since this is one of the more expensive components in a digital system, there will only be one or two of these for each imaging modality in a radiology department.

A workstation provides the controls that cannot only access images, but can be used to manipulate the image quality, and the delete to add patient information. The control console of a CT or MRI unit can be classified as a workstation. The workstation will normally have one or two high-resolution (2000 x 2000) CRT monitors and a keyboard input device to enable the numerous pre-processing and post-processing functions that may be permitted. After the desired images have been obtained, the operator will save the selected images to the picture archiving and communication system (PACS) for their storage. Usually, workstations are also connected to a multiformat camera or other device with the capacity to print out hard copies of images.

Display Station

The main difference between a workstation and a display station is in the number of activities that can be performed. The display station is generally limited to the display of stored images. There is no ability to manipulate or change the image qualities, nor to print out hard copies of images. An example of a display station would be a simple CRT at the radiologist's home for teleradiography transmissions. Because these units are rarely used to obtain a primary diagnosis on a patient, display stations are often designed with CRT monitors with a lower resolution than in the workstation. This change can lower the costs of these units to a small fraction of the workstation making the system more accessible to off site centers within the network.

The entire system of image acquisition devices, centralized computers, workstations, and display stations is referred to as the *network*. Each input, output or manipulation station within the network where information can be accessed, whether on a CRT screen or by hard copy output, is referred to as a *node* of the system.

CONCLUSION

In the next few decades digital imaging techniques and PACS storage devices will replace the more familiar hard copy imaging systems and file rooms used today. The ability of a well-designed digital imaging system to allow physicians to view images closer to the point of service (ER, OR) and obtain a diagnosis in a timelier manner are the main reason why this changeover are inevitable. One of the factors that must be considered before attempting to eliminate the film from the imaging process is the degree of acceptance by the physicians to filmless form. At the present time this is the main practical limiting factor of the totally filmless department.

SUMMARY

1. The greatest overall advantage to computerizing the imaging department is improved patient care due to the dramatically improved *accessibility* of all types of images and files. The greatest contribution of computed radiography to the quality of the image is enhanced *detectability* of low subject-contrast structures.

2. The use of the photostimulable phosphor plate has made computed radiography the most popular form of direct digital imaging because it preserves the image qualities and feasibility of a cassette receptor system and an area beam.

3. *Pixel size* in an image is inversely proportional to matrix size and directly proportional to the display field of view. As pixel size becomes smaller, spatial resolution (sharpness) increases.

4. Pixel brightness or gray shade is determined in CR by the *attenuation coefficient* (x-ray beam absorption) of elongated voxels of tissue that extend from the front to the back of the patient.

5. The number of different brightness shades that can be assigned to a pixel is dependent upon the *dynamic range* of the ADC, which in current technology is well beyond the capacity of the human eye. Thus, the gray scale of CR images is now comparable to that of conventional radiographs.

6. Although the *spatial resolution* of the CR image is slightly less than that of conventional radiographs, due to the advantages of *contrast enhancement*, this is no longer considered an important limitation.

7. The *spatial resolution* of the CRT monitor display is determined by number of scan lines (vertical resolution) and the bandpass frequency (horizontal resolution). These must both be much higher for diagnostic imaging than typical television screens can provide.

8. The *contrast resolution* abilities of computed radiography allow demonstration of tissues that have only 1 percent subject contrast between them, whereas conventional radiography requires a minimum 10 percent contrast between tissues in order to demonstrate them.

9. Doubling the mAs is often required to reduce the "grain" or noise of CR images to acceptable levels. CRT monitors must have a signal-to-noise ratio of 1000:1, much higher than conventional televisions.

10. When exposed, a photostimulable phosphor plate traps ionized electrons

at **F** centers in the molecules, composing the latent image. Scanning by red laser light releases these electrons back into their atoms, resulting in the emission of blue-violet light from the plate. This light passes through photomultiplier tubes and is converted into amplified electrical pulses. This electricity is digitized by the ADC into numerical values that can be stored in the computer.

11. The PSP plate can be re-used after the charges are completely "erased" by the CR reader. Plates that have not been used for more than 24 hours must be *erased* by the CR reader prior to use, in order to remove accumulated charges from background radiation.

12. *PSP plates* must be loaded into the cassettes with the "emulsion"-side up, so it will face the x-ray beam.

13. At the workstation, through windowing, frequency processing, and dynamic range controls, CR images may be manipulated to smooth or enhance edges, adjust window width for higher contrast or longer gray scale, or adjust window level to increase or reduce brightness.

14. Even though overexposures of as much as 120 percent and underexposures of as much as 60 percent can be corrected for brightness by *normalization* procedures, these do *not* result in high image quality.

15. Just as with conventional radiography, sufficient penetration and adequate signal-to-noise ratios must be achieved for computed and digital radiography, and the radiographer must still have a comprehensive understanding of *radiographic exposure principles*.

16. *Workstations* allow manipulation of the image as well as printing to hard copy, while *display* stations are usually limited only to displaying the image.

REVIEW QUESTIONS

1. To magnify a portion of the digital image, the display field of view must be (reduced or expanded)?

2. Name at least 6 imaging fields that acquire or process images in a digital form:

3. Contrast resolution is defined as the ability to detect tissues having _____.

4. Which device is required for the display of a digital image?

5. The modification of an analog image into a digital form which can be understood by the computer is accomplished by a device called a _____?

6. The term applied to modification of the image characteristics by the pre-programmed software programs in a digital imaging system is _____ processing.

7. As the display field of view is increased, pixel size _____ (increases or decreases) and spatial resolution _____ (increases or decreases).

8. A pixel or picture element is best defined as:

9. Each frame of the television display of a digital image consists of a discreet number of columns and rows of picture elements called the:

10. To eliminate the majority of the noise in a CR system the video system (TV camera and monitor) will require a minimum signal-to-noise ratio of about:

11. The contrast appearing on the digital image is strongly related to these three

factors:

12. The principal limiting factor for the perception of contrast in an analog imaging system is:

13. After a digital image has been acquired, it is possible to change the image brightness and contrast through the use of which two controls?

14. The principal advantage of an area beam compared to a fan beam is in its ability to:

15. What is the digital equivalent of the optical image density?

16. The release of trapped energy in a meta-stable **F** center of a BaFBr crystal is triggered by the exposure to a laser beam of what color?

17. A photomultiplier tube is incorporated into the acquisition system of a computed radiographic system to amplify and convert _____ into _____.

18. Computed radiography is a digital imaging technique, which involves acquisition of data directly from what type of image receptor?

19. The contrast resolution abilities of computed radiography allow the visualization of tissues with only _____ percent subject contrast between them.

20. The horizontal resolution of a CRT image is determined by the electrical _____.

21. The image on a photostimulable phosphor plate is not permanent and will fade at a rate of about _____ percent in 8 hours.

22. The images in a computed radiographic system can be recorded of displayed in which ways?

23. The term which refers to the process by which trapped electrons are released back into their atoms resulting in the emission of blue-violet is:

24. During the reading or acquisition cycle, the direction in which the photostimulable phosphor plate moves during the scanning phase is called the:

25. The "reading" of the latent image on a photostimulable phosphor imaging plate is normally accomplished by a _____ beam.

26. Why is normalization of grossly over-exposed or underexposed images not recommended?

27. What is the difference between a workstation and a display station?

28. The axis of the movement of the laser across the image plate during the acquisition process is known as the _____ (fast or slow) scan direction.

29. What windowing adjustment would be made to obtain an image on the CRT which is *darker*?

30. On a CR image, a combination of increased window width and lower window level would be used to demonstrate what type of tissues?

Part VI

PROCESSING THE RADIOGRAPH

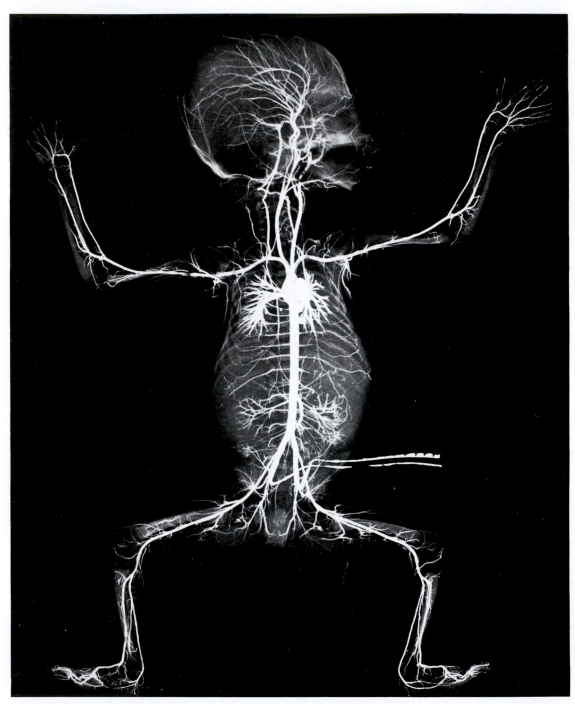

Figure 36-10. Arteriogram of a 5-month-old expired fetus. Injection was made with barium sulfate.

Chapter 37

PROCESSING STEPS AND CHEMISTRY

EVEN THOUGH the efficiency of the x-ray apparatus may be high and the best exposure practice employed, the radiograph will bc of inferior quality if the processing of the exposed x-ray film is carelessly or slovenly executed. The greatest error in the production of a radiograph often may be a flagrant disregard of the simplest of processing rules. Hence, one of the important operations is the processing procedure that brings about the physical and chemical changes to render visible the latent image created by the x-rays. This procedure requires the assistance of photographic chemistry.

STEPS IN PROCESSING PROCEDURE

Processing x-ray film to a radiograph involves at least six procedures:

1. Storing and Handling X-ray Film

The proper storage and handling of x-ray film is an important aspect of radiography. Since film is a delicate material, the manner in which it is stored and handled determines whether the radiograph will be free of artifacts.

2. Mixing and Replenishing Solutions

The manner in which the various chemical solutions used in processing are mixed and replenished (replaced) is important, since good quality radiographs are only produced when these solutions operate efficiently. Recommended methods for mixing and rates of replenishment should be carefully followed.

3. Development Process

Development of the x-ray film changes the silver bromide crystals containing the latent image to black metallic silver that constitutes the visible image. The solution used to effect this change is called a developer.

4. Fixing Process

The fixing process involves two activities and is the procedure for removing the unexposed and undeveloped silver bromide from the emulsion and for hardening the soft gelatin emulsion containing the metallic silver image. The chemical solution employed for these purposes is known as the fixing solution.

5. Washing Process

Washing is the process whereby the soluble fixing bath and silver salts are removed from the film emulsion by means of clean, flowing water.

6. Drying Process

Drying is the treatment of drying the wet radiographs for permanency and for use by the radiologist.

All of these processes must be completed in some fashion, whether using auto-matic processors or manual processing technique, to fully develop a radiographic image which may be preserved in a rela-tively permanent manner. Processing cen-ters around the chemical interactions of the developing and fixing processes. Before discussing the specific procedures for auto-matic and manual processing, a basic understanding of the chemical constituents and functions of the developing and fixing solutions is necessary.

DEVELOPER CONSTITUENTS

Conversion of the silver bromide to metallic silver must be accomplished by the many chemicals contained in the devel-oping solution and it is necessary that the developer formula be standardized with all chemicals in balance so that the results will always be the same. Each film manufactur-er recommends formulae that produce the best results with that manufacturer's film.

An x-ray developer usually contains six types of ingredients (Table 37-1).

1. SOLVENT. Chemical reactions that occur in development require that all chemicals be dissolved in water. Besides acting as a solvent for the chemicals and as a means for their ionization, water aids in softening the gelatin emulsion.

2. REDUCERS. The purpose of a reducing agent is to convert the exposed silver bro-mide crystals to black metallic silver. A reducing agent cannot be a developer unless it reacts more rapidly with *exposed* silver bromide crystals than those that are unexposed. However, the exposure must be of a degree that will cause a satisfactory image to be formed in a given develop-ment period at a given temperature. In a properly exposed radiograph, this action is usually completed upon full development and *before* the unexposed crystals have an opportunity to develop to any perceptible degree. Reducing agents commonly employed are elon, metol, phenidone and hydroquinone.

Elon or *metol* is used only in manual developer solution. Their function is to develop the medium-range gray tones of the image, providing image scale. These gray densities are developed quickly, in the first one-half of the developing time. Manual developer is often called *MQ devel-oper*. The abbreviation refers to the metol (M) and the hydroquinone (Q) which typi-cally make up manual developer. Both metol and elon are unpredictable in their chemical action at temperatures above 75° Fahrenheit (24°C). Since automatic pro-cessing utilizes high temperatures to short-en processing time, a more reliable chemi-cal had to be found for use at these tem-peratures.

Phenidone replaces elon or metol as the functional agent for developing the gray tones and radiographic scale of the image in automatic processing. For this reason, automatic developer solution is often referred to as *PQ developer* (phenidone-hydroquinone). Phenidone is designed for reliable and predictable functioning at the high temperatures (84-98°) used in auto-

Table 37-1
CONSTITUENTS OF AN X-RAY DEVELOPING SOLUTION AND THEIR FUNCTIONS

Chemical	General Function	Specific Function	
Phenidone (automatic), Elon or Metol (manual)	Developing or reducing agents.	Builds up gray densities quickly in first half of development period.	Developing agents reduce exposed silver bromide crystals in emulsion to black metallic silver constituting the image.
Hydroquinone		Builds up contrast slowly during development period.	
Sodium sulfite	Preservative	Prevents rapid oxidation of developers.	
Sodium carbonate	Alkali or activator	Governs reducing activities of developing agents; provides necessary alkaline medium and swells gelatin emulsion so that reducing agents can attack exposed silver bromide crystals.	
Potassium bromide	Restrainer	Controls activity of reducing agents and tends to prevent fog.	
Glutaraldehyde	Hardener	Controls the swelling and softening activity of the alkali, so that the emulsion is not torn off by sticking to automatic rollers.	
Water	Solvent	Provides medium into which the other chemicals may be dissolved in solution.	

matic processors.

Hydroquinone is employed in both automatic PQ and manual MQ developing solutions. Its function is to develop the maximum densities in the image, bringing out the *blacks* of the image. Thus, it is responsible for the full development of the image contrast. Hydroquinone acts upon the silver bromide crystals in the emulsion at a very slow rate, requiring the full development time to complete its function. For this reason, films which are immersed in the developer solution for too short a time demonstrate a loss of contrast and a *washed-out* appearance. The activity of

these chemicals requires their presence in an alkaline* solution. Together, the reducers produce an image with satisfactory contrast in a minimum of time provided the temperature of the solution remains in the optimum range. Reducers are not stable in the presence of oxygen, for they can readily absorb it from the air or the water.

3. ACTIVATOR. The *activator* or alkali *softens* the gelatin of the emulsion and provides the necessary alkaline medium to the solution, so that the developing agents can diffuse into the gelatin emulsion and attack the exposed silver bromide crystals. In general, the more alkaline the developer the more powerful and rapid is its action. The chemicals most frequently used are sodium carbonate and kodalk.

Sodium Carbonate. Sodium carbonate is

*In chemistry, there are two types of solutions–alkaline and acid. Developers are usually alkaline in solution: and fixers, acid in solution.

the alkali usually found in regular x-ray developer. It has been used for many years but there are some disadvantages to be recognized in its use. When a film is processed in a warm x-ray developer containing sodium carbonate and then transferred to a cool acid fixing bath, tiny bubbles of carbon dioxide gas may form in the soft gelatin. As the bubbles escape, they form tiny craters or pits in the emulsion thereby breaking up the normal character of the silver image. The finished film or radiograph then is said to have been blistered. To overcome this occurrence when sodium carbonate developers are employed, the temperatures of developer, rinse, and fixer solutions should be approximately the same.

Kodalk. Kodalk is a highly alkaline chemical activator (sodium metaborate) found in rapid x-ray developer. It has the same function as sodium carbonate. It is more capable of being used when high temperatures are encountered since it does not cause gas formation in the emulsion when the film is immersed in a cooler fixer. It is the most efficient activator available today.

4. PRESERVATIVE. The function of the preservative is to retard the activity of the reducing agents to within controlled limits so that the "life" of the developing solution is maintained over a reasonable period of time. As mentioned previously, the reducing agents react quickly with oxygen and if this reaction is not controlled, the developing solution would not last very long. The chemical, *sodium sulfite*, is used as a preservative since it serves to retard oxidation of the reducing agents and prevents the formation of stain on the film. It has an affinity for oxygen and reacts with the oxygen of the air or solution forming sodium sulfate thereby extending the life of the reducing agents.

5. RESTRAINER. The restrainer is employed to limit the action of the reducing agents to the breaking up of the *exposed* silver bromide crystals only, without attacking the unexposed crystals in the emulsion during the normal course of development. This function is quite important if a satisfactory image is to be produced, for if the restrainer is omitted the unexposed crystals would also develop, and a veil of "fog" (silver deposit) would be deposited over the image. *Potassium bromide* is, therefore, added to the developing solution as a restrainer.

However, the restrainer need only be added when mixing the *initial* batch of developer solution from which the deep tanks in the processor or manual tank will be filled. The restrainer is not included in the replenishment solution. The active restraining ingredient is the bromine. Each time a film is developed, bromine from the silver bromide in the emulsion is deposited into the developer solution, leaving only silver on the film. Therefore, the active restraining ingredient is automatically replenished as films are developed, and bromine is not needed in replenishment solutions. Because it is only used when mixing the initial batch of developer, the restrainer is often referred to as *starting solution* or *starter*.

6. HARDENER. A hardener must be added to automatic PQ developer solution in order to control the action of the alkali and water, which soften and swell the emulsion so that the developing agents can penetrate into it and act on the crystals. Without the hardener, the emulsion becomes so soft that it will stick to the automatic processor rollers, peeling off and damaging the film. Gluteraldehyde is the chemical commonly used as the hardener for automatic developer solutions. It is not necessary for manual development because the films do not

touch any surfaces during manual processing.

Table 37-1 summarizes the functions of the various chemicals in developer solution.

REDUCTION AND OXIDATION

The "active ingredients" for developer solution are called *reducers* because this word describes the chemical action they have upon the silver atoms in the film emulsion. While these chemicals *reduce* the silver bromide in the film, the film *oxidizes* the developer solution.

A chemical compound is reduced when another chemical *donates electrons* to it. A compound is oxidized when electrons are *removed* from it by another chemical. So, reduction and oxidation are really mirror images of each other, and always occur together.

In the process of chemical development, the reducing agents donate electrons to the silver bromide crystals in the film emulsion. Silver ions (Ag^+) are thus electrically neutralized to form silver atoms, as shown in the following basic chemical equation:

$$Ag+ \quad + electron \quad \rightarrow \quad Ag$$

Silver	Silver
ion	atom

It is said that the silver ions have been *reduced* into black metallic silver. The same interaction may be thought of as the silver ions *removing* electrons from the solution. The developer solution is *oxidized* by the film, and thus becomes chemically weaker as it is used. The oxygen in normal room air also tends to "steal" electrons from the developer solution over a period of time, and processing chemicals must be protected from exposure to air as much as possible in order to preserve their effectiveness. Thus, developer solution becomes oxidized and weakened *both* by room air and by the films passing through it, and it must be chemically replenished to maintain its useful strength.

Since reducing agents in the developer solution contribute electrons to the silver ions in each exposed silver bromide crystal, these silver ions become neutral and are no longer tonically attracted to the bromine atoms in the crystal (see Figure 15-2 in Chapter 15). The chemical bonds between the silver and the bromine are broken by the reducing agents. The bromine atoms are attracted by other chemicals in the developer solution and they migrate out of the film emulsion into the solution.

The silver atoms, remaining in the emulsion, coagulate or "clump" together with the partial silver deposit already formed by radiation exposure at the sensitivity speck site, as described in Chapter 15. Continued build-up of silver at exposure centers produces the final visible or manifest image.

FIXER CONSTITUENTS

The constituents of a fixing solution and their functions in the fixation process are as follows (Table 37-2).

1. SOLVENT. The solvent employed in mixing the chemicals of a fixing solution is *water*.

Table 37-2
CONSTITUENTS OF AN X-RAY FIXING BATH AND THEIR FUNCTIONS

Chemical	General Function	Specific Function
Ammonium thiosulfate (hypo)	Clearing agent	Dissolves unexposed silver bromide crystals. Does not affect reduced metallic silver of image.
Sodium sulfite	Preservative	Maintains equilibrium of chemicals in solution.
Aluminum chloride or potassium alum	Hardening agent	Shrinks and hardens emulsion.
Acetic acid	Acidifier	Provides acid medium and neutralizes developer carried over in film.
Water	Solvent	Provides medium into which the other chemicals may be dissolved in solution.

2. ACIDIFIER. *Acid* serves a double purpose for it permits the use of potassium alum as a hardening agent and neutralizes any alkaline developer that may be carried over from the developing solution.

This latter action quickly stops development and prevents the formation of stain. The acid usually employed is *acetic acid.*

3. CLEARING AGENT. The function of the *clearing agent* is to change the residual unexposed and undeveloped silver bromide crystals in the emulsion to soluble silver salts that are readily removed by washing the film in water. This is accomplished without damage to the silver image. If the film is not properly cleared, the remaining silver bromide crystals will darken on exposure to light and obscure the radiographic image. The usual chemical employed for this purpose is *ammonium thiosulfate* or sodium thiosulfate–commonly known as "hypo." The clearing action involves a chemical reaction between the sodium or ammonium thiosulfate and silver bromide in the emulsion wherein silver thiosulfate is formed and remains in solution.

4. HARDENING AGENT. The *hardening agent* is used to decrease the possibility of physical injury to the gelatin emulsion. A swollen emulsion is easily scratched or distorted by physical means during the washing and drying processes. The hardener restrains swelling of the gelatin and hardens it so that it can withstand the normal

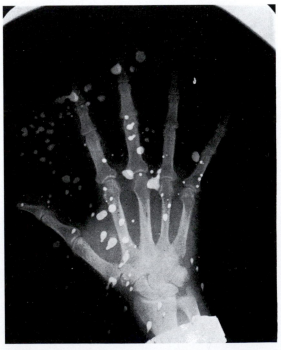

Figure 37-1. Radiograph exhibiting areas of translucence caused by fixer splash on film prior to development. The fixer dissolved out the silver emulsion.

effects of processing. The hardener also helps reshrink the emulsion to its original thickness. The hardened emulsion is protected from injury after development is completed, as a small portion of the hardener is retained by the emulsion. The two most common chemicals used as hardeners in the fixing solution are aluminum chloride and potassium alum. Chrome alum or aluminum sulfide may also be used.

5. PRESERVATIVE. The *preservative* prevents decomposition of the clearing agent by the acid with a resultant precipitation of sulfur at normal temperatures. It assists in clearing the film and prevents the residual developer carrier over in the film from oxidizing and discoloring the fixing bath. The chemical used is *sodium sulfite.*

The constituents of fixer are the same for both automatic and manual solutions. They are summarized in Table 37-2.

Developer solution is a relatively strong alkaline chemical, while fixer solution is a fairly weak acid, which accounts for their strong odors. Alkalis and acids are chemical opposites. When mixed together, they neutralize each other's chemical activity. When handling them, care must be taken not to splash fixer solution into developer tanks or containers and vice versa. Figure 37-1 demonstrates how splashing fixer solution (or any other chemical, including water) onto a film prior to processing can have a deleterious effect.

SUMMARY

1. The *development* process is designed to reduce exposed areas on the radiograph to black metallic silver, clear off of the film the unexposed silver bromide crystals, and harden and fix the permanent image for preservation.

2. *Developer* solution consists of solvent, reducers, an activator, a preservative, restrainer if it is a fresh batch, and a hardener if it is automatic solution.

3. *Fixer* solution consists of solvent, a clearing agent, an acidifier, a hardener and a preservative.

4. *PQ developer* is used in automatic processing. Its reducers are phenidone and hydroquinone, and it includes a hardening agent, gluteraldehyde, to prevent film from sticking to rollers. *MQ developer*, usually containing metol and hydroquinone as reducers, is used for manual processing.

5. Chemical *reduction* occurs when a compound gains electrons from some other compound. *Oxidation* is the loss of electrons. Developer solution is oxidized as it reduces the film emulsion.

REVIEW QUESTIONS

1. What is the function gluteraldehyde and why is it used in automatic developer solution?
2. When is "PQ" developer used?
3. Why isn't potassium bromide included in *replenisher* solution for the developer?
4. What are the two purposes of the "fix-

ing" process?
5. What is the solvent for *both* developer and fixer solution?
6. Which solution, developer or fixer, is a relatively weak acid?
7. Which densities become visible in the first few seconds of development, the

grays (gray scale) or the blacks (D-max) (maximum densities)?

8. Define "clearing" *and* state which chemical performs this function.

9. As developer solution reduces the film, what does the film do to the solution?

10. When a compound *gains* electrons from some other chemical, it undergoes _____.

Chapter 38

DEVELOPMENT VARIABLES

THE PURPOSE of development is to convert chemically the invisible latent image to the visible silver image by means of a developer solution. In the conversion of the exposed silver bromide crystals to metallic silver, the film is immersed in an alkaline developer solution that softens and swells the gelatin so that ionization of the exposed silver bromide crystals occurs and the reducing agents transform the silver ions into clumps of black metallic silver. The unexposed silver bromide is unaffected by this treatment during the development period required by the exposed crystals.

INFLUENCE OF DEVELOPMENT TIME

The time of development given to an exposed x-ray film materially affects the amount of silver deposited on the radiograph. As the time of development increases up to a certain point, the amount of silver deposit increases; as the time decreases, the quantity decreases. In general, the time required to develop a film in a given developer depends upon the emulsion and its thickness. The influence of the *time* of development on the latent image at a given temperature is illustrated in Figure 38-1. A series of ten (10) correctly exposed hand radiographs was made employing identical x-ray exposure factors. Films were developed manually at one-minute intervals at a constant temperature of 68°F in *regular* x-ray developer, Figure 38-1.

1. Radiograph 1, developed for 1 minute, shows only slight traces of silver deposit. Image detail is lacking and the contrast is low. Note the streaked background density which is characteristic of the underdeveloped radiograph.

2. No. 2, developed for 2 minutes, shows some of the important features of the image and a greater overall deposit of silver may be noted. Image detail and contrast are somewhat improved.

3. No. 3, developed for 3 minutes, shows more silver deposited but the image is still somewhat weak.

4. No. 4, developed for 4 minutes, shows a fairly well defined image.

5. No. 5, developed for 5 minutes, shows all essential details, for the maximum practical amount of silver has been deposited on the film. The x-ray exposure was such as to provide a satisfactory image when developed for 5 minutes. The amount of silver deposit with longer development times, however, is not sufficient to justify extension of the development time beyond the basic 5-minute period.

6. Nos. 6-10, developed for 6 to 10 minutes, show little gain in density.

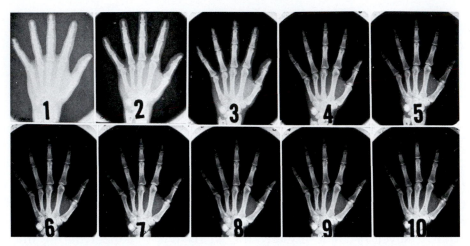

Figure 38-1. Radiographs manually processed in regular developer solution for 1 to 10 minutes at 68 degrees F. The number of minutes of development time is marked on each film.

INFLUENCE OF DEVELOPER SOLUTION TEMPERATURE

Chemical reactions are stimulated or retarded with temperature. Since processing is essentially a series of chemical reactions, the temperature of the solutions assumes major importance. Variations in temperature require adjustment in the development time factor so that uniform densities may be maintained. Temperatures should never be estimated and a good thermometer is essential to determine the correct solution temperature.

The influence of developer *temperature* on the density of the radiograph is demonstrated in a series of radiographs of the hand (Fig. 38-2), top, when times of exposure and development are held constant.

1. Radiograph A was developed for 5 minutes at 60° F. Note the weak image and the lack of silver deposit (density), as well as the low contrast within the image.

2. Radiograph B was correctly developed for 5 minutes at 68° F. Note the satisfactory gradation of densities and contrast of the image.

3. Radiograph C was developed for 5 minutes at 75° F. Note the higher density.

4. Radiograph D was developed for 5 minutes at 80° F. Note the excessive density of the image. The presence of excessive density and fog tends to produce unsatisfactory radiographic quality.

In Figure 38-2, bottom, radiographs D-F demonstrate that temperature differences require adjustment of the development time to secure comparable densities. These radiographs exhibit approximately the same overall density.

1. Radiograph A was developed at 60° F for 8½ minutes. Note that density is almost comparable to that of radiograph B.

2. Radiograph B was developed for 5 minutes at 68° F and exhibits normal density and contrast.

3. Radiograph C was developed for 3½ minutes at 75° F and is comparable to B.

4. Radiograph D was developed for 2 minutes at 80° F. Note that the image is fairly comparable to B, yet a slightly higher density is present because of the greater activity of the developer at this tempera-

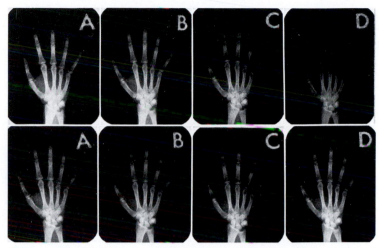

Figure 38-2. (*Top*) Radiographs developed for the same period of time, but with increasing solution temperatures from left to right, showing: (A) 60 degrees, (B) 68 degrees, (C) 75 degrees, and (D) 80 degrees. Note increased density due to higher temperatures. (*Bottom*) Radiographs developed at the same temperatures as above, increasing left to right, but with corresponding reductions in development time to compensate: (A) 8.5 minutes, (B) 5 minutes, (C) 3.5 minutes and (D) 2 minutes. Note balancing of densities.

ture and, as the solution ages, chemical fog would accrue to increase the density.

TIME COMPENSATION FOR TEMPERATURE CHANGES

Although manual solutions should be maintained at the optimum of 68°F, for the best quality, there are occasions when it is necessary to process films at other temperatures. Some compensation can be made for temperature variations *within limits* by increasing or decreasing the time of development. For higher temperatures, shorter developing times are necessary to maintain uniform radiographic density. The ideal method is to employ the time-temperature system that accurately compensates for temperature differences with the correct time of development. It is true that x-ray film may be manually developed satisfactorily without special treatment at any tem-

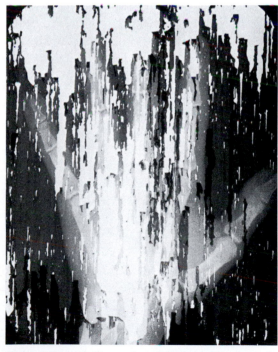

Figure 38-3. Radiograph exhibiting melted emulsion from excessively high temperature processing.

perature between 60° and 75° as long as the temperature differences are compensated by appropriate development times. The lower temperatures in this optimum range require longer development times and the higher temperatures, although permitting shorter development times, are closer to the zone where processing defects may begin to appear on the radiograph. Generally, a change of 2° will change the resulting density by 15 percent.

Figure 38-3 demonstrates how extreme solution temperatures can melt film emulsion.

INFLUENCE OF DEVELOPER SOLUTION CONCENTRATION

If developer solution is initially mixed to be too weak from excessive dilution with water or from inadequate amounts of active ingredients, the darker black areas of the radiograph will fail to be fully developed in the standard time. Therefore, not only will insufficient density develop in the image but also image contrast will be low because of the lack of dark black shades. The same effect occurs when solution is weakened due to contamination from fixer solution or other chemicals, or due to exhaustion from air oxidation or unreplenished usage. Only the lighter-gray shades are developed, and the finished radiograph has a washed-out, noncontrasty appearance.

At the ideal concentration level, attained by carefully following the manufacturer's directions in mixing the solution components, optimum contrast levels and medium overall density will be achieved.

The solution may become too concentrated from high levels of evaporation of the water when excessive ambient temperatures are present or when it is allowed to sit uncovered for extended periods of time. Hyperconcentration can also occur from improper mixing. A developer solution which is too strong will attack the *unexposed* silver bromide crystals in the film emulsion as well as the exposed crystals, so that areas that should have demonstrated a white or clear shade will develop to a gray shade, and information will be lost from the ensuing lack of contrast.

When the film is overdeveloped because of hyperconcentrated solution, the resultant loss of image contrast is referred to as *chemical fog*. It will be recalled that a fogged film can either appear too light or too dark. Either the failure to develop the very dark areas of the radiograph or the very light areas of the radiograph results in a loss of recorded information. For this reason, optimum concentration levels must be carefully monitored in the darkroom.

FIXING PROCESS

The development process reduces only a portion of the silver bromide emulsion to metallic silver. The remaining unused silver bromide must be removed, for it would impair the diagnostic and photographic character of the silver image. Subsequent chemical treatment known as the fixing process serves to *clear* the film of this unwanted silver bromide without damage to the image and, to *harden* the gelatin emulsion.

When the film is placed in the fixing

solution it is milky in appearance because of the residual unexposed and undeveloped silver bromide crystals but, as it is moderately agitated until both film surfaces are completely bathed by the solution, this milkiness gradually disappears. The action of the acidifier immediately neutralizes the residual alkaline developer and any continuing development action ceases. Since the gelatin is still swollen and porous, the clearing agent dissolves out the unexposed and undeveloped silver bromide crystals, leaving untouched the developed silver image. This is the *clearing action.* As clearing abates, the *hardening action* begins, resulting in shrinking and hardening of the gelatin emulsion containing the silver image. This hardening action is most important, since it prevents swelling of the emulsion to any marked degree in the later washing operation. It is advisable not to turn on the white light in the processing room until the film is entirely clear; otherwise it will become fogged.

INFLUENCE OF FIXER SOLUTION TEMPERATURE

As with most chemical reactions, the higher the temperature the greater the speed of fixation; the lower the temperature, the slower the speed of fixation. In fixer solutions, however, there is an optimum range of temperatures that should be used. With higher temperatures, a fixing solution tends to sulfurize thereby shortening its life. It must, therefore, be specially treated when high temperatures prevail.

INFLUENCE OF FIXATION TIME

The duration of fixation is dependent upon several factors, such as the strength and nature of the fixer employed, the temperature of the solution, the amount of film agitation, the volume of fixing solution as related to the number or surface area of the films being fixed, and the emulsion thickness. The total *fixing time* is made up of the duration of time needed to *clear* the film and that required to harden the film. For manual processing, the film should remain in the fixing bath at least for *twice* the time necessary to clear the film.

INFLUENCE OF FIXER CONCENTRATION

Alterations in the chemical concentration of the fixer solution have essentially the same effects upon the film as the corresponding changes in fixer solution temperature or fixation time. The fixation process is not a controlling factor over the essential image qualities of density, contrast, and geometrical integrity. The clearing portion of the cycle is necessary for the removal of the image *noise* which would result from failure to strip the unexposed areas of the emulsion from the film, leaving various possible artifacts. The fixing portion of the cycle is exclusively designed to ensure adequate protection and preservation of the permanent image.

Insufficient fixer concentration can result from improper solution mixing, either inadequate amounts of water or too much active ingredients. Exhaustion of the solution can occur from air oxidation when the solution is left uncovered for extended periods of time or from unreplenished usage. Insufficient fixation can leave the film emulsion sticky or wet and thus result in emulsion damage when handled. It can also result in some of the developer solution being left in the emulsion, which may demonstrate a *milky* appearance or turn the emulsion brown or yellow.

Too much fixer concentration, resulting from improper mixing or from evaporation of the water in the solution, can make the film too brittle. The emulsion would then begin to crack and deteriorate with handling and storage.

Optimum fixer concentration must be monitored to ensure a long lifetime for the permanent image. Otherwise, film damage can result which can have serious medical and legal implications.

TYPES OF IMAGE QUALITIES AFFECTED

1. Increasing development *time* increases image density. It also increases image contrast to a certain point, beyond which excessive development time will turn the entire film black, destroying contrast.
2. Increasing developer solution *temperature* increases image density. It also increases image contrast to a certain optimum level, beyond which excessive temperatures chemically fog the film, destroying contrast.
3. A 10° temperature change can be *compensated* for by adjusting development time by a factor of 2. A 2° temperature change can be compensated with a 15 percent adjustment in development time.
4. Increasing chemical *concentration* of the developer solution increases image density. It also increases image contrast to a certain optimum level, beyond which excessive concentration chemically fogs the film, destroying contrast.
5. Insufficient *fixation* time, temperature or chemical concentration can result in emulsion damage and discoloration. Excessive fixation time, temperature or chemical concentration makes the film too brittle. In either case, the archival life of the radiograph is lost and artifacts may result.
6. Film processing has no relation to geometrical or recognizability functions in the image.

REVIEW QUESTIONS

1. How will excessive development time, temperature or concentration (replenishment) affect image *contrast*?
2. The standard development time and temperature for a particular facility is 60 seconds at 68°F. If the solution temperature should climb to 74°F, how long should you develop?
3. Overfixation (or inadequate washing) will cause what problem in preserving the radiograph?
4. At solution temperatures below 60°F, which reducer fails to function properly?

Chapter 39

AUTOMATIC PROCESSORS

THE FIRST FULLY AUTOMATIC processing systems were announced in 1957. An electromechanical transport system used a series of rollers to immerse the film into and through the development tank so that the time of development became a standard factor based upon the speed at which the rollers turned. The same system then transported the film from one tank to the next and finally through a blow-dryer compartment. An electrical thermostat and heating system allowed for a self-correcting high temperature to be maintained in the solutions so that development time could be dramatically reduced. Because of the high temperatures, the chemical *phenidone* replaced metol or elon as the reducing agent designed to develop the gray scale in the image. Metol and elon become unpredictable at high temperatures. Hydroquinone was still used to develop the maximum densities in the image, so that the automatic developer solution came to be known as *PQ* (phenidone-hydroquinone) developer. The most serious problem to overcome was that the softened emulsion making contact with the rollers would stick to them and be pulled off of the film. This was resolved by adding a precise amount of the hardener *gluteraldehyde* to the automatic developer solution. The gluteraldehyde counterbalances the effect of the activator, so that the emulsion is allowed to swell and soften enough for adequate penetration of the developer chemicals into the emulsion, yet not so much as to stick to the rollers.

With time and temperature both stabilized, replenishment of the solution concentration became the primary variable in controlling image quality. Electromechanical replenishment pumps were connected to reserve solution tanks, allowing a precise rate of replenishment to be established as films were detected passing through the feed rollers. This replenishment rate could be increased or decreased to control image quality.

The resulting advantages of automatic processing were dramatic in magnitude: First, processing time was greatly reduced. While older processors required seven minutes for the entire cycle from development to drying to be completed, modern processors produce dry films in 1-4 minutes, depending on the type. Second, because the processor monitors its own internal environment, maintaining temperature, circulation, concentration and time, the quality control of radiographic images was vastly improved. In short, more consistent results are obtained in much less time.

Although some portions of an automatic processor should not be tampered with by radiographers who have no training in electronics, radiographers should understand enough about automatic processors to be able to diagnose problems and make minor corrections and repairs.

There are five interrelated electromechanical systems in the automatic

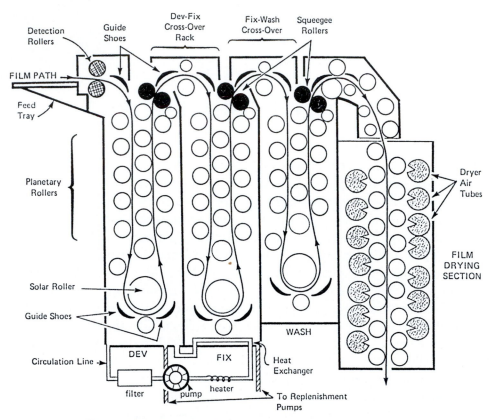

Figure 39-1. Diagram of automatic processor components.

processor which provide all of the functions of manual processing. They include the transport system, the circulation/filtration system, the replenishment system, the tempering system and the drying system.

A diagram of the main components of an automatic processor is provided in Figure 39-1. The path of the film is shown as it enters from the feed tray and is directed by the various rollers and guide shoes of the transport system through the development tank, the fixing tank, the wash tank and finally the dryer compartment. Parts of the circulation/filtration and tempering systems can be seen at the bottom of the diagram. Also, note the tubes from the replenishment system coming into the developer and fixer tanks at the bottom. You may wish to refer to this diagram frequently as you read the following sections.

THE TRANSPORT SYSTEM

All of the rollers in the automatic processor are interconnected with drive chains, elastic drive belts or intermeshing gears so that all turn at exactly the same rate. The entire transport system is driven by a master drive shaft consisting of several worm-gears (Fig. 39-2). This drive shaft is turned by a small motor, to which it is connected by a drive chain (Fig. 39-3). The rollers are arranged into four different types of racks.

The *detection rack* or *feed rack* is the first rack of rollers that the film comes into contact with as it is slid in from the feed tray (Fig. 39-1). It typically consists of two ribbed detection rollers and a guide shoe plate which turns the film downward into the development tank. As the film is pulled between the detection rollers, it separates

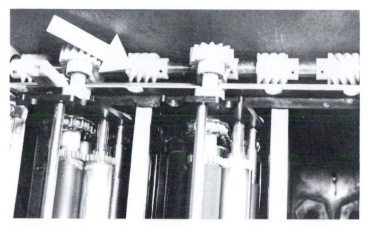

Figure 39-2. Automatic processor main drive shaft pointing out worm gears used to turn all of the racks of rollers to transport the film.

them, pushing one upward. The movable roller is connected to a microswitch on each end, so that when the film separates the rollers, the microswitch is also separated from its counterpart on the wall of the processor (Fig. 39-4). When the microswitch is separated, the replenishment system is activated to pump fresh replenisher solution into both the developer and fixer tanks. As soon as the film passes through the detection rollers, the upper one falls back down from gravity plus the magnetic attraction of the microswitch, and the switch closes to shut off the replenishment system. Hence, the longer the film being fed into the processor, the longer the replenishment system will be activated. In this way, the actual replenishment is kept roughly proportional to the total film area being processed on a daily basis. If the detection rollers were flat, the thin film would not be able to separate them sufficiently to activate the microswitch. By using ribbed rollers, the separation effect of

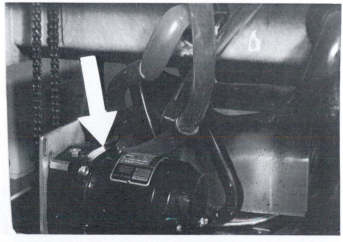

Figure 39-3. Drive motor and chain for automatic processor transport system.

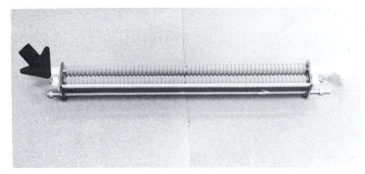

Figure 39-4. Detection rack showing ribbed rollers which separate when film is fed through them to activate replenishment pump microswitch (arrow).

the film is exaggerated so that the microswitch will work (Fig. 39-5).

The *deep racks* (used in the developer, fixer and wash tanks) consist of alternating phenolic (compressed paper and resin) rollers designed to smoothly transport the film through the tank. At the bottom of each rack, the film direction is reversed by the use of a large phenolic roller and guide shoes. The guide shoes are ribbed to prevent wet film from sticking to a flat surface and jamming up in the processor. For each deep rack, the large roller at the bottom is frequently called the *solar* roller and the smaller ones are called *planetary* rollers, comparing them with the sun and its smaller planets.

At the end of each deep rack is a set of *squeegee* rollers set flush against each other and typically consisting of one metallic roller and one rubber roller or two rubber rollers (Figs. 39-1 & 39-6). The squeegee rollers are necessary to prevent excessive amounts of solution from being carried by the film over into the next tank or, in the case of the wash rack, to prevent excess moisture on the film as it enters the drying system. Thus, the squeegee rollers replace the manual function of draining the films before placing them in the next tank.

Crossover racks consist commonly of a pair of phenolic rollers and two guide shoes (Figs. 39-1 & 39-7) and are designed to transport the film from one deep tank into the next, making a 180-degree turn.

Finally, the *dryer rollers,* usually phenolic, are alternated to transport the film through the blow-dryer system with maximum surface exposure to the drying air and deposit it in the external catch bin.

FILM

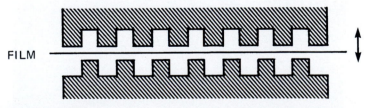

Figure 39-5. Diagram of exaggerated separation of ribbed detection rollers when a film is fed into an automatic processor which is necessary to sufficiently move the replenishment microswitch .

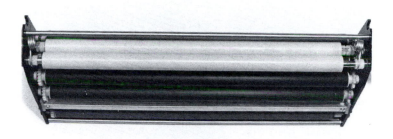

Figure 39-6. Deep solution tank rack showing pair of (lighter colored) squeegee rollers at film exit point.

THE CIRCULATION/ FILTRATION SYSTEM

Both the developer and the fixer solutions must be constantly circulated through the deep tanks to ensure even coverage across the film emulsion and eliminate air bubbles clinging to the film. The circulation system replaces the manual function of agitation. Further, it ensures consistent development of films run through both the right and the left sides of the tanks by constantly stirring the solution. The proper circulation is provided by separate pumping systems attached to the developer and the fixer tanks (Fig. 39-8). A filter may also be added to the circulation lines for the purpose of cleaning out emulsion gelatin particles, dirt, foreign particles and algae (Fig. 39-9). The thermostat and heater of the tempering system may also be found within the circulation lines (Fig. 39-10).

Figure 39-1 illustrates only the circulation line for the developer tank, with filter, pump and heater. After heating, the line passes through the bottom of the fixer tank, serving as a heat exchanger so that the fixer solution temperature is maintained slightly less than the developer solution temperature. The fixer tank has its own circulation

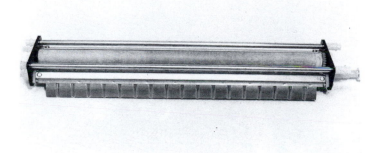

Figure 39-7. Crossover rack with ribbed guide shoes to turn film from one deep tank into the next.

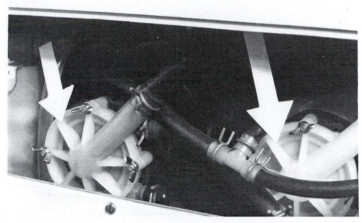

Figure 39-8. Circulation pumps for developer and fixer lines in an automatic processor.

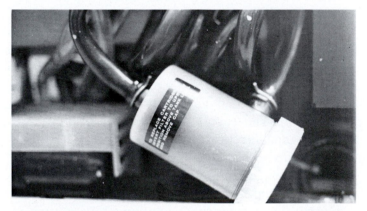

Figure 39-9. Filter placed in developer line to remove debris.

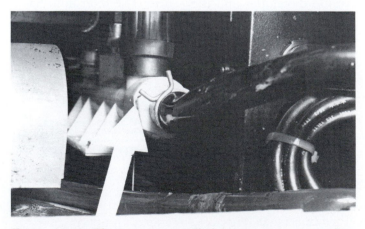

Figure 39-10. Thermostat-controlled heater coil surrounding developer line.

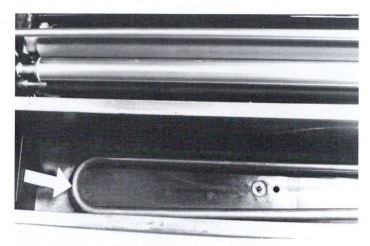

Figure 39-11. Heat exchanger pipe (arrow) carrying heated developer solution through fixer tank.

line, not shown in the diagram, but does not have its own heating element. The circulation system operates continually whenever the processor is turned on.

THE TEMPERING SYSTEM

Most automatic processors utilize a tempering system in which only one chemical solution is physically heated, and then that solution is used to transfer heat to the other tanks. In the most common example, the developer circulation line includes a thermostat and a heating coil surrounding the line. Each time the temperature reaches a minimum allowable, the thermostat activates the heater. Obviously, the temperature does not remain at an exact level but fluctuates up and down within a small range as the heater turns on and off, overcompensating slightly each way. However, this fluctuation is restricted to such a short range that temperature changes are not a significant factor in controlling image quality.

Once a solution is heated, its lines may be passed through the other tanks (Figs. 39-1 & 39-11) so that the heat is transferred out of its pipes to the other solutions. This is

called a *heat exchanger* system. Other variations of this system may initially heat a different specific solution or use a different pipe arrangement, but the principle is the same. It is recommended that the fixer and wash temperatures be maintained slightly less than or equal to the developer but never more than the developer temperature. For this reason, it is best to initially heat the developer and use it in the heat exchanger system.

In addition, thermostatic mixing valves are usually used to control the temperature of incoming water to the wash tank (Fig. 39-12). This water may pass on through and out the drain or it may be recycled and filtered to save costs.

Developer temperature may be set and adjusted by a small screw in the electrical box of the processor, but, as a rule, this should not be tampered with once it has been set at an optimum level. It is better to use replenishment rates to control image quality.

Three- and four-minute processors typically set the developer temperature in a range of 84-86°F, and the faster 90-second processors typically use temperatures of 92-96°F.

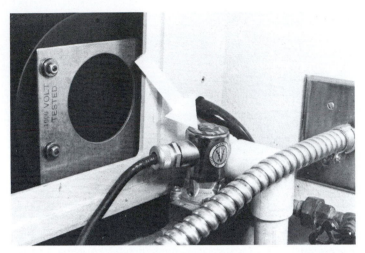

Figure 39-12. Thermostatic mixing valve on incoming water line.

THE REPLENISHMENT SYSTEM

As described in the transport system section, the replenishment microswitches are turned on each time a film passes through the detection rollers from the feed tray (Fig. 39-4). These switches activate the replenishment pumps for both the fixer and the developer (Fig. 39-13). The solution is pumped up from external reserve tanks into the bottom of the appropriate deep tank. Older developer at the top of the tank is sloughed off through an overflow funnel to one side of the deep tank and down a drain tube. The circulation system ensures that the solution within the tank remains well mixed. The reserve replenishment tanks should always have solution in them, because the pumping of air through the replenishment lines not only oxidizes the

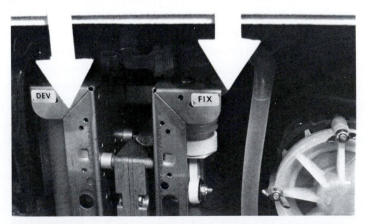

Figure 39-13. Automatic replenishment pumps of diaphragm type which pump developer and fixer solutions from replenishment tanks into deep tanks each time a film passes through the detection rollers.

solutions in the deep tanks but can damage the pumps. Floating lids, which sit directly on the solution surface in the replenishment tanks should be used, in addition to the regular tank lids, to help prevent oxidation of the replenishment solution over time.

The replenishment rate is set by a small screw on the side of the replenishment pump cam (Fig. 39-14) which adjusts the position of the pumping diaphragm relative to the cam. Although the specific replenishment rate must be determined either from the manufacturer or sensitometrically, typical replenishment rates for a 14 x 17-inch film-fed, crosswise range from 50 to 100 cc for developer and from 90 to 150 cc for fixer. Recall that in manual development, the total fixing time is double the developing time when concentration and replenishment are equivalent. Twice as much fixing is required than developing. In automatic processing, the time during which the film is immersed in each solution is equal. For example, in a 90-second processor, it spends about 20 seconds in each deep tank. Since, the time and the temperature are equivalent, the replenishment rate for the fixer must be considerably greater than that for the developer. A high level of fixer concentration allows the solution to both clear and harden the film sufficiently in only 20 seconds. The higher replenishment rates of the fixer require that fresh fixer replenishment solution be added to the reserve tank almost twice as often as the developer.

The specific replenishment rates set are based upon an average width of film passing through the detection rollers, which would be about 11 inches. The only dimension the detection rollers can *measure* is the length of the film being fed. While this procedure is entirely functional for normal work loads in a radiography department,

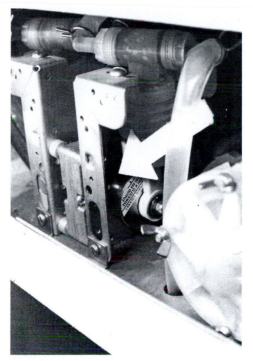

Figure 39-14. Location of replenishment rate adjustment screw on cam of replenishment pump.

specialized departments must consider adjustments in replenishment rates to account for extremes in film size. For example, in an angiography department with its own processor, most films developed are of the 14 x 14-inch size. Furthermore, whole series of angiography films are processed sequentially. Replenishment rates will most likely need to be adjusted upward in comparison with a general diagnostic department.

In the case of the wash tank, one to three gallons of water should pass through the tank per minute to provide adequate replenishment and circulation.

THE DRYER SYSTEM

The drying system is composed of a blower (Fig. 39-15), which takes in external room air and directs it under pressure

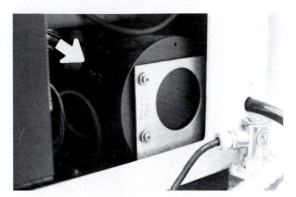

Figure 39-15. Air blower for drying system in automatic processor.

through a compartment full of heating elements (Figs. 39-1 & 39-16) The heated air is then directed down a series of tubes which surround both sides of the film as it passes through the dryer rollers. Each of the dryer tubes has a narrow slit along one side, the side facing the film, through which the heated air is forced (Fig. 39-17), as well as an insert which narrows the effective diameter of the tube in a direction away from the blower. The air pressure decreases with distance away from the blower and would result in uneven drying of the film, with the near side drying long before the far side. By narrowing the inside of the tube away from the blower, the air pressure is maintained equally across the surface of the film.

A thermostat on the side of the processor away from the heating elements adjusts the heating coil to obtain the actual temperature set for the dryer (Fig. 39-18). For a given average work load, the dryer temperature should be set at the minimum necessary to completely dry the films. The most commonly used dryer setting is about 120°F.

An outlet must be provided for the used air as it cools. On the side of the processor away from the heating elements, a duct directs the air out of the processor and preferably out of the building (Fig. 39-19). It should always be remembered that the efficiency of such an exhaust system is lost with every additional bend and turn in the duct, and as direct a route as possible should be provided to the outside.

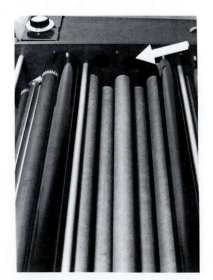

Figure 39-16. Compartment containing heating elements for dryer system showing opening (arrow) for heated air to pass down dryer tubes.

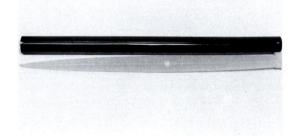

Figure 39-17. Heater tube showing slit through which air is directed toward the film surface, and plastic insert (*bottom*) which gradually narrows air passage toward the far end of the tube in order to maintain equal pressure.

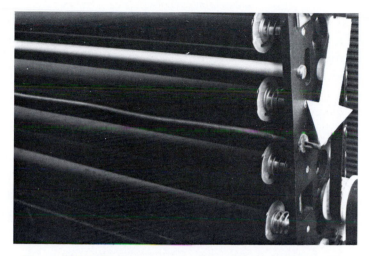

Figure 39-18. Thermostat at far side of dryer rack assembly.

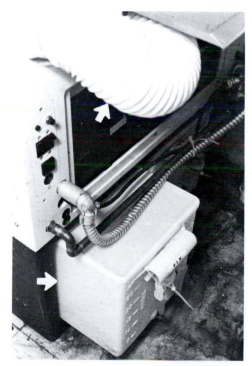

Figure 39-19. Heater exhaust duct. Replenishment tanks are visible below.

PROCESSOR MAINTENANCE

Unlike manual processing facilities, the deep tanks in an automatic processor cannot have separate covers, because of the roller arrangement, and share a common lid in the processor cover. Chemicals evaporating upward may precipitate from the lid back into the other tanks and cross-contaminate each other. For this reason, it is recommended that the lid on an automatic processor be opened slightly during periods of nonuse.

Rollers must be cleaned periodically to prevent the buildup of chemical deposits and dirt which cause artifacts as shown in the next section. During periods of nonuse, wash tanks should be drained to prevent the growth of algae. All gears and moving parts should be cleaned often to ensure smooth function. Care must also be taken not to bend or misalign any of the guide shoes or support bars on the deep racks. Even slight misalignments in rollers and guides can lead to film jamups in the processor.

COMMON AUTOMATIC PROCESSING ARTIFACTS

In addition to the fogging, static discharges, reticulation, crescent marks, stains and other artifacts which may be caused on a radiograph from rough handling or improper manual processing, there are a few artifacts that are peculiar to automatic processing.

Scratches appear as clear or *white* lines because emulsion is removed from the film base. When such scratches are straight and run in a direction *parallel* to the travel of the film through an automatic processor (Fig. 39-20) they are indicative of guide shoes that are out of alignment or not properly seated in the processor. Improperly seated dryer tubes or roller racks may also cause parallel scratching. In all of these cases, a sharp corner of metal or plastic is brought into contact with the film as it passes through the processor, damaging the emulsion.

If a guide shoe (Fig. 39-7) is set at too steep an angle, the tips of all of the ribs impressed in it will tear emulsion off of the film. The resulting artifact is a series of scratches that are parallel to the direction of the film travel and at equal intervals across the film.

Pi lines are dark linear densities running across the film *perpendicular* to the direction of film travel through the processor. They occur at regular intervals (Fig. 39-21). Pi lines are the result of chemical or dirt deposits on processor rollers. Each time a dirty roller turns, the pressure of the deposit against the film sensitizes the emulsion and turns it dark. The distance of the intervals between the pi lines is equal to the circumference of the roller causing them. The circumference of a roller is equal to 3.14 (pi) multiplied by the diameter of the roller. Hence, an aid in locating the roller causing the artifact is to divide the interval distance between the pi lines by 3.14 to derive the size of the roller. To eliminate the artifact, the rollers must be thoroughly cleaned and the deep tank solution levels checked.

Figure 39-22 is an example of *hesitation marks*. Hesitation marks are one of the most common artifacts in automatic processing. They are caused when there is a pause in the smooth transfer of the film through the various rollers of the transport system. There are several possible causes for the film to stop, including misalignment of guide shoes or rollers, the breaking of a roller gear so that a roller fails to rotate, breaking of the drive chain or a drive shaft gear, transport motor failure, or even an accidental switching off of the processor by personnel. In any case, when the film pauses, lines of altered density are created across the film wherever it is in contact

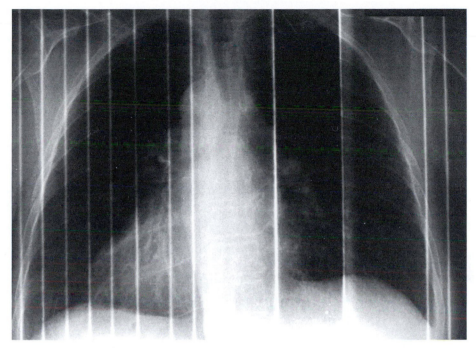

Figure 39-20. Radiograph exhibiting guide shoe scratches from misalignment of guide shoes in an automatic processor. Scratches run parallel to direction of film travel.

with rollers because, while the developer or fixer solution continues to act upon the rest of the film, the solution cannot get to the areas that are in direct contact with a roller. These lines will always lie *crosswise* to the direction of film travel. But, unlike pi-lines, they are usually at *uneven intervals.* Because many different rollers may be in contact with the film at the same time, there are different distances between deep

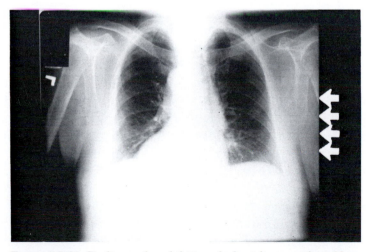

Figure 39-21. Radiograph exhibiting dark pi lines artifact. Note regular intervals of distance between lines indicative of roller size involved. Pi lines run perpendicular to direction of film travel.

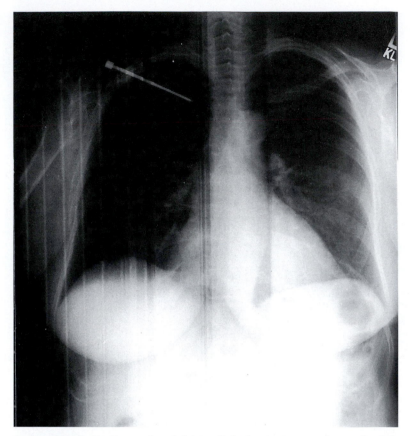

Figure 39-22. Radiograph exhibiting light hesitation marks on the left side from momentary failure of transport system. Lines run perpendicular to direction of film travel, where contact with rollers protect the emulsion from continued development. Note that some lines have a darker line to either side due to lessened pressure of the roller.

rack rollers and crossover rollers, and some of the rollers may be different sizes.

Hesitation lines may be light in color, or, more commonly, they may consist of a triple line–a light line with a dark density line along either side. *Any marks on the film caused by pressure effects, such as hesitation lines, pi lines, or crescent marks (discussed in the next chapter) may be either lighter or darker than the background density of the film. It is the amount of pressure that determines the color of the mark: Slight pressure sensitizes the film emulsion, causing it to turn dark. High pressure compresses and damages the emulsion, leaving a lighter area.* Hesitation marks most com-

monly show a light area in the middle where the pressure of the roller was greatest and where solution was prevented from reaching the film, with a dark line to either side where the pressure of the roller was diminished.

Uneven or streaky sheen on the surface of the film may be caused by uneven drying from dirty or improperly seated dryer tubes or by poor alignment of squeegee rollers, leaving the film excessively waterlogged as it enters the dryer.

Failure to transport may result from overlapping films, broken drive gears, or improperly seated, warped, or dirty roller

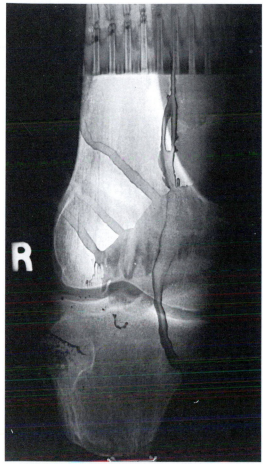

Figure 39-23. Radiograph exhibiting detection roller marks (*top*) and chemical splashes, caused by pulling film back out of an automatic processor after its leading edge had submerged into the developer solution tank.

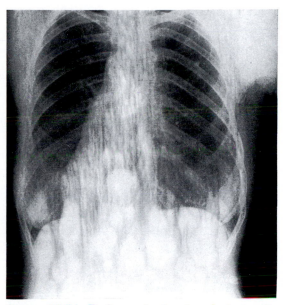

Figure 39-24. Radiograph showing dark streaks caused by dirty developer solution or by spillage of one solution into another while the film was submerged.

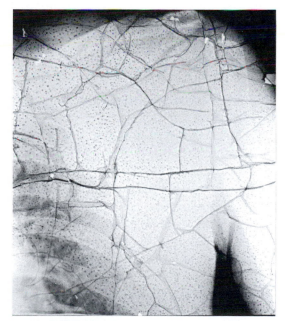

Figure 39-25. Radiograph exhibiting reticulation from excessive changes between processing solutions.

racks, guide shoes or tubes.

To avoid film jam-ups in the processor, always wait until the buzzer sounds indicating that the previously fed film is fully into the system and the film path is clear; And, alternately use the sides of the feed tray to guide the film straight into the rollers. When a film is fed crooked, students are sometimes tempted to pull a film back out of the processor. If the leading edge of the film has reached the developer solution, just a couple of inches past the detection rollers, pulling it back out will result in the artifact illustrated in Figure 39-23, as developer solution is dragged through the detection rollers and splashed onto the feed tray. The feed tray and detection rollers must be cleaned immediately after such an accident.

Figure 39-24 demonstrates the classic appearance of a radiograph that has been processed in dirty developer or fixer solution. Such a film indicates the need for an immediate cleaning of the processor tanks and the addition of fresh solutions. This is also the appearance caused if one solution is somehow spilled into a different solution tank while the film is in the tank. Figure 39-25 shows an example of film *reticulation*, a network of fine cracks in the film emulsion. Reticulation is caused when the temperature is quickly and drastically changed during processing, with the film passing either from a very cold solution into a very warm solution or vice versa. In automatic processing, this would indicate a failure within the tempering system.

SUMMARY

1. *Automatic processors* reduce total processing time to as little as 90 seconds by using high solution temperatures and ensure consistency in processing.
2. The *transport* system controls development time by its speed, while specialized rollers squeegee the film after it passes through each solution and detect inserted films to trigger the replenishment system.
3. The *circulation/filtration* system ensures uniform chemical distribution across the film and clean solution.
4. The *tempering* system uses thermostat control and heat exchangers to maintain proper solution temperature.
5. The *replenishment* system maintains proper solution concentration by adding new solution each time a film is detected. Since time and temperature are relatively fixed in automatic processing, the primary *control* for development is the replenishment rate set on the replenishment pumps.
6. The *dryer* system shrinks and dries the emulsion for permanence.

7. Parallel scratches, pi lines, and uneven sheen are examples of artifacts specific to automatic processors. Once fed, films should not be pulled back out of the processor.
8. Dark streaks are caused by dirty solutions or solutions contaminated during processing. *Reticulation* is a network of cracks caused by sudden changes in solution temperature.
9. *Hesitation marks* are light lines running *crosswise* to the direction of film travel, which usually have a dark line on either side. Anything which causes the film to temporarily stop during development will leave a lighter lines where the rollers were in contact with the film preventing the solutions from reaching it, with darker lines where the roller pressure was less.
10. *Pressure artifacts* of various types appear dark when pressure is slight and sensitizes the emulsion, and appear light when pressure is great enough to damage the emulsion.

REVIEW QUESTIONS

1. Name the two main advantages of automatic processing over manual:

2. What was the primary variable change that made it possible for automatic film processors to develop radiographs so quickly ?

3. What problem would result if gluteraldehyde were not added to automatic developer solution?

4. Why are detection rollers ribbed?

5. What replaces the function of the "rinse bath," "stop bath," or draining the film in an automatic processor?

6. How does an automatic processor compensate chemical replenishment for different sizes of films?

7. What is the purpose of guide shoes?

8. What automatic processor system replaces the function of agitating films in manual solutions?

9. In what temperature range should the developer solution be maintained for most 90-second automatic processors?

10. What are the typical replenishment rate ranges for developer and fixer in an automatic processor (per 14" film)?

11. What undesirable results occur when replenishment tanks are allowed to run out of solution?

12. In manual processing the fixing time is double the developing time. Why can the automatic processor use 20 seconds for *both*?

13. What replenishment effect would it have on automatic solutions if, at average replenishment rates, dozens of small films were processed in sequence with no large films being run?

14. What is usually the ideal air temperature for drying x-ray films in the automatic processor?

15 What can result if rack braces, guide shoes, tubes, or rollers are carelessly bent during cleaning?

16. What causes scratches, at regular intervals, in straight lines parallel to film travel?

17. Which direction do both pi lines and hesitation lines lie in relation to the direction of film travel?

Chapter 40

FILM HANDLING AND DUPLICATION PROCEDURES

X-RAY FILM is a delicate material and it should not be handled carelessly or roughly. It is sensitive to treatment of any kind—and heat, light, x-rays, radium, chemical fumes, pressure, rolling, bending, etc., are capable of adversely affecting the emulsion. Fortunately, it can be handled safely and swiftly in accordance with all the various radiographic needs as long as the radiographer knows what he must do to avoid the production of foreign marks (artifacts) on the film. The increased speed of film in late years has made it a bit more sensitive to handling operations, and greater care must be exercised.

Safety x-ray film is in common use today. It represents no greater hazard in the stock, radiographic, processing or filing rooms than would an equal quantity of paper records. Radiographs made with this film can be stored on open shelves, in manila envelopes. Discarded film boxes may be stood on end and employed for filing radiographs.

PACKING

X-ray film is packed in a hermetically sealed bag and paper wrappings to protect it from light and moisture. Each unit quantity is placed between cardboard and wrapped in black protective plastic. The package is hermetically sealed under conditions that insure approximately 50 percent humidity *inside* the package. The package is then inserted in a cardboard carton.

STORAGE

Unexposed and unprocessed x-ray film should always be kept in a cool, dry place. It should never be stored in basements or near steam pipes or other sources of heat. In extremely warm climates, only small quantities of film should be ordered at one time, so that a rapid turnover takes place.

HEAT

High temperatures exert injurious effects on the emulsion causing loss of contrast and the production of fog (Fig. 40-1). Unexposed x-ray film should not be expected to be usable more than a few weeks after subjection to temperatures of 90° to 100°F, or more than a few days at 110° to 120°F. A relatively brief period of excessive heat in transit or storage may ruin the film regardless of how well it is protected during the major portion of its life. Because x-ray film is packed in hermetically sealed containers does not mean that it no longer requires care or protection. Such packing does protect film from moisture, both from humid air or actual water immersion, and from other contaminants—as long as the package is *unbroken.* However, it does *not* provide protection from high temperatures.

An approximate guide to usability of film under various temperature storage conditions and approximately 60 percent humidity is as follows. If film is to be used in 2 months, it can withstand temperatures up to 75°F. without deterioration. If stored at 60°F, it can be kept 6 months in storage; at 50°F, for 1 year. Ideal storage conditions will prevail at temperatures of 50° to 70°F and 40 to 60 percent relative humidity.

X-RADIATION

Film must be suitably protected from the unwanted action of x-rays or radium by lead-lined walls or chests (see Fig. 40-2). Film bins located in the processing room should be protected by sheet lead.

FUMES

X-ray film must never be stored in drug rooms or other places containing fumes of any kind. Illuminating gas, formalin, ammonia, volatile oils, sewer gas, etc., will fog film in opened packages if it is stored in an atmosphere containing these substances.

PRESSURE

Film should never be subjected to extreme pressure such as wrinkling, bending, or rolling because changes take place in the emulsion which, upon development, appear as artifacts on the finished film. To avoid pressure markings, packages of

Figure 40-1. Radiograph exhibiting fog produced during storage of film in a hot basement.

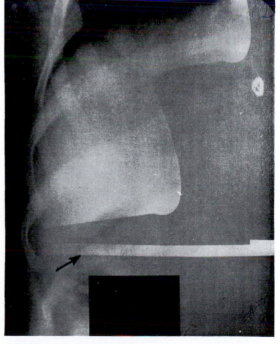

Figure 40-2. Radiograph made with film from a box that had been exposed to x-rays in a laboratory. Note radiographic image of lead foil band that was incorporated in cardboard box.

unexposed x-ray film should always be stored on edge; they should never be stacked one upon another.

EXPIRATION DATE

All film should be used before its expiration date because film aging causes loss in speed and contrast.

REFRIGERATION

Storage of unopened packages of x-ray film in refrigerators is satisfactory provided packages are removed 24 to 36 hours before they are used. This procedure is necessary to avoid the production of condensing moisture on the film when each sheet is removed from the package under high atmospheric temperatures. Open boxes of x-ray film should not be stored in refrigerators wherein conditions of high humidity usually prevail. Once a box of film is opened it should be used as soon as possible. If opened boxes of film must be contained in refrigerators, no other materials should be stored therein and some type of dehydrator should be placed in the refrigerator to reduce the humidity.

THE DARK ROOM

The construction of a "dark room" must take into account the necessity for protecting film stored there from heat, radiation, and fumes. If it is located adjacent to radiation exposure areas, the walls must have an appropriate lead equivalency. The room must be well ventilated and temperature-controlled at less than 70 degrees F (21°C), both to protect the film and to assure a healthy working environment for technicians working there. Humidity must be maintained between 40 and 60 percent to prevent static discharges on film when it is moved across counters, into and out of cassettes and into the processor feed tray.

Of course, the dark room must be made as light-proof as possible. Weatherstripping can be used around the edges of the processor and door, and a rotating door or double door will assure a light-tight entrance. Electrical interlocking systems now available for film bins and are highly recommended when regular entrances are used. These systems either lock the film bin any time the entryway door is not fully closed, or sound a warning buzzer if the door is ajar and the film bin is opened.

In constructing dark rooms, it is a mistake to use colored Formica®, tile, or paint. Loading benches must be white so that films lying on them can be recognized, and all other surfaces should be white so as to reflect the small amount of light coming from the red safelight and maximize general visibility. The loading bench should be removed, preferably opposite, from the processor and any chemical storage.

HANDLING

In handling x-ray film, the radiographer should avoid touching the film surfaces. Film should be held as near the edges as possible with clean dry hands. X-ray film is very sensitive to almost all forms of energy. When it is properly handled, exposed, and

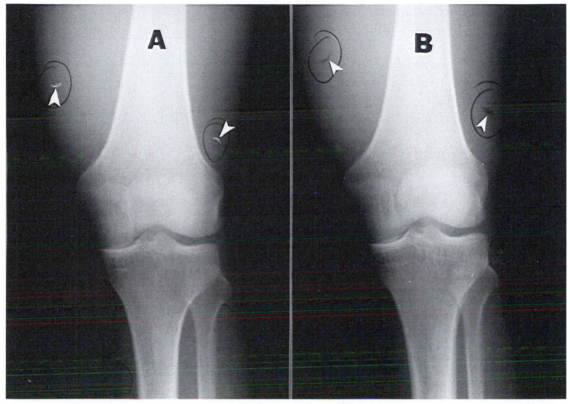

Figure 40-3. Knee radiographs demonstrating crescent (crinkle) marks from rough handling before or after exposure. Marks can be white (A) when pressure is great, or black (B) when less pressure is applied.

processed, a satisfactory image free of artifacts will result.

When films are carelessly handled in loading and unloading cassettes, they may be bent around the tips of the fingers, damaging the emulsion. The resulting artifacts are called *crescent marks* or *crinkle marks* and are semi-circular in shape.

Figure 40-3 demonstrates that crescent marks can either be light or dark. Dark crescent marks are caused when the pressure applied to the film is slight. In this case, the pressure sensitizes the film emulsion, causing the silver bromide crystals to develop a latent image and process as dark images. Light marks are caused when greater pressure is applied to the film, so that the emulsion is actually compressed and damaged, such that crystals are pushed to the side.

It is well to remember that any form of white light creeping into a processing room through cracks around the edges of partitions, windows, doors, or open film bins may fog x-ray film. Be sure that all white light is turned off in the processing room when handling film. When white light is on, film bins should be tightly closed and the tops secure on all film boxes. White light should never be turned on while films are developing because films will be fogged in the tank.

SAFELIGHT ILLUMINATION

X-ray films are sensitive to white light and must be handled either in darkness or under safelight illumination of the proper quality. The processing room should be adequately provided with both white-light and safelight illumination. White-light is necessary to perform many activities such as the mixing of chemicals, cleaning of tanks, caring for intensifying screens, placing films in the dryer, and unloading film hangers. Fixtures for white-light should be properly located to afford general illumination when films are not being developed.

Safelight illumination should be furnished in the working areas by hanging "direct" or "indirect" type lamps. Film exposed with x-ray intensifying screens is approximately 8 times more sensitive to safelight illumination than unexposed film. Because films are subjected to safelight illumination at the loading bench for a longer period than in any other zone, direct-type safelight lamps over this area are liable to raise the amount of postexposure fog to an undesirable degree. For this reason, the loading bench should be illuminated by an indirect safelight lamp. No film should be exposed to the safelight lamp for a period longer than it takes to unload a film and place it in the processor.

Safelight illumination is designed to give enough visibility in the processing room for the radiographer to accomplish all necessary duties in connection with the handling and processing of x-ray film without harmful effect to any unprocessed film that may be exposed. No safelight is safe if the standards of safety are abused. Film left out under a safelight lamp too long will fog (Fig. 40-4). If film cannot be processed at once, it should be stored in a light-tight container. *Exposed* films being more sensitive to safelight illumination should be set to one side away from the direct beam of a safelight lamp or, better still, placed under or behind a protective screen. If the films cannot be covered, the safelight lamp nearest the stacked films should be turned off.

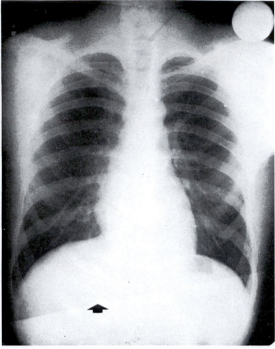

Figure 40-4. Radiograph exhibiting safelight fog because exposed film was laid on loading bench too long and partially covered by a piece of paper (below arrow).

Improper safelight illumination is a common cause of film fog. Excessive examination of films under a safelight during development as well as holding them too close to the safelight causes aerial fog and/or light fog on film. Therefore, certain considerations must be kept in mind in connection with safelight lamps and safelights.

1. The illumination will be safe only if bulbs of the wattage indicated on each lamp are used.

2. All safelight filters are safe only as long as specific conditions prevail. The standard of safety for all safelights is such that unexposed x-ray film may be safely handled in the light at a distance of 3 feet, for 1 minute. These factors apply to the use of safelights with 6B or GBX filters and unexposed film.

Safelight Lamps

Safelight lamps are an indispensable item in every processing room. Safelights, (Fig. 40-5), are lamphouses equipped with filters that provide photographically *safe* illumination in a processing room while handling and developing unprocessed film. The light emitted by a safelight is of such spectral quality and intensity that it does not fog film handled under it for a reasonable handling period and yet the illumination provided by it is as high as possible consistent with safe handling of the film. As far as practicable, the general illumination should be made indirect by suspending from the ceiling one or more safelight lamps of appropriate design and size. If the walls and ceiling are painted with a light-colored paint, the entire room will be well lighted with safe illumination. For light in specific sections of the processing room, there are safelight lamps of various designs. The choice and arrangement of safelight lamps should depend upon the amount of illumination desired and the angle at which it must fall.

Blackout conditions in the permanent processing room are neither necessary from a technical standpoint nor desirable from a psychologic one. A dark-colored wall finish will absorb much of the safelight illumination. If the quality of the light from a safelight lamp is "safe," the illumination reflected from any surface is also "safe" regardless of its color. Nor does the reflected light gain in intensity over the direct or incident light beam. The wall finish, should, therefore, reflect the maximum amount of safelight illumination and the color should be pleasant. In order to appear bright, the wall color must reflect rather than absorb light from the safelight lamp.

To avoid an excessive rate of safelight exposure to the film during darkroom handling, light bulbs of greater than 15 watts should never be used in the safelight. For regular film designed for use with calcium tungstate screens, the Wratten Series 6B safelight filter is recommended. This filter allows only those wave lengths of light in the yellow to red portion of the spectrum to be emitted. Since regular x-ray film is most sensitive to the blue-violet end of the light spectrum, this color of light in the darkroom will take a relatively long time to fog the film and is therefore considered *safe*.

Special consideration is needed for departments using the newer rare-earth technologies. Orthochromatic film must be

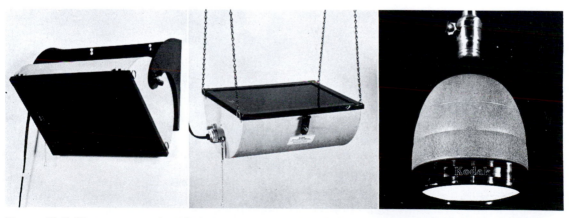

Figure 40-5. Various types of safelight lamps employed in darkrooms, equipped with 6B or GBX filters.

used with rare-earth screens because it is designed for high sensitivity to the green light which these screens emit. Since green light is closer to the red end of the light spectrum than is blue light, orthochromatic films are much more sensitive to the yellow-red light emitted by regular safelight filters and fog much faster. The *GBX* filter has been designed to emit only the darkest red portion of the spectrum and must be used in all darkrooms where orthochromatic film is developed. Maximum reflection under safelight illumination is achieved if the wall finish is either a color within this same spectral range, or a light enough shade of any other color. It is desirable also to have a color that is pleasing under white light as well as safelight illumination. In permanent installations, the ceiling and the upper 18 inches of the side walls should be painted white to provide maximum reflection of white light. For the remainder of the side walls, warm tones such as ivory, cream, or pale shades of any desired color, are generally more pleasing than white, which is apt to be too glaring and shows soil quickly.

Checking Safelight Illumination

A simple method of checking the safety of illumination is to cover part of an unexposed film and expose sections of the remainder for different lengths of time in the place where films will be uncovered in handling. This test film is then given standard development. If no fog shows on the parts that receive a reasonably long exposure, as compared with the covered part, the lighting may be assumed to be safe. If fog does appear, the distance of the safelights from the film should be increased. All safelight lamps should be tested periodically for white light leaks, fading of filter, and excess wattage of bulbs.

STATIC DISCHARGES

Every precaution in the manufacture and packing of x-ray film is employed to avoid the accumulation of static electricity on the film surfaces. Whenever two dissimilar surfaces are pressed together and separated, static electric charges develop. The electric charge becomes appreciable when one or both surfaces are nonconductors and when the atmospheric humidity is low. The quantity of the charge depends partly upon the electrical storage capacity possessed by the total surface of the area involved and the spacing of the charged parts and the insulating strength of the intervening medium.

A static electric discharge emits visible light capable of exposing the film, and the resulting artifacts assume various shapes (Fig. 40-6). They are usually treelike or bushlike in appearance (the point of discharge always has the greatest density) with fingerlike processes emanating outward from the point of discharge. Often static

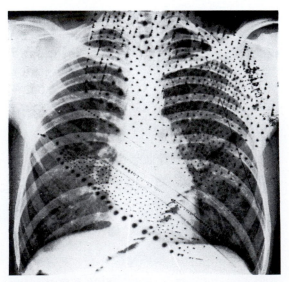

Figure 40-6. Radiograph exhibiting "smudge" type artifacts from static electricity discharges during handling. Static artifacts can also appear as "tree" or "crown" marks with branching points.

marks assume the character of black smudges. Discharges are most likely to occur in cold, dry periods and it is then that particular care must be taken to handle film carefully and avoid friction on its surface. The loading bench in the processing room should be grounded so that in the handling of the cassette any static charges that are built up can be dissipated before the cassette is opened.

Prevention of static sparks can be effected by grounding the location where static charges may develop and by increasing the humidity. To raise the humidity of the air in the x-ray and processing rooms, the use of a commercial humidifier will assist in maintaining a satisfactory humidity level. Remember that the danger point for static production occurs when the humidity is 40 percent or less. As the humidity gets less and less, static electric accumulations grow.

In the emulsion-coating operation during manufacture, static electricity is removed by ingenious and complicated methods so that static charges have no opportunity to accumulate on the film and lead to artifacts on the finished radiograph. The fact that the film is coated and dried in an atmosphere free of dust and at an optimum and constant temperature and humidity, serves to keep the formation and production of static electricity to a minimum.

REMOVAL OF FILM FROM CARTON

When obtaining x-ray film from a new carton, rapid movement should be avoided as a protection against the production of static electricity or pressure artifacts. The box of film is placed on the loading bench, the retaining strip at the edge of the cover is pulled and the cover lifted from the box top. All white light in the processing room is turned off and the safelight illumination provides ample light for opening the film box. When the cover of the box is removed, the edge of the heat sealed bag is exposed. One side of the box near its top is scored so that about one inch of the box can be folded down. This will help to remove the films later. The flap on the bag should be stripped by tearing it and stripping the top away to each side. The film then becomes visible. The two cardboard stiffeners are removed and the film may then be easily removed.

LOADING AND UNLOADING FILM

There are two types of containers in which medical x-ray films can be held during exposure—direct exposure holders and cassettes. The choice depends upon the exposure technic to be employed. In the direct exposure technic, the film is placed in the exposure holder which comprises a light-tight envelope. In the double-intensifying-screen technic, the film is placed between two x-ray intensifying screens that are mounted in a cassette. In loading and unloading x-ray film, all white light must be extinguished in the processing or loading room.

In loading, the film is placed in the open exposure holder; next, the large flap of the envelope is turned down, then the side flaps are brought over, followed by the end flap. It is most important that this procedure for protection of the film be followed if light-fog is to be avoided. The holder is now ready for use.

LOADING THE CASSETTE

When the film is removed from its carton, it should be held vertically at the middle of the top border with the fingertips of the right hand. It is then placed in the cassette on the front intensifying screen. The lid carrying the back screen is gently closed and locked by means of the back springs. When placing the film in the cassette, care should be exercised to avoid scraping or sliding the film over the edges of the cassette or surface of the screen. Be sure that in this operation the hands are dry and chemically free and that they do not come in contact with the x-ray intensifying screens.

FILM IDENTIFICATION

There are two common types of devices used to print patient identification information onto each radiograph. For both devices, a paper card with patient information is inserted into the device, and a flash of light is projected through the card, exposing the film. Regular typed ink will absorb the light and thus appear as white print on the finished radiograph.

The older *film flasher* is still widely used, but is restricted to the dark room. In the dark room after exposure, each film is removed from its cassette, and the corner of the film must be fully inserted forward and sideways into the flasher slot. The top of the flasher is then depressed, closing the device on the film and activating the light source. When a red indicator light at the top of the flasher turns off, the flash expo-

sure is complete and the film can be fed into the processor.

Many newer cassette systems use *identification cameras* which can be used in the light, and are placed into each radiographic procedures room. These systems require special cassettes with a "window" in a corner on the back cover. The window is covered with a sliding panel. Just prior to or after each exposure, the window corner of the cassette is placed into the camera, with the window facing up. A mechanism in the camera slides the window panel to the side, a flash of light prints the information onto the film, and the panel is closed.

When using identification cameras, the radiographer must be sure to slide the cassette fully into the slot of the camera, and hold it there until the entire cycle is completed, indicated by the cessation of noise from the device. If the cassette is pulled from the camera before this sound stops, the window will be open and the identification area on the film will be completely fogged.

Proper, accurate radiograph identification is essential for both legal and medical reasons. If a film is flashed with the wrong information, it can frequently be corrected by placing the correct card into the flasher and reflashing the film three times. If this procedure results in illegible print, or if the identification area is otherwise fogged, a paper sticker with *all* of the correct information should be applied to the film.

DAYLIGHT CASSETTE LOADING SYSTEMS

Mechanized cassette loading and unloading systems have been developed that are designed to preclude the need for a dark room technician or for the radiographer to perform any functions in the dark. These *daylight processing* systems are partic-

ularly useful for small departments frequently staffed by a single radiographer. The radiographer need only feed the cassette into the appropriate slot of the daylight system; he or she may then proceed with positioning or other duties while the system automatically extracts the film from the cassette, processes it, and reloads the cassette. This is done with a series of mechanical levers (to unlatch the cassette), suction cups, and rollers.

The primary advantage to daylight processors is the short time required of the radiographer, only a few seconds to insert the cassette into the machine and to retrieve it after reloading. Modern systems use microprocessor monitors and controls to detect the cassette size and load the right film. Film jam-ups in these systems can sometimes result in wasting several films and can be expensive but are rare enough that the convenience of the system far outweighs the risk of jam-ups.

CASSETTELESS DAYLIGHT SYSTEMS

Some radiographic units are provided with conveyor belt systems that retrieve films from a storage compartment and bring them directly into the bucky mechanism of the table. A pressure plate system then closes the (permanently installed) intensifying screens against the film and the exposure is made. Following exposure, the screens are opened and conveyor belts carry the film through a tunnel directly into an adjoining automatic processor.

These units might properly be called *cassetteless daylight* systems, since they, too, preclude the need for a dark room. There is an enhancement of efficiency for the radiographer similar to that for cassette daylight systems, accompanied by similar disadvantages: The conveyor belts result in static electricity discharges along the sides of each film which sometimes impinge upon the useful image, and costly film jam-ups can occur.

DUPLICATION AND SUBTRACTION PROCEDURES

Special film and duplication devices are necessary for the duplication or subtraction of radiographs. Duplication film usually has a violet coloration to it and has emulsion on only one side. The emulsion side can be recognized in three ways: First, it has a flat, low-gloss appearance and does not reflect light well. The nonemulsion side appears very glossy, and this can be seen under safelight illumination. Second, the emulsion side also *feels* rougher than the glossy non-emulsion side. Third, most duplication film manufacturers cut a notch into one side of the film near a corner. When the film is held with this notch at the top edge and toward the right corner, the emulsion side is facing you.

Duplication devices typically use ultraviolet light exposure, to which the duplication film is sensitive. The original radi-ograph and duplication film are placed on a glass plate over the ultraviolet bulbs and a lid closed over the top of the films (Fig. 40-7). The original radiograph should be placed onto the glass plate first. The duplication film is then placed on top of the radiograph by swinging the bottom edge away from you so that the emulsion side faces downward toward the radiograph and light source. If this is done properly, the notch in the duplication film will then be on the edge closest to you and toward the right corner. The films must be *registered* correctly, that is, all edges must be aligned perfectly. It may be advisable to use tape over the edges so that the films do not slide out of place when closing the lid.

It is important to remember that the exposure process used in duplication is *reversed* as compared to normal radiogra-

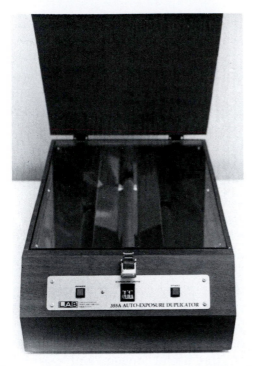

Figure 40-7. Radiographic duplicator showing glass plate over ultraviolet light source on which films are placed.

results in one-half the density.

When the lid is closed and the exposure button depressed, an indicator light comes on to indicate exposure. When the light shuts off, the exposure is terminated and the lid may be opened. The duplication film is then processed as any other radiograph.

The great advantage to duplication is its potential for saving additional patient exposure when overexposed radiographs are produced. An overexposed radiograph may be duplicated with the exposure control set to lighten up the density. The resulting duplicate may be of sufficient diagnostic value to preclude the necessity for repeating exposure of the patient. Duplicators can be of no assistance, however, with underexposed radiographs, since no information is available in the original image to be duplicated.

Subtraction Technique

For subtraction radiographs, special subtraction mask film and subtraction print film is required. The emulsion of the subtraction film is located in the same way as for duplication film.

Subtraction is only useful in contrast media procedures. The objective is to subtract or erase all of the background anatomy so that only the bolus of contrast media is seen. This may be helpful to the radiologist at times when contrasty anatomy is superimposing the bolus of contrast media and the visibility of some details of interest is hampered. It should be realized, nonetheless, that subtraction technique cannot add any information to the radiograph which was not already present, and its usefulness is therefore limited to the occasional improvement of the certainty of an already suspected diagnosis.

A scout film must be taken without any

phy. Duplication film is designed so that longer exposure times result in *less* density (Fig. 40-8). A duplication film that was not exposed will come out of the processor pitch black. Where ultraviolet exposure takes place, emulsion crystals are removed in processing and lighter densities result. The duplicator exposure control is marked off in 0.1 second *exposure units*. Although most duplication requires from 8 to 16 exposure units to obtain a density level equal to the original radiograph, the actual value to be used for a given set of equipment and film must be derived by experimentation. Once this base value is found, however, further changes in exposure time can be trusted to follow an inversely proportional relationship with density. An exposure of 2 units duration will produce a duplicate that is twice as dense as an exposure of 4 units. Doubling the exposure units

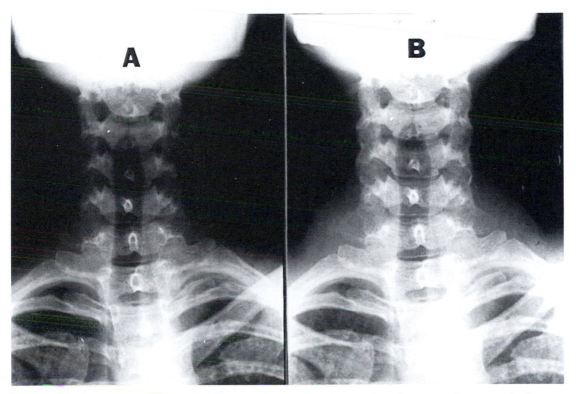

Figure 40-8. Duplicated radiographs of the cervical spine showing the relationship between duplication exposure time and image density: (A) 15 exposure units, (B) 30 exposure units. Note that density *decreases* with longer exposures.

contrast media. The patient must not move position for the remainder of the procedure after the scout film is taken. After the procedure is completed, subtraction images may be produced from any of the contrast radiographs taken by following a two-step procedure: First, a *mask* image is made from the *scout* radiograph using subtraction mask film. The scout film is placed onto the duplicator plate first, followed by the subtraction mask film placed with the emulsion side down and carefully registered. After exposure, the mask film is processed. The resulting image will be a positive, with bones appearing dark instead of light. It has been reversed from the negative image of a normal radiograph (Fig. 40-9).

For the second exposure, three films are used. A regular *contrast* radiograph from the procedure is selected to subtract and

placed on the duplicator plate first. This is followed by the *mask* film with its reversed image, carefully registered so that all background anatomy is reduced to a medium-gray shade and seems to disappear. A subtraction *print* film is then placed emulsion side down over the other two and an exposure is made. On the processed print film, only the bolus of contrast media will show well, with all other anatomy eliminated by the superimposition of positive and negative images (Fig. 40-10).

Solarization

When duplication or subtraction films are grossly overexposed, a phenomenon called *solarization* may occur, whereby the image is reversed from a negative image to a positive image. In the positive image, bones will appear black instead of white, against a gray background (Fig. 15-6 in Chapter 15). To correct the problem, the repeated duplication must be done at reduced exposure levels.

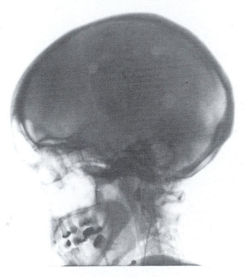

Figure 40-9. Positive image mask film produced from scout radiograph of a lateral cerebral arteriogram.

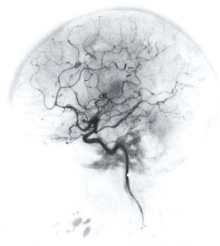

Figure 40-10. Subtraction radiograph of lateral cerebral arteriogram produced when the mask film in Figure 40-9 was superimposed over a regular radiograph with contrast media present, and then the subtraction film was exposed through both in a duplicator.

SILVER RECOVERY

Silver is a very valuable mineral, and radiology departments can recover thousands of dollars in film costs by capturing the silver removed from x-ray films in the fixer solution, rather than allowing the fixer solution to carry this silver down the drain with it. Silver reclaiming attachments can be connected to the fixer drain line for this purpose. There are two basic types of silver reclaiming units: chemical replacement units and electrolytic units.

The chemical replacement unit is a simple canister containing iron in the form of steel wool or other similar metal wools. As the fixer solution passes through the steel wool, the silver atoms are chemically attracted to the iron atoms and they attach to the wool. Later, the heavier silver-iron compounds drop off of the wool and fall to the bottom, forming *sludge*. This silver sludge may then be sold to silver reclaiming companies. Test papers for pH may be used to test solution *leaving* the container for excess silver content, indicating the need to change to a new canister. The efficiency of this method in separating silver out of the fixer solution ranges from 75-90 percent, and the canisters are replaced at a very low cost. The use of two canisters can increase the efficiency to as much as 95 percent.

The electrolytic unit utilizes an electrical cathode in the form of a drum which is negatively charged. This drum is immersed into a positively charged canister and is rotated by a motor to ensure even coating. Silver ions, repelled by the canister and attracted by the cathode, attach to the drum forming a fine coating. When the coating of silver exceeds about one-eighth of an inch in thickness, the drum should be removed and allowed to dry. After drying, the silver may be gently tapped off of the drum with a mallet to obtain a very pure silver powder. Care must be taken not to dent the drum, or to use too high of an electrical charge during reclaiming which burns the silver. Although the electrolytic method involves a considerable initial expense, the efficiency of silver recovery is 95-98 percent and there is no replacement cost once the system is operable.

SUMMARY

1. X-ray *film* should be *stored* at temperatures of 50-70° F, and 40-60 percent humidity, and protected from fumes, radiation, pressure and rough handling.
2. *Safelights* in the darkroom should not exceed 15 watts, should be filtered with a GBX or 6B filter, and should be at least 3 feet away from the loading counter and film bin. Film should be able to be exposed under these conditions for up to one minute without developing substantial fog.
3. Static discharges and other *artifacts* result from rough film handling in the darkroom.
4. When *duplicating* or subtracting radiographs, longer exposure times in the duplicator result in decreased density.
5. For *subtraction* technique, a mask film must be made from a scout radiograph, using subtraction mask film. This mask is then sandwiched between a contrast radiograph and a subtraction print film in the duplicator to produce a subtraction radiograph.
6. Electrolytic or chemical *silver recovery*

systems can save thousands of dollars in reclaiming silver from used fixer solution.

7. The dark room must be light-proof, well ventilated, temperature controlled, and generally white in color.

8. Proper radiograph identification is essential. The two general types of identification devices are film flashers and cassette ID "cameras."

9. Daylight cassette loading systems provide rapid loading and unloading of cassettes and can enhance work efficiency. Cassetteless daylight systems convey the film into the Bucky mechanism and into the processor automatically.

10. Solarization is due to overexposure upon duplicating a radiograph.

REVIEW QUESTIONS

1. State the ideal temperature and humidity ranges for x-ray film storage.

2. Describe the cause of dark crinkle marks or crescent marks.

3. What is the maximum wattage recommended for dark room safelight bulbs?

4. What is the recommended safelight filter for darkrooms storing blue-sensitive film?

5. What is the most common cause of static electricity artifacts on radiographs?

6. In darkroom lighting, how do you recognize which side of a duplication film is emulsion-coated?

7. When duplicating a film, doubling the exposure units will change the resulting density to _____ the original.

8. Define "mask film" in regard to subtraction.

9. What percentage of silver will be reclaimed from spent fixer solution using the chemical replacement method?

10. List the order in which the three films are stacked (from bottom up) for producing a subtraction radiograph.

11. State the two different reasons why dark rooms must be well ventilated.

12. What color should the loading bench be?

13. When a film is flashed with the wrong ID information, can it usually be reflashed to correct the information?

14. List the 5 required components for a daylight cassette loading system.

15. What artifact always appears on films from a cassetteless daylight system?

Chapter 41

SENSITOMETRY AND DARKROOM QUALITY CONTROL

S ENSITOMETRY is the quantitative measurement of the response of x-ray film to exposure and processing conditions. Such quantification of image qualities is important, because it allows us to monitor changes in radiographic variables and diagnose equipment problems long *before* they become bad enough to cause repeated exposures to patients. When exposure and processing conditions are ensured to be consistent, sensitometric monitoring will indicate changes in the characteristics of the film being used or of changes in the receptor system as a whole. When film, screens and exposure conditions are maintained as a constant, sensitometric monitoring will indicate changes in processing conditions. Sensitometric equipment is much more sensitive than the human eye, so that trends in processing conditions may be detected and corrected before they create visible changes in radiographic quality.

Sensitometric measurements are limited to the *visibility* functions of the image: density, contrast and noise in the form of fog. All three of these qualities are reflected in a graph of the density response of a film to exposure. Referred to as a *characteristic* curve, a sensitometric curve, or an *H and D* curve (named after Hurter and Driffield who developed it for photographic analysis), this graph may be produced by exposing a film and plotting the various density levels against the logarithm of the various exposure levels that produced them (Fig. 41-3).

A controlled exposure is required for sensitometry. There are three methods of obtaining such an exposure. The simplest and least expensive method is to use a step-wedge penetrometer and a medium exposure. The steps on the image are each measured on a densitometer and plotted on graph paper. The primary disadvantage to this technique is that the results may be affected by variations in the exposure caused by electrical fluctuations in the x-ray machine. For best results, all such variables must be eliminated except the one under study (usually film characteristics or processing conditions).

The *sensitometer* was developed to eliminate exposure variables in sensitometry (Fig. 41-1). The sensitometer is a light-exposure device which automatically adjusts for changes in electrical current to ensure that each exposure made is uniform. It is set to always deliver the same amount of light to the film. If there is a decrease in electrical current, dimming the light emitted, it will extend the exposure time until the proper amount of light strikes the film. An x-ray film is placed in the sensitometer in the same fashion as a cassette. When the exposure button is depressed, a red light indicates that exposure is taking place. After this light is extinguished, the film is removed and processed. The resulting image is similar to that obtained from a step-wedge, but the measurements taken are much more reliable.

A third method of obtaining sensitome-

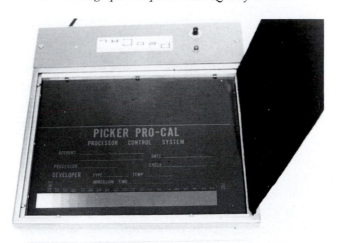

Figure 41-1. Photograph of a sensitometer used to expose films for processor monitoring. Note step-wedge optical attenuator at bottom.

try exposures is to use pre-exposed test strips. These film strips are prepared by the manufacturer to simply be stored in the film bin and run through the processor when needed. This eliminates the need for a sensitometer, but it must be taken into account that if these strips are stored in the film bin for time periods longer than regular boxes of film are stored, they may accumulate excessive levels of fog from aging and safelight exposure and will then not be reliable as an indicator of *current* conditions.

THE H AND D CURVE

The graph obtained from plotting measured densities against the relative exposure levels (corresponding to the step numbers in the step-wedge image, Fig. 41-2) will show a sigmoid-shaped curve (Fig. 41-3). The ascending portions of the curve are referred to as the *toe*, *body*, and *shoulder*, respectively.

It will be noted that the toe and shoulder portions of the curve level out to a nearly horizontal line. The *toe* represents the minimum density producible on the radiograph. It is never at zero for two reasons: First, the base of most x-ray film has a blue dye added to it to enhance the visualization of contrast. This blue tint attenuates some of the light passing through the film.

Second, a small level of fog accumulated during the manufacture and storage of x-ray film is inevitable. Hence, all x-ray film has an inherent base density before it is exposed radiographically. This density is called the *base-plus-fog*.

The shoulder portion of the curve represents the maximum density level producible on the radiograph. It levels off because there is a finite amount of silver available in the emulsion of an x-ray film to produce density. When all of the silver crystals in a particular area of the film are used up, no more density can be obtained. This level may vary somewhat from one type of film to another, but it is always well beyond what the human eye perceives as

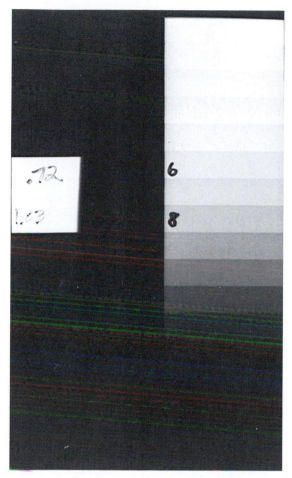

Figure 41-2. Radiograph of step wedge from which H & D curve measurements are taken. In this case, *speed* would be measured at step number 8 because it is closest to a density of 1.2, while *contrast* would be determined by subtracting step 6 from step 8.

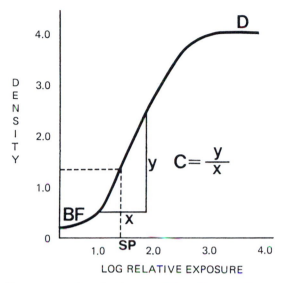

Figure 41-3. Graph of normal H & D curve showing base-plus-fog (BF), speed (SP), contrast (C), and D-max (D) for an exposure.

pitch black. The level portion of the shoulder of the curve is referred to as the *D-Max*

These two measurements, the base-plus-fog and the D-Max, are simply read off of the density axis of the graph. Normal base-plus-fog values range from 0.18 to 0.22 on the density scale for well-protected film.

The base-plus-fog should generally not exceed 0.25, which would then indicate unacceptable levels of darkroom or storage fogging. Average D-Max levels vary around 3.8 on the density scale.

The *slope* of the body portion of the H and D curve is indicative of the *contrast* of the film. This slope is determined by the ratio of the magnitude of a density change over the magnitude of the exposure change which caused it. For example, two exposure levels may be selected along the exposure axis of the graph for comparison. Remembering that these represent different portions of the *remnant* beam of radiation, the lighter exposure might be considered as that occurring under a bone, while the greater exposure would be that occurring under soft tissue (Fig. 41-3). By extending a line upward from these two numbers to the plotted curve and then over to the density axis, the two densities produced on the radiograph for bone and for soft tissue may be obtained. The differences between the two densities and the two exposures are both found by subtracting the lesser from the greater. The density difference is divided by the exposure difference to obtain a measurement of contrast, as expressed in the formula:

$$\text{Contrast} = \frac{\text{D1 - D2}}{\text{E1 - E2}}$$

where D is the density and E is the relative exposure. If the body of the H and D curve lay at a 45° angle, the density change would equal the exposure change and the above ratio would come out as 1.0 for the film contrast. If the slope is steep enough so that the density increases by four times when the exposure is doubled, the contrast would be 2.0. *The steeper the slope, the higher the contrast.*

Since the two exposure levels chosen to obtain a contrast measurement are arbitrary, such measurements may be manipulated somewhat. Film manufacturers and sales representatives often refer to the *gamma* of a film as an indicator of contrast. The film gamma is actually the most ideal contrast measurement that can be obtained from the H and D curve, taken over a small area near the middle of the body. A broader measurement which represents the performance of the film over the entire range of diagnostically useful densities is more valuable to the radiographer. The useful range of densities in diagnostic imaging is considered to be from 0.25 to 2.5. The overall contrast of the film should be measured between the densities 0.25 *plus* base-fog and 2.0 *plus* base-fog. This broader contrast measurement is called the *average gradient* of the film. Typical average gradients range around 2.92.

Film *speed* is obtained in a very different manner. Sensitometrically, speed is defined as the relative exposure required to produce a density of 1.0 *plus* base-fog on the radiograph. Therefore, the density level 1.0 plus base-fog is first found on the graph, and a line is then extended from that point over to the curve and down to the exposure axis. The *less* the relative exposure producing this density level, the *higher* the film

speed. To obtain actual film-speed numbers, the log relative exposure number must be inverted algebraically. If a log relative exposure of 1.0 is required, the speed will be 100. If a log relative exposure of 0.5 is required, the speed will be 200. At 0.25, the speed is 400, and so on. Conversely, a log relative exposure of 2.0 translates to a speed of 50.

The primary value of the H and D curve is in comparing different types of films or different types of processing chemicals or conditions. Figure 41-4 shows two different H and D curves for comparison of film types. Film *A* has greater speed than film *B* because the entire curve, including the body portion at 1.0 plus base-fog, is to the left of the film *B*, indicating that less exposure is required to achieve equivalent densities. However, film *B* has higher inherent contrast than film *A*, because the slope of the curve for film *B* is much steeper. If the

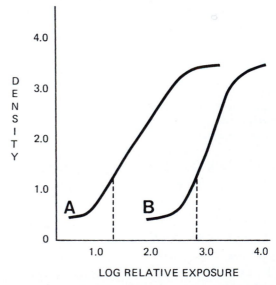

Figure 41-4. Graph of H & D curves for two different types of radiographic films. Film A is a faster speed film because its speed point is to the left of Film B. However, Film B has higher contrast since the slope of its body is steeper than that of Film A.

same film is used, two such curves could also indicate image changes from processing temperature, time or concentration changes.

On a daily basis, the primary interest in the radiology department in sensitometric quality control is in monitoring the changing *trends* of speed, contrast and base-plus-fog over time. The H and D curve does not provide a *chronological* record of these qualities. The speed, the contrast and the base-plus-fog may be separated into daily measurements and monitored over time by using a different kind of graph called the *processing control chart.*

PROCESSING CONTROL CHARTS

The most valuable application of sensitometric monitoring is found in the use of processing control charts. In effect, these charts break the H and D curve into three separate components so that each one can be individually monitored over time. As long as the same film type is used and there are no drastic variations in electrical equipment factors, these graphs will represent variations in processing conditions. It is important that processing conditions be so monitored because it is in the processor that the greatest degree of variation occurs.

The three sensitometric graphs are for speed, contrast and base-plus-fog (Fig. 41-5). The days of the week or of the month are noted across the graphs. Measurements should be taken each day at the same time after the processor has warmed up and is in regular use.

In the case of processing control charts, the *speed* is measured somewhat differently than with an H and D curve: The density value found at 1.0 plus the base-fog is recorded as a starting point on the speed graph. This value is sometimes called the *medium density*, abbreviated *MD*, and usually falls around 1.22. This value is written at the vertical mid-point on the graph. A heavier line or mark should be made on the graph at density points of 0.1 above and below this value. These are the acceptable limits for speed variation from day to day—plus or minus 0.1 from the medium density level. Variation upward or downward from day to day is normal. However, when a continuing trend persists over several days, corrective action should be taken *before* the speed crosses over these limits.

The contrast is often called the *density difference* and abbreviated *DD*. When chemistry has been freshly mixed, this value should be measured and recorded at the vertical mid-point of the contrast graph as a starting point for comparison. Like the density, the contrast levels should not surpass plus or minus 0.1 from the initial value. Contrast is actually obtained for processing control charts by subtracting the step with the density closest to 1.0 from the density two steps darker than it (if using a 21-step penetrometer image). On preexposed sensitometry strips, the measurement taken from a labeled *minimum-density* area is subtracted from that of a labeled *maximum-density* area. Typical contrast measurements fall around 1.8.

Base-plus-fog is measured at the thickest step of the wedge or the lightest density area. The initial value is measured and recorded at the vertical mid-point on the graph just after fresh chemistry is mixed. Base-plus-fog should not vary more than plus or minus 0.03 from the initial value without corrective action being taken.

In addition to the three sensitometric

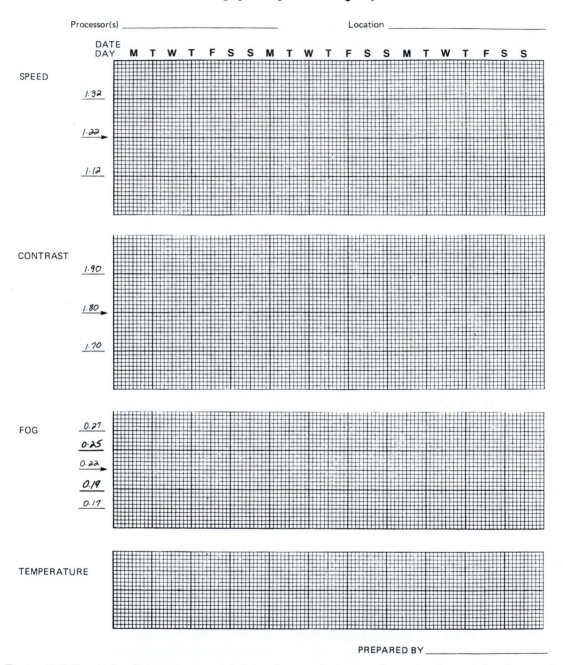

Figure 41-5. Example of processor control charts for speed, contrast, base-plus-fog and developer solution temperature as they would be set up after an initial test exposure (with fresh chemistry) yielding a speed of 1.22, a contrast of 1.80, a base-plus-fog of 0.22 and an average temperature. Unacceptable deviation limits are set at plus and minus 0.1 for speed and contrast, and at plus and minus 0.03 for base-plus-fog.

graphs, a processing solution *temperature* chart should also be used to monitor fluctuations in developer temperature from day to day, (Fig. 41-5). This practice allows any deviations in the other three graphs to be narrowed down to one interpretation and diagnosis, rather than being left with two or three possible problems that might have caused the deviation and having to investigate each of them. Recall that there are three basic variables in processing: time, temperature, and concentration. In automatic processing, the time is constant unless mechanical damage occurs to the transport system. For most problems, time may therefore be eliminated as a possible cause, leaving temperature and concentration. By monitoring the developer solution temperature daily, which can be done quickly by using a digital probe thermometer immersed in the developer for only 5-10 seconds, and by plotting the temperature variations along with the other sensitometric plots, temperature can be eliminated at a glance as a possible cause of deviations. That is, if the other sensitometric plots deviate past the acceptable levels and yet the temperature is seen to have remained constant, the problem is almost certainly being caused by improper chemical concentration. Deviation in the concentration of the chemicals could be caused by improper replenishment rates, blocked replenishment lines or broken replenishment pumps, exhaustion or contamination of the solutions.

DIAGNOSING DEVIATIONS

Figure 41-6 demonstrates the typical trends apparent on control charts for underreplenishment, overreplenishment, increasing or decreasing temperatures, and for sudden contamination of developer solution. When underreplenishment occurs, speed and contrast both tend to decrease while the base-plus-fog and temperature remain constant. For overreplenishment, the speed and fog both increase, the contrast decreases, and the temperature remains constant. When solution temperature is increasing, the speed, fog, and temperature charts will all show an increase. The contrast chart will show an increase at first, but as the temperature continues to climb, contrast will reach a peak and begin to decrease. With a loss of heat, the speed, contrast and temperature graphs will show a decrease, while the fog graph may show a slight increase or remain level. When the film bin is light-fogged or when solutions are contaminated due to human error, the graphs will change in the same directions as for over-replenishment, but the change will be acute, spiking suddenly, so that the nature of the problem is obviously human error or complete failure of a processor component such as the heater.

When processing control charts are used faithfully, and deviations are corrected before they exceed the acceptable limits, repeat rates can often be reduced by as much as 35 percent. Not only does this repeat reduction save almost one-third of all unnecessary patient exposure, but it also can save the radiology department thousands of dollars in film costs. It is to our professional, ecological, and economical advantage to use such a simple and beneficial scientific method of quality control.

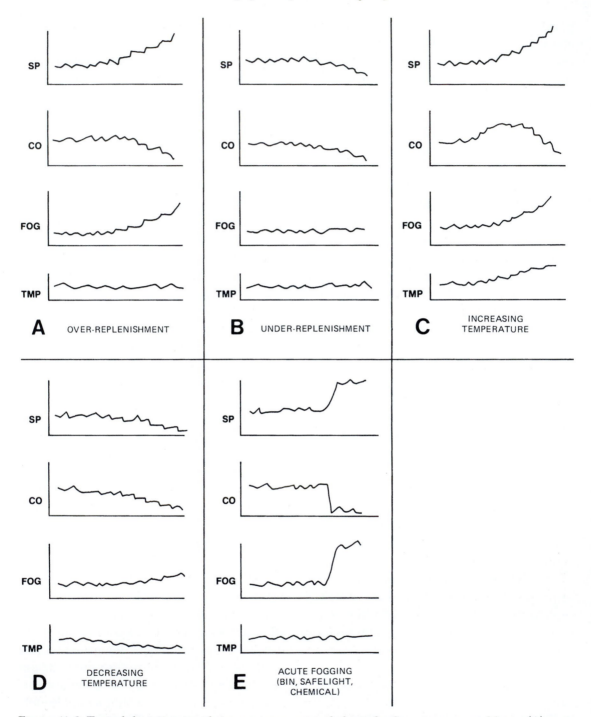

Figure 41-6. Typical deviation trends on processor control charts for five common problems: (A) over-replenishment, (B) underreplenishment, (C) increasing solution temperature, (D) decreasing solution temperature, (E) fim bin fogging or sudden contamination of solutions.

SUMMARY

1. *Sensitometry* is the quantitative measurement of film response to exposure and processing conditions.
2. The *H and D curve* is useful in comparing different image receptor systems or processing variables. It shows the base-plus-fog (toe), the D-Max (shoulder), the contrast (slope of body) and the speed points obtained.
3. *Processing control charts* allow deviations in processing conditions to be detected and corrected *before* they cause repeated exposures. Typically, the base-plus-fog should be around 0.2, the speed around 1.2 and the contrast around 1.8.
Speed and contrast should not deviate more than 0.1 from the standard, and base-plus-fog should not deviate more than 0.03 from the standard.
4. Since in automatic processing the development time is fixed and the temperature can be monitored, the *combined trends* in processing control charts can be used to diagnose the cause of deviations (replenishment, temperature or acute fogging) with fair accuracy.
5. Quality control of processing can reduce *repeated exposures* by more than 35 percent.

REVIEW QUESTIONS

1. Define sensitometry:
2. Who were Hurter and Driffield?
3. In monitoring processing conditions, why is it better to use a sensitometer than a penetrometer?
4. What is the typical range for base-plus-fog measurements?
5. What is the typical D-max level of density for most films?
6. Define average gradient:
7. The slope of the H & D curve, measured as either gamma or as average gradient, indicates the level of what image quality?
8. At a density of 1.0 plus the base-fog on an H & D graph, the curve for film B lies to the *right* of the curve for film A. What does this mean in comparing the characteristics of these two films?
9. What is the *formula* for calculating film contrast from an H & D curve?
10. Which portion of the H & D curve would give an indication of the total amount of silver available in the emulsion to produce density in the image?
11. For processing control charts, the starting point for measuring speed is found by taking the density of that step on the "step wedge" which measures closest to what value?
12. For processing control charts, the contrast should not deviate from the base value by more than plus-or-minus _____.
13. What is the maximum allowable deviation for base-plus-fog?
14. On a set of processor control charts, if the measured solution temperature has been stable, yet the contrast, speed and fog all changed, which of the three major processing variables is almost certainly responsible?
15. Over a period of time the speed is seen to be rising, the contrast is dropping and the fog is rising, but the temperature remains steady. What is causing

this trend?

16. Describe what the speed, contrast, fog and temperature charts would look like if the solution temperature was gradually decreasing.

Appendix I

BLANK TECHNIQUE CHARTS

A. Manual Exposure (2 pp)
B. Automatic Exposure Control

ABBREVIATIONS: GD = Grid
NG = Non-Grid

TORSO / SKULL CHART

PROCEDURE	Notes	VIEW	kVp	Ave CM	Total MAS by PART SIZE								
					-6cm	-4cm	-2cm	AVE	+2cm	+4cm	+6cm	+8cm	+10cm
GRID	72"	PA/AP	106	22									
CHEST		LAT	116	30									
NON-GRID	72"	AP	80	22									
CHEST		LAT	90	30									
SUPINE CHEST 40" NG		AP	80	22									
RIBS / Sternum	72"	AP↑Diap	60	22									
		OBL↑Dia	64	24									
	72"	AP↓Diap	76	22									
ABDOMEN /	GD	AP/PA	80	22									
IVP		30°OBL	80	24									
PELVIS / HIP	GD	AP	80	22									
HIP (Unil or Groin)	GRID	LAT	80	22									
SACRUM		AP / Coccyx All	76	20									
	GD	LAT	80	28									
LUMBAR SPINE		AP	80	22									
		45°OBL	80	26									
	GD	LAT	80	30									
		L5/S1 SP	*90	30									
THORACIC	GD	AP	76	22									
SPINE		Breathing LAT	60	30									
TWINING C/T	GD	LAT	76	28									
CERVICAL SPINE	40" GD	AP/Odon	76	13									
	72"**GD**	OBL/LAT	76	13									
	72"**NG**	OBL/LAT	76	13									
SKULL	GD	PA/Cald	80	19									
		LAT	76	15									
		Townes	80	22									
SINUSES / FACIAL BONES	GD	PA/Cald	76	19									
		Waters	80	20									
		Lat	76	15									
AIR CONTRAST U.G.I. / B.E.	GD	AP/PA	90	22									
		OBL/SIG	90	24									
		LAT	90	30									
SOLID-COLUMN U.G.I. / B.E.	GD	AP/PA	110	22									
		OBL/SIG	110	24									
		LAT	110	30									

EXTREMITY CHART

PROCEDURE	Notes	VIEW	kVp	mAs
HAND	PA /All Fingers		54	
	SFS EXTCAS	OBL	54	
		Fanned Lat	54	
WRIST	SFS EXTCAS	PA	60	
		OBL	60	
		LAT	60	
FOREARM	SFS EXTCAS	AP	64	
		LAT	64	
ELBOW	SFS EXTCAS	AP	64	
		OBL	64	
		LAT	64	
HUMERUS	SFS EXTCAS	AP	72	
		LAT	72	
TOES	SFS/EXT	All	60	
FOOT	SFS EXTCAS	AP	64	
		OBL	64	
		LAT	64	
CALCANEUS	SFS EXTCAS	PD	68	
		LAT	68	
ANKLE	SFS EXTCAS	AP/OBL	64	
		LAT	64	
LEG	SFS EXTCAS	AP	68	
		LAT	68	
TABLETOP KNEE	EXTCAS	AP	70	
		LAT	70	
TBLTOP KNEE REG		All	70	
BUCKY KNEE	GD	AP/OBL	70	
		LAT	70	
FEMUR	GD	AP / LAT	76	
HIP	GRID	FRG/GROIN	80	
SHOULDER	GD	AP/Transax	76	
		Transthoracic	90	
CLAVICLE	GD	AP/PA	74	
SCAPULA	GD	AP	74	
		LAT	74	

ABBREVIATIONS: GD =Grid, NG =Non-Grid. SFS
=Small Focal Spot, EXTCAS =Extremity Cassette,
REG =Regular Cassette, PIGOST = Pig-O-Stat$_{TM}$

FACIAL CHART

PROCEDURE	Notes	VIEW	kVp	mAs
MANDIBLE	GD	PA	76	
		OBL LAT	66	
	NON-GRID OBL LAT		60	
ORBIT Rheese	GD	PA OBL	76	
SINUSES	GD	SMV	80	
ZYG. ARCH	EXTCAS	SMV	62	
NASAL BONE	EXTCAS	LAT	54	

PEDIATRIC CHART

PROCEDURE	Notes	VIEW	kVp	mAs
"PREMIE" CHEST	40" NG	AP	54	
		LAT	54	
INFANT CHEST	40" NG	AP	60	
		LAT	68	
2-YEAR CHEST	72" PIGOST	PA	66	
		LAT	76	
6-YEAR CHEST	72" NG	PA	70	
		LAT	80	
ABDOMEN / IVP / PELVIS SPINES	INFANT NG		62	
	2-YEAR GD		68	
	6-YEAR GD		74	
CERVIC. SP	2-YEAR	All	64	
SKULL (PA/AP)	INFANT NG		62	
	2-YEAR GD		68	
	6-YEAR GD		74	
UPPER EXTREMITY	INFANT EXTCAS		54	
	2-YEAR EXTCAS		58	
	6-YEAR EXTCAS		62	
LOWER EXTREMITY	INFANT EXTCAS		58	
	2-YEAR EXTCAS		62	
	6-YEAR EXTCAS		66	

A E C TECHNIQUE CHART

PROCEDURE	VIEW	kVp	mA	BACKUP TIME (mAs)	DETECTOR SELECTION	DENSITY SETTING	NOTES
CHEST	PA/AP	106			▫▫ ▫		
CHEST	LAT	116			▫▫ ▫		
6-YR CHEST	PA	90			▫▫ ▫		
RIBS ↑DIAPH	AP/OBL	60			▫▫ ▫		
RIBS ↓DIAPH	AP	76			▫▫ ▫		
ABDOMEN	AP	80			▫▫ ▫		
IVP	AP/OBL	80			▫▫ ▫		
G.B. / Coned	AP/OBL	80			▫▫ ▫		
PELVIS	AP	80			▫▫ ▫		
HIP Unilateral	AP/LAT	80			▫▫ ▫		
LUMBAR SPINE	AP	80			▫▫ ▫		
LUMBAR SPINE	OBL	80			▫▫ ▫		
LUMBAR SPINE	LAT	80			▫▫ ▫		
LUMBAR SPINE	L5/ S1	90			▫▫ ▫		
THORACIC SPINE	AP	74			▫▫ ▫		
THORACIC SPINE	LAT	60			▫▫ ▫		
TWINING C/T	LAT	76			▫▫ ▫		
CERVICAL SPINE	AP	76			▫▫ ▫		
CERVICAL SPINE	Odontd	76			▫▫ ▫		
CERVICAL SPINE	Lat/Obl	76			▫▫ ▫		
SKULL (SINUS) (FACIAL)	PA/Cald	80			▫▫ ▫		
SKULL (SINUS) (FACIAL)	Waters	80			▫▫ ▫		
SKULL (SINUS) (FACIAL)	Townes	80			▫▫ ▫		
SKULL (SINUS) (FACIAL)	LAT	76			▫▫ ▫		
Mastoid/Coned	LAT	76			▫▫ ▫		
SHOULDER	AP	76			▫▫ ▫		
FEMUR	AP/LAT	76			▫▫ ▫		
KNEE / LEG	All	70			▫▫ ▫		
U.G.I.	All				▫▫ ▫		
B.E.	AP/OBL				▫▫ ▫		
B.E.	Sigm/Lat				▫▫ ▫		

Appendix II

ANSWERS TO EXERCISES

EXERCISE #1

1. 5 mAs
2. 80 mAs
3. 4 mAs
4. 25 mAs
5. 60 mAs
6. 210 mAs
7. 12 mAs
8. 7.5 mAs
9. 16 mAs
10. 6.4 mAs
11. 132 mAs
12. 15 mAs
13. 350 mAs
14. 150 mAs
15. 4.8 mAs

EXERCISE #2

1. 750 milliseconds
2. 300 ms
3. 125 ms
4. 40 ms
5. 83 ms
6. 33.3 ms
7. 5ms
8. 1.2 ms
9. 0.2 second
10. 0.167 sec
11. 0.25 sec
12. 0.035 sec
13. 0.07 sec
14. 0.015 sec
15. 0.008 sec
16. 1.2 sec

EXERCISE #3

1. 2.5 mAs
2. 50 mAs
3. 3.5 mAs
4. 0.8 mAs
5. 40 mAs
6. 25 mAs
7. 9.9 mAs
8. 1.8 mAs
9. 100 mAs
10. 32 mAs
11. 2.5 mAs
12. 90 mAs

EXERCISE #4

1. 5 mAs
2. appx. 12 mAs
3. appx. .8 mAs
4. appx. 16 or 17 mAs
5. 2.5 mAs
6. 40 mAs
7. 5 mAs
8. appx. 1.6 or 1.7 mAs
9. 5 mAs
10. 20 mAs
11. 12 mAs
12. 120 mAs (6 sets of 20)
13. appx. 48-50 mAs (4 sets of 12 or 12.5)
13. appx. 35 mAs (5 sets of 7)

EXERCISE #5

1. appx. 14 mAs (2 sets of 7)
2. 15 mAs (3 sets of 5)
3. 120 mAs
4. 70 mAs
5. 160 mAs (2 sets of 80)
6. 45 mAs (3 sets of 15)

EXERCISE #6

1. 2 sets of 40
2. 3 sets of 15
3. 2 sets of 33
4. 3 sets of 25
5. 3 sets of 60
6. 3 sets of 40 OR 2 sets of 60
7. 2 sets of 80 OR 4 sets of 40
8. 3 sets of 80 OR 4 sets of 60
9. 3 sets of 30
10. 4 sets of 80

EXERCISE #7

1. 1/40 second
2. 1/15
3. 1/30
4. 1/60
5. 1/80
6. 1/120
7. 1/20
8. 1/5 second
9. 1/40
10. 2/15 (2 sets of 7)
11. 1/15
12. 1/120
13. 3/20 (3 sets of 15)
14. 4/5 (4 sets of 60)
15. 3/5 (3 sets of 80)

EXERCISE #8

1. 0.025 second
2. 0.07
3. 0.033
4. 0017
5. 0.4
6. 0.025
7. 0.125
8. 0.025
9. 0.0125
10. 0.7
11. 0.17
12. 0.02
13. 0.07
14. 0.6
15. 0.6

EXERCISE #9

1. 4
2. 2.5
3. 10.5
4. 16.5
5. 6.75
6. 9
7. 102 kVp
8. 64.5 kVp
9. appx. 58 kVp
10. appx. 118 kVp
11. appx. 37 kVp
12. appx. 87 kVp
13. appx. 65 kVp

EXERCISE #10

1. 24 inches
2. 15
3. 10
4. 4
5. 6
6. 10
7. 30
8. 60
9. 15
10. 18

EXERCISE #11

1. 10 mAs
2. 5
3. 15
4. 7.5
5. 15

EXERCISE #12

1. 1/3 or 0.33
2. 5 times
3. 0.7
4. 3-4 times
5. 3 times
6. 5/3 or 1.67
7. 5/4 or 1.25
8. 1-14

EXERCISE #13

1. 1/4 (.25)
2. 25 x
3. 2x
4. 1/2 (.5)
5. 5x
6. 3/4 (.75)
7. 1/5
8. 150 x
9. 5x
10. 0.625x
11. 2 x
12. 1/200

EXERCISE #14

1. 0.31
2. 0.69
3. 1.93
4. 0.56

EXERCISE #15

1. 7.2 mAs
2. 8.1 mAs
3. 0.28 mAs
4. 1.17 mAs
5. 4.3 mAs
6. 8.1 mAs
7. 32 inches
8. 30 inches

EXERCISE #16

1. 75 mAs
2. 30 mAs
3. 30 mAs
4. 30 mAs
5. 15 mAs
6. 15 mAs
7. 10 mAs
8. 25 mAs
   (45" is halfway to doubling 30")

EXERCISE #17

1. 16 inches
2. 8 inches
3. 3.3 inches
4. 8 inches
5. 180 inches
6. 24 inches
7. 15 inches
8. 30 inches
9. 1.5 inches
10. 32 inches
11. 40 cm.
12. 7.5 cm.
13. 18 cm.
14. 40 inches
15. 90 inches

EXERCISE #18

Series I:	A.	3x
	B.	2x
	C.	1/2

Series II:	A.	4x
	B.	2x
	C.	1/3

EXERCISE #19

	Density	Contrast	Sharpness	Magnification	Distortion
Increase mA	+	0	0	0	0
Increase Exp. Time	+	0	−	0	0
Increase kVp	+	−	0	0	0
Increase Filtration	−(0)*	−(0)*	0	0	0
From 1-Phase to 3-Phase	+	−(0)*	0	0	0
Increase Field Size	+	−	0	0	0
Increase Motion	0	−	−	0	0
Increase Patient Size	−	−	0(−)**	0(+)**	0
Increase Grid Ratio	−	+	0	0	0
Increase Screen Speed	+	+	−†	0	0
Increase Size of Focal Spot	0	0	−	0	0
Increase SID	−	0	+	−	0
Increase OID	−	+	−	+	0
Misalign or Misangle Beam	0	0	0	0	+

*Although a slight decrease in these qualities may be measurable, it is not generally visible (see text).

**Although a decrease in these qualities would occur if larger patient size would inevitably place the part of interest further away from the film, it would make no difference at all if the part was superficial enough to be kept adjacent to the film through proper positioning.

†This is a general rule which applies only when screen emulsion is increasing in thickness, but not when phosphor chemicals are changed to obtain higher speeds.

EXERCISE #20

1. 1 and 1/2 times.
2. Three times.
3. Same technique.
4. Double (1.5-2x)
5. Four times (3.5-4x)
6. Same technique.
7. Double.
8. Same mAs plus about 6-8 kVp.
9. Double.
10. 1/4.
11. Double or increase 8 kVp.
12. Same technique.

EXERCISE #21. Explanation. First, complete the even columns of the lumbar spine section using the 4 cm rule to double or halve the mAs values, then simply split the differences to fill in the odd columns. Next, use proportional anatomy to derive the average skull, shoulder, and knee techniques as follows: Note that the original 16 mAs for an AP lumbar spine is equal to a Townes skull— The PA skull is 2/3 this technique, yielding about 10 mAs. The lateral skull is 1/2 the PA, the shoulder is equal to the lateral skull, both at 5 mAs. The knee is 6 kVp less than the shoulder, with the same mAs. Finally, use the 4 cm rule again to complete the remaining skull, shoulder, and knee columns.

Procedure	Projection	kVp	Ave CM	MAS						
Lumbar Spine	AP	80	22	18 cm 8	20 cm 12	22 cm 16	24 cm 24	26 cm 32	28 cm 48	30 cm 64
	Oblique	80	26	22 cm 16	24 cm 24	26 cm 32	28 cm 48	30 cm 64	32 cm 96	34 cm 128
	Lateral	80	30	26 cm 32	28 cm 48	30 cm 64	32 cm 96	34 cm 128	36 cm 192	38 cm 256
Skull	PA	76	19	15 cm 5	17 cm 7.5	19 cm 10	21 cm 15			
	Lateral	76	15	11 cm 2.5	13 cm 3.7	15 cm 5	17 cm 7.5			
Shoulder	AP	76	14	10 cm 2.5	12 cm 3.7	14 cm 5	16 cm 7.5			
Knee	AP	70	12	8 cm 2.5	10 cm 3.7	12 cm 5	14 cm 7.5			

VARIABLE TIME CHART:
Divide 200 mA into the original mAs values:

Procedure	KVP	mA	Time for ea. view		
			PA	OBL	LAT
WRIST	60	200	.025	.035	.05

VARIABLE KVP CHART:
Apply the 15 per cent rule:

Procedure	mAs	kVp for each view		
		PA	OBL	LAT
WRIST	5	60	64	68

INDEX